KU-351-464

Oxford Handbook of
Clinical Dentistry

Fifth edition

Laura Mitchell
and
David A. Mitchell

with contributions from

Lorna McCaul

OXFORD
UNIVERSITY PRESS

OXFORD
UNIVERSITY PRESS

Great Clarendon Street, Oxford OX2 6DP

Oxford University Press is a department of the University of Oxford.
It furthers the University's objective of excellence in research, scholarship,
and education by publishing worldwide in

Oxford New York

Auckland Cape Town Dar es Salaam Hong Kong Karachi
Kuala Lumpur Madrid Melbourne Mexico City Nairobi
New Delhi Shanghai Taipei Toronto

With offices in

Argentina Austria Brazil Chile Czech Republic France Greece
Guatemala Hungary Italy Japan Poland Portugal Singapore
South Korea Switzerland Thailand Turkey Ukraine Vietnam

Oxford is a registered trade mark of Oxford University Press
in the UK and in certain other countries

Published in the United States
by Oxford University Press Inc., New York

© David A. and Laura Mitchell, 1991, 1995, 1999, 2005, 2009

The moral rights of the authors have been asserted
Database right Oxford University Press (maker)

First published 1991
Second edition 1995
Third edition 1999
Fourth edition 2005
Fifth edition 2009

All rights reserved. No part of this publication may be reproduced,
stored in a retrieval system, or transmitted, in any form or by any means,
without the prior permission in writing of Oxford University Press,
or as expressly permitted by law, or under terms agreed with the appropriate
reprographics rights organization. Enquiries concerning reproduction
outside the scope of the above should be sent to the Rights Department,
Oxford University Press, at the address above

You must not circulate this book in any other binding or cover
and you must impose this same condition on any acquirer

British Library Cataloguing in Publication Data
Data available

Library of Congress Cataloging in Publication Data

Mitchell, Laura, 1958-
Oxford handbook of clinical dentistry/Laura Mitchell and David A. Mitchell; with
contributions from Lorna McCaul. — 5th ed.
   p. ; cm.
David A. Mitchell's name appears first on prev. ed.
Includes bibliographical references and index.
ISBN 978–0–19–955330–3 (alk. paper)
1. Dentistry—Handbooks, manuals, etc. I. Mitchell, David A. II. McCaul, Lorna.
III. Title. IV. Title: Handbook of clinical dentistry.
[DNLM: 1. Mouth Diseases—therapy—Handbooks. 2. Tooth Diseases—therapy—
Handbooks. 3. Dentistry—methods—Handbooks. WU 49 M6810 2009]
RK56.M58 2009
617.6—dc22   2009015155

Typeset by Cepha Imaging Private Ltd., Bangalore, India
Printed in Italy on acid-free paper by Rotolito Lombarda SpA

ISBN 978–0–19–955330–3

10 9 8 7 6 5 4 3 2 1

Preface to the first edition

Dental students are introduced to real live patients at an early stage of their undergraduate course in order to fulfil the requirements for clinical training, with the result that they are expected to absorb a large quantity of information in a relatively short time. This is often compounded by clinical allocations to different specialities on different days, or even the same day. Given the obvious success of the Oxford handbooks of clinical medicine and clinical specialities, evidenced by their position in the white coat pockets of the nation's medical students, the extension of the same format to dentistry seems logical. However, it is hoped that the usefulness of this idea will not cease on graduation, particularly with the introduction of Vocational Training. While providing a handy reference for the recently qualified graduate, it is envisaged that trainers will also welcome an aide mémoire to help cope with the enthusiastic young trainee who may be more familiar with recent innovations and obscure facts. We also hope that there will be much of value for the hospital trainee struggling towards FDS.

The *Oxford Handbook of Clinical Dentistry* contains those useful facts and practical tips that were stored in our white coat pockets as students and then postgraduates; initially on scraps of paper, but as the collection grew, transferred into notebooks to give a readily available reference source.

The dental literature already contains a great number of erudite books which, for the most part deal exclusively, in some depth, with a particular branch or aspect of dentistry. The aim of this handbook is not to replace these specialist dental texts, but rather to complement them by distilling together theory and practical information into a more accessible format. In fact, reference is made to sources of further reading where necessary.

Although the authors of this handbook are not the specialized authorities usually associated with dental textbooks, we are still near enough to the coal-face to provide, we hope, some useful practical tips based on sound theory. We were fortunate whilst compiling this handbook in being able to draw on the expertise of many colleagues; the contents, however, remain our sole responsibility. The format of a blank page opposite each page of text has been plagiarized from the other Oxford handbooks. This gives space for the reader to add his own comments and updates. Please let us know of any that should be made available to a wider audience.

We hope that the reader will find this book to be a useful addition to their white coat pocket or a companion to the BNF in the surgery.

Preface to the second edition

It would appear that our 'baby' is now a toddler and rapidly outgrowing his previous milieu. Caring for such a precocious child is hard work and therefore we have again relied on the help of understanding friends and colleagues who have contributed their knowledge and expertise.

The pace of change in dentistry, both scientifically and politically, is so fast that although the first edition was only published in 1991, this second edition has involved extensive revision of all chapters. Advances in dental materials and restorative techniques have necessitated major revision of these sections and we are indebted to Mr Andrew Hall, who has helped update the chapter on restorative dentistry.

Since the first edition was published, political changes in the UK have resulted in a shift towards private dentistry. This changing emphasis is reflected in the practice management chapter, which now includes a new page on independent and private practice. In addition recent developments in cross-infection control and UK health and safety law have been included.

That old favourite, temporomandibular pain dysfunction syndrome, has also been given the treatment and is now situated on a newly devised page in the chapter on oral medicine. Non-accidental injury, guided tissue regeneration, AIDS, ATLS, and numerous other topical issues have been expanded in this edition.

One aspect of this developing infant remains, however, unchanged. The sole purpose of this book is to enable you, the reader, to gain easy access to the sometimes confusing conglomerate of facts, ideas, opinions, dogma, anecdote, and truth that constitutes clinical dentistry. To this framework you should add, on the blank pages provided, the additional information which will help you treat the next patient or pass the next exam, or more importantly the practical hints and tips which you will glean with experience. It is the potential for that interaction which makes this book distinctive in clinical dentistry. It is participating in that interaction which makes your book unique.

Preface to the third edition

Like any proud parents we are surprised and delighted with the continued development of our 'baby', and we are grateful to all those who have helped or provided positive feedback. We are also grateful to our colleagues who have helped with the 'baby-care'.

Of course, now being of school age, peer group rivalry has arrived, but ours is a robust child and despite being the first kid on the block welcomes both competition and change.

Some of this change is reflected by bringing in a new contributor who has overseen a complete overhaul of the restorative dentistry chapters and a large number of new contributions to reflect dentistry in the late 1990s.

Our own areas of (increasingly erudite) specialist expertise have grown apace but we think we have curbed the temptation to dwell on these in what is, after all, a generalist text for the earlier years; we trust the odd excursion will be forgiven.

We hope that the new sections, which include: evidence-based medicine/dentistry; the new NHS complaints procedure, objective structured clinical examinations, the 1997 Advanced Life Support Guidelines, and the completely revised restorative chapters will prove helpful and informative. We would, however, like to remind you that the blank pages are there for your additional notes—and it is this that makes your copy of this Handbook unique. Please do not hesitate to share these annotations with us, we would be happy to include the best we receive in the next edition and to acknowledge the contributor.

As always while we are grateful for the contributions of our colleagues the contents and the brickbats remain our sole responsibility.

Preface to the fourth edition

A new millennium means new technology and new challenges.

So the time has come to update the *Oxford Handbook of Clinical Dentistry*. In fact the pace of change is such that all chapters in this new edition have been completely revised. To continue the analogy of earlier prefaces: our teenager is keen on exploring new avenues, so we are going to indulge this by expanding our horizons into new attitudes and technology with a section on Dentistry and the World Wide Web, and also a section on web-based learning. This new, twenty-first century edition has the added bonus of colour plates and more diagrams to aid understanding.

We are, as ever, indebted to contributors past and present. The new recruits bring both knowledge and enthusiasm to their areas of expertise as well as to the book as a whole, and build on the work of previous contributors. To all we are greatly indebted. The ultimate responsibility for errors or oversights remains, as always, ours.

Please keep sending us feedback—this is the best way for us to improve future editions.

Let's just hope the teenager doesn't rebel!!

Preface to the fifth edition

The first draft of this book was started in 1989, the year the Berlin wall came down and the first edition appeared in 1991 making our 'child' legal by this, the fifth, edition.

As an eighteenth birthday present this edition includes, as well as the usual extensive rewrite and update of the text, a substantial improvement in the quality of the illustrations, which are now in colour and integrated into the text. This will mean less space for making your own notes in the blank pages but we suspect you will be willing to make the trade-off.

In keeping with previous practice new contributors have been included in order to ensure the material is as up to date as possible and we have tried to avoid overemphasizing our current areas of sub-specialization. As before, this book is the sum of its previous incarnations helped by feedback from readers from all parts of the world and the input of contributors. As always, responsibility for any errors or omissions lies with us.

Acknowledgements

In addition to those readers whose comments and suggestions have been incorporated into the fifth edition, we would like to thank the following for their time and expertise: Mr K. Abdel-Ghalil, Dr A. Dalghous, Mr S. Fayle, Dr H. Gorton, Ms J. Hoole, Ms E. McDerra, Dr I. McHenry, Dr L. Middlefell, Mr L. Savarrio, Ms Y. Shaw. We must also acknowledge the hard work and expertise of Katherine Grice, the medical artist responsible for improving our amateur diagrams beyond recognition.

In addition, this book is the sum and distillate of its previous incarnations, which would not have been possible without Mr B. S. Avery, Mr N. Barnard, Ms F. Carmichael, Mr N. E. Carter, Mr P. Chambers, Mr M. Chan, Mrs J. J. Davison, Dr R. Dookun, Ms S. Dowsett, Dr I. D. Grime, Dr C. Flynn, Dr H. Gorton, Ms V. Hind, Mr A. Hall, Mr H. Harvie, Dr J. Hunton, Mr D. Jacobs, Mr W. Jones, Ms K. Laidler, Mr C. Lloyd, Mr P. J. Knibbs, Mr M. Manogue, Professor J. F. McCabe, Dr B. Nattress, Mr R. A. Ord, Dr J. E. Paul, Professor A. Rugg-Gunn, Professor R. A. Seymour, Professor J. V. Soames, Ms A. Tugnait, Dr D. Wood, and Professor R. Yemm.

We are grateful to the editor of the *BMJ*, the *BDJ* and Professor M. Harris, the Royal National Institute of the Deaf, Laerdal, and the Resuscitation Council UK for granting permission to use their diagrams, and VUMAN for allowing us to include the Index of Orthodontic Treatment Need.

Once again the staff of OUP deserve thanks for their help and encouragement.

Note Although this is an equal opportunity publication, the constraints of space have meant that in some places we have had to use 'he' or 'their' to indicate 'he/she', 'his/hers', etc.

Contents

Detailed contents

4 Orthodontics *119*

7 Prosthetics and gerodontology *293*

8 Oral surgery *339*

9 **Oral medicine** *395*

Symbols and abbreviations

Some of these are included because they are in common usage, others because they are big words and we were trying to save space.

▶	this is important
Δ	diagnosis
$	supernumerary
–ve	negative
+ve	positive
&/or	and/or
↑	increased
↓	decreased
<	lesser than
>	greater than
~	approximately
#	fracture
μ	micro (e.g. μg, μm)
?	question/ask about (when ? appears alone)
∴	therefore
1°	primary
2°	secondary
3°	tertiary
$\overline{5}$; $\overline{inc}$	lower second premolar, lower incisor
$\underline{2}$; $\underline{inc}$	upper lateral incisor, upper incisor
ACS	American College of Surgeons
ACTH	adrenocorticotrophic hormone
ADH	antidiuretic hormone
ADJ	amelo-dentinal junction
Ag	antigen
AIDS	acquired immune deficiency syndrome
ALS	advanced life support
AOB	anterior open bite
AP	antero-posterior
APPT	activated partial thromboplastin time
ARF	acute renal failure
ASAP	as soon as possible
ATLS	advanced trauma life support
AZT	3'-azido-3'-deoxythimidine

BCC	basal cell carcinoma
bd	twice daily
BDA	British Dental Association
BDJ	British Dental Journal
BIPP	bismuth iodoform paraffin paste
BLS	basic life support
b/w	bitewing radiograph
BMA	British Medical Association
BNF	British National Formulary
BP	blood pressure
BRON	bisphosphonate related osteonecrosis
BSS	black silk suture
Ca^{2+}	calcium
C&S	culture and sensitivity
CDS	Community Dental Service
CEJ	cemento-enamel junction
C/I	Contraindication
Class I	Class I relationship
Class II/1	Class II division 1 relationship
Class II/2	Class II division 2 relationship
Class III	Class III relationship
CLP	cleft lip and palate
cm	centimeter
CMV	cytomegalovirus
CNS	central nervous system
C/O	complaining of
COPD	chronic obstructive pulmonary disease
CP	chronic periodontitis
CPD	Continuing Professional Development
CPR	cardiopulmonary resuscitation
CSF	cerebrospinal fluid
CSM	Committee on Safety of Medicines
CT	computed tomography
CVA	cerebro-vascular accident
CVS	cardiovascular system
CXR	chest X-ray
DCP	Dental Care Professional (previously Professional Complementary to Dentistry)
dl	deciliter
DMARD	disease modifying antirheumatic drug
DMF	decayed, missing, filled

DN	dental nurse
DNA	did not attend
DOH/DH	Department of Health
DPB	Dental Practice Board
DPF	Dental Practitioner's Formulary
DPT	dental panoramic tomogram (politically correct: OPT/OPG)
DVT	deep venous thrombosis
EBA	ethoxy benzoic acid
EBM/D	evidence-based medicine/dentistry
EBV	Epstein–Barr virus
ECG	electrocardiograph
EDTA	ethylene diamine tetraacetic acid
e.g.	for example
EMD	enamel matrix derivative
EMLA	eutectic mix of lignocaine and prilocaine
ENT	ear, nose, and throat
EO	extra-oral
EOT	extra-oral traction
ESR	erythrocyte sedimentation rate
EUA	examination under anaesthesia
F	female
F/-	full upper denture (and -/F for lower)
FA	fixed appliance
FABP	flat anterior bite plane
FB	foreign body
FBC	full blood count
Fe	iron
FESS	functional endoscopic sinus surgery
fl	femtolitre
FNAC	fine-needle aspiration cytology
f/s	fissure sealant
FWS	freeway space
g	gram
GA	general anaesthesia
GAP	generalized aggressive periodontitis
GDC	General Dental Council
GDP	general dental practitioner
GDS	General Dental Services
GI	glass ionomer
GKI	glucose, potassium, insulin

GMP	general medical practitioner
GP	gutta-percha
GTR	guided-tissue regeneration
h	hour
H2	histamine 2 receptor antagonist
Hb	haemoglobin
HBeAg	hepatitis B e antigen (high-risk marker)
HBsAg	hepatitis B surface antigen
HDU	high dependency unit
Hep B/C	hepatitis B/C
Hg	mercury
HIV	human immunodeficiency virus
HLA	human leucocyte antigen
HPV	human papilloma virus
HRT	hormone replacement therapy
HSV	herpes simplex virus
ICP	intercuspal position
ICU	intensive care unit
ID	inferior dental
IDB	inferior dental block
IDN	inferior dental nerve
i.e.	that is
IE	infective endocarditis
Ig	immunoglobulin (e.g. IgA, IgG, etc.)
IM	intramuscular
IMF	intermaxillary fixation
inc	incisor
INR	International Normalized Ratio
IO	intra-oral
IRM	Intermediate Restorative Material®
ITP	idiopathic thrombocytopenic purpura
IU	international units
IV	intravenous
JP	juvenile periodontitis
K^+	potassium
KCT	kaolin–cephalin clotting time
kg	kilogram
kV	kilovolt
l	litre
LA	local anaesthesia

LAP	localized aggressive periodontitis
LFH	lower face height
LFT	liver function test
LLS	lower labial segment
LMA	laryngeal mask airway
m	metre
M	male
mand	mandible/mandibular
MAOI	monoamine oxidase inhibitor
max	maxilla/maxillary
MCQ	multiple choice question
MCV	mean corpuscular volume
MEN	multiple endocrine neoplasia
mg	milligram
MHz	megahertz
MI	myocardial infarction
micromol	micromoles
min	minute
ml	milliliter
mm	millimeter
mmHg	millimeters of mercury
mmol	millimole
MMPA	maxillary mandibular planes angle
MRI	magnetic resonance imaging
MST	slow release morphine
MSU	mid-stream urine
MTA	mineral trioxide aggregate
NAD	nothing abnormal detected
NAI	non-accidental injury
NGT	naso-gastric tube
NHS	National Health Service
nm	nanometer
nocte	at night
NSAID	non-steroidal anti-inflammatory drug
NUG	necrotizing ulcerative gingivitis
O_2	oxygen
o/b	overbite
OCP	oral contraceptive pill
od	once daily
OD	overdenture

O/E	on examination
OH	oral hygiene
OHCM	Oxford Handbook of Clinical Medicine
OHI	oral hygiene instruction
OHP	overhead projector/projection
o/j	overjet
OMF	oral and maxillofacial
OP	out-patient
ORIF	open reduction and internal fixation
OSCE	objective structured clinical examination
OTC	over the counter
OVD	occlusal vertical dimension
P/-	partial upper denture (and -/P for lower)
PA	posteroanterior
PCA	patient-controlled analgesia
PCR	polymerase chain reaction
PCT	Primary Care Trust
PDH	past dental history
PDL	periodontal ligament
PEA	pulseless electrical activity
PEG	percutaneous endoscopic gastrostomy
PFM	porcelain fused to metal (crown)
PJC	porcelain jacket crown
PM	premolar
PMH	past medical history
PMMA	polymethylmethacrylate
PO	per orum (by mouth)
ppm	parts per million
PR	per rectum
prn	as required
PRR	preventive resin restoration
PTFE	(poly)tetrafluoroethene
PU	pass urine
qds	four times daily
RA	relative analgesia
RAS	recurrent aphthous stomatitis
RBC	red blood cell count
RCCT	randomized controlled clinical trial
RCP	retruded contact position
RCT	root canal treatment/therapy

RIG	radiologically inserted gastrostomy
RMGIC	resin-modified glass ionomer composite
RRF	retrograde root filling
Rx	treatment
SC	subcutaneous
SCC	squamous cell carcinoma
sec	second
SF	sugar free
SLE	systemic lupus erythematosus
spp	species
SS	stainless steel
STD	sexually transmitted diseases
TANI	target average net income
TB	tuberculosis
TC	tungsten carbide
tds	thrice daily
TENS	transcutaneous electrical nerve stimulation
TIBC	total iron binding capacity
TMA	titanium molybdenum alloy
TMJ	temporomandibular joint
TMPDS	temporomandibular pain dysfunction syndrome
TNF	tissue necrosis factor
TTP	tender to percussion
ULS	upper labial segment
URA	upper removable appliance
URTI	upper respiratory tract infection
US (S)	ultrasound (scan)
UTI	urinary tract infection
U&Es	urea and electrolytes
VF	ventricular fibrillation
Xbite	crossbite
X-rays	either X-ray beam or radiographs
yr	year
ZOE	zinc oxide eugenol

History and examination

Contents

> **Relevant pages in other chapters** It could, of course, be said that all pages are relevant to this section, because history and examination are the first steps in the care of any patient. However, as that is hardly helpful, the reader is referred specifically to the following: dental charting, 📖 p. 734; medical conditions, Chapter 11; the child with toothache, 📖 p. 60; pre-operative management of the dental patient, 📖 p. 538; the cranial nerves, 📖 p. 508; orthodontic assessment, 📖 p. 126; pulpal pain, 📖 p. 220.

> **Principal sources** Experience.

Listen, look, and learn

Much of what you need to know about any individual patient can be obtained by watching them enter the surgery and sit in the chair, their body language during the interview, and a few well-chosen questions (Chapter 16). One of the great secrets of health care is to develop the ability to actually listen to what your patients tell you and to use that information. Doctors and dentists are often concerned that if they allow patients to speak rather than answer questions, history-taking will prove inefficient and prolonged. In fact, most patients will give the information necessary to make a provisional diagnosis, and further useful personal information, if allowed to speak uninterrupted. Most will lapse into silence after 2–3min of monologue. History-taking should be conducted with the patient sitting comfortably; this rarely equates with supine! In order to produce an all-round history it is, however, customary and frequently necessary to resort to directed questioning, here are a few hints:

- Always introduce yourself to the patient and any accompanying person, and explain, if it is not immediately obvious, what your role is in helping them.
- Remember that patients are (usually) neither medically nor dentally trained, so use plain speech without speaking down to them.
- Questions are a key part of history-taking and the manner in which they are asked can lead to a quick diagnosis and a trusting patient, or abject confusion with a potential litigant. Leading questions should, by and large, be avoided as they impose a preconceived idea upon the patient. This is also a problem when the question suggests the answer, e.g. 'is the pain worse when you drink hot drinks?' To avoid this, phrase questions so that a descriptive reply rather than a straight yes or no is required. However, with the more reticent patient it may be necessary to ask leading questions to elicit relevant information.
- Notwithstanding earlier paragraphs, you will sometimes find it necessary to interrupt patients in full flight during a detailed monologue on their grandmother's sick parrot. Try to do this tactfully, e.g. 'but to come more up to date' or 'this is rather difficult—please slow down and let me understand how this affects the problem you have come about today'.

Specifics of a medical or dental history are described on 📖 pp. 6 and 4. The object is to elicit sufficient information to make a provisional diagnosis for the patient whilst establishing a mutual rapport, thus facilitating further investigations and/or treatment.

Presenting complaint

The aim of this part of the history is to have a provisional differential diagnosis even before examining the patient. The following is a suggested outline, which would require modifying according to the circumstances:

C/O (complaining of) in the patient's own words. Use a general introductory question, e.g. 'Why did you come to see us today? What is the problem?'

Avoid 'What brought you here today?' unless you want to give them the chance to make a joke about transport or car parking.

If symptoms are present:

Onset and pattern When did the problem start? Is it getting better, worse or staying the same?

Frequency How often, how long does it last? Does it occur at any particular time of day or night.

Exacerbating and relieving factors What makes it better, what makes it worse? What started it?

If pain is the main symptom:

Origin and radiation Where is the pain and does it spread?

Character and intensity How would you describe the pain: sharp, shooting, dull, aching, etc. This can be difficult, but patients with specific 'organic' pain will often understand exactly what you mean whereas patients with symptoms with a high behavioural overlay will be vague and prevaricate.

Associations Is there anything, in your own mind, which you associate with the problem?

The majority of dental problems can quickly be narrowed down using a simple series of questions such as these to create a provisional diagnosis and judge the urgency of the problem.

The dental history

It is important to assess the patient's dental awareness and the likelihood of raising it. A dental history may also provide invaluable clues as to the nature of the presenting complaint and should not be ignored. This can be achieved by some simple general questions:

How often do you go to the dentist?
> (this gives information on motivation, likely attendance patterns, and may indicate patients who change their GDP frequently)

When did you last see a dentist and what did he do?
> (this may give clues as to the diagnosis of the presenting complaint, e.g. a recent RCT)

How often do you brush your teeth and how long for?
> (motivation and likely gingival condition)

Have you ever had any pain or clicking from your jaw joints?
> (TMJ pathology)

Do you grind your teeth or bite your nails?
> (TMPDS, personality)

How do you feel about dental treatment?
> (dental anxiety)

What do you think about the appearance of your teeth?
> (motivation, need for orthodontic treatment)

What is your job?
> (socio-economic status, education)

Where do you live?
> (fluoride intake, travelling time to surgery)

What types of dental treatment have you had previously?
> (previous extractions, problems with LA or GA, orthodontics, periodontal treatment)

What are your favourite drinks/foods?
> (caries rate, erosion)

The medical history

There is much to be said for asking patients to complete a medical history questionnaire, as this encourages more accurate responses to sensitive questions. However, it is important to use this as a starting point, and clarify the answers with the patient.

Example of a medical questionnaire

QUESTION   YES/NO

Are you fit and well?

Have you ever been admitted to hospital?

   If yes, please give brief details:

Have you ever had an operation?

   If so, were there any problems?

Have you ever had any heart trouble or high blood pressure?

Have you ever had any chest trouble?

Have you ever had any problems with bleeding?

Have you ever had asthma, eczema, hayfever?

Are you allergic to penicillin?

Are you allergic to any other drug or substance?

Have you ever had:
- rheumatic fever?
- diabetes?
- epilepsy?
- tuberculosis?
- Jaundice?
- hepatitis?
- other infectious disease?

Are you pregnant?

Are you taking any drugs, medications, or pills?

   If yes, please give details: (see Chapter 12)

Who is your General Medical Practitioner (GMP)?

▶ Check the medical history at each recall.

▶ If in any doubt contact the patient's GMP, or the specialist they are attending, before proceeding.

NB A complete medical history (as required when clerking in-patients) would include details of the patient's family history (for familial disease) and social history (for factors associated with disease, e.g. smoking, drinking, and for home support on discharge). It would be completed by a systematic enquiry:

Cardiovascular chest pain, palpitations, breathlessness.

Respiratory breathlessness, wheeze, cough—productive or not.

Gastrointestinal appetite and eating, pain, distension, and bowel habit.

Genitourinary pain, frequency (day and night), incontinence, straining, or dribbling.

Central nervous system fits, faints, and headaches.

Screening for medical problems in dental practice

Certain conditions are so commonplace and of such significance that screening (specifically looking for asymptomatic markers of disease) is justifiable. Whether or not it is appropriate to use the dental practice environment to screen for hypertension, smoking or drug and alcohol abuse is very much a cultural, personal and pragmatic decision for the dentist.

What is crucial is that if you choose to initiate say a screening policy for hypertension in practice (i.e. you measure every adult's blood pressure) you must ensure you are adequately trained in the technique, are aware of and avoid the risk of inducing disease (people get anxious at the dentist and may have 'white coat hypertension' which is of no significance) and act on significant results in a meaningful way. Generating a cohort of 'worried well' who then overload their GMP is hardly helpful whereas detecting significant hypertension in an unsuspecting middle age man who then has this corrected, could be.

Medical examination

For the vast majority of dental patients attending as out-patients to a practice, community centre, or hospital, simply recording a medical history should suffice to screen for any potential problems. The exceptions are patients who are to undergo general anaesthesia and anyone with a positive medical history undergoing extensive treatment under LA or sedation. The aim in these cases is to detect any gross abnormality so that it can be dealt with (by investigation, by getting a more experienced or specialist opinion, or by simple treatment if you are completely familiar with the problem). This is a summary, for more detail see 'In-patients' Chapter 11.

General Look at sclera in good light for jaundice & anaemia. Cyanosis, peripheral: blue extremities, central: blue tongue. Dehydration, lift skin between thumb and forefinger.

Cardiovascular system Feel and time the pulse. Measure blood pressure. Listen to the heart sounds along the left sternal edge and the apex (normally 5th intercostal space midclavicular line on the left), murmurs are whooshing sounds between the 'lup dub' of the normal heart sounds. Palpate peripheral pulses and look at the neck for a prominent jugular venous pulse (this is difficult and takes much practice).

Respiratory system Look at the respiratory rate (12–18/min), is expansion equal on both sides? Listen to the chest, is air entry equal on both sides, are there any crackles or wheezes indicating infection, fluid, or asthma? Percuss the back, comparing resonance.

Gastrointestinal system With the patient lying supine and relaxed with hands by their sides, palpate with the edge of the hand for liver (upper right quadrant) and spleen (upper left quadrant). These should be just palpable on inspiration. Also palpate bimanually for both kidneys in the right and left flanks (healthy kidneys are not palpable) and note any masses, scars, or hernia. Listen for bowel sounds and palpate for a full bladder.

Genitourinary system Mostly covered by abdominal examination above. Patients with genitourinary symptoms are more likely to go into postoperative urinary retention. Pelvic and rectal examinations are neither appropriate nor indicated and should not be conducted by the non-medically qualified.

Central nervous system Is the patient alert and orientated in time, place, and person? Examination of the cranial nerves, 📖 p. 508. Ask the patient to move their limbs through a range of movements, then repeat passively and against resistance to assess tone, power, and mobility. Reflexes: brachioradialis, biceps, triceps, knee, ankle, and plantar are commonly elicited (stimulation of the sole normally causes plantar flexion of the great toe).

Musculoskeletal system Note limitations in movement and arthritis, especially affecting the cervical spine, which may need to be hyperextended in order to intubate for anaesthesia.

Examination of the head and neck

This is an aspect of examination that is both undertaught and overlooked in both medical and dental training. In the former, the tendency is to approach the area in a rather cursory manner, partly because it is not well understood. In the latter it is often forgotten, despite otherwise extensive knowledge of the head and neck, to look beyond the mouth. For this reason the examination below is given in some detail, but so thorough an inspection is only necessary in selected cases, e.g. suspected oral cancer, facial pain of unknown origin, trauma, etc.

Head and facial appearance Look for specific deformities (📖 p. 170), facial disharmony (📖 p. 168), syndromes (📖 p. 725), traumatic defects (p. 458–62), and facial palsy (📖 p. 426).

Assessment of the cranial nerves is covered on 📖 p. 508.

Skin lesions of the face should be examined for colour, scaling, bleeding, crusting, palpated for texture and consistency and whether or not they are fixed to, or arising from, surrounding tissues.

Eyes Note obvious abnormalities such as proptosis and lid retraction (e.g. hyperthyroidism) and ptosis (drooping eyelid). Examine conjunctiva for chemosis (swelling), pallor, e.g. anaemia or jaundice. Look at the iris and pupil. Ophthalmoscopy is the examination of the disc and retina via the pupil. It is a specialized skill requiring an adequate ophthalmoscope and is acquired by watching and practising with a skilled supervisor. However, direct and consensual (contralateral eye) light responses of the pupils are straightforward and should always be assessed in suspect head injury (📖 p. 456).

Ears Gross abnormalities of the external ear are usually obvious. Further examination requires an auroscope. The secret is to have a good auroscope and straighten the external auditory meatus by pulling upwards, backwards, and outwards using the largest applicable speculum. Look for the pearly grey tympanic membrane; a plug of wax often intervenes.

The mouth, 📖 p. 10.

Oropharynx and tonsils These can easily be seen by depressing the tongue with a spatula, **the hypopharynx and larynx** are seen by indirect laryngoscopy, using a head-light and mirror, and the **post-nasal space** is similarly viewed. Skill with a flexible nasendoscope is essential for those (e.g. OMF trainees) who examine this area in detail regularly.

The neck Inspect from in front and palpate from behind. Look for skin changes, scars, swellings, and arterial and venous pulsations. Palpate the neck systematically, starting at a fixed standard point, e.g. beneath the chin, working back to the angle of the mandible and then down the cervical chain, remembering the scalene and supraclavicular nodes. Swellings of the thyroid move with swallowing. Auscultation may reveal bruits over the carotids (usually due to atheroma).

TMJ Palpate both joints simultaneously. Have the patient open and close and move laterally whilst feeling for clicking, locking, and crepitus. Palpate the muscles of mastication for spasm and tenderness. Auscultation is not usually used.

Examination of the mouth

Most dental textbooks, quite rightly, include a very detailed and comprehensive description of how to examine the mouth. These are based on the premise that the examining dentist has never before seen the patient, who has presented with some exotic disease. Given the constraints imposed by routine clinical practice, this approach needs to be modified to give a somewhat briefer format that is as equally applicable to the routine dental attendee who is symptomless as to the new patient attending with pain of unknown origin.

The key to this is to develop a systematic approach, which becomes almost automatic, so that when you are under pressure there is less likelihood of missing any pathology. As any abnormal findings indicate that further investigation is required, the reader is referred to the page numbers in parenthesis, as necessary.

EO examination (📖 p. 9). For routine clinical practice this can usually be limited to a visual appraisal, e.g. swellings, asymmetry, patient's colour, etc. More detailed examination can be carried out if indicated by the patient's symptoms.

IO examination
- Oral hygiene.
- Soft tissues. The entire oral mucosa should be carefully inspected. Any ulcer of >3 weeks' duration requires further investigation (📖 p. 444).
- Periodontal condition. This can be assessed rapidly, using a periodontal probe. Pockets >5mm indicate the need for a more thorough assessment (📖 p. 182).
- Chart the teeth present (📖 p. 734).
- Examine each tooth in turn for caries (📖 p. 26) and examine the integrity of any restorations present.
- Occlusion. This should involve not only getting the patient to close together and examining the relationship between the arches (📖 p. 124), but also looking at the path of closure for any obvious prematurities and displacements (📖 p. 152). Check for evidence of tooth wear (📖 p. 268).

For those patients complaining of pain, a more thorough examination of the area related to their symptoms should then be carried out, followed by any special investigations (📖 p. 14).

Investigations—general

▶ Do not perform or request an investigation you cannot interpret.
▶ Similarly, always look at, interpret, and act on any investigations you have performed.

Temperature, pulse, blood pressure, and respiratory rate These are the nurses' stock in trade. You need to be able to interpret the results.

Temperature (35.5–37.5°C or 95.9–99.5°F) ↑ physiologically post-operatively for 24h, otherwise may indicate infection or a transfusion reaction. ↓ in hypothermia or shock.

Pulse Adult (60–80 beats/min; child is higher (up to 140beats/min in infants). Should be regular.

Blood pressure (120–140/60–90mmHg) ↑with age. Falling BP may indicate a faint, hypovolaemia, or other form of shock. High BP may place the patient at risk from a GA. An ↑ BP + ↓ pulse suggests ↑ intracranial pressure (📖 p. 456).

Respiratory rate (12–18 breaths/min) ↑ in chest infections, pulmonary oedema, and shock.

Urinalysis is routinely performed on all patients admitted to hospital. A positive result for:

Glucose or ketones may indicate diabetes.

Protein suggests renal disease especially infection.

Blood suggests infection or tumour.

Bilirubin indicates hepatocellular and/or obstructive jaundice.

Urobilinogen indicates jaundice of any type.

Blood tests (sampling techniques, 📖 p. 542) Reference ranges vary.

Full blood count (EDTA, pink tube) measures:

Haemoglobin (M 13–18g/dl, F 11.5–16.5g/dl) ↓ in anaemia, ↑ in polycythaemia and myeloproliferative disorders.

Haematocrit (packed cell volume) (M 40–54%, F 37–47%). ↓ in anaemia, ↑ in polycythaemia and dehydration.

Mean cell volume (76–96fl) ↑ in size (macrocytosis) in vitamin B12 and folate deficiency, ↓ (microcytosis) iron deficiency.

White cell count (4–11 × 10⁹/l) ↑ in infection, leukaemia, and trauma, ↓ in certain infections, early leukaemia and after cytotoxics.

Platelets (150–400 × 10⁹/l) See also 📖 p. 492.

Biochemistry Urea and electrolytes are the most important:

Sodium (135–145mmol/l) Large fall causes fits.

Potassium (3.5–5mmol/l) Must be kept within this narrow range to avoid serious cardiac disturbance. Watch carefully in diabetics, those in IV therapy, and the shocked or dehydrated patient. Suxamethonium (muscle relaxant) ↑ potassium.

Urea (2.5–7mmol/l) Rising urea suggests dehydration, renal failure, or blood in the gut.

Creatinine (70–150micromol/l) Rises in renal failure. Various other biochemical tests are available to aid specific diagnoses, e.g. bone, liver function, thyroid function, cardiac enzymes, folic acid, vitamin B_{12}, etc.

Glucose (fasting 4–6mmol/l) ↑ suspect diabetes, ↓ hypoglycaemic drugs, exercise. Competently interpreted proprietary tests, e.g. 'BMs' equate well to blood glucose (📖 p. 532).

Virology Viral serology is costly and rarely necessary. If you must, use 10ml clotted blood in a plain tube.

Immunology Similar to above but more frequently indicated in complex oral medicine patients; 10ml in a plain tube.

Bacteriology

Sputum and pus swabs are often helpful in dealing with hospital infections. Ensure they are taken with sterile swabs and transported immediately or put in an incubator.

Nasal and axillary swabs are used to screen for MRSA is certain patients undergoing hospital based procedures (e.g. gastrostomy).

Blood cultures are also useful if the patient has septicaemia. Taken when there is a sudden pyrexia and incubated with results available 24–48h later. Take two samples from separate sites and put in paired bottles for aerobic and anaerobic culture (i.e. four bottles, unless your lab indicates otherwise).

Biopsy See 📖 p. 373.

Cytology With the exception of smears for candida and fine-needle aspiration, cytology is little used and not widely applicable in the dental specialties.

Investigations—specific

Sensibility testing It must be borne in mind when vitality testing that it is the integrity of the nerve supply that is being investigated. However, it is the blood supply which is of more relevance to the continued vitality of a pulp. Test the suspect tooth and its neighbours.

Application of cold This is most practically carried out using ethyl chloride on a pledget of cotton wool.

Application of heat Vaseline should be applied first to the tooth under test to prevent the heated GP sticking. No response suggests that the tooth is non-vital, but an ↑ response indicates that the pulp is hyperaemic.

Electric pulp tester The tooth to be tested should be dry, and prophy paste or a proprietary lubricant used as a conductive medium. Most machines ascribe numbers to the patient's reaction, but these should be interpreted with caution as the response can also vary with battery strength or the position of the electrode on the tooth. For the above methods misleading results may occur:

False-positive	*False-negative*
Multi-rooted tooth with vital + non-vital pulp	Nerve supply damaged, blood supply intact
Canal full of pus	Secondary dentine
Apprehensive patient	Large insulating restoration

Test cavity Drilling into dentine without LA is an accurate diagnostic test, but as tooth tissue is destroyed it should only be used as a last resort. Can be helpful for crowned teeth.

Percussion is carried out by gently tapping adjacent and suspect teeth with the end of a mirror handle. A positive response indicates that a tooth is extruded due to exudate in apical or lateral periodontal tissues.

Mobility of teeth is ↑ by ↓ in the bony support (e.g. due to periodontal disease or an apical abscess) and also by # of root or supporting bone.

Palpation of the buccal sulcus next to a painful tooth can help to determine if there is an associated apical abscess.

Biting on to gauze or rubber can be used to try and elicit pain due to a cracked tooth.

Radiographs (📖 pp. 16, 18, 752)

Area under investigation	Radiographic view
General scan of teeth and jaws (retained roots, unerupted teeth)	DPT
Localization of unerupted teeth	Parallax periapicals
Crown of tooth and interdental bone (caries, restorations)	Bitewing
Root and periapical area	Periapical
Submandibular gland	Lower occlusal view
Sinuses	Occipito-mental, DPT
TMJ	DPT, MRI
Skull and facial bones	Occipito-mental
	PA and lateral skull
	Submento-vertex

Local anaesthesia can help localize organic pain.

Radiology and radiography

Radiography is the taking of radiographs, **radiology** is their interpretation. Referring to a radiologist as a radiographer ensures upset.

Radiographic images are produced by the differential attenuation of X-rays by tissues. Radiographic quality depends on the density of the tissues, the intensity of the beam, sensitivity of the emulsion, processing techniques, and viewing conditions.

Intra-oral views

Uses a stationary anode (tungsten), direct current ↓ dose of self-rectifying machines. Direct action film (↑ detail) using D or E speed. E speed is double the speed of D hence ↓ dose to patient. Rectangular collimation ↓ unnecessary irradiation of tissues.

Periapical shows all of tooth, root, and surrounding periapical tissues. Performed by:

1 Paralleling technique Film is held in a film holder parallel to the tooth and the beam is directed (using a beam-aligning device) at right angles to the tooth and film. Focus-to-film distance is increased to minimize magnification; the optimium distance is 30cm. Most accurate and reproducible technique.

2 Bisecting angle technique Older technique which can be carried out without film holders. Film placed close to the tooth and the beam is directed at right angles to the plane bisecting the angle between the tooth and film. Normally held in place by patient's finger. Not as geometrically accurate a technique as more coning off occurs and needlessly irradiates the patient's finger.

Bitewings shows crowns and crestal bone levels, used to diagnose caries, overhangs, calculus, and bone loss <4mm. Patient bites on wing holding film against the upper and lower teeth and beam is directed between contact points perpendicular to the film in the horizontal plane. A 5° tilt to vertical accommodates the curve of Monson.

Occlusals demonstrate larger areas. May be oblique, true, or special. Used for localization of impacted teeth, salivary calculi. Film is held parallel to the occlusal plane. Oblique occlusal is similar to a large bisecting angle periapical. True occlusal of the mandible gives a good cross-sectional view.

Key points
- Use paralleling technique
- Use file holders
- Rectangular collimation
- E-speed film

Extra-oral views

Skull and general facial views use a rotating anode and grid which ↓ scattered radiation reaching the film but ↑ dose to patient. Screen film is used for all extra-orals (intensifying screens are now rare earth, e.g. gadolinium and lanthanum). X-rays act on screen which fluoresces and the light interacts with emulsion. There is loss of detail but ↓ the dose to patient.

Dark-room techniques and film storage are affected due to the properties of the film.

Lateral oblique Largely superseded by panoramic but can use dental X-ray set.

PA mandible Patient has nose to forehead touching film. Beam perpendicular to film. Used for diagnosing/assessing # mandible.

Reverse Townes position, as above, but beam 30° up to horizontal. Used for condyles.

Occipitomental Nose/chin touching the film beam parallel to horizontal unless OM prefixed by, e.g., 10°, 30°, which indicates angle of beam to horizontal.

Submentovertex Patient flexes neck vertex touching film, beam projected menton to vertex. ↓ use due to ↑ radiation and risk to cervical spine.

Cephalometry (📖 pp. 128, 130) uses cephalostat for reproducible position. Use Frankfort plane or natural head position. Wedge (aluminium or copper and rare earth) to show soft tissues. Lead collimation to reduce unnecessary dose to patient and scatter leading to ↓ contrast. Barium paste can be used to outline soft tissues.

Panoramic Generically referred to as DPT (dental panoramic tomograph), sometimes by make, e.g. OPT/OPG. The technique is based on tomography (i.e. objects in focal trough are in focus, the rest is blurred). The state of the art machine is a moving centre of rotation (previously two or three centres) which accommodates the horseshoe shape of the jaws. Correct patient positioning is vital. Blurring and ghost shadows can be a problem (ghost shadows appear opposite to and above the real image due to 5–8° tilt of beam). Relatively low-dose technique and sectional images can be obtained. Useful for gross pathology but less so for subtle changes such as early caries.

Lead aprons (0.25mm lead equivalent)
The 10-day rule is now defunct for dental radiology. In well-maintained, well-collimated equipment where the beam does not point to the gonads the risk of damage is minimal. Apply all normal principles to pregnant women (use lead apron if primary beam is directed at fetus), but otherwise do not treat any differently.

There is no risk in dentistry of deterministic/certainty effects (e.g. radiation burns). Stochastic/change effects are more important (e.g. tumour induction). The thyroid is the principal organ at risk. Follow principles of ALARP, 📖 p. 720.

Parallax technique involves 2 radiographs with a change in position of X-ray tube between them (e.g. DPT and periapical). The object furthest from the X-ray beam will appear to move in the same direction as the tube shift.

Advanced imaging techniques

Computed tomography (CT)

Images are formed by scanning a thin cross-section of the body with a narrow X-ray beam (120kV), measuring the transmitted radiation with detectors and obtaining multiple projections, which a computer then processes to reconstruct a cross-sectional image ('slice'). Three-dimensional reconstruction is also possible on some machines. Modern scanners consist of either a fan beam with multiple detectors aligned in a circle, both rotating around the patient, or a stationary ring of detectors with the X-ray beam rotating within it. The image is divided into pixels which represent the average attenuation of blocks of tissue (voxels). The CT number (measured in Hounsfield units) compares the attenuation of the tissue with that of water. Typical values range from air at −1000 to bone at +400 to +1000 units. As the eye can only perceive a limited greyscale the settings can be adjusted depending on the main tissue of interest (i.e. bone or soft tissues). These 'window levels' are set at the average CT number of the tissue being imaged and the 'window width' is the range selected. The images obtained are very useful for assessing extensive trauma or pathology and planning surgery. The dose is, however, higher compared with conventional films and the National Radiological Protection Board recommends that all radiologists be made aware of the high-dose implications.

Magnetic resonance imaging (MRI)

The patient is placed in a machine which is basically a large magnet. Protons then act like small bar magnets and point 'up' or 'down', with a slightly greater number pointing 'up'. When a radio-frequency pulse is directed across the main magnetic field the protons 'flip' and align themselves along it. When the pulse ceases the protons 'relax' and as they re-align with the main field they emit a signal. The hydrogen atom is used because of its high natural abundance in the body. The time taken for the protons to 'relax' is measured by values known as T1 and T2. A variety of pulse sequences can be used to give different information. T1 is longer than T2 and times may vary depending on the fluidity of the tissues (e.g. if inflamed). MRI is not good for imaging cortical bone as the protons are held firmly within the bony structure and give a 'signal void', i.e. black, although bone margins are visible. It is useful, however, for the TMJ and facial soft tissues.

Problems are: patient movement, expense, the claustrophobic nature of the machine, noise, magnetizing, and movement of instruments or metal implants and foreign bodies. Cards with magnetic strips (e.g. credit cards) near the machine may also be affected.

Digital imaging

This technique has been used extensively in general radiology, where it has great advantages over conventional methods in that there is a marked dose reduction and less concentrated contrast media may be used. The normal X-ray source is used but the receptor is a charged coupled device linked to a computer or a photo-stimulable phosphor plate which is scanned by a laser. The image is practically instantaneous and eliminates the problems of processing. However, the sensor is difficult to position and smaller than normal film, which means the dose reduction is not always obtained. Gives ↓ resolution. Popular in some European countries and gaining popularity in the UK.

Ultrasound (US)

Ultra-high frequency sound waves (1–20MHz) are transmitted through the body using a piezoelectric material (i.e. the material distorts if an electric field is placed across it and vice versa). Good probe/skin contact is required (gel) as waves can be absorbed, reflected, or refracted. High-frequency (short wavelength) waves are absorbed more quickly whereas low-frequency waves penetrate further. US has been used to image the major salivary glands and the soft tissues.

Doppler US is used to assess blood flow as the difference between the transmitted and returning frequency reflects the speed of travel of red cells. Doppler US has also been used to assess the vascularity of lesions and the patency of vessels prior to reconstruction.

Sialography

This is the imaging of the major salivary glands after infusion of contrast media under controlled rate and pressure using either conventional radiographic films, or CT scanning. The use of contrast media will reveal the internal architecture of the salivary glands and show up radiolucent obstructions, e.g. calculi within the ducts of the imaged glands. Particularly useful for inflammatory or obstructive conditions of the salivary glands. Patients allergic to iodine are at risk of anaphylactic reaction if an iodine-based contrast medium is used. Interventional sialography is now possible, e.g. for stone retrieval.

Arthrography

Just as the spaces within salivary glands can be outlined using contrast media, so can the upper and lower joint spaces of the TMJ. Although technically difficult, both joint compartments (usually the lower) can be injected with contrast media under fluoroscopic control and the movement of the meniscus can be visualized on video. Stills of the real-time images can be made although interpretation is often unsatisfactory.

Positron Emission Tomography (PET)

This relies on the detection of emitted beta particles. Applications in the head and neck are in tumour detection, particularly when coupled with a metabolite—fluorodeoxyglucose (FDG-PET). Software can allow superimposition of a CT scan onto the FDG-PET image which has a major potential role in the detection of active malignancy after non surgical treatment or the detection of occult cancers.

Differential diagnosis and treatment plan

Arriving at this stage is the whole point of taking a history and performing an examination, because by narrowing down your patient's symptoms into possible diagnoses you can, in most instances, formulate a series of investigations &/or treatment that will benefit them.

Suggested approach

- History and examination (as above).
- Preliminary investigations.
- Differential diagnosis.
- Specific investigations which will confirm or refute the differential diagnoses.
- Ideally, arrive at the definitive diagnosis(es).
- List in a logical progression the steps which can be undertaken to take the patient to oral health.
- Then carry them out.

Simple really!

This is the ideal, but life, as you are no doubt well aware, is far from ideal, and it is not always possible to follow this approach from beginning to end. The principles, however, remain valid and this general approach, even if much abbreviated, will help you deal with every new patient safely and sensibly.

An example

Mr Ivor Pain, 25, an otherwise healthy young man has 'toothache'.

C/O Pain, left side of mouth.

HPC Lost large amalgam ⌐5 3 weeks ago. Had twinges since then which seemed to go away, then 2 days ago tooth began to throb. Now whole jaw aches and can't eat on that side. The pain radiates to his ear and is worse if he drinks tea. He has a foul taste in his mouth. Little relief from analgesics.

PMH Well. Medical history NAD, i.e. no 'alarm bells' on questionnaire.

PDH Means well, but is an irregular attendee, 'had some bad experiences', 'don't like needles'.

O/E

EO Medical examination inappropriate in view of PMH. Some swelling left side of face due to left submandibular lymphadenopathy. Looks distressed and anxious.

IO Moderate OH, generalized chronic gingivitis, no mucosal lesions, caries

$$\frac{7\,6\quad|\,4\,6}{7\,6\,5\,|\,5\,7}$$

partially erupted ⌐8 with pus exuding, ⌐5 large cavity, but seems periodontally sound, no fluctuant soft tissue swelling. Otherwise complete dentition with Class I occlusion.

General investigations Temperature 38°C.

Differential diagnoses
- Acute apical abscess $\overline{5}$.
- Acute pericoronitis $\overline{8}$.
- Chronic gingivitis? Periodontitis.
- Caries as charted.

Specific investigations
- Vitality test $\overline{5}$ (non-vital).
- Periapical X-ray $\overline{5}$ (patent canal, apical area).

Rx plan
- Drain $\overline{5}$ via root canal (does not require LA as pulp is necrotic, hence won't unduly distress anxious patient, but will relieve pain and infection).
- Irrigate operculum of $\overline{8}$.
- Antibiotics (as patient is pyrexic with two sources of infection: usually due to mixed anaerobic/aerobic organisms therefore use amoxicillin and metronidazole) and analgesics (NSAID for 24–48h).
- Explain the problems and arrange a review appointment for OHI, periodontal charting, and a DPT.

Future plan
- OHI, scaling.
- RCT $\overline{5}$.
- Plastic restorations as indicated.
- Post/core crown $\overline{5}$.
- Remove third molars as indicated (clinically and from DPT).

Treatment at the first visit is kept at a minimum to relieve patient's pain and thereby gain his trust and future attendance.

Preventive and community dentistry

Contents

Relevant pages in other chapters Plaque control, 🕮 p. 198; prevention of secondary caries, 🕮 p. 226; prevention of trauma to anterior teeth, 🕮 p. 95.

Principal sources and further reading British Society for Disability and Oral Health guidelines and policy documents ᔕ www.bsdh.org.uk. British Society of Paediatric Dentistry guidelines and policy documents ᔕ www.bspd.co.uk. DOH 2007 *Delivering Better Oral Health – An evidence-based toolkit for prevention* ᔕ www.dh.gov.uk. J. J. Murray 2003 *Prevention of Oral Disease (4e)*, OUP. Scottish Intercollegiate Guideline Network (SIGN) guidelines 47 and 83 (preventing dental caries) ᔕ www.sign.ac.uk. R.R. Welbury 2005 *Paediatric Dentistry (3e)* OUP.

Dental caries

Dental caries (Figure 2.1) is a sugar-dependent infectious disease.[1] Acid is produced as a by-product of the metabolism of dietary carbohydrate by plaque bacteria, which results in a drop in pH at the tooth surface. In response, calcium and phosphate ions diffuse out of enamel, resulting in demineralization. This process is reversed when the pH rises again. Caries is therefore a dynamic process characterized by episodic demineralization and remineralization occurring over time. If destruction predominates, disintegration of the mineral component will occur, leading to cavitation.

Enamel caries The initial lesion is visible as a white spot. This appearance is due to demineralization of the prisms in a sub-surface layer, with the surface enamel remaining more mineralized. With continued acid attack the surface changes from being smooth to rough, and may become stained. As the lesion progresses, pitting and eventually cavitation occur. The carious process favours repair, as remineralized enamel concentrates fluoride and has larger crystals, with a ↓ surface area. Fissure caries often starts as two white spot lesions on opposing walls, which coalesce.

Dentine caries comprises demineralization followed by bacterial invasion, but differs from enamel caries in the production of secondary dentine and the proximity of the pulp. Once bacteria reach the ADJ, lateral spread occurs, undermining the overlying enamel.

Rate of progression of caries Although it has been suggested that the mean time that lesions remain confined radiographically to the enamel is 3–4 years,[2] there is great individual variation and lesions may even regress.[3] The rate of progression through dentine is unknown; however, it is likely to be faster than through enamel. Progression of fissure caries is usually rapid due to the morphology of the area.

Arrested caries Under favourable conditions a lesion may become inactive and even regress. Clinically, arrested dentine caries has a hard or leathery consistency and is darker in colour than soft, yellow active decay. Arrested enamel caries can be stained dark-brown.

Susceptible sites The sites on a tooth which are particularly prone to decay are those where plaque accumulation can occur unhindered, e.g. approximal enamel surfaces, cervical margins, and pits and fissures. Host factors, e.g. the volume and composition of the saliva, can also affect susceptibility.

Saliva and caries Saliva acts as an intra-oral antacid, due to its alkali pH at high flow-rates and buffering capacity. Also:

- ↓ plaque accumulation and aids clearance of foodstuffs.
- Acts as a reservoir of calcium, phosphate, and fluoride ions, thereby favouring remineralization.
- Has an antibacterial action because of its IgA, lysozyme, lactoferritin, and lactoperoxidase content.

1 E. A. M. Kidd 1987 *Essentials of Dental Caries: The Disease and its Management*, Wright.

2 N. B. Pitts 1983 *Comm Dent Oral Epidemiol* **11** 228.

3 N. B. Pitts 1991 *BDJ* **171** 313.

An appreciation of the importance of saliva can be gained by examining a patient with a dry mouth.

Chewing sugar-free gum regularly after meals does appear to ↓ caries, but the reduction is small.

Root caries With gingival recession root dentine is exposed to carious attack. Rx requires, first, control of the aetiological factors and for most patients this involves dietary advice and OHI. Topical fluoride may aid remineralization and prevent new lesions developing. However, active lesions will require restoration with GI cement (📖 p. 233).

Caries prevention

Classically three main approaches are possible:

- Tooth strengthening or protection.
- Reduction in the availability of microbial substrate.
- Removal of plaque by physical or chemical means.

In practice this means dietary advice, fluoride, fissure sealing, and regular toothbrushing (which is also important in the prevention of periodontal disease). The relative value of these varies with the age of the individual.

Of equal importance with the prevention of new lesions is a preventive philosophy on the part of the dentist, so that early carious lesions are given the chance to arrest and a minimalistic approach is taken to the excision of caries where primary prevention has failed.

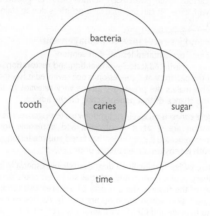

Fig. 2.1 The factors involved in the development of caries.

Caries diagnosis

As caries can be arrested or even reversed, early diagnosis is important.

Aids to diagnosis

- Good eyesight (and a clean, dry, well-illuminated tooth). Magnification between x2 and x6 (leaning forward with the naked eye magnifies the image but you can only get so close to your patient); loupes are better!
- A blunt probe should only be used to horizontally dredge plaque away from the fissures (as a sharp probe may actually damage an incipient lesion).
- Bitewing radiographs are useful in the detection of occlusal and approximal caries. They are best approached systematically viewing 'approximal–occlusal–approximal' surface for each tooth, first in enamel then dentine, first with the naked eye and then with a viewing box (magnification and external light blackened out). The clinical situation is more advanced than the radiographic appearance. However, it is thought that the probability of cavitation is low when a lesion is confined to enamel on X-ray.
- Fibreoptic transillumination (FOTI) probes with a 0.5mm tip are useful for detecting dentinal lesions at approximal sites. FOTI is considered to be an adjunct to bitewing radiographs.[1]
- Diagnodent is a laser-based instrument which uses fluorescent properties of the carious lesion to produce a quantitative reading of infected carious tissue, particularly dentine caries. Diagnodent should be used with care—it can produce false positives due to stain or dental materials.

Diagnosis and its relevance to management

▶ Remember: precavitated lesion— prevention
cavitated lesion— prevention and restoration

▶ Counsel the patient that if the lesion is not cavitated it has the potential to arrest. This makes the preventive advice very relevant to the patient, increasing the chance of that patient acting on the advice.

Smooth surface caries is relatively straightforward to diagnose. The chances of remineralization are ↑ as it is obvious, and accessible for cleaning. Restoration is indicated if prevention has failed and the lesion is cavitated, or if the tooth is sensitive or aesthetics poor.

Pit and fissure caries is difficult to diagnose reliably, especially in the early stages. A sharp probe is of limited value as stickiness could be due to the morphology of the fissure. The anatomy of the area also tends to favour spread of the lesion, which often occurs rapidly. As fissure caries is less amenable to fluoride and OH, fissure sealing is preferable to watching and waiting. Occlusal caries evident on b/w radiographs should not always be excised. If the tooth is fissure-sealed or restored, check the margins very carefully, and if intact monitor the lesion radiographically. If marginal integrity not intact, investigate the area with a small round bur. The 'cavity' can be aborted if no caries found and the surface sealed.

---

1 Faculty of General Dental Practitioners 2004. *Selection Criteria for Dental Radiography*, RCS (Eng).

Approximal caries Currently accepted practice:
- If lesion confined to enamel on b/w, institute preventive measures and keep under review.
- If lesion has penetrated dentine radiographically, a restoration is indicated unless serial radiographs show that it is static.

If in doubt whether an approximal lesion has cavitated or not, fit an elastic orthodontic separator for 3–7 days so the surfaces can be visualized.

Recall intervals[1]

This subject has evoked considerable controversy, some arguing that regular attendance puts a patient more at risk of receiving replacement fillings, while others contend that regular and frequent check-ups are necessary to monitor prevention. In fact, it would appear that only a minority of the British public attend for 6-monthly check-ups. The available evidence suggests that there is no clear benefit for recall intervals of less than 1yr for *healthy* patients, although the at-risk patient often needs to be seen more frequently.[2] In addition, as changing dentist ↑ the likelihood of replacement restorations the profession has to re-examine its criteria for replacement.

In the UK, guidance from the National Institute of Clinical Excellence (NICE) recommends that dental recall intervals ('oral health review' intervals) should be determined by the needs of the individual patient based on a risk assessment of existing disease progressing or new disease developing. For adult patients this interval can be between 3 and 24 months and for children 3 and 12 months.[1]

1 NICE 2004 *Clinical guideline on dental recall (CG19)* (↻ www.nice.org.uk).
2 N.B. Pitts 1992 *BDJ* **172** 225.

Fluoride

The history of fluoride is covered well in other texts.[1]

Mechanisms of the action of fluoride in reducing dental decay

Enamel deposition → Enamel maturation → Eruption into oral
and calcification   environment

↑   ↑   ↑

Fluoride in blood   Fluoride in tissue   Fluoride in saliva fluid
                                    fluid   and cervicular fluid

The concentration of fluoride in enamel ↑ with ↑ fluoride content of water supply and ↑ towards the surface of enamel.

Pre-eruptive effects Enamel formed in the presence of fluoride has:
- Improved crystallinity and ↑ crystal size, and therefore ↓ acid solubility.
- More rounded cusps and fissure pattern, but the effect is small.

Discontinuation of systemic fluoride results in an ↑ in caries, therefore pre-eruptive effects must be limited.

Post-eruptive effects **NB** Newly erupted teeth derive the most benefit.
- Inhibits demineralization and promotes remineralization of early caries. Fluoride enhances the degree and speed of remineralization and renders the remineralized enamel more resistant to subsequent attack.
- Decreases acid production in plaque by inhibiting glycolysis in cariogenic bacteria.
- An ↑ concentration of fluoride in plaque inhibits the synthesis of extracellular polysaccharide.
- It has been suggested that fluoride affects pellicle and plaque formation, but this is unsubstantiated.

At higher pH fluoride is bound to protein in plaque. A drop in pH results in release of free ionic fluoride, which augments these actions.

NB Fluoride is more effective in ↓ smooth surface than pit and fissure caries.

Safety and toxicity of fluoride

Fluoride is present in all natural waters to some extent. Many simple chemicals are toxic when consumed in excess, and the same is true of fluoride.

Fluoride is absorbed rapidly mainly from the stomach. Peak blood levels occur 1h later. It is excreted via the kidneys, but traces are found in breast milk and saliva. The placenta only allows a small amount of fluoride to cross, therefore pre-natal fluoride is relatively ineffective.

Fluorosis (or mottling) occurs due to a long-term excessive consumption of fluoride. It is endemic in areas with a high level of fluoride occurring naturally in the water. Clinically, it can vary from faint white opacities to severe pitting and discoloration. Histologically, it is caused by ↑ porosity in the outer third of the enamel.

---

1 J. J. Murray 2003 *Prevention of Oral Disease* (4e), OUP.

Concentration of fluoride (ppm) in water supply	Degree of mottling
<0.9	+
0.9	+
2	++
>2	++++

Toxicity

Safely tolerated dose (STD) Dose below which symptoms of toxicity are unlikely = 1mg/kg body weight

Potentially lethal dose (PLD) Lowest dose associated with a fatality. Patient should be hospitalized = 5mg/kg body weight

Certainly lethal dose (CLD) Survival unlikely = 32–64mg/kg body weight

Fluoride concentration in various products

Standard fluoride toothpastes:

   1000ppm F (parts per million fluoride) = 1mg F/ml

   1500ppm F = 1.5mg F/ml

Daily fluoride mouthrinse 0.05% NaF=0.023% F=0.23mg F/ml

APF gel 1.23% F=12.3mg/ml

Fluoride varnish 5% NaF=2.26% F=22.6mg/ml

To reach the 5mg F/kg threshold (requiring hospitalization) a 5yr-old (about 19kg) would have to ingest 95 (1mg F) tablets, 63ml of 1500ppm toothpaste, or 7.6ml of 1.23% of APF gel.

Antidotes: <5mg F/kg body weight—large volume of milk. >5mg F/kg body weight—refer to hospital quickly for gastric lavage. If any delay give IV calcium gluconate and an emetic.

▶ Advice about managing fluoride overdose can be sought from the National Poisons Information Service (0870 6006266).

Health benefits vs risks of fluoride. A number of detailed systematic reviews have been conducted to investigate the efficacy and safety of fluoride, especially in the context of public water fluoridation schemes[1–3]. These have all essentially come to the same conclusions:

1) Water fluoridation is beneficial in reducing dental caries.

2) Whilst a link with cancer (specifically osteosarcoma) has been suggested by some authors, all major systematic reviews have concluded that no conclusive evidence of such a link exists.

3) ↑ the level of fluoride in water supplies to optimal levels is accompanied by an ↑ prevalence of dental fluorosis, mostly mild and not considered to be of aesthetic concern.

4) Most systematic reviews have concluded that fluoridation has little or no effect on the prevalence of bony fractures.

1 E. G. Knox 1985 *Fluoridation of water and cancer: a review of the epidemiological evidence.* HMSO, London.

2 M. McDonagh et al. 2000 *A systematic review of public water fluoridation* University of York NHS Centre for Reviews and Dissemination.

3 Australian National Health and Medical Research Council 2007. Australian Government.

Planning fluoride therapy

Most important action of fluoride is to favour remineralization of the early carious lesion. Although fluoride incorporated within developing enamel results in a high local concentration following acid attack, the maximum benefit appears to be derived from frequent low-concentration topical administration.[1]

Systemic fluoride

▶ To minimize the risk of mottling only one systemic measure should be used at a time.

Water fluoridation at 1ppm (1mg F per litre) reduces caries by 50%. Main advantages are systemic and topical effect; no effort is required on the part of the individual; and the low cost. Yet despite this only 10% of the UK population has fluoridated water. In some countries school water has been fluoridated, but a concentration of 5ppm is required to offset the less frequent intake.

Fluoride drops and tablets Regimen (mg F per day) depends upon drinking water content (see table opposite). This approach can be almost as effective as fluoridated water, but this requires good parental motivation. Unfortunately, compliance is generally poor, so benefit as a public health measure questionable.

Milk with 2.5–7ppm F has been tried successfully.

Salt is cheap and effective for rural communities in developing countries where water fluoridation is not feasible.

Topical fluoride

Professionally applied fluorides Variety of solutions, gels, and application protocols are available. Overall, caries ↓ of 20–40%. If applied in trays without adequate suction the systemic dosage can be high therefore it is better to apply to a few, well-isolated teeth at a time. Fluoride varnish (e.g. Duraphat®) is useful for applying directly to individual lesions to aid arrest, and regular (2-4 times per year) site-specific application has been shown to be effective at ↓ caries incidence in children[1]. However, it should be applied carefully and sparingly, especially in young children as it contains 23 000ppm fluoride.

Rinsing solutions C/I in children <7yrs. The concentration depends upon the frequency of use: 0.2% fortnightly/weekly or 0.05% daily. Daily use is the most beneficial. Caries reductions of 16–50% have been reported with rinsing alone. The most widely used solution is sodium fluoride.

Toothpastes aid tooth cleaning, but, most importantly, provide fluoride. In the UK they contain abrasives (to a specified abrasivity standard), detergents, humectants, flavouring, binding agents, preservatives, and active agents, including:
1) Fluoride. Most toothpastes contain sodium monofluoro-phosphate &/or sodium fluoride, in concentrations of 1000–1450ppm (i.e. 1–1.45mg

1 DOH 2007 Delivering Better Oral Health—An evidence-based toolkit for prevention (⅍ *www.dh.gov.uk.*)

per 1cm of paste). Caries reductions of 15% (in fluoridated areas) to 30% (in non-fluoridated areas) are reported. Low-dose formulations for children <7yrs containing <500ppm are available, to ↓ risk of mottling.
2) Anticalculus agents, e.g. sodium pyrophosphate, can ↓ calculus formation by 50%.
3) De-sensitizing agents, e.g. 10% strontium or potassium chloride, or 1.4% formaldehyde.
4) Antibacterial agents, e.g. triclosan.

Recommended daily fluoride supplementation (mg F)[1-3]

For children considered to be at high risk of caries and who live in areas with water supplies containing less than 0.3ppm:

Age	mg F per day
6 months to 3yrs	0.25
3yrs to 6yrs	0.5
>6yrs	1.0

Toothpaste[1]
- Brush bd with a >1000ppm fluoride toothpaste. >3yrs and those at ↑ risk of developing caries use 1350–1500ppm fluoride toothpaste.
- Children <3yrs of age should use a 'smear' and >3 yrs a small pea-size blob (<0.3ml) of toothpaste.
- Spit out well, but not rinse, after brushing.
- Brushing with fluoride toothpaste should start as soon as the first teeth erupt (about 6 months of age). Parents should supervise brushing up to at least 7yrs of age to avoid over-ingestion of toothpaste and ensure adequate plaque removal.

Fluoride supplement (drops and tablets)

May be prescribed for children deemed to be at risk of developing caries living in areas with less than optimal fluoride in the water supply. Compliance with self-administered F supplements is often poor (i.e. parents often forget to administer them regularly).
Fluoridation of water still remains the most cost-effective method.

Other products

Casein Phosphopeptide/amorphous calcium phosphate—based on concentrated milk proteins shows promise for both caries prevention and enamel remineralization.

Chlorhexidene varnish has also been shown some efficacy in preventing approximal caries.

1 DOH 2007 *Delivering better oral health: An evidence-based toolkit for prevention.* (ℜ www.dh.gov.uk)
2 BDA/BSPD/BASCD 1997 *BDJ* **182** 6.
3 R. Holt et al. *Int J Paed Dent* 1996 **6** 139.

Bacterial plaque and dental decay

Evidence for role of bacteria in dental caries
1) *In vitro.* Incubating teeth with plaque and sugar in saliva results in caries.
2) Animal experiments e.g. germ-free rodents fed a cariogenic diet do not develop caries, but following the introduction of *Streptococcus mutans* caries occurs.
3) Epidemiological evidence showing that a supply of bacterial substrate results in caries.
4) Clinical experiments e.g. stringent removal of plaque ↓ decay.

A correlation has been found between the presence of *Strep. mutans* and caries. This is not surprising, because this organism is acidophilic, can synthesize acid rapidly from sugar and produces a sticky extracellular polysaccharide which helps bind it to the tooth. However, caries can develop in the absence of *Strep. mutans*, and its presence does not inevitably lead to decay e.g. root caries has been associated with *Strep. salivarius* and *Actinomyces* species. *Lactobacilli* are also acidophilic and have been implicated in fissure caries. In addition, plaque prevents acid diffusing away from the enamel and hinders the neutralizing effect of salivary buffers.

Methods of preventing caries by bacterial control
Physical removal of plaque
1) By a professional. If sufficiently frequent it can ↓ caries[1], but is impractical as a population-based approach.
2) By the individual. Unfortunately, at the standard employed by the majority of the general public, toothbrushing *per se* is not an effective method of caries control. However, brushing with a fluoridated toothpaste provides regular topical fluoride. Also ↓ gingivitis.

Chemical removal of plaque To achieve more than a transitory effect, an antiseptic needs to be retained in the mouth. The only chemical capable of this at present is chlorhexidine, a positively charged bactericidal and fungicidal antiseptic, which is attracted to the negatively charged proteins on the surface of teeth and oral mucosa and in saliva from where it gradually leaches out. It is available as a 0.2% mouthwash and a 1% gel (Corsodyl®) which are cheaper over the counter than by prescription. Although the main application of chlorhexidine is in the management of gingivitis, it has been shown to be effective at ↓ caries when used regularly.[2] While its widespread use for this purpose is not practical, it can be helpful in the management of handicapped patients or those with ↓ salivary flow. Unwanted effects include staining, disturbance of taste, and parotid swelling (which is reversible). It is less effective in the presence of a large build-up of plaque and is inactivated by commercial toothpastes.

1 J. Lindhe 1975 *Comm Dent Oral Epidemiol* **3** 150.
2 H. Loe 1972 *Scand J Dent Res* **80** 1.

A variety of pre-brushing rinses are now available. Research suggests that these do have a small beneficial effect if used in conjunction with toothbrushing.[1]

Immunization against caries As no vaccine is completely safe, the ethics of vaccinating against caries, an avoidable non-lethal disease, have been hotly debated.[2] Yet, despite considerable research, efforts to produce a viable vaccine have been unsuccessful due to a number of problems:

1) Which species of *Strep. mutans* to target, and whether pathogenicity would then shift to another species.
2) Differing modes of action in monkeys and rodents, therefore? relevance of experiments to humans.
3) Cross-reactivity with heart muscle in animal experiments.
4) Duration of effect and acceptance by public. Some patients may prefer caries to repeated injections of a vaccine.

1 H. V. Worthington 1993 *BDJ* **175** 322.
2 W. Sims 1985 *Comm Dent Health* **2** 129.

Fissure sealants

Pits and fissures provide a sheltered niche for bacterial proliferation. Toothbrush bristles are too wide to fit into these areas, making complete plaque removal impossible. A fissure sealant (f/s) is a material that provides an impervious barrier to the fissure system to prevent the development of caries.

Historical Several approaches to ↓ fissure caries have been tried:
- Chemical Rx of the enamel, e.g. with silver nitrate.
- Prophylactic odontotomy. This involved restoring the fissure with amalgam (hardly a preventive approach!).
- Sealing of the fissures. Several materials have been tried, including black copper cement (not retained), cyanoacrylate (toxic), polyurethane, and GI cement. The most common type of fissure sealant is a composite resin used with an acid-etch technique.

Is there a need for sealants? In developed countries ↓ in caries seen in recent years has not been uniform for all tooth surfaces. Part of this ↓ is due to an ↑ availability of fluoride, leading to a greater reduction in approximal, rather than in pit and fissure caries. Therefore the need for a method of occlusal caries is even more pressing.

Are sealants effective? To be effective, need to be carefully applied to susceptible teeth. Most valuable in recently erupted (especially first) molars, but moisture control is difficult. Therefore sealants should be monitored and replaced if lost. For maximum benefit, teeth should be sealed as soon as practicable after eruption and certainly within 2yrs. Guidelines for placement of f/s have been described.[1]

Patient selection f/s should be provided for 6s in:
- children with impairments;
- those with extensive caries in the primary dentition (dmfs is 2 or more).

Children with caries-free primary dentitions do not need routine f/s of 6s but should be monitored regularly. f/s of primary molars is not normally recommended.

Tooth selection

For children who fulfil the criteria above:
- All susceptible fissures of permanent teeth should be sealed—occlusal, fissures and cingulum, buccal, and palatal pits. Teeth should be sealed as soon as sufficiently erupted for adequate moisture control.
- Where occlusal caries affects one 6 the remaining caries-free permanent molars (6s and 7s) should be f/s.

If there is doubt about a stained fissure, a bitewing X-ray should be taken. If the lesion is in enamel, f/s and monitor clinically and radiographically. If in doubt, carry out an enamel biopsy. If the lesion extends to dentine place a PRR, providing the cavity does not extend to more than one-third of the occlusal surface, in which case a conventional restoration is required. Composite resin-based sealant retention: >85% after 1yr and >50% after 5yrs.[1]

1 BSPD 2000 *Int J Paed Dent* **10** 174.

Discussion of the cost-effectiveness of sealants compared to restoration has been well aired over the years, which is surprising given that the end results are not comparable. However, recent studies which have indicated that amalgam restorations have a rather more finite life than was once assumed (📖 p. 236), has deflated this debate.

Types of fissure sealant Sealants can be classified by polymerization method (light- or self-cure), resin system (Bis-GMA or urethane diacrylate), colour (clear or tinted), and whether they are filled or unfilled. The choice is one of personal preference; however, it has been pointed out that coloured/opaque sealants are more readily obvious to the patient. The retention rates of the different types are similar: success depends upon maintaining an absolutely dry field during application.

GI sealants do release fluoride but have poorer retention than resin sealants. They are useful for high caries-risk children as a temporary sealant where adequate isolation for successful placement of resin-based sealants is not possible; e.g. partially erupted teeth/poor cooperation.

Fissure sealant technique
1) Prophylaxis (this may be omitted if the tooth is already relatively free from plaque).
2) Isolate and dry the tooth.
3) Etch for the time recommended by the manufacturer (usually 20–40sec) with 30–50% phosphoric acid.
4) Wash thoroughly, re-isolate, and dry very, very well. If salivary contamination occurs, re-etch.
5) Application of a suitable enamel bonding agent may improve retention
6) Apply f/s (method depends upon delivery system).
7) After polymerization try to remove the sealant. If satisfactory, occlusal adjustment is usually not required unless a large volume has inadvertently been applied or a filled resin is used.

Follow up f/s should be monitored clinically and where appropriate, radiographically (bitewings). Defective sealants should be replenished to maintain their marginal integrity.

1 National Institutes of Health 1984 *J Am Dent Assoc* **108** 233.

Sugar

Sugar—is used to refer to the mono- and disaccharide members of the carbohydrate family. Monosaccharides include glucose (dextrose or corn sugar), fructose (fruit sugar), galactose, and mannose. Disaccharides include lactose (in milk), maltose, and sucrose (cane or beet sugar). Polysaccharides (starch) are chains of glucose molecules and are not readily broken down by the oral flora. Dietary sugars have been classified as intrinsic when they are part of the cells in a food (vegetables and fruit) or extrinsic (milk sugar or, the real baddy, non-milk extrinsic sugar, e.g. table sugar). Both intrinsic and extrinsic sugars may cause decay, although non-milk extrinsic sugars are most cariogenic.

Evidence for the role of sugar in dental caries[1]

1) Epidemiological evidence:
   • World-wide comparison of sugar consumption and caries levels.
   • Low caries experience of people on low-sugar diet, e.g. wartime diet; patients with hereditary fructose intolerance.
   • ↑ caries experience following ↑ availability of sugar, e.g. Eskimos
   • Cross-sectional studies relating caries experience to sugar intake.
2) Clinical studies, e.g. Vipeholm study, Turku sugar study (xylitol).
3) Plaque pH studies, *in vivo* and *in vitro*. See Stephan curve, Figure 2.2.
4) Animal experiments e.g. rats fed by stomach tube do not develop caries.

Sucrose is considered a major culprit—most commonly available sugar and able to facilitate production of extracellular polysaccharide in plaque. However, other sugars can also cause caries. E.g. frequent consumption of fruit-based drinks is known to be a key factor in the development of early childhood caries (ECC). In ↓ cariogenicity:

1) Sucrose, glucose, fructose, maltose (honey).
2) Galactose, lactose.
3) Complex carbohydrate (e.g. starch in rice, bread, potatoes).

The frequency of sugary intakes and the interval between them, the total amount of sugar eaten in the diet, and the concentration of sugar and stickiness of a food have been shown to be important. The acidogenicity of a sugar-containing food can be modified by other items in the food or meal. Foods that stimulate salivary flow can speed the return of plaque pH to normal, e.g. cheese, sugar-free gum, salted peanuts.

Sugar and health In 1989 the COMA panel on Dietary Sugars and Human Disease reported that dental decay is positively associated with the frequency and amount of non-milk extrinsic sugar consumption. However, while sugar may contribute to the excess calorific intake which causes obesity and predisposes towards diabetes or coronary heart disease, there is no direct evidence linking sugar intake and these medical conditions.[2]

---

1 A. Rugg-Gunn 1993 In *Nutrition and Dental Health*, OUP.
2 COMA 1989 *Dietary Sugars and Human Disease*, HMSO.

Prevention of caries by ↓ the availability of microbial substrate in food
This approach aims to take into account the modern habit of 'snacking' (also known as 'grazing'):
1) Remove sugar from selected foods.
2) Substitute non-cariogenic sweeteners.
3) Modify sugar-containing foods so that they are less cariogenic.

Modification of only a restricted number of snack foods would probably be insufficient to have a significant effect.

Figure 2.2 is a Stephan curve showing the pH drop that occurs after a sugary drink is consumed (shown by arrow). The dashed line indicates the critical pH; below this pH demineralization will occur. The shape of the curve is affected by a number of factors, including the type of sugary food, buffering potential of the saliva, and foods or drinks ingested after the sugary challenge.

Fig. 2.2

Alternative sweeteners
(In this table sweetness of sucrose = 1)

Sweetener	Type	Sweetness	Cariogenicity	Comments
Sorbitol	Bulk sweetener	0.5	Low	Isocalorific to sugar
Mannitol	Bulk sweetener	0.7	Low	
Xylitol	Bulk sweetener	1	None	Diarrhoea
Isomalt	Bulk sweetener	0.5	Low	
Lycasin*	Bulk sweetener	0.75	Low	
Acesulfame	Intense	130	None	
Aspartame	Intense	200	None	C/I in phenylketonuria
Saccharin	Intense	500	None	Bitter aftertaste
Thaumatin	Intense	4000	None	

* Lycasin® is the trade name for hydrogenated glucose syrup (which didn't fit in the table!).

The bulk sweeteners (largely polyols) can cause osmotic diarrhoea if consumed in large amounts and are therefore C/I in small children. However, it is probably wise to avoid all artificial sweeteners in pre-school children. The bulk sweeteners are isocalorific with sucrose, whereas the intense sweeteners are low calorie.

Recommendations for ↓ the risk of caries
1) Reduce frequency of consumption of sugar-containing foods and drinks, especially between meals.
2) Reduce frequency of consumption of fruit-based drinks, even those labeled 'no added sugar'.
3) A few snack foods are 'safe' (e.g. nuts and cheese), but foods containing artificial sweeteners may be less decay-producing.
4) Foods containing starch and sugar in combination (e.g. cakes, biscuits) and carbonated sugary drinks are especially decay-producing.

Dietary analysis and advice

Diet can affect teeth:

Pre-eruptively Fluoride is the most important. The effect of calcium, phosphate, vitamins, and sugar is unclear, but is unlikely to be great.

Post-eruptively Again, fluoride is important, as is sugar. Acidic foods or drinks can cause erosion (📖 p. 268).

Dietary analysis

Aim To ↓ the time for which the teeth are at risk of demineralization and increase the potential remineralization period.

Indications (i) high caries activity (ii) unusual caries pattern (iii) suspected dietary erosion.

Dietary advice should be tailored to the individual. This is most easily done after analysing the patient's present eating pattern.

Method A consecutive 3 or 4 day analysis (including at least one weekend day) is the most widely used, with the patient recording the time, content, and quantity of food/drink consumed. In addition, toothbrushing and bedtime should be indicated. When the form is returned the entries should be checked with the patient.

Analysis

1) Ring the main meals. If in any doubt, identify those snacks that contain complex carbohydrate. Assess nutritional value of meals.
2) Underline all sugar intakes in red.
3) Identify between-meal snacks and note any associations, e.g. following insubstantial meals or at school.
4) Decide on a maximum of three recommendations.

Dietary advice should include an explanation of the effect of between-meals eating and sugary drinks. It must also be personal, practical, and positive! The suggestion that a child should select crisps when friends are buying sweets is more likely to be followed than total abstinence.
Some helpful hints:

- Save sweets to be eaten on 1 day, e.g. Saturday dinnertime, or to be eaten at the end of a meal.
- All-in-one chocolate bars are preferable to packets of individual sweets.
- Foods which ↑ salivary flow (e.g. cheese, sugar-free chewing gum) can help to reverse the pH drop due to sugar if eaten afterwards.
- Treacle, honey, and fruit (especially fruit juice) are cariogenic.
- Artificial sweeteners should be avoided in pre-school children.
- Fibrous foods, e.g. apples, are preferable to a sucrose snack, but they can still cause decay and there is no evidence that they can clean teeth.

Where the nutritional content of meals is inadequate considerable tact is necessary. It may be possible to suggest that larger meals would reduce the temptation to eat snacks. For children who are 'picky' eaters snacks and sweets saved until the end of a meal can act as an encouragement to consume more food at mealtimes.

BUT Remember that while cheese, peanuts, and crisps may constitute a safe snack in dental terms, they are all high in fat, and peanuts can be inhaled by small children. Also, 'diet' cola is sugar-free, but can still cause erosion if large quantities are drunk.

Therefore, dental dietary advice should be given in the wider context of the general health of the individual, i.e. ↓ consumption of sugars and fats, and ↑ consumption of fibre-rich starchy foods, fresh fruit, and vegetables. Meals provide a better nutritional balance than snacks. Hence good eating/drinking at mealtimes and avoiding between meals snacking is healthy.

Dental health education

What is it? The objective of dental health education is to influence the attitude and behaviour of the individual to maintain oral health for life and prevent oral disease.

Primary prevention: seeks to prevent the initial occurrence of a disease or disorder and is aimed at healthy individuals.

Secondary prevention: aims to arrest disease through early detection and Rx.

Tertiary prevention: helps individuals to deal with the effects of the disease and to prevent further recurrence.

Who should give it? All health professionals. In practice, many patients relate better to advice from a hygienist or nurse.

What information should be given? It is important that the information given is factual and that different sources do not give conflicting advice. In order to unify the profession's approach, the Health Education Authority has published a policy document[1] laying out four simple messages:

- Restrict sugar-containing foods to mealtimes.
- Clean teeth and gums thoroughly twice daily with a fluoride toothpaste.
- Attend the dentist regularly.
- Water fluoridation is beneficial.

How? The way in which the advice is imparted is as important as its content. There are three main routes:

1) The mass media. This is an expensive alternative and, whilst commercial advertisers tempt the consumer, the success of a dental health education message which is exhorting the public to stop doing something they find pleasurable is not guaranteed.
2) Community programmes. These need to be carefully planned, targeted, and monitored.
3) One-to-one in the clinical environment. This is usually the most successful approach, because the message can be tailored to the individual and reinforcement is facilitated. However, it is expensive in terms of manpower.

Individual dental health education Because many patients find the dental surgery threatening, it may be better to choose a more neutral environment, e.g. a dental health or preventive unit. It is important that the information is given by someone the patient trusts and can relate to—this is not always the dentist! It is important also to have adequate time, as a hurried approach is of dubious value, and to choose words that the patient will understand.

The following approach has been used successfully:

1) Define the problem and its aetiology. For example, poor OH which has resulted in periodontal disease—is it because the patient lacks motivation or the appropriate skills? This stage includes questioning the patient to discover how often and for how long he brushes.

---

1 DOH Health Development Agency 2004 *The Scientific Basis of Dental Health Education* 4th ed.

2) Set realistic objectives. It is better to start with trying to motivate the patient to brush well once a day rather than teaching them how to floss.
3) Demonstrate on the patient, as this makes the advice more relevant, and more likely to be remembered.
4) Monitor by comparing plaque scores before and after. This not only enables you to monitor improvement but also allows improvements in the patient's oral hygiene behaviour to be reinforced.
5) Remember that everyone responds well to praise, so if a patient is doing well, tell him.

Keys to successful dental health education
- Relevant to the individual, their life-style and problems
- Keep the message simple. Too much information may be counter-productive.
- Repetition of message.
- Positive reinforcement.

Where to go for help or information Advice on preparing a talk on dental health education, setting up a preventive unit, or even a health programme can be obtained from:
1) Local Health Education (or Promotion) Unit. These centres will be happy to provide leaflets, educational packs, slides, videos, or just advice.
2) Consultant in Dental Public Health, or nearest Department of Post-graduate Dental Education.

Provision of dental care

Delivery of care

General Dental Service This is the main source of dental care for the majority of the population (whether NHS or private).

Salaried Dental (Community) Service The Community Dental Service (CDS) was formed from the School Dental Service in 1974.

In 1989 the remit of the CDS was expanded (the guidance being updated in 1997) to cover the following:

- Provision of oral health promotion.
- Rx for patients for whom there is evidence they would not otherwise seek Rx from the GDS, e.g. patients with special needs.
- Rx of patients who have experienced difficulty obtaining Rx from the GDS (normally termed the 'safety net' function).
- Provision of Rx which may not be generally available in the GDS.
- Dental health screening of children in state schools and other vulnerable groups with particular special needs.
- Epidemiology to assist the planning of local health services and as part of coordinated national surveys.
- Community Dental Services, Salaried General Dental Services and/or Emergency Dental Services have, in many areas of the UK, recently been managerially amalgamated and are now known as *Salaried Primary Dental Care Services*.

Hospital Service The role of the consultant service is to provide specialist advice and Rx, in addition to postgraduate training.

Receipt of care

Two factors are important:

1) Availability and accessibility of dental services. Research shows that a greater proportion of the public visit the dentist regularly where the dentist to population ratio is high. This ratio tends to follow a geographical pattern, with the greatest number of dentists in the south-east.
2) Social class affects both the incidence of dental disease and the uptake of dental care. Interestingly, the differences in caries experience between the social classes are much lower in fluoridated regions.

Because dentists have traditionally preferred to practise in leafy suburbs rather than poor inner city areas, these effects are often compounded.

As part of a government initiative in 1999, Dental Access Centres were established in some areas with the aim of increasing the provision of NHS dental care. Such development was reinforced in 'Modernizing Dentistry— Implementing the NHS Plan'.[1] Further changes outlined in the document 'Options for Change'[2] also aim to address patient access issues.

Barriers to the uptake of dental care[3]

Aside from the problems experienced by patients accessing NHS dental care, research has shown that the two main barriers to regular uptake of dental care by the general public are anxiety and cost.

Anxiety This manifests as fear of pain or a particular procedure, or a feeling of vulnerability brought about by relinquishing control to the dentist in the sensitive area of the mouth. A patient's first impressions are important as the reception they receive from staff and the environment in which they wait to be seen could either allay or reinforce their anxieties. The attitude of the dentist is also a significant factor: a 'good' dentist has a friendly, personal touch and explains what treatment is going to involve.

Cost The perception still exists that dental Rx is expensive. Patients often find the way in which the charges are calculated confusing, but welcome an estimate of the costs prior to Rx.

Furthermore the pattern of attendance varies throughout life, with children now enjoying a visit to the dentist, but adolescents breaking the habit of regular attendance due to apathy &/or other pressures on their time. A return to the dentist may be triggered by pregnancy and desire to provide a good example to the children, or a need for urgent Rx and a fear of becoming edentulous.

1 DOH 1999 *Modernizing Dentistry—Implementing the NHS Plan* (🖱 www.dh.gov.uk)
2 DOH 2002 *NHS Dentistry—Options for Change* (🖱 www.dh.gov.uk)
3 K.B Hill *et al.* 2003 *BDJ* **195** 654.

Dentistry for the disabled

A disabled person is someone with a physical or mental impairment which has a substantial and long-term adverse effect on his ability to carry out normal day-to-day activities.

Intellectual impairment (mental handicap/learning difficulty) Prevalence 3%. Classified into mild (IQ 50–70) and severe (IQ <50).

Many cases lack well-defined aetiology but there are some subgroups where cause/diagnosis is known:
- Down syndrome; Fragile–X syndrome.
- Cerebral palsy, birth anoxia.
- Meningitis, rubella.
- Autism, microcephaly.

Physical impairment Most common is cerebral palsy, which is the motor manifestation of cerebral damage. Many patients with cerebral palsy have normal IQs, but ↑ muscle tone and hyperactive reflexes can make Rx difficult. Many can be treated by GDS provided there is wheelchair access.

Medical impairment 1% of children have either heart disease, bleeding disorders, diabetes, or kidney disease.

Sensory impairment i.e. blindness, deafness (Figure 2.3).
Many have more than one type of impairment.

The above groups are general disabilities. We also need to consider those that are orally disabled, i.e. have gross oral problem or deficit which necessitates special dental Rx (e.g. cleft lip &/or palate).

Disability Discrimination Act 1995—this requires that:
- Employers must not discriminate against disabled employees.
- Service providers (including dentists) have to consider making reasonable adjustments to the way they deliver services so that disabled people can access them.

Problems

It is difficult to generalize, but usually mental disability provides the biggest challenge. Difficulties ↑ in patients with >1 impairment.
- Delivery of care. This has three aspects: (i) ↓ demand, due to low priority placed on dental health; (ii) lack of provision made to provide the necessary care; (iii) practical difficulties in carrying out dental work.
- In general, disabled patients have ↓ plaque control and ↑ periodontal problems.
- Although caries incidence is not significantly ↑ compared to the normal population, the amount of untreated caries is.
- Long-term sugared medications.
- Prevalence of hepatitis in institutionalized patients.
- Dentures may be impractical therefore extractions not a realistic solution to the problems of providing dental Rx.
- Consent (☐ see p. 654).

Management

Difficult to generalize. Patients with less severe disabilities can be treated in GDS along with other members of the family. Those with severe medical &/or mental impairments are probably best managed by a specialist who will have ↑ access to specialist facilities.

Rx planning An initial plan should be formulated ignoring the disability. This can then be discussed with the patient, parent, or carer and modified for the individual. Where treatment needs are not urgent, it is advisable to start with OHI and prevention, then re-assess Rx requirements in the light of the response. For those patients for whom a satisfactory standard of OH is not possible, restorative Rx should aim to ↓ plaque accumulation. Excellent guidelines for the dental care of patients with disability and impairment have been produced by the British Society for Disability and Oral Health.[1]

OHI Those patients who can brush their own teeth should be encouraged to do so. Modification of toothbrush handles (📖 p. 336) or purchase of an electric one may be helpful. Where patients are unable to brush their teeth, instruction should be given to their carer. The best method is to stand behind the patient and cradle the head with one arm, leaving the other free to brush. However, if possible this should be supplemented with regular professional cleaning. Chemical control of plaque with chlorhexidine may be helpful.

Restorative care Greatest problems are posed by mentally impaired. Kind but firm restraint may be necessary—ideally, get the patient's carer to help. A prop (e.g. McKesson rubber) may be needed. It is often easier to use intraligamentary LA technique. Sedation may help reduce the spontaneous movements of cerebral palsy. In some cases there is no alternative but to carry out examination and Rx under GA. In addition, for those patients who can tolerate out-patient Rx, but only a little at a time, it may be kinder to clear a backlog under GA, thus allowing concentration on prevention subsequently. However, this approach requires special facilities and no medical C/I.
Down syndrome, 📖 p. 727.

The Royal National Institute for the Deaf
STANDARD MANUAL ALPHABET

A B C D E

F G H I J K

L M N O P Q

R S T U V

W X Y Z

Fig. 2.3 The Standard Manual Alphabet. Reprinted by kind permission of the RNID (✆ www.rnid.org.uk)

1 British Society for Disability and Oral Health. (✆ www.bsdh.org.uk)

Dental Care Professionals (DCPs)

Dental Care Professionals (previously known as Professions Complementary to Dentistry) are a growth area in dentistry. With increasing demand for dental Rx and restraints on health care costs, the advantages of delegating more routine tasks to dental auxiliaries is obvious. There is also improved job satisfaction for all members of the dental team.

The GDC now register and regulate DCPs. This has resulted in a number of changes:

- Any registrant is able to own a practice and 'carry out the business of dentistry'.
- Lists of 'permitted duties' have been replaced by a requirement for all registrants to work within their training and competence.
- Registrants have to attain certain skills and competences before registration in a certain group and will be able to develop additional ones during their career. There are however, some skills which registrants in a particular group would not develop without becoming a different type of registrant because those skills are 'reserved' to other groups.
- All registrants have to undertake CPD. DCPs have to do 150h in every 5-year cycle and of these 50h must be verifiable (📖 p. 714)[1].
- All registrants need to have professional indemnity cover.

The following classes of DCP are recognized and regulated by the GDC[2]:

- *Dental nurses*—provide clinical or other support to patients and other registrants. They are not permitted to diagnose disease or treatment plan
- *Dental hygienists*—help patients maintain their oral health. They are not permitted to undertake any of the skill areas reserved to dental technicians, clinical dental technicians and dentists
- *Dental therapists*—carry out certain items of dental treatment under the prescription of a dentist. They are not permitted to undertake any of the skill areas reserved to dental technicians, clinical dental technicians and dentists.
- *Orthodontic therapists*—carry out certain parts of orthodontic treatment under the prescription of a dentist. They are not permitted to diagnose disease or treatment plan or activate archwires. This grade of auxiliary is widely employed in many countries, including the USA and Scandinavia where their permitted duties may differ.
- *Dental technicians*—make dental devices under prescription from a dentist or Clinical Dental Technician. They may also repair dentures direct to the public. They do not provide treatment or advice for patients as ascribed to hygienist, therapists, orthodontic therapists or dentists.

1 GDC 2008 *Continuing Professional Development for DCPs.* (🖰 www.gdc-uk.org)
2 GDC 2009 *Scope of Practice.* (🖰 www.gdc-uk.org)

- *Clinical Dental Technicians*—provide complete dentures directly to patients and other dental devices on prescription from a dentist. They are also qualified dental technicians. Patients with natural teeth or implants must see a dentist before the Clinical Dental Technician can begin treatment. They do not provide treatment or advice for patients as ascribed to hygienist, therapists, orthodontic therapists or dentists. It is fair to say that there has been some resistance to the recognition of this grade of DCP from other members of the dental profession!

Lies, damn lies, and statistics

Sugar

- The UK per capita consumption of sugar is >0.5kg/week.
- UK children receive about $\frac{1}{5}$ to $\frac{1}{4}$ of their energy intake from sugars. Of these $\frac{2}{3}$ are added sugars, >$\frac{2}{3}$ of which come from sweets, table sugar, and soft drinks.[1]
- 65% of all soft drink sales are to <15-yr-olds.
- Low-income families consume more sugar/person/day than higher-income families.

Fluoride

- Water fluoridation ↓ caries experience, and increases the proportion of children free of caries by between 5% and 64%.
- A cup of tea may contain up to 6ppm of fluoride. (1 in 3 people in UK take teabags abroad with them on holiday!)
- At equivalent concentrations there is no difference in the efficacy of sodium fluoride or sodium monofluorophosphate-containing toothpastes.[2]

Caries

- A reduction of 10–60% in the caries experience of developed countries has been widely reported. This is thought to be due to a variety of factors, including: fluoride toothpaste, increased public awareness, changes in infant feeding practices, ↓ sugar consumption, and antibiotics in the food chain.
- In addition, there has been a change in the pattern of carious attack, with a greater ↓ in smooth surface than fissure caries (perhaps reflecting the influence of fluoride).
- Small occlusal lesions appear to be becoming the predominant type of lesion.[3]
- **BUT**: there is some evidence to suggest that the ↓ in caries may have halted in Britain, especially in young children.[4]

Adult dental health in the UK[5, 6]

A marked regional variation was noted, with Scotland and N. Ireland having the smallest number of sound untreated teeth (13 and 12.6, respectively). The average number of filled teeth was highest in southern England (9.1).

1 A. J. Rugg-Gunn et al .1986 *Human Nutrition: Applied Nutrition* **40A** 115.

2 *American Journal of Dentistry*, Special Issue,1993.

3 A. Sheiham 1989 *BDJ* **165** 240.

4 R. Welbury (ed.) 2005 *Paediatric Dentistry*, OUP.

5 OPCS Monitor 1990 *Adult Dental Health United Kingdom*, HMSO.

6 M. Kelly et al. 2000 *Adult Dental Health Survey: Oral Health in the United Kingdom 1998*, HMSO.

	1978	*1988*	*1998*
Proportion of adults edentulous	30%	21%	13%
Average condition of teeth:			
Missing	9 teeth	7.8 teeth	7.2 teeth
Decayed	1.9 teeth	1 tooth	1.5 teeth
Filled	8.1 teeth	8.4 teeth	7 teeth
Sound	13 teeth	14.8 teeth	15.7 teeth

Periodontal disease

- Prevalence in UK:

	17–24yrs	25+ yrs
Gingivitis	77%	87%
Periodontitis	3%	64%

- Recent estimates indicate that approximately 10–15% of adults may be at high risk of developing progressive periodontal disease.

Child dental health

- The proportion of caries-free 5-yr-olds in England and Wales rose from 29% in 1973 to 55% in 1993, thus achieving one of the goals set by the WHO for the year 2000.[1] No statistically significant change in decay prevalence was seen in either 5- or 8-yr-olds between 1993 and 2003, but the proportion of decayed primary teeth that had been filled had ↓ significantly.[2] Hence, in many parts of the UK, approximately half of 5-yr-olds still have decay experience. The distribution of caries is also highly skewed, with about 80% of caries occurring in 20% of the population[3].
- Reductions in levels of dental caries among children in the UK since 1983 were substantially greater in the permanent dentition than those found in primary dentition. However, levels of caries are still substantial. In 2000/01 38% of 12-yr-olds in England and Wales had caries experience in the permanent dentition[4].
- 54% of 9-yr-old children are in need of orthodontic Rx.

Indices

DMFT	decayed, missing, and filled permanent teeth.
dmft	decayed, missing, and filled deciduous teeth.
deft	decayed, exfoliated, and filled deciduous teeth.
dft	decayed and filled deciduous teeth.
DMFS	decayed, missing, and filled surfaces in permanent teeth.
Care index	Proportion of dmft that has been treated by filling (ft/dmft).

---

1 M. O'Brien 1994 *Childrens' Dental Health in the UK 1993*, HMSO.

2 R. Harker and J. Morris 2004 *Childrens Dental Health in England 2003*, HMSO.

3 N. B. Pitts *et al.* 2003 *Comm Dent Health* **20** 45.

4 N. B. Pitts *et al.* 2002 *Comm Dent Health* **19** 46.

Paediatric dentistry

Contents

Principal sources and further reading R. Andlaw 1996 *A Manual of Paedodontics*, Churchill Livingstone. J. O. Andreasen 2007 *Textbook and Color Atlas of Traumatic Injuries to the Teeth* (4e), Blackwell Publishing. COPDEND/DOH 2007 Child Protection and the Dental Team ℬ www.cpdt.org.uk. M. S. Duggal et al. 2002 *Restorative Techniques in Paediatric Dentistry*. Dunitz. R. R. Welbury 2005 *Paediatric Dentistry* (3e), OUP. BSPD policy documents and clinical guidelines ℬ www.bspd.co.uk. International Association of Dental Traumatology guidelines ℬ www.iadt-dentaltrauma.org.

The child patient

▶ Treat the patient not the tooth.

Principal aims of Rx

- Development and maintenance of healthy and attractive 1° and 2° dentitions.
- Freedom from pain and infection.
- A happy and cooperative patient.
- Prevention is priority.

Points to remember

- Praise good behaviour (reinforcement, 📖 p. 58), ignore bad.
- Involve parents (they determine whether child will return).
- Do not offer choice where there is none. Avoid rhetorical questions (Would you like to sit on my chair?).
- Children have short attention spans (↑ with age).
- Children have ↓ sensory acuity (may confuse pressure with pain, sensibility tests less reliable).
- Children have ↓ manual dexterity, therefore need help with tooth-brushing <7yrs.
- Formulate a comprehensive Rx plan, which should address both operative and preventive care.
- Start with easy procedures (e.g. OHI) and progress, at child's pace, to more complicated Rx.
- Set attainable targets for each visit and attain them.

The first visit

- Children should first visit a dentist as soon as they have teeth (i.e. about 6 months of age). For young children, watching other members of the family receive Rx prior to their turn may be preferable.
- Let parent accompany child: check medical history and reason for attendance.
- Talk to child: communication is the key to success!
- Show patient chair, mirror, light, and explain purpose (tell, show, do, 📖 p. 58).
- Count the patient's teeth.
- If good progress, polish a few teeth, but don't tire child by attempting too much.
- Show parent child's teeth and what has been done that visit.
- If child in pain, the source of this needs to be determined and dealt with as quickly as possible.
- Younger children can be more successfully examined if a parent sits with child facing and then lowers child back on to his/her arm or the dentist's lap.

Treatment planning for children

Diagnosis Dental caries is often a rapidly progressing condition in children. It is essential to secure an accurate Δ before making a Rx plan. This is achieved by taking a history, doing an examination, and, where possible, taking bitewing radiographs.

▶ Bitewings are important for an accurate Δ unless approximal surfaces of the primary molars can be visualized (i.e. the dentition is spaced).

Rx plan The ultimate aim in dentistry for children is for the child to reach adulthood with good dental status and a positive attitude towards dental health and dental Rx. The final Rx plan will take into account the following considerations:
* Behaviour management (📖 p. 58).
* Prevention (Chapter 2).
* Restorative Rx (📖 p. 80).

▶ *Remember to consider the developing occlusion:*
* Long-term prognosis for first permanent molars (📖 p. 137).
* Palpate for 3|3 at age 9–10yrs (📖 p. 142).
* Beware disturbances in eruption sequence (📖 p. 62) and asymmetry.
* Early referral to specialist for skeletal discrepancies, and for any abnormal findings.

The Rx plan is drawn up visit by visit. Each visit has both a preventive and operative component (delivering one preventive message per visit).

As it is considered to be easier to administer LA for maxillary teeth, these teeth are usually treated before mandibular teeth.

Restorative care (i.e. repair) without prevention is of limited value. Dental caries is treated by 'preventive' measures; restoration purely repairs the damage caused by the carious process.

Children with caries in primary molars treated by prevention alone are likely to experience toothache/infection, especially if the child is young when the caries is first diagnosed. Therefore a combination of prevention and restoration/extraction is indicated for most children with caries in the 1° dentition.

Other considerations

Pain or evidence of infection may influence the order of the Rx plan.

Temporization (i.e. hand excavation and dressing) of open cavities at the start of Rx:
* gives a good introduction to dentistry;
* helps to minimize the risk of pain before Rx is completed;
* improves comfort (e.g. during brushing and eating);
* reduces salivary *Streptococcus mutans* count;
* produces a preliminary coronal seal, enhancing the chances of pulpal recovery and survival;
* may provide slow release of fluoride in the short term if a GI cement is used.

Delivery of care

Once the Rx plan has been decided upon:

- Discuss with parent and patient the Rx options.
- LA/sedation/GA—consider and discuss risks vs. benefits of each (📖 p. 59).
- Plan operative care at a pace appropriate to the child's ability to cope.
- Be prepared to reconsider method of delivery of care (e.g. sedation/GA) if patient proves unable to accept Rx using original delivery strategy.

Look out for any signs of underlying medical or social problems which may modify the Rx plan:
- small stature;
- failure to thrive;
- systemic disease;
- NAI (📖 p. 96).

The anxious child

Techniques for behaviour management

Most of these are fancy terms to describe techniques that come with experience of treating children over a period of time.

General principles

- Show interest in child as a person.
- Touch > facial expression > tone of the voice > what is said.
- Don't deny patient's fear.
- Explain—why, how, when.
- Reward good behaviour, ignore bad.
- Get child involved in Rx, e.g. holding saliva ejector.
- Giving the child some control over the situation will also help them to relax, e.g. raising their hand if they want you to stop for any reason.

Tell, show, do Self-explanatory, but use language the child will understand.

Behaviour shaping Aim to guide and modify the child's responses, selectively reinforcing appropriate behaviour, whilst discouraging/ignoring inappropriate behaviour.

Reinforcement This is the strengthening of patterns of behaviour, usually by rewarding good behaviour with approval and praise. If a child protests and is uncooperative during Rx, do not immediately abandon session and return them to the consolation of their parent, as this could inadvertently reinforce the undesirable behaviour. It is better to try and ensure that some phase of the Rx is completed, e.g. placing a dressing.

Modelling Useful for children with little previous dental experience who are apprehensive. Encourage child to watch other children of similar age or siblings receiving dental Rx happily.

Desensitization Used for child with pre-existing fears or phobias. Involves helping patient to relax in dental environment, then constructing a hierarchy of fearful stimuli for that patient. These are introduced to the child gradually, with progression on to the next stimulus only when the child is able to cope with previous situation.

Should parent accompany child into surgery? Essential on first visit, thereafter depends upon child's age. If in doubt ask child's preference. However, if parent is dental phobic, their anxiety in the dental environment may be unhelpful, so in these cases it is probably wiser to leave mum or dad in the waiting room. Some children will play up to an over-protective parent in order to gain sympathy or rewards, and may prove more cooperative by themselves. However, many parents wish to be involved in, and informed about, their child's Rx. Ideally parents should be motivated positively and instructed implicitly to act in the role of the 'silent helper'.

Sedation

Sometimes indicated for the genuinely anxious child who wishes to cooperate and also may help children with over-active gag reflexes and those where analgesia additional to LA may be needed (e.g. for difficult extractions such as 6s).

Oral: Drugs such as midazolam and chloral hydrate can be used, although specialized knowledge and skills are required.

Intramuscular: rarely used in children.

Intravenous: rarely used in children.

Per rectum: popular in some Scandinavian countries.

Inhalation: uses nitrous oxide/oxygen mixture to produce RA and is most popular technique for use with children. Effective for ↓ anxiety and ↑ tolerance of invasive procedures in children who wish to cooperate but are too anxious to do so without help. It is a good idea not to carry out any Rx during the visit when the child is introduced to 'happy air'. Let child position nose-piece themselves. Further details see chapter 13.

Hypnosis

Hypnosis produces a state of altered consciousness and relaxation, though it cannot be used to make subjects do anything that they do not wish.[1] Attendance at a course is necessary to gain experience with susceptible subjects. It can be described as either a way of helping the child to relax, or as a special kind of sleep.

General anaesthesia

Allows dental rehabilitation &/or dental extractions to be achieved at one visit. GA should only be used for dental Rx when absolutely necessary (i.e. when other methods of management, e.g. local analgesia or sedation, are deemed unsuitable). Alternative strategies and the risks of GA must be discussed to enable parents to make an informed decision. From December 2001 dental GA in the UK can only be provided in a hospital setting.[2]
The risk of unexpected death of a healthy person:
- under GA has been estimated to be about 3 or 4 in 1 million;
- under sedation has been estimated to be about 1 in 2 million.

Other behaviour problems and their management

- The questioner attempts to delay Rx by a barrage of questions. Firm but gentle handling is needed. Tell the patient that you understand their anxieties and that you will explain as you go along.
- The temper tantrum: Try to establish communication. Praise good and ignore bad behaviour. Set an easily achievable goal e.g. brushing teeth and make sure it is achieved—comment on the positive outcome, rather than what was not achieved.

1 J. Hartland 1982 *Medical and Dental Hypnosis*, Baillière Tindall.
2 HMSO 2000 '*A Conscious Decision*'—*A Review of the Use of Dental General Anaesthetic and Sedation Services in Primary Dental Care*.

The child with toothache

When faced with a child with toothache the dentist has to use his clinical acumen to try and determine the pulpal state of the affected tooth/teeth, as this will decide the Rx required. To that end the following investigations may be employed:

History Take a pain history (📖 see p. 220) from the child and parent. Beware of variations in accuracy; anxious children may deny being in pain when faced with an eager dentist, whereas parents who feel guilty for delaying seeking dental Rx may exaggerate pain. Remember some pathology is painless, e.g. chronic periradicular periodontitis.

Examination Swelling, temperature, lymphadenopathy. Intraorally look for caries, abscesses, chronic buccal sinuses, mobile teeth (? due to exfoliation or apical infection) and erupting teeth.

Percussion Can be unreliable in children. Care needed to establish a consistent response.

Sensibility testing Again, this is unreliable in primary teeth, but for permanent teeth a cotton-wool roll, ethyl chloride, and considerable ingenuity may provide some useful information. In older children electric pulp testing may be helpful.

Radiographs Bitewing X-rays are most useful, because not only are they less uncomfortable for small mouths than periapicals, but they also show up the bifurcation area where most 1° molar abscesses start.

Remember, the only 100% accurate method is histological!

Diagnosis

Fleeting pain on hot/cold/sweet stimuli = reversible pulpitis.
Longer-lasting pain on hot/cold/sweet stimuli = irreversible pulpitis.
Spontaneous pain with no initiating factor (no mobility, not TTP) = irreversible pulpitis.
Pain on biting and pressure &/or swelling and tenderness of adjacent tissues, mobility = acute periradicular periodontitis.

With a fractious child keep examination and operative intervention to a minimum, doing only what is necessary to alleviate pain and win child's trust.

If extractions under a GA are required consider carefully the long-term prognosis of remaining teeth to try and avoid a repeat of the anaesthetic in the near future.

Other common potential causes of toothache:
• Dentoalveolar trauma (📖 p. 94).
• Mucosal ulceration (📖 p. 404).
• Teething (📖 p. 62).

Diagnosis	Emergency management	Definitive management
Reversible pulpitis	LA Excavate soft caries: If exposed and vital—dress ledermix Restore temporarily with a zinc oxide/eugenol cement	Pulpotomy or extraction
Irreversible pulpitis	LA Excavate soft caries: If exposed and vital—dress ledermix. Restore temporarily with a zinc oxide/eugenol cement	Pulpotomy/pulpectomy or extraction
Acute periradicular periodontitis	LA (may not be necessary if loss of vitality is certain) Excavate soft caries until pulp chamber accessed— dress pulp chamber with formocresol or ledermix on cotton wool. Seal with temporary dressing	
Acute periodontitis with facial swelling If: • No or mild pyrexia (<38° C) • Localized acute erythematous tender soft tissue swelling • No significant involvement of 'danger areas' (see below) • Not otherwise systemically unwell	Antibiotics and analgesics Ensure adequate fluid intake Establish drainage via tooth (and dress) if possible Review every 24h to ensure resolution	Extraction of tooth (or pulpectomy in selected cases) once acute phase has resolved
If: • Significant pyrexia >38° C • Poorly localized, spreading infection • Systemically unwell: dehydration, lethargy, nausea, and vomiting • Swelling involving a 'danger area', i.e. floor of mouth	Aggressive antibiotic Rx (e.g. amoxicillin and metronidazole) Immediate referral to specialist centre	Extraction of tooth &/or intra-/extra-oral drainage

Abnormalities of tooth eruption and exfoliation

Natal teeth are usually members of the 1° dentition, not supernumerary teeth, and so should be retained if possible. Most frequently occur in lower incisor region and because of limited root development at that age, are mobile. If in danger of being inhaled or causing problems with breast-feeding, they can be removed under LA.

Teething As eruption of the 1° dentition coincides with a diminution in circulating maternal antibodies, teething is often blamed for systemic symptoms. However, local discomfort, and so disturbed sleep, may accompany the actual process of eruption. A number of proprietary 'teething' preparations are available, which usually contain a combination of an analgesic, an antiseptic, and anti-inflammatory agents for topical use. Having something hard to chew may help, e.g. teething ring.

Eruption cyst is caused by an accumulation of fluid or blood in the follicular space overlying an erupting tooth. The presence of blood gives a bluish hue. Most rupture spontaneously, allowing eruption to proceed. Rarely, it may be necessary to marsupialize the cyst.

Failure of/delayed eruption

▶ Disruption of normal eruption sequence (see Figure 3.1) and asymmetry in eruption times of contralateral teeth >6 months warrants further investigation.

It must be remembered that there is a wide range of individual variation in eruption times. Developmental age is of more importance in assessing delayed eruption than chronological age.

General causes Hereditary gingival fibromatosis, Down syndrome, Gardner syndrome, hypothyroidism, cleidocranial dysostosis, rickets.

Local causes
- Congenital absence. Is the most likely cause for failure of appearance of 2 (📖 p. 64).
- Crowding. Rx: extractions.
- Retention of primary tooth. Rx: extraction of 1° tooth.
- Supernumerary tooth. Is the most likely reason for failure of eruption of 1 (📖 p. 64).
- Dilaceration (📖 p. 70).
- Dentigerous cyst.
- Trauma to 1° tooth leading to apical displacement of 2° incisor.
- Abnormal position of crypt. Rx: extraction or orthodontic alignment. See options for palatally displaced 3 (📖 p. 142).
- Primary failure of eruption usually affects molar teeth. The aetiology is not understood. Although bone resorption proceeds above the unerupted tooth, they appear to lack any eruptive potential. Refer for advice, ultimately extraction may be necessary.

Infraoccluded (ankylosed) primary molars Occur where the 1° molar has failed to maintain its position relevant to the adjacent teeth in the developing dentition and is therefore below the occlusal level of adjacent teeth.

Caused by preponderance of repair in normal resorptive/repair cycle of exfoliation. This is usually self-correcting (if the permanent successor is present and not ectopic) and the affected tooth is exfoliated at the normal time.[1] However, where the premolar is missing or where the infraoccluded molar appears in danger of disappearing below the gingival level, extraction may be indicated.

Ectopic eruption of the upper first permanent molars resulting in an impaction of the tooth against the E occurs in 2–5% of children. It is an indication of crowding. In younger patients (<8yrs) it may prove self-correcting ('jump'). If still present after 4–6 months ('hold') or in older children, insertion of an orthodontic separating spring (or a piece of brass wire tightened around the contact point) may allow the 6 to jump free. More severe impactions should be kept under observation. If the E becomes abscessed or the 6 is in danger of becoming carious then the 1° tooth should be extracted. The resulting space loss can be dealt with later as part of the overall orthodontic Rx plan.

Premature exfoliation Most common reason for early tooth loss is extraction for caries. Traumatic avulsion is less common. More rarely, systemic disease such as leukaemia may result in an abnormal periodontal attachment and thus premature tooth loss. Alveolar bone loss in a young child is a serious finding and warrants referral.

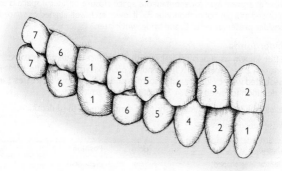

Fig. 3.1 Normal sequence of eruption (permanent dentition).

1 J. Kurol 1985 *Am J Orthod* 87 46.

Abnormalities of tooth number

Anodontia

Means complete absence of all teeth. Rare. Partial anodontia is a misnomer.

Hypodontia (Oligodontia)

Developmental absence of one or more teeth.

Prevalence 1° dentition: 0.1–0.9%, 2° dentition: 3.5–6.5%.[1] In Caucasians most commonly affected teeth are 8 (25–35%), 2 (2%), lower 5 (3%). Affects F > M and is often associated with smaller than average tooth size in remainder of dentition. Peg-shaped 2 often occurs in conjunction with absence of contralateral 2 **NB** 3 migrates down guided by the distal aspect of 2. When 2 is absent, peg-shaped, or small-rooted, it is important to monitor the maxillary canine for signs of ectopic eruption.

Aetiology Often familial—polygenic inheritance. Also associated with ectodermal dysplasia and Down syndrome.

Rx: 1° dentition—none. 2° dentition—depends on crowding and malocclusion.

8—none.

2— see p. 112.

5— (**NB** 5 sometimes develop late). If patient crowded, extraction of E, either at around 8yrs for spontaneous space closure or later if space is to be closed as a part of orthodontic Rx. If lower arch well-aligned or spaced, consider preservation of E, and bridgework later.

Hyperdontia

Better known as supernumerary teeth. *Prevalence* 1° dentition 0.8%, 2° dentition 2%.[1] Occurs most frequently in premaxillary region. Affects M>F. Associated with cleido-cranial dysostosis and CLP. In about 50% cases $ in 1° dentition followed by $ in 2° dentition, so warn mum!

Aetiology Theories include: offshoot of dental lamina, third dentition.

Classification either by

Shape	or	Position
Conical (peg-shaped)		Mesiodens
Tuberculate (barrel-shaped)		Distomolar
Supplemental		Paramolar
Odontome		

Effects on dentition and treatment
- No effect. If unerupted keep watch if erupts—extract.
- Crowding. Rx: extract; if supplemental, extract tooth with most displaced apex.
- Displacement. Can cause rotation &/or displacement. Rx: extraction of $ and fixed appliance, but tendency to relapse.

1 A. H. Brooks 1974 *J Int Assoc Dent Child* **5** 32.

- Failure of eruption. Most likely cause of <u>1</u> to fail to erupt. Rx: extract $ and ensure sufficient space for unerupted tooth to erupt. May require extraction of primary teeth &/or permanent teeth and appliances. Then *wait*. Average time to eruption in these cases is 18 months.[1] If after 2yrs unerupted tooth fails to erupt despite sufficient space may require conservative exposure and orthodontic traction.

1 D. DiBiase 1971 *Dental Practitioner* **22** 95.

Abnormalities of tooth structure

Disturbances in structure of enamel

Enamel usually develops in two phases, first an organic matrix and second mineralization. Disruption of enamel formation can therefore manifest as:

Hypoplasia

Caused by disturbance in matrix formation and is characterized by pitted grooved, or thinned enamel.

Hypomineralization

Hypocalcification is a disturbance of calcification. Affected enamel appears white and opaque, but post-eruptively may become discoloured. Affected enamel may be weak and prone to breakdown. Most disturbances of enamel formation will produce both hypoplasia and hypomineralization, but clinically one type usually predominates.

Aetiological factors (not an exhaustive list)

Localized causes: Infection, trauma, irradiation, idiopathic (see enamel opacities, 📖 p. 72).

Generalized causes:
(i) Environmental (chronological hypoplasia).
   (a) Pre-natal, e.g. rubella, syphilis.
   (b) Neo-natal, e.g. prolonged labour, premature birth.
   (c) Post-natal, e.g. measles, congenital heart disease, fluoride, nutritional.
(ii) Hereditary
   (a) Affecting teeth only—amelogenesis imperfecta.
   (b) Accompanied by systemic disorder, e.g. Down syndrome.

Chronological hypoplasia

So called because the hypoplastic enamel occurs in a distribution related to the extent of tooth formation at the time of the insult. Characteristically, due to its later formation, <u>2</u> is affected nearer to the incisal edge than <u>1</u> or <u>3</u>.

Fluorosis, 📖 p. 28

Treatment of hypomineralization/hypoplasia depends on extent and severity:

Posterior teeth Small areas of hypoplasia can be fissure-sealed or restored conventionally, but more severely affected teeth will require crowning. SS crowns (📖 p. 86) can be used in children as a semi-permanent measure.

Anterior teeth Small areas of hypoplasia can be restored using composites, but larger areas may require veneers (📖 p. 250) or crowns. For Rx of fluorosis, 📖 see p. 72.

Molar incisor hypomineralization (MIH) (Figure 3.2)

- Aetiology unknown. Prevalence ↑ over the past two decades in developed countries.
- Primarily affects 6s, but significant proportion also have defects on permanent incisors.
- Affected 6s have hypomineralized defects of enamel, varying from discoloration to severe enamel dysplasia with post-eruptive

breakdown. Sensitivity ↑, secondary caries ↑. Defects may affect anything from one to all 6s.

- Yellow/white opacities on buccal surface of affected incisors. Distribution often asymmetrical. No clear chronological pattern. Incisors less prone to enamel breakdown than 6.

Rx options include intracoronal restoration, SS crowns, or extraction (📖 p. 137). Consider partial composite veneering for incisors.

Amelogenesis imperfecta

Many classifications exist, but generally these are classified by the type of enamel defect &/or the mode of inheritance.

Main types:

Hypoplastic—Enamel may be thin (smooth or rough) or pitted. Most commonly autosomal dominant inheritance.

Hypocalcified—Enamel is dull, lustreless, opaque white, honey, or brown coloured. Enamel may breakdown rapidly in severe cases. Sensitivity ↑, calculus ↑ common. May be autosomal dominant or recessive.

Hypomaturation—mottled or frosty looking white, opacities, sometimes confined to incisal third of crown ('snow-capped teeth').

Usually both 1° and 2° dentitions and all the teeth are affected. The different subgroups give rise to a wide variation in clinical presentation, ranging from discoloration to soft &/or deficient enamel. It is therefore difficult to make general recommendations, but it is wise to seek specialist advice for all but the mildest forms. Rx: in more severe cases, SS crowns and composite resin can be used to maintain molars and 2° incisors, prior to more permanent restorations when child is older.

Disturbances in the structure of dentine

Disturbances in dentinogenesis include dentinal dysplasias (types I and II), regional odontodysplasia, vitamin D-resistant rickets, and Ehlers–Danlos syndrome—all of which are rare.

Dentinogenesis imperfecta (hereditary opalescent dentine) is more common affecting 1 in 8000. Both 1° and 2° dentitions are involved, although later-formed teeth less so. Main types:

I—associated with osteogenesis imperfecta.

II—teeth only.

Affected teeth have an opalescent brown or blue hue, bulbous crowns, short roots, and narrow flame-shaped pulps. The ADJ is abnormal, which results in the enamel flaking off, leading to rapid wear of the soft dentine. Rx: along similar lines as for severe amelogenesis

▶ Early recognition and Rx of amelogenesis and dentinogenesis imperfecta important to prevent rapid tooth wear.

Disturbances in the structure of cementum

Hypoplasia and aplasia of cementum are uncommon. The latter occurs in hypophosphatasia and results in premature exfoliation. Hypercementosis is relatively common and may occur in response to inflammation, mechanical stimulation, or Paget's disease, or be idiopathic. *Concrescence* is the uniting of the roots of two teeth by cementum.

Fig. 3.2 Upper first permanent molar in a patient with molar incisor hypomineralization, prior to restoration.

Abnormalities of tooth form[1]

Normal width $\underline{1}$ = 8.5mm, $\underline{2}$ = 6.5mm.

Double teeth

Gemination occurs by partial splitting of a tooth germ.

Fusion occurs as a result of the fusion of two tooth germs. As fusion can take place between either two teeth of the normal series or, less commonly, with a $ tooth, then counting the number of teeth will not always give the correct aetiology.

As the distinction is really only of academic interest, the term 'double teeth' is to be preferred. Both 1° and 2° teeth may be affected and a wide variation in presentation is seen. The prevalence in the 2° dentition is 0.1–0.2%.

Rx for aesthetics should be delayed to allow pulpal recession. If the tooth has separate pulp chambers and root canals, separation can be considered. If due to fusion with a $ tooth, the $ portion can be extracted. Where a single pulp chamber exists either the tooth can be contoured to resemble two separate teeth or the bulk of the crown reduced.

Macrodontia/megadontia

Generalized macrodontia is rare, but is unilaterally associated with hemifacial hypertrophy. Isolated megadont teeth are seen in 1% of 2° dentitions.

Microdontia

Prevalence 1° dentition <0.5%. In 2° dentition overall prevalence is 2.5%. Of this figure 1–2% is accounted for by diminutive $\underline{2}$. Peg-shaped $\underline{2}$ often have short roots and are thought to be a possible factor in the palatal displacement of $\underline{3}$ (📖 p. 142). $\underline{8}$ also commonly affected.

Dens in dente

This is really a marked palatal invagination, which gives the appearance of a tooth within a tooth. Usually affects $\underline{2}$, but can also affect premolars. Where the invagination is in close proximity to the pulp, early pulp death may ensue. Fissure sealing of the invagination as soon as possible after eruption may prevent this, but is often too late. Conventional RCT is difficult and extraction is usually required.

Dilaceration

Describes a tooth with a distorted crown or root. Usually affects $\underline{1}$. Two types seen, dependent upon aetiology.

Developmental[2]	*Traumatic*
Crown turned upward and labially	Crown turned palatally
Regular enamel and dentine	Disturbed enamel and dentine
Usually no other affected teeth	formation seen
Affects F > M	

1 A. H. Brooks 1974 *J Int Assoc Dent Child* **5** 32.

2 D. J. Stewart 1978 *BDJ* **145** 229.

The traumatically induced type is caused by intrusion of the 1° incisor, resulting in displacement of the developing 2° incisor tooth germ. The effects depend upon the developmental stage at the time of injury.

Rx: depends upon severity and patient cooperation. If mild it may be possible to expose crown and align orthodontically provided the apex will not be positioned against the labial plate of bone at the end of the Rx, otherwise extraction indicated.

Turner tooth

Term used to describe the effect of a disturbance of enamel and dentine formation by infection from an overlying 1° tooth therefore usually affects premolar teeth. Rx: as for hypoplasia, ⌨ p. 66.

Taurodontism

Of academic interest only, but seems to crop up on X-rays in exams much more frequently than in clinical practice. Means bull-like, and radiographically an elongation of the pulp chamber is seen. Rx: none required.

Abnormalities of tooth colour

Extrinsic staining

By definition this is caused by extrinsic agents and can be removed by prophylaxis. Green, black, orange, or brown stains are seen, and may be formed by chromogenic bacteria or be dietary in origin. Chlorhexidine mouthwash causes a brown stain by combining with dietary tannin. Where the staining is associated with poor oral hygiene, demineralization and roughening of the underlying enamel may make removal difficult. Rx: a mixture of pumice powder and toothpaste or an abrasive prophylaxis paste together with a bristle brush should remove the stain. Give OHI to prevent recurrence.

Intrinsic staining

This can be caused by:
- Changes in the structure or thickness of the dental hard tissues, e.g. enamel opacities.
- Incorporation of pigments during tooth formation, e.g. tetracycline staining (blue/brown), porphyria (red).
- Diffusion of pigment into hard tissues after formation, e.g. pulp necrosis products (grey), root canal medicaments (grey).

Enamel opacities

Are localized areas of hypomineralized (or hypoplastic) enamel. Fluoride (🕮 p. 28) is only one of a considerable number of possible aetiological agents.

Treatment Four possible approaches:

1) Acid pumice abrasion technique is used only for surface enamel defects. Two approaches (take pre-op photos to monitor improvement):

Hydrochloric acid technique (quicker)

A mixture of 18% hydrochloric acid and pumice is applied to the affected area using a wooden stick. The mixture is rubbed into the surface for 5sec and then rinsed away. These two steps are repeated (max. 10 times—removing <0.1mm enamel) until the desired colour change is achieved. The enamel is then polished and a fluoride solution applied.[1]

Phosphoric acid technique (slower but potentially safer)

A number of variations of this technique are in use. A commonly used method is to etch with 30–50% orthophosphoric acid for 1–2min, wash, then pumice slurry (pumice and water) on rubber prophy cup for 1min (take care not to overheat the tooth). Wash. Repeat etch and pumice stage twice more, washing between. Dry tooth and apply topical fluoride solution (avoid pigmented varnishes). May be repeated up twice more, but leave at least 6 weeks before each repeat to check for improvement.

▶ Rubber dam, protective eyewear, bicarbonate of soda placed around teeth to be treated, and care, essential.

---

1 T. P. Croll 1986 *Quintessence Int* **17** 81.

2) Bleaching, 📖 p. 274.
3) Veneers, 📖 p. 250.
4) Crowns, 📖 p. 242.

Anatomy of primary teeth (& relevance to cavity design)

Primary teeth differ in several respects from permanent teeth, affecting both the sequelae of dental disease and its management (Figure 3.3).

Thinner enamel (1) Enamel in 1° teeth is approximately 1mm thick, which is ½ that of 2° teeth.

Larger pulp horns (2) The pulp chamber in 1° teeth is proportionately larger, with more accentuated pulp horns. DE—three pulp horns MB, DB, and palatal. DE—four pulp horns MB, ML, DB, and DL. These features mean that caries will affect the pulp sooner and there is a greater likelihood of pulp exposure during cavity preparation. Aim for 0.5–1.0mm penetration of dentine only.

Pulpal outline (3) follows the amelo-dentinal junction more closely in 1° teeth, therefore cavity floor should follow external contour of tooth sinuously to avoid exposure.

Narrower occlusal table Greater convergence of the buccal and lingual walls results in a proportionately narrower occlusal table. This is more pronounced in D than E therefore, over-extension of an occlusal cavity or lock can lead to weakening of the cusps.

Broad contact points (4) This makes detection of interproximal caries more difficult, and means that in 1° molars divergence of the buccal and lingual walls towards the approximal surface is necessary to ensure cavity margins are self-cleansing. Isthmus should not extend >½ intercuspal distance.

Bulbous crown (5) 1° molars have a more bulbous crown form than 2°, molars, making matrix placement more difficult.

Inclination of the enamel prisms (6) In the cervical ⅓ of 1° molars the enamel prisms are inclined in an occlusal direction so there is no need to bevel the gingival floor of a proximal box.

Cervical constriction (7) is more marked in 1° molars, therefore if the base of the proximal box is extended too far gingivally it will be difficult to cut an adequate floor without encroaching on the pulp.

Alveolar bone permeability This is increased in younger children, thus it is usually possible to achieve local anaesthesia of 1° mandibular molars by infiltration alone, up to 6yrs of age.

Thin pulpal floor and accessory canals (8) may explain the greater incidence of inter-radicular involvement following pulp death.

Root form (9) 1° molars have proportionately longer roots than their permanent counterparts. They are also more flared to straddle the developing premolar tooth. The roots are flattened mesio-distally, as are canals within.

Radicular pulp (10) follows a tortuous and branching path, making complete cleansing and preparation of the root canal system almost impossible, although instrumenting canals is often easier than suggested in some texts.

In addition, as the roots resorb, a different approach to RCT is needed for the 1° dentition, pure zinc oxide and eugenol being the obturation material of choice.

Fig. 3.3 Cross-sections of second deciduous molar showing features of anatomy of primary molars.

Extraction versus restoration of primary teeth

Despite a welcome reduction in the prevalence of dental decay, the dilemma of whether to restore or extract a primary tooth is still all too familiar. In making a decision a number of factors should be considered:

Age This will influence the likely cooperation for restorative procedures, the expected remaining length of service of the affected tooth, and the severity of sequelae following early tooth loss (as the earlier the tooth is lost the greater the potential for space loss).

Medical history Possible sources of recurrent bacteraemia should be avoided in the immunocompromised patient (hence pulp therapy is inappropriate and extractions should be carried out under antibiotic cover). In haemophiliacs, extractions should be avoided and 1° teeth preserved, if possible, until their exfoliation. Prevention is particularly important in these patients.

Motivation and cooperation of parents As it is the parents that bring the child to the surgery, we must explain to them the benefits of maintaining the primary dentition. Unfortunately, a small proportion of the population still regard a dentist that fills primary teeth with suspicion—after all, everyone knows that baby teeth fall out!

Caries rate In a child with an otherwise caries-free mouth every attempt should be made to preserve an intact dentition. Where there is extensive caries, restoration of Es and loss of Ds can be an acceptable compromise.

Pain If a child is suffering pain from one or more teeth, this needs to be alleviated as soon as possible. If symptom-free, then the dentist will have more time to explore the extent of the lesion(s) and the child's cooperation.

Extent of lesion(s) In 1° molars destruction of the marginal ridge indicates a high probability of pulpal involvement.[1] If several 1° molars require pulp therapy, and cooperation/motivation is poor, serious thought should be given to extraction rather than restoration.

Position of tooth Although early loss of 1° incisors will have little effect, extraction of C, D, or E will, in a crowded patient, lead to localization of the crowding. Extraction of Es, particularly in the upper arch, should be deferred, if possible, until the first permanent molar has erupted.

Presence/absence of permanent successor Bear in mind the amount of crowding present and the likelihood of spontaneous space closure.

Malocclusion If still undecided, it is worth considering the occlusion. In a particularly crowded case, restoration of a decayed tooth may be indicated if further space loss would mean that extraction of more than one premolar per quadrant would be required. Much has been written about compensating (same tooth in opposing arch) and balancing

---

1 M. S. Duggal 2002 *Eur J Paed Dent* **3** 112.

(contralateral tooth) extractions, although this is still an area of some controversy.[1] The rationale is that a symmetrical problem is easier to deal with later, but if taken to its logical conclusion, gross caries of $\underline{D|}$ and $|\overline{E}$ will result in a clearance! In general, loss of Cs in a crowded patient should be balanced to prevent a centre-line shift.

So much for the theory; in practice, it should be remembered that a happy and cooperative patient is more important long term. For some children this may mean that the extraction of several carious teeth at the one visit is preferable to prolonged open combat in the dental chair. For most, restoration is better than running the risk of a GA, which in itself may be a distressing experience. Inevitably, the wrong decision will sometimes be made, but we are all human.

1 W. P. Rock 2002 *Int J Paed Dent* **12** 151.

Local analgesia for children

Although there is no scientific evidence to suggest that 1° teeth are less sensitive than 2° teeth, clinically it is often possible to complete cavity preparation without LA, provided extensive dentine removal is not required. However, Walls et al. found that restorations placed without LA did not survive as long as those where LA was used.[1]

General principles

- Explain to patient in terms they will understand what you are trying to do and why.
- Use flavoured topical anaesthesia (20% benzocaine).
- Warm anaesthetic solution to room temperature only.
- Use fine-gauge disposable needle.
- Always have dental nurse to assist.
- Hold mucosa taut.
- Use slow rate of injection.
- Warn about post-op numbness and avoidance of self-inflicted trauma (e.g. lip chewing).

Choice of anaesthetic agent

1st choice: lidocaine 2% with 1:80 000 adrenaline. Maximum dose = 4.4mg/kg.

2nd choice: prilocaine 3% with felypressin (0.03IU/ml)—gives less profound anaesthesia. Maximum dose = 6.6mg/kg.

In both cases maximum dosage equates to (i) 2.2ml for a healthy 10kg 1.5-yr-old child and (ii) 4.4ml for a healthy 20kg 5-yr-old (i.e. 1× 2.2ml cartridge per 10kg). This may need to be reduced for children with certain medical conditions.

Infiltration injection

Used for maxillary teeth, mandibular incisors and lower primary molars before lower first permanent molar has erupted. After 6yrs of age bone permeability is reduced and an IDB is required. Technique as for adults (📖 p. 586). In children, the malar buttress overlies 6, so it is often advisable to deposit some solution over the more permeable bone mesial and distal to this tooth.

Block injection

Inferior dental block Using thumb and forefinger, find the shortest width of ramus. Penetrate about 1cm into lingual tissues from internal oblique ridge, on a line between thumb and finger. An aspirating syringe is essential.

Posterior superior alveolar block is rarely required in children. If necessary due to failure of infiltration for 6, the technique should be modified by depositing solution distal to the zygomatic buttress and massaging it backwards towards the posterior superior alveolar foramen (maxillary molar block).[2]

1 A. W. G. Walls 1985 *BDJ* **158** 133.
2 A. K. Adatia 1976 *BDJ* **140** 87–92.

Alternative techniques

Intraligamentary injection These purpose-designed syringes have an ultra-short needle and a 'gun' or 'pen' appearance. This makes it helpful for children with a needle phobia, or as a more acceptable alternative or adjunct to an IDB. In addition, as the lips and tongue are not anaesthetized it is useful for young or disabled children, in whom there is a greater risk of post-operative soft-tissue trauma.

Jet injection In this technique a jet syringe (e.g. Syrijet or Injex™) is used to inject LA solution under pressure through mucosa and bone to a depth of about 1cm. Useful for producing soft-tissue analgesia prior to conventional LA injection or for infiltration analgesia, and for patients who will not contemplate LA using a needle.

Computer-controlled delivery (e.g. The Wand) Allows carefully controlled slow delivery via a line and needle resembling an IV giving set. Especially useful for direct palatal analgesia.

Restoration of carious primary teeth

Making an accurate pre-operative Δ (including appropriate radiographs) and Rx plan is essential. This will enable Rx to be provided as efficiently as possible (📖 p. 56)

Local anaesthesia, 📖 p. 78.

Isolation Ideally, rubber dam should be used routinely for all restorative procedures. It not only protects the airway, but also improves moisture control and visibility, and aids in patient management. It is essential for all root canal and pulp therapy for permanent teeth, and advisable for restoration of primary teeth. If placement of rubber dam is not possible, plastic disposable salivary ejectors are better tolerated than the metal flange type.

Instruments

Burs High-speed; pear-shaped bur numbers 330 and 525, and short fissure bur number 541. Slow-speed: a selection of pear-shaped and round burs are most useful. For access use a small bur and for caries removal use the largest round bur which fits into the cavity.

Handpiece A miniature-head handpiece is invaluable. Some children are apprehensive of the aspirator tip, making use of a high-speed, water-cooled handpiece difficult; others find the vibration of the slow-speed handpiece distressing, and may confuse it with pain. In these cases a vivid imagination and considerable ingenuity help. It is possible, but time-consuming, to complete cavity preparation with hand instruments.

Material selection for intracoronal restorations

Amalgam Despite toxicity and environmental pollution concerns, this still remains an acceptable and durable material for class I and II restorations in 1° molars.

GI cement Has advantages of adhesion and fluoride release, but more technique sensitive and less wear resistant than amalgam. Useful in non-load bearing class III and V cavities, temporization of 1° teeth in young, pre-cooperative children, or teeth near to exfoliation.

Compomer A modified composite-type material with some of the properties of GI cement. More technique and moisture sensitive than amalgam, but studies suggest similar longevity.

Composite resin Early studies suggested poor performance in 1° teeth, but modern materials placed with good isolation (i.e. rubber dam) should perform similarly to compomers, although little recent data on performance in 1° molars exists.

▶ Plastic, intracoronal restorations perform best in 1° molars with small class I and II cavities. SS crowns (📖 p. 86) give superior longevity where lesions are more extensive.

Principles of cavity design

Outline form Should include any undermined enamel. Extension for prevention is now outmoded, but any suspect adjacent fissures should be included. Do not cross transverse marginal ridges unless they are undermined.

Caries removal Caries should be excavated from the ADJ first. If necessary, you may need to re-establish outline form to improve access to ensure ADJ is caries free. Then progress to carefully removing caries from floor.

Resistance form/retention form The completed restoration must be able to adequately resist dislodgement. Usually a 90° cavosurface angle and caries removal suffice.

Reasons for failure of restorations in primary teeth

- Recurrent caries, often due to failure to adequately complete caries removal because of flagging patient cooperation or failure to use adequate LA. If unable to finish cavity it is better to place a temporary dressing and try again at another visit.
- Cavity preparation does not satisfy the mechanical requirements of the filling material.
- Inadequate moisture control, especially true of GI cements, compomers and composites.
- Presence of occlusal high spot.

Many others, but these are the most common.

Useful tips

- Let the child participate by 'looking after' the saliva ejector or cotton wool.
- If the child is nervous give them some control by asking them to signal, e.g. by raising their hand, if they want you to stop.
- If the child's cooperation runs out before the cavity is completed, try and ensure all caries is removed from the ADJ and place a dressing of either zinc oxide or GI cement. This can then be left for several visits, until you are ready to try again.
- Vibration is less of a problem with lower teeth, therefore if possible start with a lower tooth.
- However, giving LA is easier in the maxilla.
- Don't try to do too much at one visit—quadrant conservation is not really feasible in an 8-yr-old!

Communication

▶ It is important to explain to the child what you are trying to do, and why, in terms they can understand.

It may be helpful to describe some of the instruments we use in ways that can make them seem less threatening to a child, e.g.

slow-speed handpiece	Mr Buzz/buzzy bee/bumble bee
high-speed handpiece	Mr Spray/wizzy brush/tooth tickler
handpiece and prophylaxis cup	electric toothbrush/tooth polisher
aspirator tip	vacuum cleaner/hoover
rubber dam	tooth raincoat
saliva ejector	straw
	curly-wurly (coiled type only)
air from 3-in-1	wind
fissure sealant	plastic coating
etchant solution	tooth shampoo/cleaner
	lemon juice
cotton wool roll	snowman
dental light	the sun/car light

Class I in primary molars

📖 See p. 74 for anatomy of 1° molars and effect upon cavity design. Have all necessary instruments and filling materials ready so that appointment is kept as short as possible. (Figure 3.4.)

- Explain and show child (and parent) what you are trying to do.
- LA if required (📖 p. 78).
- In small cavity will need to gain access and this is most easily done with a high-speed handpiece and pear-shaped bur. The outline can then be established and caries removed.
- In larger cavities an excavator or large round bur can be used to start caries removal from the walls. Any undermined enamel should be cut back.
- If caries deep, stop and re-assess whether pulpotomy (📖 p. 91) required.
- Check retention and walls are caries free.
- Wash and dry cavity.
- Line with hard-setting calcium hydroxide if using amalgam.
- Place amalgam incrementally. GI or composite are also acceptable.
- Check occlusion.
- This is usually a good opportunity to reinforce any preventive advice, but keep it brief.

▶ Praise child, and if bribery has not been used don't forget the sticker/badge/toothbrush.

Polishing of amalgam restorations in 1° molars is unnecessary.

Fig. 3.4 Cross-sectional view of class I restoration (bucco-lingually).

Class II in primary molar—amalgam

📖 See p. 74 for anatomy of 1° molars and effect upon cavity preparation. Class II cavities (Figure 3.5) are designed for the Rx of inter proximal caries and consist of three parts.

Occlusal key is designed to retain the restoration and eliminate any occlusal caries. Should be prepared first and is identical to class I cavity preparation, 📖 p. 82. This component is essential for class II amalgam restorations, but can be omitted for minimal cavities restored with adhesve materials.

Isthmus joins the occlusal key with the interproximal box. It is the part of the filling most prone to fracture. Dimensions of the isthmus are a balance between:

adequate depth		*adequate width*
without risking	——————	without weakening
pulpal exposure	Δ	cusps
(1.5–2mm)		(⅓ – ½ distance between cusps)

Approximal box To allow access for caries removal. Ideally should just extend into embrasures and walls should converge occlusally.

Minimal caries with marginal ridge intact (usually diagnosed on pre-operative b/w radiographs).
- Follow steps for small occlusal cavity.
- When occlusal cavity (key) complete, extend it towards approximal surface. Most texts advise retaining some enamel inter-proximally to protect adjacent tooth, but this is often easier said than done.
- Establish floor of box, taking care not to extend beyond maximum bulbosity of tooth.
- Fracture away remaining approximal enamel with hand instruments.
- Complete preparation of box following external contours of tooth and 90° cavosurface angle.
- Remove all caries. If exposure, then pulp Rx.
- Check retention.
- If amalgam, place hard-setting lining; if adhesive material, no lining needed.
- Position narrow matrix band and wedge.
- Place material and shape/carve with matrix in place. Light cure if necessary.
- Check occlusion.

More advanced approximal caries (marginal ridge broken down—likelihood of pulpal involvement).
   Plastic restorations perform best in class I and small class II cavities. In extensive cavities &/or where pulp Rx is necessary, SS crowns provide a more durable restoration.

Fig. 3.5 Cross-section of D̄| mo restoration (mesio-distally).

Stainless steel crowns

▶ SS crowns are the most durable restoration for 1° molars with extensive caries and those where pulp Rx has been performed.

▶ SS crowns do contain small traces of nickel and are therefore not suitable for patients with a known nickel allergy.

Indications

- Badly broken down 1° molar.
- After pulp therapy in 1° molars.
- As interim measure for 2° molars, where crowns are required but the patient is too young.
- Temporary coverage during preparation of cast crown for premolar or 2° molar.
- Developmental anomalies.
- Severe tooth loss due to bruxism/erosion.

Instruments High-speed tapered diamond bur (e.g. 582) and diamond occlusal wheel. Straight handpiece and a stone. Slow-speed handpiece and burs as required. Crown scissors, dividers, selection of suitable crowns and Adam's pliers. Johnstone contouring pliers (no 114) and Abel pliers (no 112) are also useful.

Technique

SS crowns rely for retention only on a tight adaptation at the gingival margin of the preparation, therefore taper of preparation walls is not critical (Figure 3.6).

1) LA and if possible rubber dam.
2) Measure M–D length with dividers to aid crown selection.
3) Remove caries.
4) Occlusal reduction (approx 1mm) with occlusal wheel, roughly following cuspal planes.
5) Approximal reduction (approx 20° from vertical) using tapered diamond, without producing a ledge at gingival margin.
6) Remove buccal and lingual bulbosities only sufficient to seat crown (often little/no reduction required).
7) Select crown. Correct size will be a 'click' fit.
8) Check height and occlusion. Minor prematurity is not a problem. If extensive blanching of surrounding tissues or over-extended, trim crown. Usually not necessary.
9) Use pliers to adapt contact points and crimp margins. Smooth trimmed margins with stone.
10) Cement with zinc polycarboxylate or GI cement.

Technique for 2° molars (Figure 3.7) is similar but more careful adjustment is necessary.

Success rates

A number of studies have demonstrated that SS crowns have a far superior longevity to other types of restoration in 1° molars.

'Hall' technique SS crown placed directly onto a carious primary molar with no caries removal or conventional preparation. Initial studies have indicated favourable results probably due to creation of an effective peri-coronal seal.[1]

1 N.P. Innes *et al.* 2007 BMC Oral Health **7** 18.

Basic technique:
- Separators placed a few days before may aid placement.
- Carious 1° molar free from obvious pulpal or peri-radicular pathology.
- Select correct-size crown, fill with a suitable cement (GI is recommended) and place on tooth.
- Get child to bite down on crown, seating it onto the tooth.

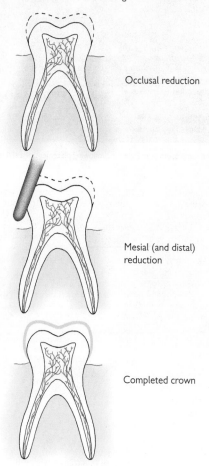

Occlusal reduction

Mesial (and distal) reduction

Completed crown

Fig. 3.6 Preparation for stainless steel crown.

Fig. 3.7 The same tooth as in Figure 3.2 following placement of a stainless steel crown.

Class III, IV, and V in primary teeth

See note regarding nomenclature p.227.

Carious 1° incisors and canines are seen less frequently than molars and are therefore indicative of a high caries rate (see Severe Early Childhood Caries 📖 p. 90).

Management Objectives are relief of pain and prevention. Aesthetics are less important.

Rx options include:
- Extraction.
- Topical 2% sodium fluoride and observation. Intervene if caries progresses.
- Discing (safer to use flat fissure No. 1 bur, than disc) plus topical fluoride.
- Restoration; usually there is insufficient hard tissue for adequate retention, therefore adhesive materials are preferable.

Class III restoration Similar technique to that used for permanent incisors, but omit incisal retention groove.

Class IV restoration If restoration is essential the greater strength of composite is required. Polycarboxylate (strip) crowns are advocated by some paedodontists, for the well-motivated child.

Class V restoration Remove caries with inverted cone and restore with GI.

Composite strip crowns Cellulose acetate crown forms for primary incisors. Enable restoration of primary incisors using composite resin.

Severe early childhood caries

Aetiology Frequent ingestion of sugar &/or reduced salivary flow.

Nursing bottle or bottle mouth caries Associated with frequent consumption of a sugar-containing drink, especially from a feeding-bottle. Also seen in some cases of prolonged on-demand breast-feeding, especially where children >1yr old suckle frequently during the night, due to the lactose in breast milk.[1] Characteristically, starts with the maxillary 1° incisors, but in more severe cases the first 1° molars are also involved. The mandibular incisors are relatively protected by the tongue and saliva.

Rampant caries A term often used to describe extensive, rapidly progressing caries affecting many teeth in the primary &/or permanent dentition.

Severe early childhood caries may also be caused by the prolonged and frequent intake of sugar-based medications, however, both pharmaceutical companies and doctors are more aware of the problem and the number of alternative sugar-free preparations is increasing. 📖 See p. 116 for list.

Radiation caries Radiation for head and neck cancer may result in fibrosis of salivary glands and salivary flow. Patients often resort to sucking sweets to alleviate their dry mouth, which exacerbates the problem.

Management

- Removal of aetiological factors (education, artificial saliva).
- Fluoride rinses for older age groups (daily 0.05%).
- 1°dentition—may need to extract teeth of poor prognosis and concentrate on prevention for permanent dentition.
- 2°dentition—need assessment of long-term prognosis for teeth. Final Rx plan should be drawn up in consultation with orthodontist.

1 G. J. Roberts 1982 *J Dentistry* **10** 346.

Primary molar pulp therapy

NB Primary molar roots resorb

Where the carious process has jeopardized pulpal sensibility there are two alternatives: (i) extraction; (ii) pulp therapy.

Indication and contraindications See Extraction versus restoration, 📖 p. 76

- Any medical condition where a focus of infection is potentially dangerous is an absolute contraindication to pulp therapy.
- Pulp therapy may be preferable to extraction in children with bleeding disorders.
- Tooth must be restorable following pulp therapy.

Diagnosis of state of the pulp can be difficult, as not only is a child's perception of pain less precise than an adult's, but the clinical picture may also be complicated by death of one root canal whilst the other(s) remain vital.

Indicators of possible pulp involvement

- Breakdown of marginal ridge.
- Symptoms.
- Tenderness to percussion, ↑ mobility, buccal swelling/sinus.
- Inter-radicular radiolucency seen radiographically.

Definitions

Pulpotomy: removal of coronal pulp and Rx of radicular pulp.

Pulpectomy: removal of entire coronal and radicular pulp.

Principles of Rx Attempting to retain the vitality of the coronal pulp in 1° molars is not recommended because (i) pulpal involvement is more likely, (ii) it is difficult to accurately determine the likely condition of the pulp and (iii) calcium hydroxide frequently leads to internal resorption. Therefore, direct pulp capping is only advisable for small traumatic exposures. Pulpotomy remains the Rx of choice for 1° molars:

Vital pulp—pulpotomy (procedure of choice)

Non-vital pulp—pulpectomy

Materials The most commonly used medicaments are:

Ferric sulfate—this is the technique currently recommended by most authorities.[1]

Formocreosol—still used by some, however, recent concerns about the toxicity and potential mutagenicity of formalin-containing compounds has led many authorities to advise against its use where suitable alternatives exist

Calcium hydroxide—time consuming to use and success not as good as ferric sulfate.

MTA (mineral trioxide aggregate)—initial trials show promise. Very expensive.

Devitalizing paste (paraformaldehyde)—has fallen out of favour (for the same reasons as formocresol).

Beechwood creosote—for non-vital pulpotomy.

Success rates over 90% for vital pulps.[2]

---

1 BSPD 2006 *Int J Paed Dent* **16** (suppl) 16.

2 V. Srinivasan et al. 2006 *Int J Paed Dent* **16** 117.

Pulp therapy techniques

Pulpotomy (for the vital primary molar pulp)

In 1° molars the relatively larger pulps result in earlier pulpal involvement, therefore amputation of the coronal pulp leaving healthy radicular pulp *in situ* (pulpotomy) gives more consistent results than techniques that attempt to retain vitality of the whole pulp e.g. indirect pulp capping.

Technique
1) Give LA and place rubber dam.
2) Complete cavity preparation and excavate caries.
3) Remove roof of pulp chamber.
4) Amputate coronal pulp with a large excavator or sterile round bur.
5) Wash chamber and arrest bleeding with damp cotton wool.
6) Place cotton wool pledget dampened with 15.5% ferric sulfate on exposed pulp stumps for at least 1min, then remove.
7) Apply dressing of reinforced ZOE cement.
8) Restore tooth, usually with a stainless steel crown (Figure 3.8).

Problems
Necrotic pulp—proceed with non-vital technique or extract.
Profuse haemorrhage—indicates more serious inflammation of the radicular pulp. Intermediate dressing with ledermix followed by non-vital technique or extraction.

Pulpectomy (for non-vital primary molar pulp)

A pulpectomy is often considered difficult in primary molars because of the complexity of ribbon-shaped canals (although instrumentation is often easier than some texts might suggest). The risk of damage to the permanent successor also needs to be considered, but if conditions are favourable it is the Rx of choice for non-vital pulps.[1] The technique can be carried out in one or two visits.
1) LA and rubber dam.
2) Remove the necrotic pulp, locate and file and irrigate canals (sodium hypochlorite 0.1%).
3) Cleanse to within 2–3mm of apex, but avoid extending beyond.
4) Fill canal with plain ZOE paste, non-setting calcium hydroxide or iodo-form paste (e.g. Vitapex®) with a spiral filler.
5) Restore with SS crown.

If there is evidence of any infection a two-stage Rx is recommended, leaving non-setting calcium hydroxide in the canals for 1–2 weeks prior to filling.

Success rate >80% at 3 years has been reported.

1 M. D. Duggal 1989 *Dental Update* **16** 26.

Pulp therapy for primary anterior teeth

Usual Rx is extraction, as <u>A</u> and <u>B</u> are exfoliated before patient is able to cooperate satisfactorily with more complicated Rx. However, <u>C</u> is exfoliated later and unilateral loss may result in centre-line shift, therefore pulp treatment is indicated for some patients. The root canal morphology is amenable to pulpectomy and the canal should be cleaned using files, with care (remember underlying successor). A resorbable filling material, e.g. calcium hydroxide or ZOE, should be used.

Stainless steel crown

Hard-setting cement

Re-inforced zinc oxide cement

Vital pulp

Fig. 3.8

Dental trauma

▶ If evidence of head injury, transfer patient to hospital immediately.

Note
- By 12yrs of age 33% of boys and 19% of girls have experienced at least one episode of dental trauma.[1]
- Prognosis ↑ with good immediate Rx, therefore see patient as soon as possible.
- Avulsed permanent teeth should be re-planted immediately.
- Child and parent may be upset, therefore handle accordingly and defer any non-urgent Rx.
- Take good notes for future reference and medico-legal purposes.
- If crown # this will have dissipated most of the energy of impact, therefore root # less likely.

History
Take a structured history as an *aide-mémoire* and for medico-legal purposes.
- Loss of consciousness? Concussion/headache (🕮 p. 456). Refer immediately to hospital.
- Accompanied by? Parent/teacher? Consider consent issues.
- When? Time interval between injury and Rx affects prognosis.
- Where? Does patient need a tetanus booster? If so, refer to GMP or hospital.
- How? Be alert to the possibilities of other injuries and NAI.
- Tooth fragments? These may have been inhaled or embedded in soft tissues (e.g. lip). If fragment/tooth not accounted for &/or loss of consciousness, a CXR is mandatory.
- PDH—Previous trauma may affect prognosis, cooperation in the dental setting.
- PMH—Check for bleeding disorder and allergy to penicillin.

Aims of Rx
1° dentition: (i) preserve integrity of permanent successor; (ii) preserve primary tooth if cooperation good and compatible with first aim.
2° dentition: (i) preserve vitality of the tooth to allow maturation of the root; (ii) restore the crown to prevent drifting, tilting, and overeruption.

Principles of Rx
Emergency Rx
- Elimination of pain.
- Protection of pulp.
- Reduction and immobilization of mobile teeth.
- Suturing of soft tissue lacerations (IO—3/0 resorbable suture (Dexon®, Vicryl®); EO—refer to hospital).
- ? antibiotics, ? tetanus, ? analgesics, ? chlorhexidine mouthwash.

---

1 B. Chadwick 2004 *Children's Dental Health in the UK*, HMSO.

Intermediate Rx
- Pulp therapy.
- Consider orthodontic requirements and long-term prognosis of damaged teeth.
- Semi-permanent restorations.
- Keep under review, usually 1 month, 3 months, and then 6-monthly for 2yrs.

Permanent Rx
- Usually deferred until >16yrs (to allow pulpal and gingival recession and ↓ likelihood of further trauma); e.g. definitive crown.

Classification of tooth injuries

Several exist; some use roman numerals, others describe the injuries sustained (WHO system):
Complicated #—pulp exposed.
Uncomplicated #—pulp intact.

Prevention

- Prevalence ↑ as the o/j ↑ (>9mm prevalence doubles) ? early orthodontics.
- Mouthguard for sports (vacuum-formed thermoplastic vinyl best, triple thickness).

Be alert for evidence of non-accidental injury (p. 96).

Non-accidental injury and neglect

▶ All professionals involved with children need to be alert to the possibility of non-accidental injury (NAI) or neglect.

NB The term NAI is now favoured over 'child abuse'

The following signs are associated with NAI:
- Usually younger children are involved.
- The presenting injuries may not match the parent's account of how they were sustained. The account may change over time.
- Delay attending at a surgery or clinic for Rx of the injury.
- Bruises/injuries of different vintages are found on examination.
- Ear pinches and frenal tears in children <1yr old are highly suspicious.
- 50% of abused children will have signs on the head &/or neck.

'Child Protection and the Dental Team' is a detailed and practical web-based resource developed by COPDEND/DOH aimed specifically at dentists and other DCPs and can be accessed at: ℰ www.cpdt.org.uk

Management

Local guidelines are produced by Local Safeguarding Children Boards (LSCBs) or Area Child Protection Committees. To find yours type 'LSCB' followed by your area into an internet search engine. A copy of the local LSCB guidance should be kept in every practice.

If NAI is suspected:
- Take a careful history and keep full records.
- Discuss concerns with an experienced/trusted colleague and decide if further action/referral is justified.
- Provide any urgent/emergency dental care.
- Talk to child and parents—tactfully explain your concerns, seeking consent to sharing of information. Rarely, if you feel informing the parents/carers may put the child or others (including yourself) at risk, you may still share information and/or refer if you believe it is in the child's best interests to do so.

Where to get help and advice (tip: write the telephone numbers of the first three on your copy of the local LSCB guidance)
- Child Protection nurse.
- Local consultant paediatrician.
- Social Services.
- Child's health visitor.
- Your defence organization.

Making a referral Referral should be made directly to Social Services and followed up in writing within 48 hours. The child's medical practitioner should also be informed. If a child presents with serious injuries which are suspicious, they should be referred to the nearest accident and emergency department, with the department informed of the situation before the child's arrival.

Tact and understanding is required when dealing with the patient's family. Try to avoid making accusations and concentrate on treating the patient's injuries, expressing the need to refer them on to experts who will be able to fully evaluate the situation and offer appropriate help.

Injuries to primary teeth

30% to 40% of 5-yr-olds have experienced dental trauma,[1] most frequently at toddler stage. As alveolar bone is more elastic the younger the child, the most common injuries are luxation or avulsion. Crown and root # are relatively rare.

Management

If radiographs are required, you may have to get mother to hold child and film. Alternatively, try placing a periapical film between the teeth (like an occlusal view) and angle the beam at 45°.

Need to consider the effect of any proposed Rx upon permanent successor.[2] Splinting of 1° incisors is exceedingly difficult and not indicated. When in doubt, extract 1° tooth! For definitions, ▣ see p. 104.

Concussion of tooth Rx: reassurance and soft diet.

Subluxation If tooth near to exfoliation, extract. Otherwise, soft diet (for about 1 week). May become non-vital, therefore keep under observation. Give appropriate advice re possible complications.

Lateral Luxation/Extrusion Extraction if loose and tooth in danger of being inhaled, or if tooth interferes with occlusion. If crown displaced labially, increased risk of damage to underlying 2° incisor.

Intrusion Most common injury (>60%). If X-ray confirms that tooth has been forced into follicle of 2° tooth, extract 1° incisor. Otherwise leave tooth and wait to see if spontaneous eruption will occur (between 1 and 6 months). Unfortunately, pulpal necrosis often follows, necessitating either pulp Rx (▣ p. 93) or extraction. Should the tooth fail to erupt, then extraction is indicated. It is prudent to warn parents about possible damage to underlying permanent tooth.

Avulsion Replantation not recommended due to risk of damage to permanent successor.

Crown Fracture Rare. Minimal # can be smoothed and left under observation. Larger # either restore with composite &/or RCT if pulp involved, or extract.

Root Fracture Provided not displaced and little mobility, advise soft diet and keep under review. If coronal fragment displaced or mobile, extract, but leave apical portion as it will usually resorb.

Sequelae of trauma

Primary dentition

If discoloration becomes grey/reddish in early post-trauma period, pulp may be vital and discoloration reversible. Greying later indicates pulp necrosis. Yellowing of tooth is suggestive of calcification of pulp—no Rx required.

---

1 B. Chadwick 2004 *Children's Dental Health in the UK*, HMSO.

2 J. O. Andreasen 2007 *Textbook and Color Atlas of Traumatic Injuries to the Teeth*, Blackwell Publishing.

Ankylosis Rx: extraction to prevent displacement of 2° incisor.

Pulp death Rx: RCT or extraction.

Permanent dentition

More than 50% of children <4yrs trauma to 1° tooth affects underlying developing successor.[1] Effect depends upon stage of development, type of injury and severity, Rx, and pulpal sequelae. Can cause hypomineralization, hypoplasia (likelihood increased if <4yrs and/or injury more severe), dilaceration, severe malformation, and arrest of development.

1 G. Roberts 1996 *Oral and Dental Trauma in Children and Adolescents*, OUP.

Injuries to permanent teeth—crown fractures

Prevalence: 26–76% of injuries.

Enamel only

For small enamel #, smooth with white stone.

Enamel and dentine

Need to protect exposed dentine, preferably with a hard-setting calcium hydroxide cement and an acid-etch retained composite. If time permits, this can be done with a crown former to restore tooth contour. Keep under review. Veneer or PJC can be considered later. If # near to pulp, treat as for pulp involvement.

Acid-etch composite tip technique

- Place rubber dam, if possible.
- Place hard-setting calcium hydroxide on exposed dentine. No need to bevel enamel.
- Using contralateral tooth as guide, select a cellulose acetate crown former.
- Trim crown former to within 1–2mm of # line.
- Etch enamel for 20sec, wash, and dry.
- Place bonding resin and cure.
- Put sufficient composite and a little extra into crown former and position.
- Allow to cure and remove crown former.
- Trim, using soflex discs. Shofu points are useful for palatal aspect.
- Check occlusion.

Enamel, dentine, and pulp

Rx depends upon size of exposure; state of root development (1 root radiographically complete 10–11yrs, histologically 14–15yrs); time since injury and other injuries (e.g. root #). If apex open ↑ blood supply to pulp, therefore likelihood of pulp death ↓. This is advantageous as Rx should be directed towards retaining vitality of radicular pulp to allow root closure to continue. If pulp non-vital, 📖 see p. 276. Otherwise, Rx alternatives are:

Pulp cap

Indications: exposure <1mm; <24hrs; complete or incomplete root development; pulp still vital. Cover exposure with calcium hydroxide (e.g. Dycal®), and place composite tip. Review vitality.

Partial (Cvek) pulpotomy

Indications: exposure >1mm; >24hrs; complete or incomplete root development, pulp still vital.
1) LA and rubber dam.
2) Slightly enlarge access at site of exposure with high speed and amputate pulp to a depth of 2–4mm into healthy pulp tissue.
3) Arrest bleeding with sterile, moist cotton wool (usually takes several minutes).
4) Cover amputation site with non-setting calcium hydroxide.

5) Seal with GI cement.
6) Restore crown.

Full coronal pulpotomy

Indications: Large, contaminated exposures; long duration; incomplete root development; coronal pulp demonstrates impaired vascularity.

1) LA and rubber dam.
2) Open up pulp chamber and amputate coronal pulp to cervical construction with sterile bur/sharp excavator.
3) Wash with sterile water.
4) Place non-setting calcium hydroxide and restore tooth with polycarboxylate or GI cement and composite.
5) Leave 6–8 weeks, then review symptoms and vitality. No need to investigate for presence or not of a calcific barrier.
6) If tooth becomes non-vital, ▱ see p. 276.

All pulpotomized teeth should be kept under long-term review as pulp necrosis and calcification are common sequelae. Success rates of 72% for cervical pulpotomies and 96% for minimal (Cvek) pulpotomies have been reported.[1]

1 M. E. J. Curzon 1999 *Handbook of Dental Trauma*, Wright.

Root fractures

Prevalence: <10% of injuries to permanent dentition.

- Where root # is suspected, two radiographic views at different angulations in the vertical plane are advisable to improve chances of visualizing the # line.
- The prognosis for this type of injury depends upon whether the # line communicates with the gingival crevice. Actual Rx depends on position of #.

Apical ⅓ Usually no Rx required unless mobility ↑ significantly. However, tooth should be kept under observation as death of coronal ⅔ of pulp may occur. Only need to prepare canal to # line as apical ⅓ usually retains vitality. Prognosis good. If extraction required, apical ⅓ can be left *in situ* to preserve bone.

Middle ⅓ In majority of cases tooth is loosened, therefore rigid splinting advisable to attempt to achieve hard-tissue union of # line. 12 weeks previously advocated, but recent evidence suggests flexible splinting for 4 weeks may give similar outcome[1]. If coronal part not displaced loss of vitality unlikely. Where coronal fragment displaced, re-position, splint, and if loss of vitality occurs, RCT to # line. Calcium hydroxide should be used as an interim dressing to limit inflammation and resorption. Delay in Rx ↓ prognosis. If extraction required, consider leaving apical portion *in situ*.

Coronal ⅓ In this group there is a high risk of direct communication with the gingival crevice, allowing ingress of bacteria into pulp. Where no obvious risk, flexible splinting for a prolonged period (up to 4 months) is advocated[1]. Where the # line extends coronally, emergency Rx is either (i) temporary stabilization or (ii) extraction of the coronal fragment. Definitive treatment usually is extraction of both parts of tooth or, preferably, removal of the coronal fragment, and appropriate RCT of remainder, followed by placement of a dressing which will prevent gingival tissues overgrowing root surface. Can use a temporary post-retained crown, but repositioning of the coronal fragment using a dentine-bonding agent and composite has been described. Permanent Rx is post and core crown.

If # extends below alveolar crest, need improved access for crown fabrication. There are two alternatives:

Ostectomy/gingivectomy	Orthodontic extrusion
Gives quicker result	Cervical circumference of
Needs post and diaphragm	crown ↓ compared to
Tend to get perio pocket	contralateral tooth
Leads to ↓ gingival width	Better crown:root ratio
	Gingival margin migrates with crown

---

1 IADT 2007 *Guidelines for treatment of injuries to permanent teeth.* (🖑 www.iadt-dentaltrauma.org)

Orthodontic extrusion can be accomplished, using a URA with a buccal arm which engages either an attachment bonded on to labial surface of temporary post and core crown or any available enamel. Gentle forces of 50–100g should be used. When sufficient extrusion has been achieved, retain for at least 3–6 months before fabricating a permanent restoration.

Oblique Provided # does not extend above alveolar crest, can treat as coronal #. Otherwise, consider extraction of coronal portion only, leaving apical portion *in situ* to preserve bone.

Vertical Extraction is often only option.

If tooth extracted, a P/- will need to be fabricated (p. 294).

Luxation, subluxation, intrusion, and extrusion

Prevalence: 15–40% of injuries.

Definitions

Concussion Injury to supporting tissues of tooth, without displacement.

Lateral Luxation Displacement of tooth (laterally, labially, or palatally).

Subluxation Actually means partial displacement, but commonly used to describe loosening of a tooth without displacement.

Intrusive Luxation Displacement of tooth into its socket. Often accompanied by # of alveolar bone.

Extrusive Luxation Partial displacement of tooth from its socket.

Treatment

Concussion Reassurance and soft diet.

Luxation Need to reposition tooth as soon as possible. Give LA and use fingers to push back into place. Then tooth should be splinted flexibly for 2–3 weeks. If there has been a delay of >24h since the injury, manual reduction is unlikely to be successful. In these cases the tooth can be repositioned orthodontically. If the displaced tooth is interfering with the occlusion an URA, with buccal capping, should be fitted as soon as possible. If root development is complete loss of vitality is a common sequelae following luxation (~70%), leading to inflammatory resorption (📖 p. 110). Teeth with immature apices have a much better chance of pulp survival. External or internal resorption and pulp canal obliteration may also occur, therefore keep under review.

Subluxation If minor, no Rx other than advising a soft diet is necessary. If mobile, splint for 1–2 weeks and watch vitality.

Intrusion[1] Teeth with immature roots frequently re-erupt and therefore no immediate Rx is required. Teeth with closed apices have a limited potential for re-eruption and will need orthodontic extrusion. This should be started as soon as possible to facilitate access for RCT. However if displacement is severe (>6mm intrusion) consider surgical repositioning (whether apex is open or closed). Surgically repositioned teeth require flexible splinting for 1–2 weeks. Pulp death &/or root resorption can ensue rapidly after injury and early pulp extirpation and placement of the calcium hydroxide dressing is advisable. Pulp death is virtually certain in teeth with closed apices, and occurs in ⅔ of immature teeth.

Extrusion The affected tooth should be repositioned under LA with digital pressure and splinted for 1–2 weeks. Again, loss of vitality is a common sequel, so the tooth should be observed for any signs of resorption or pulp death.

1 M. J. Kinirons 1998 *Int J Paed Dent* **8** 165.

If any of the above occur in conjunction with # of the alveolar bone, the splinting period should be ↑ to 3–4 weeks to aid bony healing. If, however, the socket is comminuted, splinting may need to be extended to 6–8 weeks.

Splinting

Indications

- To stabilize a loosened tooth to allow periodontal healing and improve patient comfort. In order to promote fibrous rather than bony healing (ankylosis), a short splinting time with a flexible splint is recommended: avulsion 7–14 days; luxation <3 weeks; middle third root # 4 weeks.
- To stabilize a cervical-third root # and encourage healing with calcified tissue, flexible splinting for up to 4 months is indicated.

Methods

Direct Constructed on patient. An almost infinite variety has been described, but the following are the most popular:
- Acid-etch splint with composite/acrylic/epimine resin &/or wire.
- Orthodontic attachments and sectional archwire.
- Preformed metal (titanium trauma splint).
- Lone standing teeth can be supported by sling suture[1].
- Lead foil &/or cement. Useful in Australian Outback, but better alternatives available in most dental surgeries!

Indirect This type of splint is removable, allowing an assessment of mobility or firmness, which may be of value in cases of reimplantation. The more common types are:
- URA with cribs 6⌊6 and occlusal coverage.
- Vacuum-formed thermoplastic polyvinylacetatepolyethylene (!) 'Drufomat' type.

However, this approach requires an impression of traumatized mouth and involves some delay (few hours/days) before splint can be fitted, so in practice direct splinting is usually preferred.

Factors affecting choice of splint

- Type of injury and therefore length of time splint required. For example, coronal-third root # will need up to 4 months of splinting, therefore composite and wire splint advisable. For re-planted tooth prolonged splinting should be avoided as may lead to ankylosis.
- Number of teeth injured and availability of uninjured adjacent teeth, e.g. if both 1⌊1 traumatized and no adjacent teeth full coverage acrylic splint or sling-suture may be indicated.
- Facilities and time available.

1 M. E. J. Curzon 1999 *Handbook of Dental Trauma*, Wright.

Management of the avulsed tooth

Exarticulation = avulsion. Prevalence: 0–16% of injuries.

Factors affecting prognosis Success depends upon re-establishment of a normal periodontium.

- *Time from loss to re-implantation* As PDL cells rarely survive >60min extra-orally, immediate replacement (by whoever is available at the scene) is the Rx of choice.
- *Storage medium* Prognosis saline > milk > water > air (both tap-water and dry storage rapidly damage periodontal cells.)
- *Splinting time* 7–10 days flexible splinting. Prolonged splinting may promote ankylosis.
- *Viability of pulp* Seepage of pulp breakdown products into PDL will contribute to the development of inflammatory resorption. Although re-vascularization is possible in a tooth with an open apex which is replaced within 30min, those teeth with closed apices and longer extra-alveolar times should be considered non-vital.

Immediate Rx (if avulsed tooth not already replaced)

- Avoid handling root surface. If tooth contaminated, hold crown and agitate gently in saline.
- Place tooth in socket. If does not readily seat, get patient to bite on gauze for 15–20min.
- Compress buccal and lingual alveolar plates.
- Splint a curved piece of light wire (a light twist-flex SS wire is ideal) to acid-etched enamel of affected and adjacent teeth using temporary crown material as this is less traumatic to remove than composite.
- Prescribe antibiotics, chlorhexidine mouthwash and arrange tetanus booster if necessary.

Intermediate Rx (7–10 days later)

- Review splinting. Stop if tooth appears firm, continue for further week if still mobile. If still mobile after 2 weeks, check nothing has been overlooked, e.g. root # or loss of vitality—in these cases prognosis is poor.
- If apex closed (or tooth with open apex, but extra-alveolar period >30min) extirpate pulp within 7–10 days, clean canal, and place an initial intra-canal dressing of calcium hydroxide. Some advocate an intermediate dressing of polyantibiotic/steroid (Ledermix®) paste placed for 1–2 weeks prior to placement of calcium hydroxide.
- Keep teeth with open apices under close observation, so that at the first sign of pulp death RCT can be instituted. Waiting for radiographic evidence of inflammatory resorption is too late.
- Keep tooth under review.

Prognosis If above procedure followed, medium-term survival is relatively good[1] but long-term survival is generally poor
- Incomplete root formation: 60% survive 5yrs.
- Complete root formation: 80% survive 5yrs.

Long-term survival is closely related to extra-alveolar dry-storage time. Teeth stored dry for >30min have a very poor long-term prognosis, but replantation may still be worthwhile, as failure is usually by replacement resorption which is slow (i.e. tooth may last several years) and maintains bulk of alveolus (facilitates future prosthetic replacement).

Where prognosis is deemed to be poor, premolar transplant can be considered at 10–12yrs old.

Sequelae

Surface resorption occurs as a result of minor trauma to PDL cells. Usually is self-limiting and affected areas are repaired by cementum. No Rx.

Replacement resorption (ankylosis) caused by damage to PDL cells during extra-alveolar period and promoted by prolonged splinting. It appears that the absence of vital periodontal ligament allows resorption of the root and replacement by bone. In growing child results in infra-occlusion of affected tooth. Once started is usually progressive, resulting in the eventual loss of the tooth.

Inflammatory resorption Development is dependent upon the presence of both damage to the periodontal ligament and breakdown products from pulp necrosis diffusing through the dentinal tubules to the PDL. Occurs rapidly, as soon as 1–2 weeks after injury. Once evident radiographically prognosis is poor, as it is progressive and Rx is not always successful. Inflammatory resorption can be prevented by extirpation of the pulp as soon as is practicable after injury and placement of non-setting calcium hydroxide. If resorption is halted a GP root filling can be placed.

Delayed presentation Where viability of PDL cells doubtful, Andreasen has suggested chemical Rx of the root surface with fluoride to limit resorption.[1] Following RCT with GP, the tooth is immersed in 2.4% sodium fluoride solution for 20min. Then tooth is replanted and splinted for 6 weeks. As some replacement resorption is inevitable, perhaps best limited to adults. If the extra-alveolar period is greater than 24h, leave and consider instead whether the resulting space should be maintained with a P/- (📖 p. 294).

---

1 J. O. Andreaen 1992 *Atlas of Replantation and Transplantation of Teeth*, Mediglobe.

Pulpal sequelae following trauma

Damage to the pulp can occur as a result of disruption of the apical vessels or exposure of the pulp by a crown or root #, or be caused by haemorrhage and inflammation of coronal pulp, resulting in strangulation.

Pulp death

Remember that no response to vitality testing indicates damage to the nerve supply of a tooth, but not necessarily to the blood supply. Therefore following trauma, you should assess vitality in the light of symptoms, tooth colour, mobility, presence of buccal swelling and radiographic evidence. Except where a tooth has been replanted, it is best to adopt a wait and see approach if in doubt about vitality. When pulp death has occurred, subsequent Rx depends upon whether the apex is closed or open.

RCT of teeth with immature apices

As achievement of an apical seal is difficult in a tooth with an open apex, Rx should aim to produce apexification (i.e. a hard-tissue barrier across the apex). Under rubber dam, the necrotic pulp should be extirpated. The working length is set 1–2mm short of the radiographic apex (unless vital pulp tissue is encountered earlier) and narrow files are used in order to negotiate any undercuts. The canal should then be filled with a radiopaque non-setting calcium hydroxide (e.g. Hypocal™ or Ultracal®) to the apex and sealed. The calcium hydroxide should be replaced every 3 months, until a calcific apical barrier is detectable by gentle probing with a paper point. Then the canal can be filled. Usually, because of the width of the canal, a large GP point (a conventional point upside down) is required. This should be warmed in a flame before pressing into place and then lots of laterally condensed points used to obtain a good seal. The average time for a calcific barrier to be formed is 9 months.[1] A 5-yr survival rate of 86% has been reported[2] but many teeth will fail eventually secondary to cervical root fracture. This probably results from weakening of the tooth due to large access cavity and brittleness of dentine which may be associated with long-term dressing with calcium hydroxide. Some now advocate MTA as an alternative to calcium hydroxide, allowing obturation to be achieved more quickly over fewer visits.

Resorption

Commonly seen after avulsion, luxation, intrusion, or extrusion.

Internal resorption is associated with chronic pulpal inflammation, which results in resorption of dentine from the pulpal surface. Is progressive, therefore the pulp needs to be carefully extirpated. Dressing the tooth with calcium hydroxide appears to help arrest the resorption and once controlled, a GP filling may be placed. If perforation has occurred the prognosis is ↓ considerably. Raising a flap, removal of granulation tissue, and placement of an amalgam seal are indicated.

1 I. C. Mackie 1988 *Dental Update* **15** 155.

2 I. C. Mackie 1993 *BDJ* **175** 99.

External resorption Three types are seen: surface, replacement, and inflammatory (📖 p. 109).

Calcification occurs in 6–35% of luxation-type injuries. Prophylactic endodontic Rx is not necessary as pulp necrosis occurs in only 13–16% of cases. A high rate of success (80%) has been reported for subsequent RCT, despite a hairline or no root-canal detectable on X-ray.

Management of missing incisors

1 Rarely congenitally absent; usually lost following trauma or because of dilaceration.

2 Congenitally absent in approx. 2% of population (with ↑ likelihood of displacement **3**). May also be lost following trauma.

Missing upper anterior teeth are noticed by the general public before other types of malocclusion. The aim of Rx is to provide 321|123 smile. Although Cary Grant did well enough with a missing upper central incisor, symmetry is usually preferable. The management of missing incisors involves either recovery or maintenance of space for prosthetic replacement, or orthodontic space closure. Previous studies have shown that patients were more satisfied with space closure than prosthetic replacement[1] however, with the introduction of implants and newer materials this may change.

For each patient a number of factors need to be considered:

Skeletal relationship In a class III case, space closure in the upper arch could compromise the incisor relationship, whereas in a class II/1 it would facilitate o/j ↓. Consider also the vertical relationship, as space closure is easier in patients with ↑ LFH and vice versa in ↓ LFH.

Crowding/spacing In a patient with no crowding, space closure is difficult and requires prolonged retention. Before opening space it is important to ensure that sufficient will be available at the end of Rx for an adequate prosthetic replacement (minimum width for implant to replace **2** is 6.5mm). A Kesling set-up may be useful.

Colour and form of adjacent teeth Although much can be done with veneers, composite additions and grinding, if **3** is significantly darker &/or caniform in shape, it will be difficult to turn it into convincing **2** if space closure planned. **2** can only be used to mimic **1** if root length and circumference at gingival margin are not significantly smaller.

Inclination of adjacent teeth The final axial inclination of the teeth will determine the aesthetics of the finished result.

Buccal occlusion If a good Class I buccal interdigitation exists this may C/I bringing the posterior teeth forward to close space.

Unilateral loss A symmetrical result is more pleasing, therefore maintenance or opening of space is preferable. If a **2** is missing and the contralateral tooth is peg-shaped, thought should be given to extracting this tooth to achieve symmetry.

Smile line If the patient has a high smile line then need to consider gingival level. In some cases may need gingival surgery.

Patient's wishes and cooperation Only after assessing the above factors can the patient be given an informed choice. If the patient refuses fixed appliances this may alter the Rx plan.

1 S. Robertsson 2000 *Eur J Orthodontics* **22** 697.

Kesling set-up Requires duplicate models of both arches, including at least two of the upper arch. Using a small hacksaw, the teeth which will require orthodontic movement are removed from the model and repositioned using wax. As many alternatives as desired can be tried to find the best result.

Space closure This can be facilitated by early extraction of the primary teeth on the affected side; therefore the earlier the decision is made to close space, the better. Active space closure requires FA to achieve correct axial inclination. It is better to carry out any masking procedures before orthodontic Rx, e.g. contouring 3̲ to resemble 2̲ (by removal of enamel incisally, interproximally and from the palatal aspect &/or composite addition) as this will facilitate final positioning and occlusion. Retain with a bonded retainer.

NB the average difference in width between 3̲ and 2̲ is 1.2mm, which can easily be removed mesially and distally from 3̲.

Space-maintenance/opening If an incisor is selectively extracted and space maintenance is desired, a P/- or acid-etch bridge should be fitted immediately. Where 2̲ congenitally missing, space may need to be opened orthodontically with FA. Some advocate encouraging the 3̲ to erupt adjacent to the 1̲ and then retracting it to open space to give better bone levels for implant or bridge. Following space opening, retention with a P/- for 3–6 months is advisable to allow the teeth to settle. If an acid-etch retained prosthesis is planned, ensure that there is sufficient room occlusally for the wings.

Resin bonded bridge, 📖 p. 266.

Transplantation of a lower premolar into the socket of an extracted incisor can be considered if lower arch is crowded.

Implant when growth complete, becoming more widely available (📖 p. 330).

Common childhood ailments affecting the mouth

▶ Refer any patient with an ulcer that doesn't heal within 3 weeks or with any soft-tissue lesion of unknown aetiology.

See chapter 9 Oral medicine.
Most common disease is gingivitis (📖 p. 187).

Viral

Primary herpetic gingivostomatitis Occurs >6 months of age. Symptoms: febrile, cervical lymphadenitis, vesicles → ulcers on gingiva and oral mucosa. Rx: soft diet with plenty of fluids. Self-limiting, lasts for approximately 10 days.

Secondary herpes labialis Vesicles form around the lips, and crust. Self-limiting, but 5% aciclovir cream will speed healing.

Hand, foot, and mouth disease Rash on hands and feet plus ulcers on oral mucosa and gingiva. Little systemic upset. Self-limiting.

Herpangina Febrile illness with sore throat due to ulcers on soft palate and throat. Usually lasts about 3–5 days. Rx: soft diet.

Warts Check hands. Usually self-limiting.

Also chickenpox (vesicles → ulcers), mumps (inflamed parotid duct), glandular fever (ulcers), measles.

Bacterial

Impetigo Very infectious staphylococcal (&/or streptococcal) rash. Starts around mouth and may be mistaken for 2° herpes.

Streptococcal sore throat Can contract associated streptococcal gingivitis (rare as hen's teeth!).

Necrotising ulcerative gingivitis Rare <16yrs (📖 p. 191).

Fungal

Candida Commensal of the mouth, which may become pathogenic when oral environment favours its proliferation. Two types of manifestation are seen in children. (i) **Acute pseudo-membraneous candidiasis** (thrush). Seen in newborn, under-nourished infants after prolonged use of antibiotics or steroids. Presents as white patches that rub off. Rx: miconazole (25mg/ml) and correct underlying problem. (ii) **Chronic atrophic candidiasis.** Most commonly URA and poor OH &/or high sugar intake. Rx: OHI for appliance and teeth. Chlorhexidine mouthwash or miconazole gel.

Miscellaneous

Aphthous ulceration[1] 📖 p. 404.

---

1 E. A. Field 1992 *Int J Paed Dent* **2** 1.

Common causes of oral ulceration in children (in order of frequency) aphthous; trauma; acute herpetic gingivostomatitis; herpangina; hand, foot, and mouth disease; glandular fever. If in doubt refer.

Common causes of soft-tissue swellings in children Abscess; mucocele; eruption cyst; epulides; papilloma.

▶ Oral cancer does occur in children, therefore if in doubt refer for biopsy.

Sugar-free medications

The potential cariogenic effect of long-term medication sweetened with sugar is now well-recognized. Therefore sugar-free preparations should be prescribed whenever possible. Unfortunately, there is no evidence that rinsing out or brushing the teeth after use of a sugar-based medicine will significantly ↓ the incidence of caries. Current medical advice is for liquid medicines to be given to children by disposable syringes. This approach has the advantage that an accurate dose can be directed at the back of the mouth.

Below is a list of some sugar-free medicines. It is not exhaustive and where required reference should be made to the *British National Formulary*.

Analgesics

Aspirin (>12 years)	Dispersible aspirin tablets
Paracetamol	Disprol® paediatric
	Junior Disprol® suspension/tablets
	Panadol® baby and infant elixir
	Panadol® Junior sachets
	Panadol® soluble
	Junior Panaleve®/Panaleve® elixir
Paracetamol and codeine	Panadeine® soluble
	Paracodol® dispersible tablets
	Solpadeine®
Ibuprofen	Ibuprofen oral suspension SF

Antacids

Aluminium and magnesium	Mucogel®
	Maalox® suspension
Cimetidine	Dyspamet® chewable tablets or suspension
Ranitidine	Zantac® dispersible tablets
	Zantac® suspension

Anticonvulsants

Carbamazepine	Tegretol® liquid
Phenobarbital	Phenobarbital elixir 30mg/10ml
Sodium valproate	Epilim® crushable tablets/elixir

Anti-infectives

Aciclovir	Zovirax® suspension
Amoxicillin	Amoxil® dispersible tablets SF
	Amoxil® sachets SF
Amphotericin	Fungilin® oral suspension/lozenges
Ampicillin and cloxacillin	Ampiclox® neonatal suspension
Erythromycin	Erythroped® sachets
Miconazole	Daktarin® oral gel

Respiratory agents

Salbutamol

Cobutolin® syrup
Salbutamol syrup (Evans)
Ventolin® syrup

Miscellaneous

Folic acid
Iron edetate
Vitamins A, B, C, D, and E

Lexpec® syrup
Sytron®

Orthodontics

Contents

Relevant pages in other chapters Surgical management of CLP, 📖 p. 472; abnormalities of eruption, 📖 p. 62; supernumerary teeth, 📖 p. 64; orthognathic surgery, 📖 p. 474.

Further reading BOS 1996 *Young Practitioners Guide to Orthodontics*. T.M. Graber *et al.* 2005 *Orthodontics—Current principles and techniques* (4e), Elsevier Mosby. *K.G. Isaacson et al.* 2008 *Orthodontic Radiographs—Guidelines*, BOS. L. Mitchell 2007 *An Introduction to Orthodontics* (3e) OUP. W. R. Proffit *et al.* 2007 *Contemporary Orthodontics* (4e), Mosby.

It has been said that orthodontists forget to ask the patient to open wide, thus missing any dental pathology, whilst generalists forget to ask the patient to close together, thus missing any malocclusion! The aim of this chapter is to help ensure that this is not true. A problem-orientated approach has been used (rather than by classification) for simplicity.

What is orthodontics?

Orthodontics has been defined as that branch of dentistry concerned with growth of the face, development of the dentition, and prevention and correction of occlusal anomalies.[1]

Prevalence of malocclusion Crowding approx. 60%; Class II/1 ~15–20%; Class II/2 ~10%; Class III ~3% (Figure 4.1).

Why do orthodontics? Research shows that individual motivation has more effect upon the presence of plaque than alignment of the teeth, therefore, the main indications for orthodontic Rx are aesthetics and function. Functional reasons for Rx include deep traumatic overbite; ↑ overjet especially if the lips are incompetent (↑ risk of trauma), and labial crowding of a lower incisor (as this reduces periodontal support labially). While it is accepted that severe malocclusion may affect self-esteem and psychological well-being, the impact of more minor anomalies and, indeed, perceived need, are influenced by social and cultural factors. The Index of Orthodontic Treatment Need (IOTN) has been developed to try to standardize and quantify this difficult issue (☐ p. 122).

It is important that patients realize that orthodontic Rx is not without its disadvantages. Even with good OH, a small loss of periodontal attachment is common and with poor OH this will be ↑. Decalcification (decay) will occur if there are frequent sugar intakes between meals and around 1–2mm of root resorption is associated with fixed appliance Rx and in at-risk patients (shortened/blunt root shape) this may be ↑. Therefore, the potential benefits to the patient must be sufficient to counter-balance these risks.

Who should do orthodontics? All dentists should be concerned with growth and development. Unless anomalies are detected early and any necessary steps taken at the appropriate time, then provision of the best possible outcome for that patient is less likely. Most orthodontic Rx in Europe is now carried out by trained specialist orthodontic practitioners. In the UK the hospital consultant service acts as a source of advice and a referral point for more complex and multidisciplinary problems.

When should we do orthodontics? This depends upon the particular anomaly. In the early mixed dentition, Rx is only indicated to correct incisor and/or posterior Xbites with displacement. Functional appliance Rx may be started in the mixed dentition to coincide with the pubertal growth spurt; however, the majority of orthodontic Rx is not started until the 2° dentition. Rx during the early teens is preferable because the response to orthodontic forces is more rapid, appliances are better tolerated, and, most importantly, growth can be utilized to help effect sagittal or vertical change. In adults, lack of growth; ↑risk of periodontal disease; worn, damaged and missing teeth and slower tooth movement and will limit the type of malocclusion that can be tackled by orthodontics alone. The proportion of adult orthodontic patients is ↑.

1 W. J. B. Houston 1986 *A Textbook of Orthodontics*, Wright.

▶ If in doubt, refer a patient for advice earlier rather than later, especially in cases with marked skeletal discrepancies.

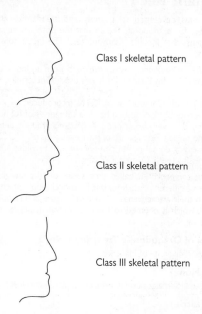

Class I skeletal pattern

Class II skeletal pattern

Class III skeletal pattern

Fig. 4.1

The Index of Orthodontic Treatment Need

The IOTN was developed to quantify and standardize an individual patient's need for orthodontic Rx, so that the potential benefits can be weighed against the possible disadvantages.[1] The Index consists of two components:

The dental health component was developed from an index used by the Swedish Dental Health Board (which was used to determine the amount of financial help that would be given by the State towards Rx costs). The Dental Health Component of IOTN (reproduced by kind permission of University of Manchester) has five categories of Rx need, ranging from little need to very great need. A patient's grade is determined by recording the single worst feature of their malocclusion. MOCDO is helpful when assessing dental health component as it provides a hierarchy of severity—Missing teeth; Overjet; Crossbite; Displacement; Overbite.

The aesthetic component is based on a series of 10 photographs of the labial aspect of different class I or class II malocclusions, which are ranked according to their attractiveness. A patient's score is determined by the photograph, which is deemed to have an equivalent degree of aesthetic impairment.

The Index of Orthodontic Treatment Need

(Copyright © University of Manchester)

Grade 1 (None)

1 Extremely minor malocclusions including displacements less than 1mm.

Grade 2 (Little)

2a Increased overjet 3.6–6mm with competent lips.
2b Reverse overjet 0.1–1mm.
2c Anterior or posterior crossbite with up to 1mm discrepancy between retruded contact position and intercuspal position.
2d Displacement of teeth 1.1–2mm.
2e Anterior or posterior openbite 1.1–2mm.
2f Increased overbite 3.5mm or more, without gingival contact.
2g Pre-normal or post-normal occlusions with no other anomalies. Includes up to half a unit discrepancy.

Grade 3 (Moderate)

3a Increased overjet 3.6–6mm with incompetent lips.
3b Reverse overjet 1.1–3.5mm.
3c Anterior or posterior crossbites with 1.1–2mm discrepancy.
3d Displacement of teeth 2.1–4mm.
3e Lateral or anterior openbite 2.1–4mm.
3f Increased and complete overbite without gingival trauma.

1 W. C. Shaw 1991 *BDJ* **170** 107.

Grade 4 (Great)

4a Increased overjet 6.1–9mm.

4b Reversed overjet greater than 3.5mm with no masticatory or speech difficulties.

4c Anterior or posterior crossbites with greater than 2mm discrepancy between retruded contact position and intercuspal position.

4d Severe displacement of teeth, greater than 4mm.

4e Extreme lateral or anterior openbites, greater than 4mm.

4f Increased and complete overbite with gingival or palatal trauma.

4h Less extensive hypodontia requiring pre-restorative orthodontic space closure to obviate the need for a prosthesis.

4l Posterior lingual crossbite with no functional occlusal contact in one or both buccal segments.

4m Reverse overjet 1.1–3.5mm with recorded masticatory and speech difficulties.

4t Partially erupted teeth, tipped and impacted against adjacent teeth.

4x Supplemental teeth.

Grade 5 (Very great)

5a Increased overjet greater than 9mm.

5h Extensive hypodontia with restorative implications (more than one tooth missing in any quadrant) requiring pre-restorative orthodontics.

5i Impeded eruption of teeth (with the exception of third molars) due to crowding, displacement, the presence of supernumerary teeth, retained deciduous teeth, and any pathological cause.

5m Reverse overjet greater than 3.5mm with reported masticatory and speech difficulties.

5p Defects of cleft lip and palate.

5s Submerged deciduous teeth.

Definitions

Ideal occlusion Anatomically perfect arrangement of the teeth. Rare.

Normal occlusion Acceptable variation from ideal occlusion.

Competent lips Lips meet together at rest.

Incompetent lips Lips do not meet together at rest.

Frankfort plane Line joining porion (superior aspect of external auditory meatus) with orbitale (lowermost point of bony orbit).

Class I The lower incisor edges occlude with, or lie immediately below the cingulum of upper incisors (Figure 4.2).

Class II The lower incisor edges lie posterior to the cingulum of the upper incisors. *Division 1* the upper central incisors are upright or proclined and the overjet is ↑ (Figure 4.3). *Division 2* the upper central incisors are retroclined and the overjet is usually ↓ but may be ↑ (Figure 4.4).

Class III The lower incisor edges lie anterior to the cingulum of the upper incisors and the overjet is ↓ or reversed (Figure 4.5).

Bimaxillary proclination Both upper and lower incisors are proclined.

Overjet Distance between the upper and lower incisors in the horizontal plane.

Overbite Overlap of the incisors in the vertical plane.

Complete overbite The lower incisors contact the upper incisors or the palatal mucosa.

Incomplete overbite The lower incisors do not contact the upper incisors or the palatal mucosa.

Anterior open bite There is no vertical overlap of the incisors when the buccal segment teeth are in occlusion.

Crossbite A deviation from the normal bucco-lingual relationship. May be anterior/posterior &/or unilateral/bilateral.

Buccal crossbite Buccal cusps of lower premolars or molars occlude buccally to the buccal cusps of the upper premolars or molars.

Lingual crossbite Buccal cusps of lower molars occlude lingually to the lingual cusps of the upper molars.

Dento-alveolar compensation The position of the teeth has compensated for the underlying skeletal pattern, so that the occlusal relationship between the arches is less severe.

Leeway space The difference in diameter between C, D, E, and 3, 4, 5. Greater in lower than upper arch.

Mandibular deviation Path of closure starts from a postured position of the mandible.

Mandibular displacement When closing from the rest position, the mandible displaces (either laterally or anteriorly) to avoid a premature contact.

Class I incisor
relationship

Class II/I incisor
relationship

Class II/2 incisor
relationship

Class III incisor
relationship

Fig. 4.2–4.5

Orthodontic assessment

Equipment A mirror, probe, a SS ruler and 'sharp' eyes.

Brief screening procedure

The purpose of this is to ensure early detection and Rx of any abnormality, prepare the patient for any later Rx and influence the management of any teeth of poor prognosis.

At every visit Once the 2° incisors have erupted and until 2° dentition is established (if in doubt refer).

- Keep the eruption sequence in mind ($\square$ p. 62). Any deviations from this should be observed for a few months only and then investigated.
- Failure of a tooth to appear >6 months after the contralateral tooth has erupted should ring alarm bells.
- Ask child to close together and look for Xbites, reverse or ↑ o/j.
- Consider the long-term prognosis of the first permanent molars ($\square$ p. 137).

From age 9yrs and until they erupt, palpate for <u>3</u> in the buccal sulcus. A definite hollow &/or asymmetry warrants further investigation.

Detailed orthodontic examination

Should be carried out in a logical sequence so that nothing is missed.
- Who wants Rx (patient or parent) and what for?
- What complexity of Rx is patient prepared to accept. Have the patient's peers worn braces and if not, will the child make a good pioneer?
- Enquire about any previous extractions and orthodontic Rx.

EO examination (with Frankfort plane horizontal)
- Assess skeletal pattern:
   (i) antero-posteriorly (max=mand—Class I; max>mand—Class II; max<mand—Class III). See Figure 4.1.
   (ii) vertically (Frankfort–Mandibular planes angle approx. 28°. Lower face height is the distance from the base of the nose to the point of the chin, and in a normally proportioned face is equal to the middle facial third eyebrow line to base of nose)
   (iii) transversely (? Asymmetry)
- Soft tissues: Lips are only competent if they meet at rest. If >2mm gap between the lips at rest then can be considered incompetent. Check the position of the lower lip relative to the <u>inc</u> and how the patient achieves an oral seal (? lip to lip; lip to tongue; or by the lower lip being drawn up behind the incisors). Note also the length of the upper lip, the amount of <u>inc</u> seen, and lip tonicity.
- Check rest position of mandible and for any displacement on closure.
- Habits? Does patient suck a thumb/finger, bite fingernails or brux?

IO examination
- Record OH, gingival condition, and teeth present. Any teeth of poor prognosis?

- LLS: Inclination to mandibular base, crowding/spacing, displaced teeth, angulation of $\overline{3|3}$.
- ULS: Inclination to maxillary base, crowding/spacing, rotations, displaced teeth, presence and angulation of $\underline{3|3}$.
- Measure o/j (mm), o/b (↑ or ↓, complete or incomplete) (Figure 4.6). Check centre lines coincident and correct within face.
- Buccal segments: crowding/spacing, displaced teeth.
- Check molar and canine relationship. Any Xbites?

X-rays

Usually a DPT is taken and, if not clearly visible on the DPT, an intraoral of the inc. A lateral skull view is indicated if the patient has a skeletal discrepancy or A–P movement of the incisors is anticipated.

- Look for unerupted, missing, displaced or $ teeth, or other pathology. Check root morphology looking for blunt or pipette-shaped roots.
- Cephalometric analysis, 📖 p. 128.

Summary

Should include a description of the patient's incisor relationship and skeletal pattern, and the main points of the malocclusion, e.g. crowding, Xbites. This gives a 'problem list' from which the aims of Rx can be derived (📖 p. 132).

Study models are not obligatory, but are advisable to facilitate treatment planning (at leisure); medico-legally; to provide evidence as to the justification for treatment; for measuring the progress and outcome of treatment and also for those bodies commissioning & paying for treatment. Study models should be trimmed so that they occlude correctly on a flat surface.

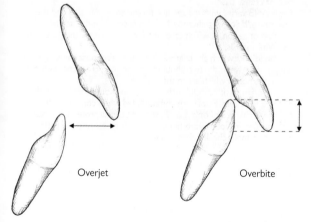

Overjet

Overbite

Fig. 4.6

Cephalometrics

Cephalometric analysis is the interpretation of lateral skull radiographs (Figure 4.7). It is not obligatory for orthodontic Δ and where the incisor position is not to be changed significantly, the X-ray exposure may not be justified for the information gained. However, where A–P movement is required, a lateral skull radiograph will back-up the clinical assessment of skeletal pattern, and help to determine the degree of difficulty and type of appliance indicated. Serial lateral skulls aid assessment of growth.

Tracing/digitizing

Although this has been done using grease-proof paper and a TV as background illumination (yes, really!), the quality of diagnostic information so obtained is limited. Tracing paper (secured to the film with masking tape), a sharp pencil (a 0.5mm propelling-pencil is ideal), and good background illumination are essential. Digital images can be digitized directly. Spotting orthodontic landmarks is infinitely easier if carried out in a darkened room. If a point is hard to see, block off the rest of the film so that only that area is illuminated. If this fails, try holding the film up to a bright spotlight, but if still not clear, make a guesstimate! Due to the slight magnification (7–8%), two images of the mandibular border are usually seen. Both should be traced and an average taken for gonion. By convention, the most prominent image should be traced, i.e. the most anterior in the face so that the difficulty of Rx is not underestimated.

Pitfalls

- Consider the cephalometric values for a particular patient in conjunction with their clinical assessment, as variation from the normal in a measurement may be compensated for elsewhere in the face or cranial base.
- Angle ANB varies with the relative prominence of nasion and the lower face. If SNA significantly ↑ or ↓ this could be due to the position of nasion, in which case an additional analysis should be used, e.g. Wits analysis.
- For landmarks which are bilateral (unless superimposed exactly) the midpoint between the two should be taken to correspond with other reference points which are in the midline.
- Tracing errors; with careful technique these should be of the order of ± 0.5° and 0.5mm. Errors are compounded when comparing tracings, therefore changes of only 1 or 2° should be interpreted with caution.
- If the values you obtain are the norms for a giraffe and the patient looks humanoid check your tracing!

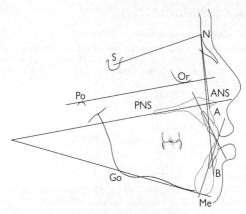

Fig. 4.7 Most commonly used cephalometric points:

S   = Sella: mid-point of sella turcica.
N   = Nasion: most anterior point on fronto-nasal suture.
Or   = Orbitale: most inferior anterior point on margin of orbit
        (take average of two images).
Po   = Porion: uppermost outermost point on bony external
        auditory meatus.
ANS   = Anterior nasal spine.
PNS   = Posterior nasal spine.
Go   = Gonion: most posterior inferior point on angle of mandible.
Me   = Menton: lowermost point on the mandibular symphysis.
A   = A point: position of deepest concavity on anterior profile
        of maxilla.
B   = B point: position of deepest concavity on anterior profile of mandibular
        symphysis.

Frankfort plane   = Po–Or.
Maxillary plane   = PNS–ANS.
Mandibular plane   = Go–Me.

Lower facial height (LFH) is the distance from anterior nasal spine to menton as a percentage of the total face height (from nasion to menton).

More cephalometrics

Analysis and interpretation

The analysis of lateral skull tracings is carried out by comparing a number of angular measurements and proportions with average values for the population as a whole. Normal values for Caucasians (UK),[1] standard deviations in parentheses:

SNA	= 81°(±3)
SNB	= 79°(±3)
ANB	= 3°(±2)
1-Max	= 109°(±6)
1̄-Mand	= 93°(±6) or 120 minus MMPA
MMPA	= 27°(±4)
Facial proportion	= 55% (±2)
Inter-incisal angle	= 133°(±10)

When interpreting a tracing bear in mind the following rules of thumb:
- 68% of values lie within 1 standard deviation of the mean
- 95% of values lie within 2 standard deviation of the mean
- >99% of values lie within 3 standard deviation of the mean

It is important to remember that the ANB difference is not an infallible assessment of skeletal pattern as it assumes (incorrectly in some cases) that there is no discrepancy in the cranial base and that A and B are indicative of basal bone position. When a cephalometric tracing seems at odds with your clinical impression it is worth doing another analysis which avoids reliance on the cranial base, such as a Wits analysis.

Before deciding on a Rx plan it is helpful to consider what factors have contributed to a particular malocclusion, e.g. in a patient with a Class II/1 incisor relationship on a Class I skeletal pattern, the prognosis for Rx is much better if the ↑ o/j is due to proclination of the upper rather than retroclination of the lower incisors. The relative contribution of the maxilla and mandible to the skeletal pattern may indicate possible lines of Rx; e.g. if an ↑ o/j is due to a retrusive mandible, a better aesthetic result may be achieved by use of a functional appliance.

As a rough guide can assume that there is ~2.5° of angular movement for every millimetre of linear movement of the incisor edge.

1 J. R. E. Mills 1987 *Principles and Practice of Orthodontics*, Churchill Livingstone.

Wits analysis

Used to assess antero-posterior skeletal pattern (Figure 4.8).

Method:

- Construct the functional occlusal plane (FOP) by drawing a line through the cusp tips of the molars and premolars or deciduous molars.
- Drop perpendiculars to the FOP from A point (to give AO) and B point (to give BO).
- Measure the distance from AO to BO.

In Class I AP relationship:

Males: BO is 1mm (±1.9mm) ahead of AO
Females: BO=AO (±1.77mm)

Functional
occlusal plane

AO BO

Fig. 4.8 Wits analysis.

Treatment planning

Problem list

Following assessment of the patient a summary should be made of the main features of the malocclusion (📖 p. 127). The problem list can then be drawn up; e.g.

- Class II/1 incisor relationship with ↑overjet
- Posterior crossbite
- Crowding

Aims of Rx

This is derived from the above problem list; e.g.

- Correct crossbite
- Relieve crowding
- Align arches
- Correct incisor relationship i.e. ↓overjet

Plan lower arch

The lower arch lies in a zone of stability between the lips, cheeks, and tongue; therefore, it is safer to consider it as immutable. This gives a starting point around which to plan Rx. The first step is to decide if the lower arch is sufficiently crowded to warrant extractions. If the crowding is likely to ↑ (patient in early teens), then extractions may be indicated (📖 p. 136). In Class 11/2 cases it may be advisable to accept a little crowding (📖 p. 147). If in doubt refer for advice.

Plan upper arch

In most cases planning will be to a Class I incisor and buccal segment relationship. Therefore, it may be helpful, in the mind's eye, to correct the upper canine into a Class I relationship with $\overline{3}$ (in corrected position if LLS crowded). This will give an indication of the space required and the amount and type of movement necessary. In the upper arch, space for retraction of $\underline{3}$ can be gained by (i) extractions, (ii) expansion (only indicated if a Xbite exists), (iii) distal movement of the upper buccal segments (📖 p. 138). (iv) a combination of these. Should extractions be indicated in both arches, mechanics are often easier if the same tooth is extracted in the upper as in the lower. However, in Class II cases it may be advantageous to extract further forward in the upper arch and vice versa in Class III.

Final Rx plan

The next step is to plan what tooth movements need to be carried out, including which appliances are to be used and in what sequence. E.g. if distal movement of $\underline{6|6}$ is to be carried out it may be wise to fit the headgear first and review in the light of progress before embarking on extractions. To every force there is an equal and opposite reaction. In orthodontic treatment the resistance to unwanted tooth movement is called anchorage and also needs to be considered when planning Rx. Retention of the final result should be included in the Rx plan and the need for compliance with wearing retention appliances explained to the patient.

The practicalities of providing Rx also warrant consideration. In some cases more than one Rx plan can be offered to the patient, with a hierarchy of complexity and finished result. If a compromise plan is chosen by the patient this should be recorded in the consent process.

The final plan for the example above may be:

- Quad helix appliance to expand upper arch.
- Extraction of all four first premolars.
- Lower fixed appliance.
- Upper fixed appliance once crossbite corrected.
- Reduce overjet.
- Retain corrected tooth movements.

Prognosis

Will the proposed Rx be stable? Beware of o/j reduction in a patient with grossly incompetent lips, or proclination of upper incisors in a Class III where there is no o/b to hold the corrected position.

Consent

The risks and benefits of the proposed plan should be carefully explained to the patient/parent. It is advisable to get written consent, including specific details of the Rx and associated risks.

▶ *Beware* if the malocclusion under consideration contains one of the following features:

- Marked skeletal discrepancy, anteroposteriorly (II or III), or vertically.
- If the o/j is increased and the upper incisors are upright.
- If the o/j is reversed and there is no o/b to retain correction of the incisor relationship.
- Severe Class II/2 malocclusions.
- Class II/1 incisor relationship, with molars a full unit Class II and a crowded lower arch.

Rx planning is the most important, and most difficult, part of orthodontics. All but the trained orthodontist are advised to seek specialist advice.

Management of the developing dentition

See also delayed eruption, 📖 p. 62.

The way in which mixed dentition problems are approached will often affect the ease or difficulty of subsequent Rx.

Normal development of dentition The 1° incisors are usually upright and spaced. If there is no spacing warn the parents that the 2° incisors will probably be crowded. Overbite reduces throughout the 1° dentition until the incisors are edge to edge. All 2° incisors develop lingual to their predecessors, erupt into a wider arc, and are more proclined. It is normal for 1|1 to erupt with a median diastema which reduces as 2|2 erupt. Later, pressure from the developing canines on the roots of 2|2 results in their being tilted distally and spaced. This has been called the 'ugly duckling stage', but it is better to describe it as normal development to parents. As the 3 erupts the 2 upright and the spaces usually close.

The majority of Es erupt so that their distal edges are flush. The transition to the normal stepped (Class I) molar relationship usually occurs during the 2° dentition as a result of greater mandibular growth &/or the leeway space.

Development of dental arches In the average (!) child, the size of the dental arch is more or less established once the deciduous dentition has erupted, except for an increase in inter-canine width (2–3mm up to age 9yrs) which results in a modification of arch shape.

Retained deciduous teeth—if deflecting eruption of 2° tooth, extract.

Infraoccluded deciduous molars Prevalence 8–14%. Provided there is a successor, an infraoccluded 1° molar will probably be exfoliated at the same time as the contralateral tooth.[1] Extraction is only indicated if there is no successor or the infraoccluded molar is likely to disappear below the gingival margin.

Impacted upper first permanent molars Prevalence 2–6%. Indicative of crowding. Spontaneous disimpaction rare after 8 yrs. Can try dislodging 6 by tightening a piece of brass wire round the contact point with E over several visits. Otherwise just observe, extracting E if unavoidable and dealing with resultant space loss in 2° dentition.

Habits Effects produced depend upon duration of habit and intensity. It is best not to make a great fuss of a finger-sucking habit. If parents concerned, reassure them (in presence of child) not to worry, as only little girls/boys suck their fingers. Appliances to break the habit may help, but most children will stop when they are ready. However, this is no reason to delay the start of Rx for other aspects of the malocclusion.

1 J. Kurol 1985 *Am J Orthod* **87** 46.

Effects of premature loss of deciduous teeth

Unfortunately, when a child attends with toothache, in the rush to relieve pain it is all too easy to extract the offending tooth without consideration of the consequences. The major effect of early deciduous tooth loss is localization of crowding, in crowded mouths. The extent to which this occurs depends upon the patient's age, degree of crowding, and the site. In a crowded mouth the adjacent teeth will move round into the extraction space, therefore, unilateral loss of a C (and to a lesser degree a D) will result in a centre-line shift. This is also seen when a C is prematurely exfoliated by an erupting 2. As correction of a centre-line discrepancy often involves fixed appliances, prevention is better than cure, so loss of Cs should always be balanced. If Es are lost the 6 will migrate forward. This is particularly marked if it occurs before eruption of the permanent tooth, so if extraction of an E is unavoidable try to defer until after the 6s are in occlusion and do not balance or compensate.

The effect of early loss of 1° teeth on the eruption of the permanent successor is variable.

Timely loss of Cs is indicated for

- 2 erupting palatally due to crowding. Extraction of C|C as the 2 erupting may allow the tooth to escape labially and prevent a X̄bite.
- Extraction of C̅|C̅ when a lower incisor is being crowded labially will help to ↓ loss of periodontal support.

Balancing extraction Extraction of the same (or adjacent) tooth on the opposite side of the arch to preserve symmetry.

Compensating extraction Extraction of the same tooth in the opposing arch.

Extractions

In orthodontics, teeth are extracted either to relieve crowding or to provide space to compensate for a skeletal discrepancy.

▶ Before planning the extraction of any permanent teeth a thorough orthodontic and radiographic examination should be carried out.

▶ In a Class I or II, it is advisable to extract at least as far forward in the upper arch as the lower; vice versa in a Class III.

Lower incisors Following the extraction of an inc, the LLS tends to tilt lingually followed by the ULS. In addition, it is difficult to arrange 6 ULS teeth around 5 LLS teeth. However, if indicated, will need FAs.

Upper incisors are never the teeth of choice for extraction, but if traumatized or dilacerated, there may be no alternative (📖 p. 112).

Lower canines should only be extracted if severely displaced, as the resulting contact between $\overline{2}$ and $\overline{4}$ is unsatisfactory.

Upper canines, 📖 p. 140.

First premolars are the most popular choice, due to their position in the arch and because a good contact point between the canine and second premolar is more likely. For maximum spontaneous improvement 4s should be extracted just as the 3s are appearing, but if appliance therapy is planned, defer until the canines have erupted.

Second premolars Preferred in cases with mild crowding, as their extraction alters the anchorage balance, favouring space closure by forward movement of the molars. FAs are required, especially in the lower arch. If 5s hypoplastic or missing there may be no choice. Early loss of an E will often lead to forward movement of the 6 and lack of space for 5s. In the upper arch this results in $\underline{5}$ being displaced palatally and provided $\underline{4}$ is in a satisfactory position, extraction of $\underline{5}$ on eruption may ↓ the need for appliance therapy. In the lower arch 5s are usually crowded lingually. Extraction of $\overline{4}$ is easier and will give $\overline{5}$ space to upright spontaneously.

First permanent molars, 📖 p. 137.

Second permanent molars Extraction of $\overline{7}$ will not alleviate incisor crowding but may relieve mild lower premolar crowding and avoid difficult extraction of impacted $\overline{8}$.

To increase likelihood of $\overline{8}$ erupting successfully to replace $\overline{7}$, need: posterior crowding and $\overline{8}$ formed to bifurcation and at an angle of between 15° and 30° to long axis $\overline{6}$. Even so, may still require appliance therapy to align $\overline{8}$ on eruption.

In the upper arch extraction of $\underline{7}$ often limited to facilitating distal movement of the upper buccal segments.

Third permanent molars Early extraction of these teeth used to be advocated to prevent LLS crowding, but as this can occur even in their absence, wisdom teeth are only a part of the aetiology. In addition, extraction of symptomless $\overline{8}$ is not advisable.

Space can also be provided in selected cases by:
- expansion (only in upper arch with a Xbite, otherwise not stable);
- distal movement of the upper buccal segments (📖 p. 138);
- reducing the width of the teeth interproximally (usually limited to LLS in selected cases).

Extraction of the first permanent molars

First permanent molars are never the first choice for extraction, as even if removed at the optimal time a good spontaneous alignment of the remaining teeth is unlikely. However, when a two-surface (or more) restoration is required in a molar tooth for a child, the long-term prognosis should be considered. A well-timed extraction may be better for the child (and your BP) than heroic attempts to restore hopeless molars. Equally well, placing a dressing and maintaining a poor-quality 6 until the 7 has erupted and the extraction can be incorporated into an orthodontic plan, may keep you on the specialist orthodontists' Christmas card list. Points to note:

- Check the remaining teeth are present and in a good position. If not, avoid extraction of 6 in affected quadrant.
- In the lower arch good spontaneous alignment is more likely following extraction $\overline{6}$ if: (i) $\overline{7|7}$ development has reached bifurcation (ii) angulation between crypt $\overline{7}$ and $\overline{6}$ is <30° (iii) $\overline{7|7}$ crypts overlap $\overline{6|6}$ roots.
- There is a greater tendency for mesial drift in the maxilla, therefore, the timing of loss of $\underline{6}$ is less critical.
- Assess the prognosis for remaining 6s. If they are all restored then extraction of all four is probably indicated. If only one poor $\underline{6}$, do not extract corresponding lower tooth. If $\overline{6}$ of poor prognosis it is advisable to extract opposing $\underline{6}$ as otherwise this tooth will overerupt and prevent $\overline{7}$ moving forward. Balancing with extraction of a corresponding sound $\overline{6}$ is inadvisable; better to deal with other side of arch on its merit.
- In Class I with anterior crowding and Class II malocclusions, $\underline{6|6}$ should, if possible, be preserved until $\underline{7|7}$ have erupted, and can be held back by an appliance and the extraction space utilized for relief of crowding and/or o/j reduction.
- In Class III, if $\underline{6|6}$ of poor prognosis try to preserve until incisor relationship corrected (to provide retention for appliance). In cases with poor quality $\overline{6|6}$, extract at optimal time to aid space closure.
- If the dentition is uncrowded, avoid extraction of 6s as space closure will be difficult.
- Extraction of 6s will relieve buccal segment crowding, but will have little effect on labial segment crowding. Impaction of 8s less likely but not impossible.

▶ In a child with poor quality 6s, remember that the premolars may well be in a similar condition 6 yrs on unless the caries rate is stabilized.

Distal movement of the upper buccal segments

This is usually thought of as an alternative to extraction, but in practice often results in the crowding being shifted distally, requiring the loss of $\underline{7}$ or $\underline{8}$. It is only applicable to the upper arch, in the following situations:

• Either Class I with mild upper-arch crowding, or Class II/1 with well-aligned lower arch and molars <1 unit Class II.
• High anchorage case where extraction of 1 tooth per quadrant does not provide sufficient space to align upper arch.

Can be achieved either using a temporary anchorage device (📖 p. 156) or more usually by headgear to molar bands on $\underline{6|6}$. As $\underline{6|6}$ move distally, will need some expansion to keep the roots in cancellous bone. The chances of success are greater in a growing child. Can expect ½ unit change in 3–4 months with good cooperation. If need unilateral distal movement, extraction of $\underline{7}$ on that side can be considered (provided $\underline{8}$ in good position). To facilitate distal movement a direction of pull parallel to the occlusal plane (aka straight pull) is advisable.

Headgear safety

There have been a number of cases where damage to the eye as a result of headgear has resulted in loss of vision. For this reason headgear should only be used by those who have received training and to avoid injury to the face, it should only be used in conjunction with safety mechanisms which prevent displacement &/or recoil of the facebow. The British Orthodontic Society recommends the use of 2 separate safety devices. If eye injury should occur immediate referral to an ophthalmologist is required.

Spacing

Uncommon in UK; crowding is the norm.

Generalized spacing

Is due either to hypodontia or small teeth &/or large jaws. Note that hypodontia is associated with small teeth (📖 p. 64). Rx of spacing is problematic; a purely orthodontic approach is liable to relapse and requires prolonged retention. In milder cases try and encourage the patient to accept the situation. In more severe cases a combined restorative/orthodontic approach will be required. This may involve composite additions or veneers to increase the width of the teeth &/or orthodontics to localize the space for provision of an implant and/or prosthesis.

Median diastema

Prevalence 6-yr-olds = 98%, 11-yr-olds = 49%, 12–18-yr-olds = 7%.

Aetiology Small teeth in large jaws; absent or peg-shaped 2|2; midline $; proclination of ULS; physiological (caused by pressure of developing teeth on upper incisor roots which resolves as 3 erupts), or due to a frenum.

The upper incisive frenum is attached to the incisive papilla at birth. As 1|1 erupt the frenum recedes, but this is less likely if the arch is spaced. A frenum contributes to a diastema in a small number of cases and is associated with the following features:

- Blanching of incisive papilla when frenum put under tension.
- Radiographically there is a V-shaped notch in the interdental bone between 1|1, indicating the attachment of the frenum.
- Anterior teeth may be crowded.

Management Always take a periapical X-ray to exclude presence of a $.

- Before 3 erupted: if diastema <3mm—review after eruption of canines as will probably ↓ unaided. If >3mm—may need to approximate incisors to provide space for canines to erupt, but care is required not to resorb roots of 2|2 against crowns of 3|3. Usually requires FA and prolonged retention.

- After 3 erupted: orthodontic closure will require prolonged retention as has high tendency to relapse. If frenum undoubtedly a major aetiological factor perform a frenectomy during closure, but retention still wise. Alternatively, measure width of 1 2, and if they are narrower than average (1 = 8.5mm, 2 = 6.5mm) consider composite additions or veneers to close space. If teeth of normal width and no other orthodontic Rx required, could try and talk patient into accepting their diastema.

Buccally displaced maxillary canines

▶ Width $\underline{3}$ > width $\underline{4}$ > width $\underline{C}$.

$\underline{3}$ is usually the last tooth to erupt anterior to $\underline{6}$. If the upper arch is crowded, $\underline{3}$ may be squeezed buccal to its normal position, in which case space needs to be created for its alignment. Usually $\underline{4}$ is the tooth of choice for extraction and, if so, this should be carried out just as $\underline{3}$ is about to erupt. If there is plenty of space it is sufficient to keep the patient under review, otherwise fit a space-maintainer.

Where $\underline{2}$ and $\underline{4}$ are in contact, extraction of $\underline{4}$ alone will not provide sufficient space to accommodate the canine and thought should be given to extracting $\underline{3}$. Less commonly, a canine may develop well forward over the root of $\underline{2}$. In this case orthodontic Rx to align $\underline{3}$ will be prolonged. If the arch is crowded it may be simpler to extract $\underline{3}$ and align remaining teeth. Cases where $\underline{3}$ has been extracted need to rotate $\underline{4}$ slightly mesio-palatally to hide palatal cusp therefore FA required.

Transposition almost exclusively involves a canine tooth. In the maxilla $\underline{3}$ is usually transposed with $\underline{4}$ and in the mandible the lateral incisor is more commonly involved. Rx options include alignment of teeth in transposed position, extraction of the most displaced tooth, or correction if transposition of root apices is not complete.

Palatally displaced maxillary canines

▶ Early detection is essential.

Width 3 > width 4 > width C.

Prevalence

Up to 2%. Occurs bilaterally in 17–25% of cases. F > M.

Aetiology

In normal development, the maxillary canine develops palatal to C and then migrates labially to erupt down the distal aspect of 2 root. The aetiology of palatal displacement is not fully understood, but some suggest a lack of guidance is the reason behind the association with missing or short-rooted 2[1] (~6% of palatal 3 associated with small 2). Others argue that it is an inherited polygenic trait and that the link with missing or short-rooted 2 is part of association with other dental anomalies including microdontia and hypodontia.[2]

Prevention

Early detection may allow corrective interceptive Rx, therefore when examining any child >9yrs, palpate for unerupted 3. If there is a definite hollow &/or asymmetry between sides, further investigation is warranted. Extraction of C may result in improvement of a displaced 3,[3] but this eliminates the possibility of maintaining C should sufficient improvement in the position of 3 not materialize; therefore confine to those cases where the 3 is not too far displaced. More markedly displaced 3 should be referred to a specialist.

Assessment

Clinically by palpation and from inclination of 2; and by X-rays. A DPT and an intra-oral view or two intra-oral views with tube shift can be used to assess the position of the canine by parallax (📖 p. 71 remember your 'pal' goes with you!). Consider also position and prognosis of adjacent teeth (including C), the malocclusion, and available space.

Management

If the canine is only very slightly palatally displaced or impacted between 2 and 4, provision of space should result in eruption. The majority of palatally displaced canines, however, do not erupt spontaneously, so hopeful watching and waiting may only result in an older patient who is less willing to undergo the prolonged Rx required to align the displaced tooth. Rx alternatives available:

- Interceptive extraction of C in mixed dentition (see above).
- Maintain C and keep unerupted canine under radiographic review. Provided no evidence of cystic change or resorption, removal of 3 can be left until GA required, e.g. for extraction of 8s. Patient must understand that C will eventually be lost, necessitating a prosthesis.

1 A. Becker 1981 *Angle Orthodontist* **51** 24.

2 S. Peck 1994 *Angle Orthodontist* **64** 249.

3 S. Ericson 1988 *Eur J Orthod* **10** 283.

- No Rx, if 2 and 4 are in contact and appearance is satisfactory, or if patient refuses other options. Again, 3 will require removal in due course.
- Exposure and orthodontic alignment only feasible if (a) canine in favourable position for orthodontic alignment; (b) sufficient space available for 3, or can be created; (c) patient willing to undergo surgery and prolonged orthodontic Rx (usually 2+yrs). Sequence is to arrange exposure, and allow tooth to erupt for 3 months, and then commence orthodontic traction to move tooth towards arch. FAs are required.
- Autotransplantation is not an instant solution, as space is needed to accommodate 3, which may involve appliances &/or extractions. Prognosis is ↑ by avoiding damage to PDL and if root formation is not complete. If apex not open should root fill <10 days. Immature apex may revascularize.

Resorption

Unerupted and impacted canines can cause resorption of incisor roots. For this to occur a 'head-on' collision between the two seems to be required. If detected on X-ray, a specialist opinion should be sought, quickly. Extraction of the canine may be necessary to limit resorption, but if extensive, removal of the affected incisor may be preferable, thus allowing the canine to erupt.

Further reading:
M. Leonardi et al. 2004 Angle Orthodontist **74** 581.
P. F. McSherry 1998 BJO **25** 209.
P. F. McSherry and A. Richardson 1999 EJO **21** 41.

Increased overjet

When is an o/j increased? This is really a matter of opinion, but provided the arches are well-aligned, an o/j <6mm is acceptable. If Rx is required for other reasons, consider reduction of o/j >4mm. If lips are grossly incompetent then risk of trauma to inc is ↑, but relapse potential also↑.

Aetiology

Skeletal pattern Increased o/j can occur in association with Class I, II, or even III skeletal patterns. If Class II, often due to a normally sized mandible being positioned posteriorly on the cranial base. Be wary of patients with vertical proportions at either extreme of the range, as they are difficult to treat.

Soft tissues The effects of the soft tissues are usually determined by the skeletal pattern, as the greater the discrepancy the less likely it is that the patient will have competent lips. Where the lips are incompetent, the way an anterior oral seal is achieved will influence incisor position; e.g. if the lower lip is drawn up behind the upper incisors this may have contributed to the increased o/j, but if the incisors can be retracted within control of the lower lip at the end of Rx the prognosis for stable o/j reduction is good. The soft tissues can also help to compensate for the skeletal pattern by proclining the lower &/or retroclining the upper incisors.

Dental Crowding may contribute to an increased o/j, therefore relief of crowding may aid stability. Digit-sucking can cause proclination of the upper and retroclination of the lower incisors, but in a growing child this will resolve once habit is stopped unless maintained by adverse soft-tissue activity.

▶ In the majority of cases skeletal pattern will determine ease of Rx, but the soft tissues will influence the stability of the end result.

Stability of overjet reduction

Provided the inc have been retracted to a position of balance within the lower lip, this should not be a problem. Nevertheless, a period of retention is usually necessary to allow for periodontal fibre and soft-tissue adaption. However, prolonged retention will not make stable an inherently unstable position. E.g. if Rx is stopped before o/j reduction is complete and as a result the lips are not competent, there is a risk that the patient will return to retracting the lower lip behind the ULS to achieve an anterior oral seal, which may lead to an ↑ o/j.

Further reading:
J. E. Harrison *et al.* 2007 Orthodontic Treatment for prominent upper front teeth in children *Cochrane Database of Systemic reviews*, Issue 3.

Management of increased overjet

(See also Functional appliances, 📖 p. 164.)

Principles

- Provision of space for o/j reduction &/or relief of crowding.
- Reduce o/b before o/j reduction (📖 p. 147).
- Tooth movements required to ↓ o/j.
- Consider stability of treated result and plan retention—aim to achieve lip competence and control of the inc by the lower lip.

Class I or mild Class II skeletal pattern

If the overjet is <6mm, alignment is acceptable and orthodontic Rx not indicated for other reasons, consideration should be given to accepting the position of the incisors, particularly if the inc are not proclined, or stability following overjet reduction is questionable.

The majority of patients in this category are managed using fixed appliances ± extractions. If the skeletal pattern is more Class II then a functional appliance can be used for growth modification prior to FA. Treatment with a functional appliance can be commenced in the late mixed dentition, otherwise it is advisable to await the 2° dentition before embarking on Rx to reduce an o/j (📖 see p. 120).

Moderate to severe Class II skeletal pattern

Approaches available:

- Modification of growth—either by restraint of maxillary growth with headgear, or by encouraging mandibular growth with a functional appliance.
- Orthodontic camouflage—by extractions in upper arch and bodily movement of inc and FA.
- Surgical correction.

Because mandibular growth predominates during teens, a greater proportion of Class II than Class III skeletal problems is amenable to orthodontic correction. Research would suggest that the amount of growth modification that can be achieved is limited, but every little helps and in practice the majority of growing children in this category are treated by a combination of growth modification and camouflage. This usually takes the form of an initial phase of functional appliance therapy, followed by FA ± extractions.

Adults whose skeletal pattern is not too severe may be treated by orthodontic camouflage, but in cases with a more severe skeletal problem &/ or an ↑ o/b a surgical correction may be the only option.

Increased overbite

Normal o/b is between ⅓ and ½ overlap of the lower incisors. It is more practical to record o/b in terms of whether it is increased, decreased, or normal, rather than to try to measure it with a ruler. Increased o/b is associated with Class II/2 incisor relationship, where typically 1|1 are retroclined and 2|2 are proclined, reflecting their relationship to the lower lip. But the o/b can also be ↑ in Class III and II/1 malocclusions. Increased o/b *per se* is not an indication for Rx, unless it is traumatic and this is relatively rare, but o/b reduction may be necessary before correction of other anomalies. In Class III cases an ↑ o/b is advantageous as this will help to retain the corrected incisor position.

Aetiology

↑ o/b occurs because the incisors are able to erupt past each other due to a combination of some or all of the following interrelated factors: ↓ LFH; high lower lip line; retroclined incisors; ↑ inter-incisal angle.

Normal inter-incisal angle is 135°. Highest acceptable angle is 145°. Above this value the tendency for the lower incisors to erupt may be inadequately resisted.

In some Class II/2 cases, the LLS teeth are trapped by the ↑ o/b behind the ULS. Freeing them by e.g. provision of a URA with a biteplane may allow the lower incisors to spontaneously procline to a new stable position. This is one of the few situations where proclination (within reason!) of the LLS is stable.

Approaches to reducing overbite

- *Extrusion/eruption of molars.* Passive eruption of lower molars occurs when an URA incorporating a biteplane is worn. Active extrusion of molars in either arch is possible using FA. However, unless the patient grows vertically to accommodate this increased dimension, the molars will re-intrude under the forces of occlusion once appliances are withdrawn. This approach is of limited value in adults.
- *Intrusion of incisors.* This is difficult, requires FA, and in most cases the major effect is extrusion of the buccal segments. More successful in growing patients.
- *Proclination of lower incisors.* Movement of the lower incisor from their position of stability within the soft tissue envelope is unstable in most cases. Active proclination should only be attempted by the experienced orthodontist, who will be better able to judge those cases where this is indicated.
- *Surgery.* Indicated in severe cases especially if associated with A–P skeletal discrepancy, and in adults.

Stability of overbite reduction

Depends upon eliminating or reducing the aetiological factors, but ↓ LFH and high lower lip line can only be altered if growth is favourable. Reduction of the inter-incisal angle is necessary to provide a 'stop' to the incisors re-erupting, but requires FA to move incisor apices lingually.

Management of increased overbite

Class II/2

It is often prudent to avoid extractions when the lower arch is mildly crowded in a Class II/2, as extractions may be followed by lingual tipping of the lower incisors resulting in a further ↓ in o/b. Cases with sufficient crowding to warrant premolar extractions in the lower arch and moderately to severely increased overbite are best treated with FA to close space by forward movement of the buccal segments and to correct the incisor relationship.

Where o/b ↓ is required, the inter-incisal angle will need to be reduced in order to achieve a stable result. Usually this necessitates FA. However, in growing patients with a skeletal II pattern an alternative approach is to procline <u>inc</u> and use a functional appliance to reduce the resultant overjet. Proclination can be done either with URA first, or with FA on ULS, or by incorporating a spring in the functional appliance.

Class II/1

o/b ↓ is required before o/j ↓. If a functional appliance is indicated for A–P correction then some o/b reduction can often be achieved during this phase by trimming the appliance in the buccal segments. If headgear is being used then it may be helpful to commence o/b ↓ with an URA clipped over the bands on the upper molars. Rx of most II/1 will need FA either as the sole Rx or following a functional appliance or headgear. Including lower second molars in the FA will aid intrusion of the LLS (by ↑ vertical anchorage), but inevitably some extrusion of the molars will occur.

Class III (📖 p. 149)

Avoid reducing o/b as it will aid retention of the corrected incisor position.

Retention

Reducing the inter-incisal angle will aid stability. Following FA Rx use of an URA type retainer with a flat anterior biteplane may be helpful. Where the incisal relationship has been changed, retention ideally should be continued until growth is complete. In some patients this is not practicable.

Further reading:
D. T. Millett et al. 2006 Orthodontic Treatment for deep bite and retroclined upper front teeth in children Cochrane Database of Systemic reviews, Issue 4.

Anterior open bite (AOB)

Vertical overlap of incisors (o/b)

←————————————————————————→

↑o/b   normal o/b   incomplete o/b   AOB

AOB can occur in Class I, II, and III malocclusions.

Aetiology

Either *skeletal*—vertical > horizontal growth (↑ LFH &/or ↑ MMPA), or *environmental*—habits, tongue thrust, iatrogenic. Or a combination of these. If the distance between maxilla and mandible is sufficiently increased such that even if incisors develop to their full potential they do not meet, an AOB will result. This is often associated with incompetent lips and a lip-to-tongue anterior oral seal, which may exacerbate the AOB. Tongue thrusts are usually adaptive and can maintain an AOB due to a habit even after the habit has stopped.

Localized failure of maxillary dento-alveolar development resulting in an open bite is seen in CLP.

Treatment

Is generally difficult except where due mainly to a habit, therefore it is wise to refer patient to a specialist for advice.

Skeletal In milder cases can align arches and accept, or try to restrain vertical development of the maxilla &/or upper molars with headgear &/or a functional appliance with posterior bite blocks. Extrusion of the incisors is unstable. For more severe cases the only alternative is surgery.

Habits Better to await natural cessation of habit, but not if that means deferring Rx for other aspects of malocclusion. Once habit stops o/b should re-establish within 3yrs, unless perpetuated by soft tissues or because it is skeletal in origin.

Tongue thrust None.

Hints for cases with ↑ vertical dimensions and ↓ o/b or AOB.
- Avoid extruding molars, e.g. cervical pull headgear to 6|6, URA with a biteplane.
- Avoid upper arch expansion as this will tip down the palatal cusps of buccal segment teeth, reducing o/b.
- Extraction of molars will not 'close down bite'.
- Space closure is said to occur more readily in patients with ↑ LFH and ↑ MMPA.

Further reading:
D. A. Lentini-Oliveira *et al.* 2007 Orthodontic and Orthopaedic treatment for anterior open bite in children *Cochrane Database of Systemic Reviews*, Issue 2.

Reverse overjet

This will include only those cases with >2 teeth in linguo-occlusion, i.e. Class III cases. For management of one or two teeth in crossbite, see p. 152.

Aetiology

Skeletal Reverse overjets are usually associated with an underlying Class III skeletal pattern. This is most commonly due to either a large mandible &/or a retrusive maxilla. Class III malocclusions occur in association with the whole range of vertical patterns. Crossbites are a common feature, due either to a large mandible or a more forward position of the mandible relative to the maxilla.

Soft tissues A patient's efforts to achieve an anterior oral seal often result in dento-alveolar compensation, i.e. retroclination of the lower and proclination of the upper incisors therefore the incisor relationship is often less severe than underlying skeletal pattern.

Dental crowding This is usually greater in the upper than the lower arch.

Assessment (p. 126)

Consider also the following:
- Patient's opinion about their facial appearance (be tactful!).
- Severity of skeletal discrepancy.
- Amount and anticipated pattern of facial growth
- Amount of dento-alveolar compensation. If upper incisors already markedly proclined, further proclination is undesirable.
- Amount of overbite. Need a positive o/b to retain corrected incisor position at the end of treatment. Remember that proclination of ULS will reduce o/b and retroclination of LLS will ↓ o/b.
- Can patient achieve an edge-to-edge contact of the incisors? If so this ↑ prognosis for correction of incisor relationship.

Treatment planning (see p. 132).

▶ Class III malocclusions tend to become worse with growth.
▶ In severe cases seek a specialist opinion before embarking on Rx or extractions, as if surgery is necessary, decompensation (i.e. correcting the position of the incisors to their normal inclination) will probably involve the reverse of orthodontic camouflage.

Major factors determining Rx approach are skeletal discrepancy and overbite:

Skeletal pattern	Normal or ↑ o/b	↓ o/b
Mild to normal	Procline ULS	Accept
Moderate	FA to procline ULS and retrocline LLS	Accept or FA to retrocline LLS ± procline ULS
Severe	Surgery	Align and accept if possible, or surgery

If child on borderline between groups, assume more severe as growth will probably prove you right.

Management of reverse overjet

(Figures 4.9 and 4.10)

Relief of crowding Extractions in the upper arch alone may run the risk of worsening the incisor relationship, therefore it is advisable to extract at least as far forward in lower arch as upper.

Moderate crowding responds best to extraction of premolars. Extraction of 5|5 will maintain 4|4 to support the ULS, but often crowding in the upper arch necessitates extraction of 4|4. Proclination of ULS, if indicated, will provide some space for relief of crowding. If using FA to recline LLS, space will be required in the lower arch to accomplish this. Distal movement of the upper buccal segments is C/I in Class III as restraint of maxillary growth is undesirable.

Practical Rx

Accept This may be the wisest option for those patients with increased LFH and reduced o/b (because of the potential problems with stability), with Rx directed towards achieving alignment within the arches only.

Growth modification This is less applicable to Class III malocclusions due to the pattern of facial growth during the pubertal growth spurt. Getting a working bite for an active functional type of appliance is difficult (think about it!). Protraction headgear or facemask can be used to apply a forward force to the maxilla and maxillary teeth, but prolonged retention is usually required as the normal growth pattern re-establishes itself.

Proclination of ULS with an URA This is only applicable as an interceptive measure in the mixed dentition for mild cases where ULS is not already proclined and where sufficient o/b will be present to retain the corrected incisor position.

Camouflage Can be achieved by retroclination of LLS ± proclination of ULS. By interchanging the position of the incisors within the neutral zone, stability is not compromised. Requires fixed appliances in both arches. Class III elastic traction from the back of the upper arch to the 3̄ region helps to retrocline LLS. However, in addition to extruding the incisors, which is desirable, also results in extrusion of the upper molars, which reduces o/b. Therefore these cases should be managed by a skilled operator.

Orthodontics and orthognathic surgery (📖 p. 168). In a proportion of cases the severity of the skeletal pattern precludes orthodontics alone and surgery is indicated. It is difficult to produce hard and fast rules, but 2 predictors from a cephalometric analysis which have been suggested are:

1) ANB value below −4°
2) lower incisor angle to the mandibular plane of <83°

Patients need to be fully informed of the risks of surgery (as well as the risks of orthodontic treatment) in order to be able to make an informed decision.

Fig. 4.9 Correction of a Class III incisor relationship by retroclination of the lower incisors increases overbite.

Fig. 4.10 Correction of a Class III incisor relationship by proclination of the upper incisors alone reduces overbite.

Crossbites

By convention the lower teeth should be described relative to the upper (📖 p. 124). Xbites can be anterior or posterior (unilateral /bilateral), with displacement, or with no displacement.

Aetiology

Xbites can be skeletal &/or dental in origin. For posterior Xbites, the skeletal component is usually the major factor. Antero-posterior discrepancies obviously play a part in anterior Xbites, but can also result in posterior Xbites in Class II (lingual Xbite) and Class III (buccal Xbite) skeletal patterns.

Displacement may occur when a premature or deflecting cuspal contact is encountered on closure and the mandible is postured either anteriorly or laterally to achieve better interdigitation. This new path of closure becomes learned and the patient closes straight into maximum interdigitation. To help detect displacement on closure, try to get the patient to close on a hinge axis by asking them to curl their tongue back to touch the back of the palate and then close together slowly, whilst guiding the mandible back via the chin. In addition, look for other clues like a centre-line shift (of lower in direction of displacement) in association with a posterior unilateral Xbite. Evidence suggests that displacing contacts may predispose to TMPDS.

Anterior crossbites

For Class III 📖 see p. 149.

Anterior Xbites can be treated interceptively in mixed dentition if associated with a displacement, provided sufficient o/b exists to retain the result. If not, probably best to defer until the 2° dentition and use FA. Upper lateral incisors that are displaced bodily will require buccal root torque for correction.

Posterior crossbites[1]

Unilateral Generally, the greater the number of teeth involved the greater the skeletal contribution to the aetiology. If only affects one or two teeth in each arch, movement of opposing teeth in opposite directions can be achieved by cross-elastics attached to attachments on the affected teeth. Unilateral Xbite from the canine region distally is usually associated with a displacement, as true skeletal asymmetry is rare. If the arches are of a similar width when the patient closes the cusps will meet so the patient displaces laterally to achieve a better interdigitation. In these cases Rx should be directed towards expanding the upper arch so that it fits around the lower, provided the upper teeth are not already buccally tilted.

Bilateral buccal crossbite This suggests a greater underlying transverse skeletal discrepancy. Is less commonly associated with displacement.

---

1 J. Harrison 2001 Cochrane Library, Issue 2, Oxford.

Correction of a bilateral Xbite should be approached with caution, because partial relapse may result in the teeth occluding cusp to cusp and development of a unilateral Xbite with displacement.

Bilateral lingual crossbite (or scissor bite) occurs due to either a narrow mandible or a wide maxilla. In milder cases only 4|4 may be involved, and if these teeth are extracted to relieve crowding or for retraction of 3|3, so much the better. Where the whole buccal segments are involved, Rx will probably involve expansion of the lower &/or contraction of the upper, therefore refer to a specialist.

Rapid maxillary expansion

Involves a screw appliance comprising bands attached to 64|46 and connected to a midline screw. The object is to expand the maxilla by opening the midline suture and is therefore more successful in younger patients. Large forces are required to accomplish this—the screw is turned 0.2mm twice a day for about 2 weeks. Over-expansion is necessary as the teeth relapse about 50% under soft-tissue pressure. Not to be attempted by the inexperienced!

Quad helix appliance

This is a very efficient fixed, slow expansion appliance. It is made of 1mm SS attached to bands on 6|6 and is W-shaped. Activated by expanding ½ tooth width per side before placement (Figure 4.11).

Fig. 4.11 Quad helix appliance.

Anchorage

Anchorage is defined as the source of resistance to the reaction from the active component(s) in an appliance. In practice, it is the balance between the applied force and the available space. E.g. in a case where 3|3 are being retracted following extraction of 4|4, an equal, but opposite force will also be acting on 65|56. The amount of forward movement of these anchor teeth will depend largely upon their root surface area and the force used.

Anchorage loss can be minimized by limiting the number of teeth being moved at any one time, applying the correct force for the movement required, and ↑ the resistance of the anchor teeth (e.g. by permitting only bodily movement). In some situations, movement of the anchor teeth is desirable, e.g. in a Class III where space is being opened up for an unerupted 3. However, it is important to assess the anchorage requirements of a particular malocclusion before embarking on treatment. If no or little movement of the anchor teeth is desirable, then anchorage should be reinforced from the start.

Reinforcing anchorage

Intra-maxillary (teeth in same arch) By including the maximum number of teeth in the anchorage unit. Applicable to both fixed and removable appliances.

Inter-maxillary (teeth in opposing arch) This is achieved by running elastics from one arch to the other. It is mainly applicable to FA, as an URA will be dislodged. The direction of elastic pull is described according to the type of malocclusion to which it is applicable.

Increased mucosal coverage By virtue of its palatal coverage an URA has more potential anchorage than an FA.

Extra-oral Anchorage is transmitted to the appliance by elastic or spring force from a head or neck strap. This involves a face-bow, which engages tubes soldered onto molar cribs (URA) or bands (FA). The direction of pull can be selected according to the malocclusion with an overall direction of pull above the occlusal plane for patients with ↑ vertical proportions (hi-pull) and vice versa for ↓ vertical proportions (cervical pull). For EO anchorage, 250g for 10h/day should suffice. For EO traction (i.e. using the headgear force to achieve movement rather than just resist it) forces in the region of 500g for 14–16h/day are necessary.

Following reports of a number of cases where eye damage (including blindness) occurred due to headgear, the use of at least two safety mechanisms is advised.

TAD 📖 see p.156.

Anchorage loss

May occur because of

1) failure to appreciate fully anchorage requirements at Rx planning stage (generally if 75–100% of space generated from extractions is required for planned tooth movement, anchorage requirements are high)

2) active force exceeding available anchorage (often due to over-activation or too many teeth being moved at a time)

3) poor patient compliance

Temporary Anchorage Devices (TAD)

Implants have been adopted in orthodontics to provide skeletal anchorage, with ↓ need for patient compliance. This has ↑ the envelope in terms of the severity of malocclusions that can be treated by orthodontics alone. Currently the term TAD is in vogue, but mini-implants, microscrews, bone anchorage devices (BAD) also used. Success rates of 80–90% have been reported.[1]

Types of implant

Osseointegrated	No osseointegration
Designed to maximize surface contact for integration	Designed for ease of placement and removal
Short body length and large diameter	Screw or plate
Surface coating	No surface coating
More difficult to place. ↑ morbidity at removal due to osseointegration	Plate design more difficult to place and remove than screw
Usually used in edentulous, retromolar, palatal areas	Can be placed in dento-alveolar bone between tooth roots
Useful when wish to replace a missing tooth after orthodontic treatment	

A screw design with no osseointegation is now the most widely used in orthodontics, because it is easy to place and remove. Typically 1–2mm wide and 6–15mm in length with a neck that protrudes through the mucosa and a head designed for attaching an orthodontic force system (e.g. elastic or coil spring).

There are 2 sub-divisions:
• Self-tapping—site is pre-drilled with specially designed handpiece prior to insertion of screw.
• Self-drilling—implant is screwed directly into bone. Better results as causes less thermal damage to bone.

Site selection

• Treatment mechanics—including direction of desired force
• Anatomy—tooth roots, other structures
• Depth of available bone including thickness of cortical plate
• Bone quality
• Access for placement
• Gingival health and quality—Good OH. Attached gingiva better

Need good X-rays.

1 S. Kuroda et al. 2007 Am J Orthod Dentofac Orthoped **131** 9.

For self-tapping screw design only need superficial anaesthesia at insertion site—an advantage as the patient will be able to alert the operator if a tooth root is inadvertently hit during placement! Advisable to get patient to rinse with chlorhexidine prior to placement. Some self-tapping types use a stent to guide placement. Screws can be inserted with a hand (screw) driver or using an engine driver i.e. a speed reduction (<30rpm) contra-angle handpiece.

Loading

Most operators load the self-tapping screws immediately in adults, but delay 2 weeks in teenagers. The osseointegrated type require a latent period for integration. Need to avoid excess force levels (<250g).

Explantation

Fancy term for removal. For osseointegrated types need to raise a flap and cut out implant. Screw designs can usually be removed without LA by unscrewing.

Problems

Success is a screw that is functional for the duration the orthodontic force is required. A screw that is slightly mobile may still be functional. If a screw contacts a root then this usually results in the screw becoming loose &/or some patient discomfort.

- Screw becomes loose—remove and replace in another site.
- Breakage—about 3–4%.
- Root damage—evidence suggests that if root is perforated then get healing by cementum.
- Mucosal discomfort—check OH.

Further reading:
J. Prabhu and R.R.J. Cousley 2006 Bone Anchorage Devices in Orthodontics *J Orthod* **33** 288.
NICE 2007 IPG238 *Mini/Micro implantation for orthodontic anchorage: guidance* (🖰 www.nice.org.uk).

Removable appliances—scope and limitations

Removable appliances are single-arch appliances that can be taken out of the mouth by the patient (see Figure 4.12). They are only capable of tilting movements of individual teeth, but can be used for moving blocks of teeth. In addition they can be used to allow differential eruption of teeth via biteplanes or buccal capping. Now used more as an adjunct to comprehensive FA treatment and for retention after FA.

Advantages of removables	Disadvantages of removables
Removable for tooth-brushing	Patient can leave appliance out
Easy to adjust—↓ chair-side time	Only tipping movements possible
Palatal coverage ↑ anchorage	Affects speech
	Good technician required
Can be used for o/b ↓	Intermaxillary traction not possible
Can transmit forces to blocks of teeth	Lower removable appliances are difficult to tolerate
	Inefficient for multiple tooth movements

Indications

Active
- Movement of blocks of teeth, e.g. correction of a buccal crossbite by expansion of upper arch.
- As an interceptive Rx in the mixed dentition, e.g. correction of an upper incisor in crossbite.
- Overbite reduction.
- In conjunction with other appliance, e.g. to facilitate distal movement of upper molar(s) with headgear.
- Elimination of occlusal interferences by addition of biteplane or buccal capping. Useful for movement of a tooth over the bite during fixed appliance Rx.
- Simple tipping movement of an individual tooth. The fulcrum for tipping is about $\frac{1}{3}$ to $\frac{1}{2}$ from the root apex. So as the crown tips away from the applied force the root apex moves in the opposite direction.

Passive
- Space maintainer, e.g. following loss of an upper central incisor due to trauma.
- Retaining appliance, e.g. following fixed appliance Rx.
- Habit deterrent.

Fig. 4.12 Upper removable appliance to expand upper arch with midline screw.
cribs 6|6 0.7mm SS
  4|4 0.6mm SS
buccal capping or FABP

Removable appliances—design

Four components need to be considered for every appliance.

Active component

Exerts force required for desired movement.

Springs

Springs (made in SS wire) are the most commonly used active component because they are versatile and cheap to construct.

The relationship between the distance (d) that an orthodontic spring is deflected on activation, the length of the spring (l), the diameter or radius (r) of the wire it is composed of, and the force generated is:

$$F \propto \frac{dr^4}{l^3}$$

In practice this means that for two identical springs in order to deliver the same amount of force:
0.5mm wire would be activated about 3mm.
0.7mm wire would be activated about 1mm.

Palatal finger springs are the most commonly used active components for mesial or distal movement along the arch. They are fabricated in 0.5mm wire and are easy to adjust and activate. If boxed out from the acrylic and made with a guard wire they are more stable in the vertical plane than a buccal spring and therefore should be used in preference.

For details of other types of spring the reader should consult a specialist text.

Elastics

Less commonly used nowadays, but are sometimes used for aligning displaced teeth, e.g. palatal canine, using an attachment bonded onto the tooth surface, to which an elastic is applied by the patient to a hook soldered onto a labial bow or crib of a VRA.

Screws

A screw appliance is useful when the teeth to be moved need to be clasped for retention (e.g. expanding the upper arch in the mixed dentition see Figure 4.12). The thread on a screw is opened (or closed) by means of a key, a quarter turn of which separates the two halves by 0.2mm. It is advisable to start patients turning the screw only once a week, progressing on to a maximum of two turns per week. If worn intermittently, a screw appliance will become progressively ill-fitting. Remember that these screws have about 18 activations and if turned more than that will part company!

Retention

This is the means by which the appliance is retained in the mouth. The best retention posteriorly is provided by the Adams crib (Figure 4.13), which is made in SS in either 0.7mm (for permanent molars) or 0.6mm (for premolars and primary molars) wire. These clasps are very technician-sensitive and no amount of adjustment will compensate for a badly made crib. Should engage about 1mm of undercut, which on a child's molar may be at, or just under, the gingival margin and in an adult may only be part-way down the clinical crown. The versatility of the crib can be increased by soldering tubes for EOT, labial bows, or buccal springs onto the bridge of the clasp.

Anterior retention can be gained by a labial bow or either an Adams or Southend Clasp. All these components are usually constructed in 0.7mm wire.

Anchorage

Resists force generated by active component(s); see p. 154.

Baseplate

Not only holds other elements together, but may also itself be active. Heat-cure acrylic is more robust than self-cure.

- A flat anterior biteplane should only be prescribed if o/b ↓ is required. Should specify the height (e.g. half the height of 1/1) and how far back the biteplane should extend (e.g. o/j =3mm). In order to ↑ the likelihood of the URA being worn the molars should only be separated by 1–2mm by the biteplane and further self-cure acrylic added as required to re-activate during Rx.
- Buccal capping frees the occlusion on the tooth being moved and allows further relative eruption of the incisors (therefore is C/I if o/b is already ↑). Should be trimmed so that the teeth to be moved are separated only by 1–2mm.

▶ The easier it is for the patient to insert and wear their URA, the more likely it is that Rx will be successful, therefore keep design simple.

Fig. 4.13 Adjustment of Adams crib.
1 Arrowhead moves horizontally towards tooth.
2 Arrowhead moves towards tooth and also vertically towards gingival crevice.

Fixed appliances

▶ FA should only be used in cooperative patients with good OH, to minimize damage to the teeth and their supporting tissues.

As the name implies, FA are attached to the teeth. They vary in complexity, from a single attachment on two opposing teeth for correction of a Xbite, to full fixed appliances in both arches. FA give precise three-dimensional control of tooth movement. They can be used to tilt, rotate, intrude, extrude, and move teeth bodily. Not surprisingly, FA have a greater propensity for things to go wrong, therefore they should only be used by those with the necessary skills and training.

Principles

- Rx planning (📖 p. 132). Need particular attention to anchorage requirements, especially if apical movement is planned.
- As FA are able to achieve bodily movement, it is possible (within limits) to move teeth to compensate for a skeletal discrepancy.
- FA can be used in conjunction with other appliances &/or headgear.
- For initial alignment flexible archwires are used, but to minimize unwanted movements, progressively more rigid archwires are necessary.
- Archwires should be based on the pre-Rx lower arch-form for stability.
- Mesio-distal movement is achieved either by: (i) sliding the teeth along the archwire with elastic force (sliding mechanics), or (ii) moving the teeth with the archwire.

Intermaxillary traction (📖 p.154) is often used to aid antero-posterior correction and increase anchorage.

Components of fixed appliances

Bands Usually used on molar teeth so that the end of the arch wire is retained even if band becomes loose. Indicated for other teeth if bonds fail or lingual attachment is required for de-rotation. If tooth contacts are tight these will need to be separated prior to band placement using an elastic doughnut stretched around the contact point for 1–7 days. Use of GI cements helps to ↓ decalcification.

Bonds are attached to enamel with (acid-etch) composite. There are two commonly used types: (i) metal (poor aesthetics); (ii) ceramic (prone to # and can cause enamel wear). There is a wide variety of designs (see Types of FA below).

Archwires Flexible nickel titanium archwires are used in the initial stages of Rx and more rigid stainless steel wires used in the later stages for the planned tooth movements. Tungsten molybdenum, and cobalt chromium alloys are also popular.

Auxillaries Elastic rings or wire ligatures are used to tie the archwire to the brackets. Forces can be applied to the teeth by auxiliary springs or elastics.

Types of fixed appliance

Almost infinite variety, but most well-known are:

Standard edgewise Now largely historical. Brackets are rectangular and wide mesio-distally for rotational control. Round wires are used initially for alignment, but rectangular wires are necessary for apical control. The intended final three dimensional position of each tooth had to be built into the archwire by bends placed in the archwire in all three planes of space.

Pre-adjusted systems These 'pre-programmed' brackets are designed with the average values for the intended final three dimensional position built into the archwire slot. Thus the amount of archwire bending required is reduced. As each tooth has its own individual bracket with a built-in prescription for that tooth, these systems are more expensive, but that is offset by savings in operator time. A number of different prescriptions are available.

Self ligating systems have a clip mechanism incorporated into the bracket to hold the archwire in place (rather than elastic or wire tie) which ↓ friction, making tooth movement quicker. This is an expanding area with new designs being developed regularly examples include Damon, Smartclip, Innovation.

Tip edge is based on the Begg philosophy which used round wires which fitted loosely into a vertical slot in the bracket, thus allowing the teeth to tip freely. Auxiliaries were required to achieve apical and rotational movements. Tip-Edge brackets also have pre-adjusted values incorporated to give the 'finish' produced by using a straight wire appliance.

Lingual appliances Popular with patients, but not widely available as access for placement and adjustment more challenging! Expensive.

Clear Aligner Therapy Known as CAT. These are vacuum-formed thermoplastic 'removable appliances'. Included here as they are popular with patients as a more aesthetic alternative to FA. Study models are scanned digitally and then the computer program designs a sequence of models with increment changes in tooth position. A series of clear plastic aligners are then made which move teeth to desired final result. The rate of tooth movement is 0.25 to 0.33mm/aligner. Only applicable to mild malocclusions treated without extractions.

More details can be found in specialist texts (naturally the reference is my own book!).[1]

1 L. Mitchell 2007 *An Introduction to Orthodontics*, OUP.

Functional appliances—rationale and mode of action

Definition Functional appliances utilize, eliminate, or guide the forces of muscle function, tooth eruption, and growth to correct a malocclusion.

Philosophy The term functional appliance dates back to a belief that by eliminating abnormal muscle function normal growth and development would follow. Nowadays, the importance of both genetic and environmental factors in the aetiology of malocclusion is acknowledged, but functional appliances are still successfully used in the Rx of Class II malocclusions by a combination of skeletal and dental effects. Functional appliances (or just 'functionals') can also be used in the management of AOB and Class III, but those approaches are beyond the scope of this text.

Mode of action In the average child the face grows forward relative to the cranial base and mandibular growth predominates. Functional appliances help to harness this change to correct Class II malocclusions by a combination of force application and force elimination. The relative contributions of each depend upon the design of appliance. Force application usually takes the form of inter-maxillary traction, i.e. a restraining effect on the maxilla and maxillary teeth and a forward pressure on the mandible and mandibular teeth. A similar effect is produced with Class II elastics (📖 p. 154). Functional appliances are ineffective for individual tooth movement.

Indications

- To achieve some antero-posterior correction for a Class II malocclusion prior to FA ± extractions. Ideally: Class II/1 with mandibular retrusion, average or reduced LFH, or upright or retroclined LLS. A useful test is to examine the profile with patient postured forward to a Class I incisor relationship, and if not improved consider another appliance.
- Can be used as sole appliance in milder cases with well-aligned arches.

Changes produced by functional appliances

Skeletal

- Research would suggest that changes seen are 25% skeletal and 75% dental.
- Optimizing of mandibular growth. The evidence would suggest that in the short term an extra 1–2mm mandibular growth results, however, long term that overall gain is small.
- Restraint of forward maxillary growth.
- Forward movement of the glenoid fossa.
- ↑ LFH.

Dental

- Palatal tipping of the upper incisors.
- Labial tipping of the lower incisors (not a consistent finding).
- Inhibition of forward movement of the maxillary molars.
- Mesial and vertical eruption of the mandibular molars.

Keys to success with functional appliances

- Cooperative and keen patient. Remember that cooperation is finite.
- Favourable growth; therefore coincide Rx with pubertal growth spurt (girls 11–13yrs, boys 13–15yrs).
- Confident operator, so that child believes appliance will work and will persevere with wearing it.

Further reading:
J. E. Harrison *et al.* 2007 Orthodontic Treatment for prominent upper front teeth in children Cochrane Database of Systemic Reviews, Issue 3.
K. D. O'Brien *et al.* 2003 Effectiveness of treatment for Class II malocclusion with the herbst or twin-block appliances: a RCCT *Am J Orthod Dentofac Orthop* **124** 128.

Types of functional appliance and practical tips

Choice of appliance

Some of the more popular types:

Twin Block Is the most commonly used design in the UK. Comprises a separate URA and a lower removable appliance which by means of sloping buccal blocks help to posture the mandible forward. Because they are individual upper and lower appliances and are retained by clasping the teeth they are well tolerated by patients and can be worn for meals. In addition, a screw can be incorporated in the upper twin block if expansion is required, as well as springs (e.g. to align 2). Need well-extended upper and lower impressions and plus a wax bite recorded with the mandible postured forwards 7–10mm (see Figures 4.14 and 4.15).

Medium opening activator (MOA) Useful in case with ↓ LFH as design allows eruption of lower molars. It is a one-piece functional therefore a preliminary phase of upper arch expansion prior to fitting the MOA is required in most patients to co-ordinate arch widths. Must be made in heat-cure acrylic as extensions to lower arch prone to fracture. Worn full-time except eating.

Herbst Is a fixed functional appliance. Comprises metal cast splints cemented onto the buccal segment teeth which are connected by metal arms in a piston arrangement which hold the mandible forward. Achieves rapid antero-posterior correction. Expensive to make.

Functionals in Class II/1 with ↑ LFH

Need appliance with molar capping to try and prevent molar eruption, encourage auto-rotation of the mandible, and thus ↓ LFH. Constructing the appliance with a greater amount of vertical bite opening is thought to result in a more forward direction of mandibular growth.[1] More effective if incorporate high-pull headgear to restrain vertical maxillary growth.

Practical tips

- Advise patient to wear appliance full-time. Only twin block appliance can be worn for eating. See every 2 months.
- Problems with appliances that fall out in bed at night are often cured by ↑ wear during the day.
- Expect at least 1mm o/j reduction per month (more with Herbst).
- Wise to continue until o/j edge-to-edge i.e. over-correct.
- Retain by wearing nights only, for about 3 months before progressing on to FA. The buccal blocks of a Twin Block can be reduced to encourage molar eruption during this phase.

---

1 S. E. Bishara 1989 *Am J Orthod Dentofac Orthop* **95** 250.

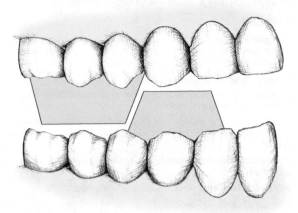

Fig. 4.14 Demonstrating how the inclined bite blocks of the Twin Block appliance hold the mandible forward in a postured position.

Fig. 4.15 Twin Block appliance.

Orthodontics and orthognathic surgery

Orthognathic surgery is the correction of skeletal discrepancies that due to their severity lie outside the scope of orthodontics. Usually deferred until active growth has slowed to adult levels.

Diagnosis and Rx planning

This is best undertaken jointly by orthodontist and maxillofacial surgeon. Require the following information:

Patient's perception of problem Are they concerned with appearance of jaws or teeth, speech, or problems with eating? Are their expectations realistic?

Clinical examination Assessment of the balance and proportions of full face and profile.[1]

Study models Needed to assess co-ordination of arches.

Radiographs require DPT and lateral skull, plus PA skull for asymmetries. It is helpful to compare patient's cephalometric tracing with the ideal (Bolton Standard) to visually assess areas of discrepancy. A number of computer programs of varying complexity and cost are available to aid in Δ and planning. However, these should not supersede clinical assessment.

Photographs Required as pre-Rx record and can also be manipulated with lateral skull for visual computer predictions.

It is important to correlate desired facial changes with patient's occlusion. Pre-surgical orthodontics will be required to decompensate teeth so that a full surgical correction is possible.

It is important (in order to obtain informed consent) that patients are fully informed of the risks of surgery, particularly mandibular procedures in addition to the orthodontic risks. The British Orthodontic Society has produced an excellent dvd which provides a well-balanced overview for prospective patients.

Sequence of Rx

Pre-surgical orthodontics Aim of this phase is to align and coordinate the arches so that the teeth will not interfere when the jaws are placed in their correct position. This usually involves decompensation, i.e. removal of any dento-alveolar compensation for the skeletal discrepancy so that the teeth are at their correct axial inclinations and a full surgical correction can be achieved. If a segmental procedure is planned space will be needed interdentally for surgical cuts. It is inefficient to carry out movements that can be accomplished more readily at surgery (e.g. expansion of upper arch if Le Fort 1 planned), or following surgery (e.g. levelling of lower arch in Class II/2). In addition, the FA provides a means of fixation at surgery.

---

1 N. P. Hunt 1984 *Br J Orthod* **11** 126.

Surgery, 📖 p. 474. Full records should be taken for final planning. For bimaxillary procedure need study models mounted on semi- or fully adjustable articulator.

Post-surgical orthodontics Lighter round wires and inter-maxillary traction are used to detail occlusion.

Retention This is the same as after conventional FA Rx.

Relapse This can be surgical or orthodontic or both. Relapse more likely in Rx of deficiencies as soft tissues are under greater tension post-operatively. Research[1] has shown the following hierarchy of stability:

Very stable	Max. up
	Mand. forward
	Chin—any direction
Stable	Max. forward
	Max. asymmetry
Stable with rigid fixation	Max. up & mand. forward
	Max. forward and mand. back
	Mand. asymmetry
Least stable	Mand. back
	Max. down
	Widening of max.

Distraction osteogenesis

A proportion of severe cases (particularly congenital craniofacial deformity) require movements beyond the scope of conventional orthognathic surgery—principally due to soft tissue restriction. Distraction osteogenesis is useful in the management of these cases as it involves slow distraction across the osteotomized bones, which stretches the surrounding soft tissues. The surgical cuts for an osteotomy are made in the usual way, but then after allowing a few days for initial callus formation, traction is applied across the bone cuts via a distractor. The healing callus is put under tension and bone is laid down in the direction of force. A period of consolidation is required after the desired surgical movements are achieved.

---

1 W. R Proffit *et al.* 2007 *Head Face Med* **3** 21.

Cleft lip and palate

Prevalence CLP varies with racial group and geographically. Occurs in 1:700 Caucasian births, but prevalence ↑. M > F. If unilateral L > R. Family history in 40% of cases.

Isolated cleft palate occurs in 1:2000 births. F > M. Family history in 20%.

Aetiology Multifactorial with both genetic and environmental factors (including maternal smoking, alcohol and phenytoin intake) involved. Can occur in isolation or as part of a syndrome.

Classification Many exist, but best approach is to describe cleft: primary &/or secondary palate; complete or incomplete; unilateral or bilateral. Submucous cleft of the palate is often missed until poor speech noticed, as overlying mucosa is intact.

Problems

Embryological anomalies Tissue deficit, displacement of segments, abnormal muscle attachments.

Post-surgical distortions Unrepaired clefts show normal growth. In repaired clefts maxillary growth is ↓ antero-posteriorly, transversely, and vertically. Mandibular growth also ↓.

Hearing and speech are impaired.

Other congenital anomalies occur in up to 20% of cases with CLP and are more likely in association with isolated clefts of palate than lip.

Dental anomalies In CLP ↑ prevalence of hypodontia and $ teeth (especially in region of cleft). Teeth adjacent to cleft are often displaced. Also ↑ incidence of hypoplasia and delayed eruption.

Management (of unilateral complete CLP)

Team usually includes cleft surgeon, ENT surgeon, health visitors, orthodontist, speech therapist, clinical psychologist, and central coordinator. Centralization of care and audit of outcome gives better results.

Birth Parents need explanation, reassurance, and help with feeding. Pre-surgical orthopaedics is now out of vogue as benefits not proven.

Lip closure Usually between 3–6 months of age. Delaire or Millard &/or modifications are the most popular. Some surgeons do Vomer flap at same time. Bilateral lips are closed either in one or two operations.

Palatal closure Usually between 9–12 months. Delaire or Von Langenbeck ± modifications are the most popular. Deferring repair until patient is older ↓ growth disturbance, but speech development is adversely affected.

Primary dentition Speech and hearing assessments. Establishment of good dental care.

Mixed dentition May be necessary to procline upper incisors if they erupt into linguo-occlusion, otherwise orthodontic Rx is better deferred until just prior to secondary bone grafting at 8–10yrs.

Alveolar bone graft If an alveolar cleft is present then this should be grafted when the canine root is ½ to ⅔ formed (around age 8½ to 10½yrs) with cancellous bone. Advantages:

- Provides bone for 3̲ to erupt through.
- Allows tooth movement into cleft site therefore may avoid prosthesis.
- ↑ bony support for alar base.
- Aids closure of oro-nasal fistulae.
- Also helps to stabilize mobile premaxillary segment in bilateral cases.

To aid surgical access and improve outcome usually need to expand collapsed arches and align the upper incisors prior to grafting. FA are usually used and care is required not to move roots of adjacent teeth into cleft. Bone usually harvested from the iliac crest.

Permanent dentition Because of the restraining effects of primary surgery upon facial growth, cleft patients often have a Class III malocclusion. If this is not significant (and/or patient doesn't want orthognathic surgery) then definitive Rx for alignment and space closure with FA can be carried out. Ideally, if 2̲ missing, Rx should aim to bring 3̲ forward to replace it, thus avoiding a prosthesis.

Late teens If orthognathic surgery is indicated (📖 p. 474) then this should be deferred until active growth has slowed to adult levels. Pre-surgical orthodontic alignment with FA will be required. If nasal revision surgery is planned then this should be carried out after bony surgery.

A proportion of cleft patients will have a skeletal discrepancy that is too severe for conventional surgical movements. In addition advancement of the maxilla may, by bringing forward the soft palate, adversely affect speech. In these cases distraction osteogenesis (p. 169) can be considered.

Periodontology

Contents

Principal sources and further reading J. Lindhe 2008 *Clinical Periodontology and Implant Dentistry* (5e), Munksgaard. *Journal of Clinical Periodontology*, Munksgaard.

Oral microbiology

The mouth is colonized by microorganisms a few hours after birth, mainly by aerobic and facultative anaerobic organisms. The eruption of teeth allows the development of a complex ecosystem of microorganisms. Around 700 different species can colonize the mouth and the healthy mouth depends on maintaining an environment in which these organisms coexist without damaging oral structures.

Microorganisms worth noting

Streptococcus mutans group Several species are recognized within this group, including *S. mutans* and *S. sobrinus*. Facultative anaerobe. Synthesizes dextrans. Colony density rises to >50% in presence of high dietary sucrose. Able to produce acid from most sugars. Most important organisms in the aetiology of caries.

Streptococcus oralis group includes *S. sanguis*, *S. mitis*, and *S. oralis*. Account for up to 50% of streptococci in plaque. Heavily implicated in 50% of cases of infective endocarditis.

Streptococcus salivarius group accounts for about half the streptococci in saliva. Inconsistent producer of dextran.

S. intermedius, S. angiosus, S. constellatus (formerly *S. milleri* group) Common isolates from abscesses in the mouth and at distant sites.

Lactobacillus Secondary colonizer in caries. Very acidogenic. Often found in dentine caries.

Porphyromonas gingivalis Obligate anaerobe associated with chronic periodontitis and aggressive periodontitis.

Aggregatibacter actinomycetemcomitans Microaerophilic, capnophilic, Gram –ve rod. Particular pathogen in aggressive periodontitis.

Tannerella Forsythia

Prevotella intermedia Found in chronic periodontitis, localized aggressive periodontitis, (juvenile periodontitis), necrotizing periodontal disease, and areas of severe gingival inflammation without attachment loss.

Prevotella nigrescens New, possibly more virulent.

Fusobacterium Obligate anaerobes. Originally thought to be principal pathogens in necrotizing periodontal disease. Remain a significant periodontal pathogen.

Spirochaetes Obligate anaerobes implicated in periodontal disease; present in most adult mouths. *Borrelia*, *Treponema*, and *Leptospira* belong to this family.

Borrelia vincenti (refringens) Large oral spirochaete; probably only a co-pathogen.

Actinomyces israelii Filamentous organism; major cause of actinomycosis. A persistent rare infection which occurs predominantly in the mouth and jaws and the female reproductive tract. Implicated in root caries.

Candida albicans Yeast-like fungus, famous as an opportunistic oral pathogen; probably carried as a commensal by most people.

Plaque

Dental plaque, which is a biofilm, is a firmly adherent mass of bacteria in a muco-polysaccharide matrix. It cannot be rinsed off but can be removed by brushing. It is the root of most dental evils.

Attachment Although it is possible for plaque to collect on irregular surfaces in the mouth, to colonize smooth tooth surfaces it needs the presence of *acquired pellicle*. This is a thin layer of salivary glycoproteins, formed on the tooth surface within minutes of polishing. The pellicle has an ion-regulating function between tooth and saliva and contains immunoglobulins, complement, and lysozyme.

Development Up to 10^6 viable bacteria per mm^2 of tooth surface can be recovered 1h after cleaning;[1] these are selectively adsorbed streptococci. Bacteria recolonize the tooth surface in a predictable sequence. *Streptococcus mutans* synthesizes extracellular polysaccharides (glucan and fructan) specifically from sucrose and promotes its early colonization this way. Cocci predominate in plaque for the first 2 days, following which rods and filamentous organisms become involved. This is associated with ↑ numbers of leucocytes at the gingival margin. Between 6 and 10 days, if no cleaning has taken place, vibrios and spirochaetes appear in plaque and this is associated with clinical gingivitis. It is generally felt that the move towards a more Gram −ve anaerobe-dense plaque is associated with the progression of gingivitis and periodontal disease.

Plaque in caries (📖 p. 24) As several oral streptococci, most notably mutans streptococci, secrete acids and the matrix component of plaque, there is a clear relationship between the two. However, various other factors complicate the picture, including saliva, other microorganisms, and the structure of the tooth surface.

Plaque in periodontal disease There is a direct correlation between the amount of plaque at the cervical margin of teeth and the severity of gingivitis,[2] and experimental gingivitis can be produced and abolished by suspending and reintroducing oral hygiene.[3] It is commonly accepted that plaque accumulation causes gingivitis, the major variable being host susceptibility. While there are numerous interacting components which determine the progression of chronic gingivitis to periodontitis, particularly host susceptibility, the presence of plaque, particularly 'old' plaque with its high anaerobe content, is widely held to be crucial, and most Rx is based on the meticulous, regular removal of plaque.

1 R. Gibbons 1973 *J. Periodont* **44** 347.
2 M. Ash 1964 *J. Periodont* **35** 424.
3 H. Loe 1965 *J. Periodont* **36** 177.

Calculus

Calculus (tartar) is a calcified deposit found on teeth (and other solid oral structures) and is formed by mineralization of plaque deposits. It can be subdivided into:

Supragingival calculus, most often found opposite the openings of the salivary ducts, i.e. 76|67 opposite the parotid (Stensen's) duct and on the lingual surface of the lower anterior teeth opposite the submandibular/sublingual (Wharton's) duct. It is usually yellow, but can become stained a variety of colours.

Subgingival calculus is found, not surprisingly, underneath the gingival margin and is firmly attached to tooth roots. It tends to be brown or black, is extremely tenacious, and is most often found on interproximal and lingual surfaces. It may be identified visually, by touch using a WHO 621 probe, or on radiographs. With gingival recession it can become supragingival.

Composition Consists of up to 80% inorganic salts, mostly crystalline, the major components being calcium and phosphorus. The microscopic structure is basically that of a randomly orientated crystal formation.

Formation is always preceded by plaque deposition, the plaque serving as an organic matrix for subsequent mineralization. Initially, the matrix between organisms becomes calcified with, eventually, the organisms themselves becoming mineralized. Subgingival calculus usually takes many months to form, whereas friable supragingival calculus may form within 2 weeks.

Pathological effect Calculus (particularly, subgingival calculus), is associated with periodontal disease. This may be because it is invariably covered by a layer of plaque. Its principal detrimental effect is probably that it acts as a retention site for plaque and bacterial toxins. The presence of calculus makes it difficult to implement adequate oral hygiene.

Aetiology of periodontal disease

Plaque is the principal aetiological factor in virtually all forms of periodontal disease. Periodontal damage is almost certainly the direct consequence of colonization of the gingival sulcus by organisms within dental plaque. However, the progression from gingivitis to periodontitis is far more complex than this statement suggests, as it involves host defence, the oral environment, the pathogenicity of organisms, and plaque maturity. It is probably easiest to regard periodontal disease as a complex multifactorial infection complicated by the inflammatory response of the host. Various elements of this process are worthy of special note:

Microbiology

The changing microbiology of dental plaque has already been referred to (📖 p. 176). The inflammatory response of gingiva to the presence of initial young plaque creates a minute gingival pocket which serves as an ideal environment for further bacterial colonization, providing all the nutrients required for the growth of numerous fastidious organisms. In addition, there is an extremely low oxygen level within gingival pockets, which favours the development of obligate anaerobes, several of which are closely associated with the progression of periodontal disease. High levels of carbon dioxide favour the establishment of the capnophilic organisms, some of which are associated with localized aggressive periodontitis (LAP).

Briefly, clinically healthy gingivae are associated with a high proportion of Gram +ve rods and cocci which are facultatively anaerobic or aerobic. Gingivitis is associated with an ↑ number of facultative anaerobes, strict anaerobes, and an increasing number of Gram −ve rods. Established periodontitis is associated with a majority presence of anaerobic Gram −ve rods.

The 1996 World Workshop in Periodontics identified 3 species as causative factors for periodontitis. These are *Aggregibacter actinomycetemcomitans* Aa (previously called *Actinobacillus actinomycetemcomitans*), *Porphyromonas gingivalis* and *Tannerella forsythia*. However these are not the only causative pathogens and there are other putative pathogens for which there is evidence. These are: *Prevotella intermedia*, *P melaninogenica*, *Fusobacterium nucleatum*, *Peptostreptococcus micros*, *Eubacterium* species, *Eikenella corrodens*, *Prevotella nigrescens*, *Treponema denticola* and *Campylobacter rectus*. There is a strong association between Aa and localized aggressive periodontitis.

Some studies have suggested that specific viruses may be responsible for the aetiology and progression of periodontal lesions.[1]

---

1 J. Slots 2005 *Periodontology 2000* **38** 33.

Immunopathology

The inflammatory response to the presence of dental plaque is detectable both clinically and histologically, and is certainly responsible for at least some of the periodontal destruction which occurs. Both inflammatory and immunologically mediated pathways can contribute to periodontal damage. Antigenic substances released by plaque organisms elicit both cell-mediated and humoral responses which, while designed to be protective, also cause local tissue damage, usually by complement activation (Bystander Damage). Non-immune mediated damage is caused by one or all of the major endogenous mediators of inflammation: vasoactive amines (histamine), plasma proteases (complement), prostaglandins and leukotrienes, lysosomal acid hydrolases, proteases, free radicals, and cytokines.

Host response

Local and systemic modifying factors influence progress of the disease.

Systemic factors include smoking, immune status, stress, endocrine function (e.g. diabetes), drugs, genetic factors, age, and nutrition.

Local factors are tooth position and morphology, calculus, overhangs and appliances, occlusal trauma, and mucogingival state.

Periodontal disease and risk for systemic disease

There is a growing body of evidence suggesting an association between periodontal disease and atherosclerotic cardiovascular disease, pregnancy complications, diabetes, respiratory disease, kidney disease and certain cancers. No conclusions can yet be drawn as to whether these are causal associations, however it highlights the importance of oral health as part of a generally healthy lifestyle.[1]

1 R. C. Williams 2008 *Curr Med Res Opin* **24** 1635.

Pathogenesis of gingivitis and periodontitis

Initial lesion: Develops as plaque accumulates around the gingival margins. At 24h there is vasodilation in the adjacent gingival tissues.

2–4 days: increased intercellular gaps therefore gingival crevicular fluid flow flushes noxious substances away and releases antibodies, complement and protease inhibitors. Polymorphs appear.

Early lesion: May persist for a long time. After several days there are increased numbers of vascular units therefore clinically there is erythema. Lymphocytes and polymorphs predominate. Fibroblasts degenerate and collagen fibres break down. The basal cells of the junctional epithelium and sulcular epithelium proliferate to form rete pegs in the adjacent connective tissue. Subgingival biofilm develops as junctional epithelium loses contact with enamel.

Established lesion: Gingival crevicular fluid flow increases. There are increased numbers of lymphocytes and plasma cells in the connective tissue and junctional epithelium. The junctional epithelium converts to pocket epithelium. The established lesion may remain stable with no progression for months or years or may convert to a destructive advanced lesion.

Advanced lesion: As the pocket deepens the biofilm continues to develop apically. Inflammatory cell infiltrate extends further apically into the connective tissues. Plasma cells dominate There is loss of connective tissue attachment and alveolar bone which represents the onset of periodontitis.

The disease is initiated and maintained by substances produced by the biofilm. Some (such as proteases) cause direct injury to host cells, some cause tissue injury by activation of host inflammatory and immune responses.

Epidemiology of periodontal disease

Epidemiology is the study of the presence, severity and effect of disease on a population. This helps identify aetiological and risk factors and effectiveness of preventive and therapeutic measures at a population level. Various scoring systems for measuring periodontal disease in a population have been developed. The value of these indices in the screening and management of individual patients soon became apparent. The following two indices fulfil both these criteria and are simple and easy to perform:

Debris or Oral Hygiene Index This can be modified for personal use by using disclosing agents.[1]
0 No debris or stain.
1 Soft debris covering not more than ⅓ of the tooth surface.
2 Soft debris covering more than ⅓ but less than ⅔.
3 Soft debris covering over ⅔ of tooth surface.

Basic Periodontal Examination (BPE) Also known as Community Periodontal Index of Treatment Needs (CPITN).[2] This technique is used to screen for those patients requiring more detailed periodontal examination. It examines every tooth in the mouth (except third molars), thus taking into account the site-specific nature of periodontal disease. A World Health Organization (WHO) periodontal probe (ball-ended with a coloured band 3.5–5.5mm from the tip) should be used (Figure 5.1). The mouth is divided into sextants, i.e. two buccal and one labial segment per arch. Six sites on each tooth are explored and the highest score per sextant recorded, usually in a simple six-box chart.
0 = No disease,
1 = Gingival bleeding but no pockets, no calculus, no overhanging restoration. Rx: OHI.
2 = No pockets >3mm, but plaque retention factors present, e.g. overhang. Rx: OHI, scaling, and correction of any iatrogenic problems.
3 = Deepest pocket 4 or 5mm. Rx: OHI, scaling, and root planing.
4 = One or more tooth in sextant has a pocket >6mm. Rx: scaling and root planing, &/or flap as required.
* = Furcation or total loss of attachment of 7mm or more. Rx: full periodontal examination of the sextant regardless of CPITN score.

Individuals identified as having areas of advanced periodontal disease will require a full probing depth chart, together with recordings of mobility, recession and furcation involvement, and radiological examination. BPE cannot be used for close monitoring of the progress of Rx.

Other techniques for assessing the levels of periodontal disease include:

Marginal bleeding index (MBI) Score 1 or 0 depending on whether or not bleeding occurs after a probe is gently run around the gingival sulcus. A percentage score is obtained by dividing by the number of teeth and multiplying the result by 100.

---

1 J. Greene 1960 *J Am Dent Assoc* **61** 172.
2 J. Ainamo 1988 *Int Dent J* **32** 281.

Plaque index (PI) This is based on the presence or absence of plaque on the mesial, distal, lingual, and buccal surfaces revealed by disclosing.

$$\text{Percentage score} = \frac{\text{number of surfaces with plaque} \times 100}{\text{total number of teeth} \times 4}$$

Both the MBI and PI can be expressed as bleeding or plaque-free scores in this way obtaining a high score is a good thing, which may be both easier for the patient to understand and a more positive motivational approach.

Although periodontal diseases are very common, severe forms affect no more than about 10–15% of the population. Overall, periodontitis accounts for between 30 and 35% of all tooth extractions; caries and its consequences account for up to 50%.[1]

The direct association between the presence of tooth surface plaque and periodontal damage has been confirmed, but the rate of destruction has been shown to vary, not only between individuals but also between different sites in the same mouth, and at different times in the same individual.

WHO probe for use in BPE/CPITN (Figure 5.1).

Black band

5.5 mm

2 mm

3.5 mm

Fig. 5.1

If black band disappears on probing pocket, perform full periodontal examination in that sextant.

1 P. Papapanou 1996 *Ann Periodontol* **1** 1.

Classification and diagnosis

Classification of periodontal disease

The currently used classification of periodontal diseases was introduced by the 1999 International Workshop for a Classification of Periodontal Diseases and Conditions.

   I Gingival diseases (non-plaque induced and plaque induced)

   II Chronic periodontitis.

   III Aggressive periodontitis.

   IV Periodontitis as a manifestation of systemic disease.

   V Necrotizing periodontal diseases.

   VI Abscesses of the periodontium.

   VII Periodontitis associated with endodontic lesions.

   VIII Development or acquired deformities and conditions.

Plaque associated periodontal disease are infections caused by microorganisms that colonize the tooth surface at or below the gingival margin.

   The primary cause is bacterial plaque but associated risk factors are: specific bacteria, cigarette smoking and diabetes mellitus. There is a two-way association between periodontitis and diabetes with more severe periodontal destruction associated with diabetes but poorer control of diabetes in patients with periodontal disease.

Diagnosis

Diagnosis of periodontal diseases is arrived at by thorough history taking, clinical and radiographic examination and special investigations. Particular features in relation to history are presence of relevant factors in medical history and smoking habit. Clinical examination allows assessment of plaque control, loss of gingival contour, swelling, recession of periodontal tissues, periodontal pocketing, furcation lesions and tooth mobility. The basic periodontal examination (□ see p. 182) provides an overview of the periodontal status. Detailed pocket charting should be carried out if advanced periodontitis is detected.

Pocketing

Periodontal pockets can be divided into the following:

False pockets are due to gingival enlargement with the pocket epithelium at or above the amelocemental junction.

True pockets imply apical migration of the junctional epithelium beyond the amelocemental junction and can be divided into suprabony and intrabony pockets. Intrabony are described according to the number of bony walls:

- Three-walled defect is the most favourable, as it is surrounded on three sides by cancellous bone and on one side by the cementum of the root surface.
- Two-walled defect may be either a crater between teeth having bone on two walls and cementum on the other two, or have two bony walls, the root cementum, and an open aspect to the overlying soft tissues.
- One-walled defects may be hemiseptal through-and-through defects, or one bony wall, two root cementum, and one soft tissue.

Pocket depths are measured from the gingival margin to the estimated base of the pocket. Attachment levels are measured from a fixed reference point: the cement–enamel junction or margin of a restoration to the base of the pocket. Pockets are therefore dependent on the position of the gingival margin.

Periodontal probes are the key instruments in detecting pockets. Numerous designs exist, and while individual preference will influence choice, it is sensible to reduce variability by selecting a single type of probe and using that type of probe throughout any one individual's Rx. The use of the WHO probe for screening using the BPE index is described on 📖 p. 182. Patients who are identified as having advanced CP should then be investigated further, including probing around each tooth. The main other indicator of periodontal disease, bleeding, is also detected using a probe (gently), and again consistency with a single type of probe is necessary.

Probing variables The depth of penetration depends upon:
- Type of probe and its position.
- Amount of pressure used.
- Degree of inflammation.[1]

It is now apparent that the measurement obtained with a probe does not correspond to sulcus or pocket depth. In the presence of inflammation a probe tip can pass through the inflamed tissues until it reaches the most coronal dento-gingival fibres, about 0.5mm apical to the apical extent of the junctional epithelium, i.e. an overestimation of the problem. The amount of penetration into the tissues varies directly with the degree of inflammation, so that, following resolution of inflammation, an underestimate of attachment levels may be given. Formation of a tight, long junctional epithelium following Rx may also give a false sense of security if probing measurements are not interpreted with a degree of caution. For this reason the term 'probing pocket depth' is preferred to pocket depth.

---

1 M. A. Listgarten 1980 *J Clin Periodont* **7** 165.

Diagnostic tests and monitoring

It is widely accepted that disease active and inactive pockets exist. Progression is episodic and more likely in susceptible patients. Bleeding on probing has traditionally been the most useful indicator of disease activity; however, only 30% of sites which bleed will go on to lose attachment.[1]

With ↑ emphasis on specific periodontopathic bacteria (📖 p. 174) and availability of assays for components of immunological response, chair-side diagnostic tests using gingival crevicular fluid have been developed. Three types exist:

- Based on detection of antibodies to specific periodontopaths, e.g. Kodak Evalusite.
- Based on components of immune response, e.g. elastase in Dentsply Prognostick.
- Based on tissue breakdown by products, e.g. aspartate aminotransferase in Colgate-Palmolive's Periogard.

These aim to predict sites of future and actual disease progression, and the first may indicate need for specific antibiotic therapy (📖 p. 202).

There is a huge amount of ongoing research into improving and refining these tests, but evidence is still required to demonstrate predictive ability and a higher level of accuracy than bleeding on probing.

Other peripheral techniques worthy of note are pocket temperature probes and computerized subtraction radiovisiography.

Radiographs are useful in comparing degree of bone loss and root surface deposits with pocket depth. Standardized sequential radiographs allow monitoring of disease.

- Horizontal bitewings provide a good view of interproximal bone, useful for relatively minor degrees of bone loss (pocketing <5mm) and to detect calculus deposits. Vertical bitewings are recommended when pocketing is >5mm.
- Full mouth periapicals (long cone technique), supplemented with vertical or horizontal bitewing, have been the radiological assessment of choice for patients with significant periodontal disease, i.e. irregular pocketing. They can clearly demonstrate root surface deposits, furcation involvement, extensive bone loss, intrabony pocketing, and perio-endo lesions. The results of a radiographic examination, clinical assessment, and assessment of pocket depth can all be marked on an updatable periodontal chart to monitor progress with Rx.

1 N. Lang 1986 *J Clin Periodont* **13** 590

Gingival diseases

Chronic gingivitis is, as the name suggests, inflammation of the gingival tissues. It is **not** associated with alveolar bone resorption or apical migration of the junctional epithelium. Pockets >2mm can occur in chronic gingivitis due to an increase in gingival size because of oedema or hyperplasia (false pockets). Different types of gingivitis are described; the commonest type is plaque induced.

Plaque-induced gingivitis This is present in virtually all mouths to some extent. The classic triad of redness, swelling, and bleeding on gentle probing are diagnostic and are usually associated with a complaint by the patient that their 'gums bleed on brushing'. False pocketing may also be present. This gingivitis occurs as a result of low-grade infection caused by the presence of undisturbed dental plaque, which is associated with a change in the flora from Gram +ve aerobes to Gram −ve anaerobes (📖 p. 176). This gives rise to inflammatory changes in the associated gingivae; these are detectable histologically prior to the appearance of overt clinical gingivitis, which is observed after about 7 days of undisturbed plaque accumulation. The inflammatory response seen comprises an alteration in the integrity of the gingival microcirculation, an ↑ in the numbers of inflammatory cells in the gingival connective tissue (i.e. plasma cells, lymphocytes, macrophages, and neutrophils), a ↓ in the number of fibroblasts, and a ↓ in collagen density. These inflammatory changes are easily reversible after institution of effective plaque control. While gingivitis is reversible, it should be remembered that calculus and other factors which promote plaque retention (e.g. overhanging restorations) will make adequate oral hygiene difficult. These factors should therefore be corrected by scaling and appropriate restorative treatment in addition to OHI. Gingivitis may be a precursor to, or marker of, chronic periodontitis, and this must be excluded by measuring probing attachment levels (looking for 'true' pockets) and excluding the presence of alveolar bone loss by radiographs, if indicated. Other forms of gingivitis include:

Gingivitis modified by systemic factors. These would include puberty-associated gingivitis, menstrual cycle-associated gingivitis, pregnancy-associated gingivitis, pyogenic granuloma, diabetes mellitus-associated gingivitis, and gingivitis associated with blood dyscrasias, e.g. leukaemia-associated gingivitis.

Gingivitis modified by medications. These would include drug-influenced gingival enlargement and drug-induced gingivitis, e.g. oral contraceptive-associated gingivitis and drug-induced gingival overgrowth due to phenytoin or ciclosporin.

Gingival disease modified by malnutrition. These would include ascorbic acid-deficiency gingivitis (scurvy) and gingivitis due to protein deficiency.

Primary herpetic gingivostomatitis, 📖 p. 398.

Acute streptococcal gingivitis Rare. Beefy, red, painful gingivae usually caused by a Lancefield A streptococcus. Rx: penicillin V 500mg qds for 7 days and OHI.

Chronic periodontitis

Chronic periodontitis can be regarded as a progression of the combination of infection and inflammation of gingivitis into the deep tissues of the periodontal membrane. All periodontitis develops out of gingivitis but not all gingivitis progresses to periodontitis. The proportion of sites that do progress in a subject or population is not known and the factors leading to progression are not well understood. Periodontitis is classified as localized when <30% of sites are affected and as generalized when >30% of sites are affected.

Severity of disease is classified as follows:
Mild: 1–2mm of probing attachment loss
Moderate: 3–4mm of probing attachment loss
Severe: ≥5mm of probing attachment loss.

Periodontitis is initiated and sustained by microbial plaque but host factors determine the pathogenesis and rate of progression of disease. In most cases progression is slow to moderate but periods of rapid tissue destruction may occur. Risk factors include plaque, age, smoking, systemic disease, stress, and genetics.

It is characterized by breakdown of periodontal fibre bundles at the cervical margin, resorption of alveolar bone, and apical proliferation of junctional epithelium beyond the amelocemental junction (Figure 5.2).

Diagnosis is based on:
- Probing to elicit bleeding (which is the single most useful indicator of disease activity), measuring pocket depth attachment levels, and detecting subgingival calculus.
- Testing teeth for mobility and vitality.
- Radiographic examination (vertical bitewings and periapicals). See radiological selection criteria, 📖 p.186.

Treatment (see 📖 pp. 196–215).

Fig. 5.2 DPT showing the typical appearance of established adult periodontitis; the patient was a diabetic who smoked.

Aggressive periodontitis

A group of rare and often severe, rapidly progressive forms of periodontitis. Often characterized by early age of onset and tending to occur in families and with non-contributory medical history. The amounts of plaque are out of proportion with the severity of periodontal destruction. Often associated with *Aggregibacter actinomycetemcomitans*. Hyper-responsive macrophage phenotype. Progression of attachment loss may be self arresting.

Two main forms:
1) Generally aggressive periodontitis (GAP): previously generalized juvenile periodontitis
2) Locally aggressive periodontitis (LAP): previously localized juvenile periodontitis)

GAP is a severe form of generalized periodontitis affecting young adults (<30 years). Generalized interproximal attachment loss affecting at least 3 permanent teeth other than first molars and incisors. Pronounced episodic nature of the destruction of attachment and alveolar bone. Poor serum antibody response to infecting agents. Affects 1–2% of the Western population with an ↑ in Afro-Caribbeans.

LAP is a severe form of localized periodontitis with onset around puberty. Localized attachment loss of at least 2 permanent teeth one of which is a first molar and involving no more than 2 teeth other than first molars and incisors.

Treatment:
1) Achievement of adequate supragingival plaque control
2) Sub-gingival instrumentation to disrupt biofilm
3) Adjunctive antibiotics: see 📖 p. 202

Necrotizing periodontal diseases

The necrotizing periodontal diseases are:

Necrotizing gingivitis (previously known as, Vincent's gingivitis, Vincent's gingivostomatitis, ulceromembraneous gingivitis, or trench mouth. It should not be confused with Vincent's angina, which is also a fusospirochaetal infection but is typically localized over the tonsils).

Necrotizing periodontitis

Necrotizing stomatitis: where the necrotizing lesion has spread to include tissue beyond the mucogingival junction.

This destructive inflammatory condition is rapid, debilitating and usually runs an acute course

Necrotizing gingivitis (NG) is characterized by painful ulcerated, necrotic papillae and gingival margins which leave a punched-out appearance. The ulcers are covered by a yellowish grey slough. Patients also often complain of a metallic taste and the sensation of their teeth being wedged apart and there is foetor oris. Interproximal craters develop and there is loss of crestal bone. Bony sequestra may develop. Loss of attachment and development of necrotizing periodontitis may occur. Regional lymphadenitis, fever, and malaise feature in some cases. It can be confused with primary herpetic gingivostomatitis. Necrotizing periodontal disease rarely occurs in children in Northern Europe and USA. Prevalence is higher in developing countries. NG is associated with poor oral hygiene, but stress and smoking act as co-factors. It is usually a limited gingival condition, but a rare and more serious form known as cancrum oris or noma is found in patients who are malnourished, and in this form can lead to extensive destruction of the jaws and face.

Microbiology Originally *Borrelia vincenti* (*refringens*) and *Fusobacterium fusiformis* were held to be the major culprits in a mixed anaerobic infection. Further research has, however, served to confuse the picture, with *Porphyromonas* spp. being implicated, as well as *Treponema* spp., *Selenomonas* spp. and *Prevotella* spp. The crucial aspect of the microbiology of NG is that it is a Gram −ve anaerobic infection which has been shown to actually invade the tissues but usually responds to local debridement. In recent years, the tendency for patients who are HIV +ve to develop severe NG, sometimes with bone necrosis, has renewed interest in it. From the practical point of view it should be remembered that NG presenting in an otherwise apparently healthy young adult may be a presenting sign of HIV infection. Consider examining the mouth for other signs of infection (📖 p. 440), and directing the patient to appropriate counselling &/or HIV testing.

Initial Rx: It is wise to get the patient to rinse with chlorhexidine gluconate 0.2% prior to ultrasonic scaling to reduce aerosol spread. Chlorhexidine rinses may also be prescribed as an adjunct to brushing, which is painful initially. In most cases local measures, i.e. thorough debridement and adequate oral hygiene will suffice; however, if there is evidence of systemic upset (lymphadenopathy) metronidazole 200mg tds for 3 days is indicated. Penicillins are also effective. Once the ulcers have healed, scaling can be carried out

Later Rx, such as gingivectomy for persistent craters, is only rarely required.

Periodontal abscess

This is a localized collection of pus within a periodontal pocket. It occurs either due to the introduction of virulent organisms into an existing pocket or ↓ drainage potential. The latter classically occurs during Rx as reduction of inflammation in the coronal gingival tissues occludes drainage by a tighter adaptation to the tooth. May also occur due to impaction of a foreign body such as a fishbone in a pre-existing pocket or even in an otherwise healthy periodontal membrane.

Clinically there may be swelling, pus from pocket or sinus, pain tenderness to percussion and signs of periodontitis.

Diagnosis Need to distinguish from apical abscess.

Apical abscess	Periodontal abscess
Non-vital	Usually vital
TTP vertically	Pain on lateral movements
May be mobile	Usually mobile
Loss of lamina dura on radiograph	Loss of alveolar crest on radiograph

Insertion of a GP point into an associated sinus and a radiograph may be helpful.

Emergency Rx: Incision and drainage under LA; systemic antibiotic, e.g. metronidazole 200–400mg tds &/or amoxicillin 250–500mg tds for 5 days if systemic involvement.

Further Rx: mechanical debridement after the problem has settled to avoid iatrogenic damage to healthy periodontal tissues adjacent to the lesion.

Follow-up: conventional Rx for periodontal pockets (📖 p. 204), combined periodontal–endodontic lesion (📖 p. 194).

Periodontitis associated with endodontic lesions

NB It is essential to vitality test any heavily restored tooth with periodontal involvement.

Given the relative frequency of both periodontal disease and periapical pathology, it is not surprising that both may occur together, which can result in diagnostic confusion. In fact, there is little evidence to support the popular notion that periodontitis leads to pulp necrosis. However, there is no doubt that pulp pathology can exacerbate periodontal problems.

Pulpal problems
Acute pulpitis 📖 p. 220.

Non-vital pulp (📖 p. 220) may cause asymptomatic periapical lesion or periapical abscess.

Lateral canal &/or non-vital pulp may mimic periodontal abscess, as can a root perforation following endodontic therapy.

Vertical root fracture &/or non-vital pulp can lead to periodontal inflammation and may mimic periodontal abscess.

Horizontal root fracture may mimic periodontal abscess.

Periodontal pathology and its effect on the pulp
Deep pocketing may encroach on lateral canals in the apical ⅓ of the root, but is otherwise unlikely to cause direct pulpal pathology.

Gingival recession is directly associated with hypersensitivity of root dentine.

Root planing and furcation procedures actively involve dentine, and can clearly lead to hypersensitivity and sometimes acute pulpal changes.

Differential diagnosis

	Primarily periodontal	*Primarily endodontic*
History	No preceding toothache	Often toothache
Percussion	TTP especially lateral	TTP especially vertical
Probing	Pocketing always	May be no pockets
Probing sinus	May lead to pocket	May lead to apex
Vitality test	Usually +ve	–ve
Radiographs	Vertical bone loss	Apical area

Combined perio-endo lesions
These may be either:
- Coexisting, but separate from each other, in which case standard endodontic and periodontal therapy are used as indicated.
- Interconnected, in which case probing both pocket and sinus will reach the apex. This can be confirmed by taking a periapical film with a GP point inserted into the pocket.

Rx of combined interconnected lesion First, resolve the acute infection and inflammation by drainage (&/or antibiotics), then treat with orthograde RCT (the greater the pulpal component the better the prognosis).

The apparent periodontal lesion will often be seen to resolve to a substantial degree over a period of months, therefore, the decision to carry out surgery should be deferred. Combined apical surgery and periodontal surgery is quite feasible but carries a poorer long-term prognosis. The worst prognosis applies to those teeth where the periapical/pulpal pathology has been due entirely to apical extension of the periodontal pocket. These are often diagnosed after the fact, when endodontics completely fails to resolve the lesion.

Principles of treatment

- Establish diagnosis.
- The overall aim could be summarized as the creation of a healthy mouth which the patient is both capable of, and willing to, maintain.
- It is often convenient to divide the principles of periodontal therapy into three phases:

1) The *initial* (cause-related) phase, where the aim is to control or elimi-nate gingivitis and arrest any further progression of periodontal disease by the removal of plaque and other contributory factors. Periodontal disease is an infection due to the presence of plaque, therefore, control of plaque is the key to success. More complex treatments will always fail in the absence of effective plaque control.

2) The *corrective* phase is designed principally to restore function and, where relevant, aesthetics. Corrective techniques include scaling, root debride-ment, periodontal access surgery, regenerative surgery, mucogingival sur-gery, selected use of local and systemic antibiotics, treatment of furcation lesions, restorative work, endodontics, and occlusal adjustment.
The aims of this phase are:
  (i) to eliminate pathological periodontal pockets, or to create a tight epithelial attachment where the pocket once existed;
  (ii) to arrest loss of, and in some cases improve, the alveolar bone support;
  (iii) to create an oral environment which is relatively simple for the patient to keep plaque-free.

3) The *maintenance* (supportive) phase aims to reinforce patient motivation so that their OH is adequate to prevent recurrence of dis-ease. This phase is receiving ↑ attention due to the relative ease with which disease activity can be monitored by probing and chair-side diag-nostic assays (📖 p. 186).

Plaque control

Following the comments on the pages covering the aetiology and epidemiology of periodontal disease, it is quite clear that dental plaque is the cause of the problem and its elimination will prevent periodontal diseases. This is easier said than done—remember most of the world's population has gingivitis &/or periodontitis. The key to prevention is regular and thorough plaque removal, therefore, OHI is probably the most useful advice you can give to your patients. Smoking exacerbates periodontal disease and adversely affects Rx outcome. Patients should be advised of this.

Oral hygiene instruction

OHI should include an explanation of the nature of the patient's disease and hence the reasons for good oral hygiene. Identify and demonstrate to the patient the disease (swollen gingivae, bleeding on probing) using a hand mirror, then demonstrate the cause (plaque), either directly, by scraping off a deposit, or by disclosing. Explain how plaque starts to grow immediately after tooth-brushing, so that regular removal is necessary, and that it cannot be rinsed away. Then demonstrate how to remove it, avoiding overt criticism of the patient's present efforts, as this is often counter-productive.

Mechanical plaque control

Tooth-brushing requires a brush, ideally with a small head and even nylon bristles (3–4 tufts across by 10–12 lengthways), which should be renewed at least monthly. Toothpaste makes the process more pleasant and is a useful medium for topical fluoride and other agents. Anticalculus pastes ↓ plaque formation by about 50%. Chlorhexidine-containing toothpastes are active against plaque microorganisms. Numerous methods can be described, based on the movement of the brush stroke: rolling, vibratory, circular, vertical, horizontal. The best is the one which works for that patient (as demonstrated by absence of plaque on disclosing after brushing) and does no harm to tooth or gingivae. The horizontal scrub is notorious for possibly exacerbating gingival recession. Modifications to toothbrushes and brushing technique are often required in children, the elderly, and those with disabling diseases.

Interdental cleaning Brushing alone is unlikely to clean the interdental spaces adequately; however, it must be mastered first by the patient, before interdental cleaning is taught. Flossing, mini interdental brushes (particularly good for concave root surfaces), and interspace brushes are available for cleaning interproximally. The use of dental floss is something of an art form and must be learned by demonstration.

Chemical plaque control

Mouthwashes may help for patients who struggle with mechanical methods. This may be because of lack of dexterity or due to mucosal conditions (e.g. aphthae, Benign Mucous Membrane Pemphigoid) or following periodontal surgery. The antiseptic of greatest proven value is chlorhexidine gluconate. This is commonly used in a 0.2% mouthwash or gel, although 0.12% mouthwash is also available. A standard regimen is 10ml of solution rinsed for 1min bd. The gel can be used instead of toothpaste. Chlorhexidine causes staining and altered taste. **NB** An interaction between conventional toothpaste and chlorhexidine reduces the antiseptic's efficacy. Other proprietary antiseptic rinses have yet to meet this 'gold standard'.

Professional preventive techniques

Regular periodic examination for periodontal disease, which is largely asymptomatic, is essential. This requires a full oral examination, including probing for pockets as part of routine examination (📖 p. 10). In patients who have been demonstrated to have periodontal disease, 3-monthly follow-ups are advisable. Routine scaling and polishing is of little value unless accompanied by intensive education and motivation of the patient (however tedious this may be), as it is the patient's efforts which will prevent the re-formation of plaque and initiation of periodontal disease. Employment of a hygienist has obvious benefits in this area. Elimination, avoidance, and Rx of iatrogenic problems such as overhanging margins on restorations, ill-fitting crown margins, poorly designed appliances, etc., are mandatory.

Where periodontal pockets do not heal after initial therapy and good plaque control has been achieved, further treatment is required in the form of root debridement.

Scaling and root debridement

Non-surgical therapy in periodontal disease consists of scaling, debridement, restorative Rx (to correct coexisting or exacerbating factors, e.g. periapical infection, overhanging margins), and the use of antiseptics and antibiotics.

Scaling is the removal of plaque and calculus from the tooth surface, either with hand instruments (e.g. sickles, curettes, hoes and chisels) or mechanically (e.g. Cavitron). Scaling can be sub- or supragingival depending upon the site of the deposits. Supra gingival scaling is usually completed first as far as initial therapy. LA is usually not necessary. Subgingival scaling may require LA and involves the removal of subgingival root deposits. Root debridement aims to remove a thin layer of endotoxin-loaded cementum in addition to the deposits. It is customary to make use of an ultrasonic scaler for the bulk of the work and finish off, particularly subgingivally, with hand instruments. The precise use of hand instruments is largely a matter of personal preference; however, it is essential to use controlled force and a secure finger-rest. Ultrasonic instruments are quicker, but they can be uncomfortable and leave an uneven root surface (though the significance of the latter is controversial). Ultrasonic scaling employs a frequency of 25–40 000 cycles/sec. Another instrument, known as a sonic scaler and vibrating at 1600–1800 cycles/sec, has been shown to be equally effective at removing calculus and may result in smoother root surfaces. With both it is essential to use a copious coolant spray. In practice it is probably impossible to differentiate between subgingival scaling and root debridement, as in both techniques plaque, calculus, root cementum, and small amounts of dentine will be removed. These are the core procedures for **all** periodontal techniques; the only real difference with formal surgery is that it allows Rx under direct vision, osseous recontouring and sculpting if desired, and repositioning of the gingiva.

Traditionally one quadrant at a time is treated under LA, partly because it is painful and partly because it is tedious when performed meticulously, which is the only worthwhile way to do it. It has been suggested, however, that a full mouth approach is preferable. This means completion of root debridement within 24h, with concurrent use of a chlorhexidine mouthwash. The aim is to reduce the bacterial load and minimize chance of reinfection by reducing bacterial load in pockets and intra oral niches. More recently, comparison of full mouth disinfection and the quadrant approach has failed to demonstrate a significant difference in outcomes. Success will allow tight adaptation of the pocket epithelium to the root, creating a *long junctional epithelium*.

The teeth are usually polished after scaling, preferably using a rubber cup and a fluoride-containing paste (e.g. toothpaste). Patients can then appreciate the feeling of a clean mouth, which they must then maintain.

Local delivery of medicaments

Due to controversy over the efficacy and unwanted effects of systemic antibiotics, methods of direct delivery into the pocket have been explored. These have included using injected pastes or gels, or by impregnated fibre. This gives a high local dose, low systemic uptake, and prolonged exposure of the pathogens to the drug. The rate of crevicular fluid turnover is such that the substantivity of these agents is low. Examples: Blackwell Dentomycin® (minocycline), Colgate-Palmolive Elyzol® (metronidazole), Actisite® (tetracycline) and PerioChip® (chlorhexidine). However, only small ↑ in attachment levels have been reported and currently local adjunctive antibiotics are only indicated for the Rx of persistent localized defects in patients with good plaque control. Root debridement must be carried out prior to placement to disrupt the biofilm.

Systemic antibiotics

There is evidence to support the use of antibiotics as an adjunct to mechanical non-surgical therapy in aggressive periodontitis and some forms of chronic periodontitis and acute periodontal infections. A review of the use of antibiotics in periodontology recommended their use for patients with recent, or a high risk of, periodontal breakdown.[1] Short-term, relatively high doses, or high locally delivered doses, are used. The two most useful drugs are:

Tetracycline. 250mg qds for 2 to 3 weeks in adults. It is active against spirochaetes, *Aggregatibacter actinomycetemcomitans*, and many other periodontal pathogens. Most useful in the Rx of LAP. Oxytetracycline and doxycycline are currently popular. In addition to being antibacterial, tetracyclines ↓ host neutrophil collagenases and ↓ bone loss. Crevicular fluid concentrations are high. Currently there is much interest in doxycycline (20mg bd for 3 months). At this dose it has no detrimental effect on the periodontal microflora and its action is mainly to reduce collagenolytic metalloproteinases.

Metronidazole. 200mg tds for 1 to 2 weeks. Effective against protozoa and strict anaerobes and capable of eliminating all the strict anaerobes found in periodontal pockets. As it does not interfere with aerobes or facultative anaerobes it is highly unlikely to allow the development of opportunist pathogens. There is frequent mention of the mutagenicity and teratogenicity of this drug in animal studies but, despite widespread use in medicine, no clinical evidence has emerged to support this. It is, in fact, an extremely safe and useful drug. When combined with mechanical pocket therapy, significant improvements in terms of probing depth have been demonstrated.[2] There is an emetic interaction with alcohol.

Recently it has been suggested that a combination of amoxicillin (250mg qds) and metronidazole (200mg qds) for 2 weeks may be effective.

1 J. Slots 1990 *J Clin Periodont* **17** 479.

2 W. J .Loesche 1984 *J Clin Periodont* **55** 325.

Periodontal surgery—1

There has been a progressive move away from pocket elimination surgery, towards the creation of a healthy periodontium which gives access for both professional and home cleaning. Recognition that periodontal disease is a localized infection due to the presence of dental plaque, and that its arrest and prevention is dependent on the removal of plaque and plaque-retaining factors, has allowed a far more rational and conservative approach to therapy to develop.

Aims:
- Provide access for scaling and root planing in deep (>5mm) pockets which have not responded to non-surgical treatment
- Create subgingival root surfaces which are accessible for cleaning, either by professionals or by the patient
- Maximize the potential for healing of damaged periodontal tissues
- Create new periodontal attachment in the case of regenerative procedures

The modified Widman flap (open flap debridement) is suitable for those patients who, despite good supragingival plaque control, still have true pockets but do not need recontouring of the gingival margins.

As smoking ↓ outcome of Rx, some periodontologists have limited Rx in those continuing to smoke. While periodontal surgery hardly has the public impact of cardiac surgery, the ethical problem is the same.

Practical tips for periodontal surgery

LA The infiltration, block &/or lingual/palatal injections required will be determined by the site of surgery. Both LA and haemostasis are improved by injecting directly into the gingival margin and interdental papillae until blanching is seen.

Suturing techniques Interrupted interproximal sutures are used when buccal and lingual flaps are being reapposed at the same level. When flaps are repositioned at different levels, a suspensory suture is used where the suture only passes through the buccal flap and is suspended around the cervical margins of the teeth.

Periodontal packs These are essential after gingivectomy to ↓ post-operative discomfort. Many favour them after all periodontal surgery to help reappose the flap to bone. Classified:
- Eugenol dressings, e.g. ZnO, have the advantage of being mildly analgesic but can cause sensitivity reactions.
- Eugenol-free dressings, e.g. Coe-Pak™, are more popular.

The modified Widman flap[1]

This is a technique which enables open debridement of the root surface, with a minimal amount of trauma. There is no attempt to excise the pocket, although a superficial collar of tissue is removed. This has the advantage of allowing close adaptation of the soft tissues to the root surface with minimal trauma to, and exposure of, underlying bone and connective tissue, thus causing fewer problems with post-operative sensitivity and aesthetics (Figure 5.3).

1 S. Ramfjord 1974 *J Periodont* **45** 601.

Technique (after Ramfjord and Nissle 1974). A scalloped incision is made parallel to the long axis of the teeth involved 1mm from the crevicular margin, except when pockets are <2mm deep when an intracrevicular incision is made. This incision is extended interproximally as far as possible, separating the pocket epithelium from the flap to be raised, and then extended mesially and distally, allowing the flap to be raised as an envelope without relieving incisions. The flap should be as conservative as possible and only a few millimetres of alveolar bone exposed by a second incision intercrevically to release the collar of pocket epithelium and granulation tissue. A third incision at 90° to the tooth separates the pocket epithelium, and this is removed along with accompanying granulation tissue with curettes and hoes. The root surface is then thoroughly scaled and root planed. Although bony defects can be curetted **no** osseous surgery is carried out. The flaps are then repositioned to cover all exposed alveolar bone and sutured into position. Post-operatively chlorhexidine 0.2% 10ml rinse bd is given.

Notes There continues to be considerable confusion about nomenclature with this type of flap. The original Widman flap described in 1918 by Leonard Widman used relieving incisions and osseous surgery, and attempted to remove the pocket. The Neumann flap used an intracrevicular incision, again attempting to excise the pocket, but the 'modified flap operation' described by Kirkland in 1931 did not require sacrifice of inflamed tissues or apical displacement of the gingival margin. The latter was, of course, the precursor of the 'modified Widman flap'.

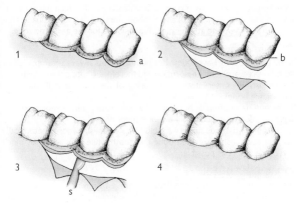

Fig. 5.3 Modified Widman flap.
1 Design of flap
  a Incision
2 Flap elevated
  b Gingival cuff to be discarded
3 Excision of supra-alveolar pocket
  s Scalpel blade
4 Flap repositioned and sutured in place

Periodontal surgery—2

Apically repositioned flap

This procedure is used to expose alveolar bone and includes the option for osseous surgery to correct infrabony defects. It allows excellent access to the root surface for debridement (Figure 5.4). The principal difference between this procedure and the modified Widman flap is the deliberate exposure of alveolar bone, and the apical repositioning of the flap with post-operative exposure of the root surfaces. This is primarily a buccal procedure, and although it can be performed on lingual pockets, it is obviously impossible on the palate where a conventional or reverse bevel gingivectomy approach has to be used.

Technique A reverse bevel incision is made in the attached gingiva angled to excise the periodontal pocket in a scalloped outline with vertical relieving incisions at either end. A split thickness flap is made down to bone and then converted to full thickness, leaving a residual collar of tissue around the root surfaces. This combination of pocket epithelium and granulation tissue is removed with a curette. If indicated the alveolar crest can be remodelled.

Advantages Include: exposure of alveolar bone with controlled bone loss; exposure of furcation area; minimal post-operative pocket depth; ability to reposition the flap; and primary closure of the wound. In addition, keratinized gingiva is preserved.

Disadvantages Exposure of root surface (leading to ↑ susceptibility to caries and sensitivity) and loss of alveolar bone height, which accompanies full exposure of the bone at operation. Not suitable for the aesthetic zone.

Osseous surgery

Bone recontouring has become less popular as it is always accompanied by some degree of alveolar resorption and therefore ↓ support for the tooth. *Osteoplasty* is conservative recontouring of the bone margin (i.e. non-supporting bone).
Ostectomy is excision of bone aimed at eliminating infra-alveolar pocketing, but unfortunately it also ↓ alveolar support.

   The aim of osseous surgery should be to establish a more anatomically correct relationship between bone and tooth while maintaining as much alveolar support as possible.

Other flap procedures

These include simple replaced flaps which give ↑ bony access compared to the modified Widman flap. Also crown-lengthening procedures, which can range from a simple gingivectomy to an apically repositioned flap ± bone removal. In addition, many periodontologists have their own modification of the aforementioned techniques.

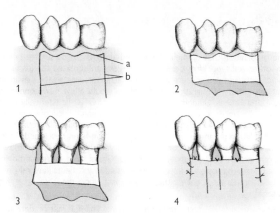

Fig. 5.4 Apically repositioned flap.
1 Design of flap
  a Reverse bevel incision
  b Relieving incisions
2 Elevating the flap. Tissue enclosing pocketing is discarded
3 Flap elevated, pockets excised. Osseous surgery can be performed at this stage
4 Flap apically repositioned and sutured in position

Gingivectomy

↓ in use. Indications: persistent deep supra-alveolar pockets (e.g. gingival hypertrophy); reshape severely damaged gingivae into an easily manageable contour; to treat gingival overgrowth; temporary crown lengthening prior to restorative procedures. It is **not** suitable for the management of deep 'true' pocketing as excision of the pocket will remove the entire thickness of keratinized gingivae. Of no value in the Rx of intrabony lesions.

Technique Pockets are delineated by use of pocket marking forceps, e.g. Crane–Kaplan forceps marking out a line of incision (either smooth or scalloped) made with a blade angled at 100–110° to the long axis of the tooth. This bevelled incision excises supragingival pockets and allows for gingival recontouring. Once the incision has been made the strip of gingiva remaining is released by an intercrevicular incision. The root surfaces are then curetted and an open area of freshly cut granulation tissue left to heal under a periodontal pack for about 1 week. Chlorhexidine mouthwash 10ml bd.

Disadvantages Loss of attached gingiva, raw wound, exposed root surface (which ↑ likelihood of sensitivity and caries). Some remodelling of alveolar bone occurs, despite there being no operative interference.

Regenerative techniques

Guided-tissue regeneration

The recognition that epithelium migrated along the root surface before any other cell type, after periodontal surgery, and created the *long junctional epithelium* which prevented new attachment, created the possibility that prevention of migration of epithelium would allow new connective tissue attachment. Guided-tissue regeneration (GTR) is essentially interposing a barrier to epithelial migration prior to completion of surgical or non-surgical therapy. Original barriers were non-resorbable. More recently, resorbable membranes (e.g Bio-gide, Vicryl) have been developed. These eliminate the need for a second stage of surgery. Bone grafts may be used in combination with a barrier membrane. Grafts from inorganic bovine bone matrix (Bio-oss) are in widespread use. Many patients have religious, cultural or personal beliefs that may impact upon the choice of graft material.

Emdogain is a product containing porcine enamel matrix derivative (EMD) proteins in a propylene glycol alginate gel. Enamel matrix proteins (e.g. amelogenin) are found in Hertwig's sheath and induce root formation in the developing tooth. Locally applied enamel matrix proteins may help form acellular cementum, the key tissue in the development of a functional periodontium.

Technique Access to the root surface is gained surgically, the cementum is mechanically cleaned, and EMD solution is applied to the root surfaces following conditioning with EDTA to remove the smear layer after instrumentation. The access flaps are then repositioned and sutured.

Outcome Regeneration of cementum, periodontal ligament, and alveolar bone appears to be possible. A Cochrane review of the use of EMD to regenerate periodontal tissue in intrabony defects has shown it to be effective.[1] Case selection is important in success of regeneration techniques. They work best in cases with 3 walled defects or grade II furcations. Good oral hygiene is essential. Smoking has an adverse effect on outcomes. Requires careful and meticulous surgical technique.[2]

Future developments in tissue engineering may allow the possibility of regeneration of replacement teeth and periodontal tissues in humans.[3]

1 M. Esposito 2004 *J Dent Educ* **68** 834.

2 G. Sharpe 2008 *Dental Update* **35** 304.

3 H. C. Slavkin 2006 *Periodontology 2000* **41** 9.

Furcation involvement

The extension of periodontal disease into the bi- or trifurcation of multi-rooted teeth is known as furcation involvement.

Diagnosis is established by probing into the furcation and by radiographs. The possibility of pulpal pathology is ↑ in teeth with furcation involvement and sensitivity testing is essential. Radiographs give a guide to the degree of alveolar bone loss both mesially and distally, and in the furcation area.

Classification

1st degree: horizontal loss of support not exceeding ⅓ tooth width. Requires scaling and root planing, possibly with furcation plasty.

2nd degree: horizontal loss of support exceeding ⅓ but not encompassing the total width of the furcation area. May require furcation plasty, &/or tunnel preparation, &/or root resection, &/or extraction. Guided tissue regeneration for mandibular molars

3rd degree: horizontal through-and-through destruction in the furcation area. May require tunnel preparation, &/or root resection, &/or extraction.

Rx techniques

Scaling and root debridement (📖 p. 200) Unless the post-Rx morphology can be kept clean by the patient it will not be successful.

Furcation plasty An open procedure involving a muco-periosteal flap to allow root debridement and scaling, followed by the removal of tooth structure in the furcation area to achieve a widened entrance to give access for cleaning. Osseous recontouring may be used if indicated. The flap is repositioned and sutured to ↑ access post-operatively. There is an obvious risk of pulpal damage and post-operative dentine sensitivity/caries.

Tunnel preparation is a similar procedure to furcation plasty using buccal and lingual flaps, the main difference being that the entire furcation area is exposed and the flaps are sutured together intra-radicularly to leave a large exposed furcation. There is a high risk of post-operative caries, dentine sensitivity, and pulpal exposure, making this a method to be used with caution. It is of most value for mandibular molars in patients with optimal OH. In many cases considered for furcation plasty or tunnelling, it may be more sensible to proceed to a more radical approach such as root resection.

Root resection Involves amputation of one (or even two) of the roots of a multirooted tooth, leaving the crown and the root stump. It is important to ensure that the root to be retained can be treated endodontically, is in sound periodontal state with good bony support, is restorable, and will be a viable tooth in the long term. At operation it is wise to raise a flap to enable direct visualization of the root surface. Resection of the root with a high-speed bur is followed by smoothing, recontouring, and restoration of any residual pulp cavity. It is sometimes not possible to proceed with root resection, despite apparently favourable radiographs, especially in maxillary molars, so warn patient pre-operatively.

Hemisection Involves dividing a two-rooted tooth in half to give two smaller units each with a single root. Again, RCT is necessary pre-operatively and restoration of the divided crown is required post-operatively.

Extraction Ensures removal of periodontal disease but carries its own problems.

Guided tissue regeneration[1] (📖 p. 208).

Enamel matrix derivatives (EMD) (📖 p. 208).

It is important to note that the techniques described above are of less significance to long-term outcome than the degree of plaque control that can be achieved and maintained by the patient. Mini interproximal brushes are a valuable aid in cleaning furcation defects and are available in a variety of sizes and shapes.

---

1 R. Ponteriero 1989 *J Clin Periodont* **16** 170.

Mucogingival surgery

Mucogingival surgery encompasses those techniques aimed at the correction of local gingival defects. The rationale for this type of surgery has been hotly debated over many years. Initially, it was felt that a margin of attached gingiva of around 3mm was required to protect the periodontium during mastication and to dissipate the pull to the gingival margin from frenal attachments. In fact, data from properly conducted experimental work have demonstrated that the width of attached gingiva and the presence or absence of an attached portion is **not** of decisive importance for the maintenance of gingival health.[1] As a result of this, the indications for mucogingival surgery have been rationalized:

- where change in the morphology of the gingival margin would improve plaque control, e.g. presence of high frenal attachments or deep areas of recession
- areas where recession creates root sensitivity or aesthetic problems
- a very thin layer of attached gingiva overlying a tooth which is to be moved orthodontically: the evidence for this is somewhat anecdotal.

Gingival recession

Gingival recession is one of the commonest reasons for carrying out mucogingival surgery. The two commonest causes are plaque-induced gingival inflammation and toothbrush trauma, revealing dehiscences in alveolar bone. Therefore, basic periodontal care and correction of faulty toothbrushing technique are the first lines of Rx. While anatomical features may contribute, these and trauma from occlusion, high frenal attachments, and impingement from restorations etc., are a secondary consideration.

Mucogingival techniques

These can be divided into two main groups:

Vestibular extension procedures essentially aim to ↑ the area of attached gingivae and deepen the buccal or labial sulcus. As they are always accompanied by a degree of bone resorption, these methods are not recommended as a therapeutic periodontal technique.

Grafting is subdivided into:

1) *Free grafts*, which are completely removed from their donor area. Free gingival grafts, commonly of palatal mucosa and connective tissue, are taken and grafted to donor sites prepared by incising between attached and alveolar mucosa. While this technique may successfully cover exposed root surfaces of around 2mm square and will certainly ↑ the width of keratinized gingiva, long-term cross-over studies suggest that in the presence of meticulous OH there is no significant difference between attachment levels in grafted and non-grafted sites with similar degrees of recession.[2]

2) *Pedicle grafts* are not separated from their blood supply. Commonly used pedicle grafts are the laterally repositioned flap, coronally repositioned flap, and the double papilla flap. These techniques may be of some value in very narrow areas of isolated gingival recession. Technically, of course, these are flaps *not* grafts.

1 J. Wenstrom 1987 *J Clin Periodont* **14** 181.

2 H. S. Dorfmann 1980 *J Clin Periodont* **7** 316.

Occlusion and splinting

All matters relating to occlusion seem to have developed a high degree of mysticism about them in the dental world; this is also true of the relationship between occlusion and periodontal therapy.

It used to be claimed that angular bony defects and ↑ mobility were directly attributable to trauma from the occlusion. This belief is less commonly held nowadays as angular defects can be found around both occlusally traumatized and non-traumatized teeth.[1] It is, however, self-evident that an already periodontally diseased tooth can change its relationship in the arch to become traumatized, or that a tooth which is already in traumatic occlusion can develop periodontal disease, and that the two factors can exacerbate one another. Occlusal trauma cannot induce periodontal tissue breakdown but may enhance the rate of progression of disease.

Tooth mobility ↑ tooth mobility may simply be a result of loss of periodontal attachment and bony support. It may also result purely as a localized effect due to a heavy occlusal loading, causing a widening of the periodontal membrane space, though this is usually iatrogenic in origin. It is now felt that the Δ of occlusal trauma should only be made where progressive increasing tooth mobility is observed, but in order to do this it is necessary to have an objective method of measuring tooth mobility. This can be done using a Mobility Index:[2]

Grade 1 = Mobility <1mm buccolingually
Grade 2 = Mobility 1–2mm buccolingually
Grade 3 = Mobility of >2mm buccolingually &/or vertical mobility.

Rx First priority should be to diagnose and treat any existing periodontal disease and correct any pre-existing iatrogenic causes, e.g. poor crowns or bridges, high restorations. If tooth mobility persists as a direct result of diagnosable occlusal trauma, occlusal adjustment is a sensible Rx modality. If the tooth is mobile as a result of lack of alveolar bone support, this is not automatically an indication for splinting (see below).

Splinting Indicated in the following situations:
- Tooth with healthy but ↓ periodontium where mobility is ↑.
- Tooth with ↑ mobility which patient finds uncomfortable during function.

It is very easy to design splints which are impossible for the patients to keep clean as all additions to the natural tooth surface will ↑ plaque retention. A wide range of different techniques and materials have been described, including orthodontic wire fastened to teeth by resin-composite, resin-composite alone, fixed bridges, partial prostheses, acid-etch retained splints, and more recently, fibre-reinforced resin-composite splinting.

1 J. Waerhaug 1970 *J Periodont* **50** 355.

2 A. Grace 1989 *Periodontal Control: An Effective System for Diagnosis, Selection, Control and Rx Planning in General Practice*, Quintessence.

Peri-implantitis

Osseo-integrated implants are now well established (📖 p. 390). Implants which have achieved full osseo-integration may fail by overloading, peri-implantitis (similar to periodontitis), or a combination of both, with failure rates being high in smokers. Implant salvage in the failing stage consists of ↓ overloading and the entire arsenal of periodontal therapies. Local antibiotics and bone-supplemented GTR may be particularly useful.

Tissue transformation using bone morphogenetic protein may also prove useful in the future.

Supportive periodontal therapy

Once corrective phase is complete a programme of supportive therapy begins. To avoid reinfection and to maintain the therapeutic benefits long term patients require monitoring and sometimes treatment to support their own home care. Maintenance visits will involve re-evaluation of plaque control, bleeding on probing, pus and furcation lesions and radiographs if required. Treatment of persistent bleeding pockets and a full mouth polish should be carried out. The first 6 months after completion of corrective treatment is the healing phase and regular professional tooth cleaning should take place. Then maintenance visits begin at 3–4 monthly intervals and may be lengthened up to 6 months if appropriate although there is no good evidence for the ideal frequency of maintenance visits. Various aspects such as plaque control, bleeding on probing and alveolar bone heights are considered and frequency decided accordingly.

Restorative dentistry

Contents

Relevant pages in other chapters Caries diagnosis, 📖 p. 26; amalgam, 📖 p. 608; resin composite, 📖 p. 610; the acid-etch technique, 📖 p. 614; dentine adhesive systems, p.616; glass ionomers, 📖 p. 618; cermets, 📖 p. 623; cements, p.624; impression materials, 📖 p. 626; casting alloys, 📖 p. 630; acid-etch tip, 📖 p. 100.

Principal sources and further reading *Operative Dentistry. Dental Update. The British Dental Journal.* B. G. N. Smith 1997 *Planning and Making Crowns and Bridges,* Dunitz. P. A. Brunton 2002 *Decision Making in Operative Dentistry,* Quintessence. J. L. Gutmann et al. 1997 *Problem Solving in Endodontics,* 3rd edn, Mosby. E. A. M. Kidd et al. 2003 *Pickard's Manual of Operative Dentistry,* 8th edn, OUP. S. J. Davies and R. J. Gray 2002 *A Clinical Guide to Occlusion,* British Dental Association. J. M. Whitworth 2002 *Rational Root Canal Treatment in Practice,* Quintessence.

To attempt to resolve the problem of caries by preparing and restoring teeth is comparable to trying to resolve the problem of poliomyelitis by manufacturing more attractive and better quality crutches, more quickly and more cheaply.

Treatment planning

A proper treatment plan can only result from a thorough patient assessment, which must include a history, an examination, relevant special tests, and ultimately, a diagnosis.

Under ideal circumstances an integrated treatment plan is formulated for each patient at the start of every course of treatment. Very often, however, the treatment plan will need to be revised in the light of clinical findings as the treatment progresses, e.g. patient cooperation, response to periodontal therapy, investigation of teeth of doubtful prognosis, etc. When dealing with patients with a range of problems it is therefore wise to formulate a treatment plan which has a number of achievable goals, and then on completion of this to reassess the patient to decide on what further treatment is necessary.

Sequence of treatment

This list is obviously an oversimplification but should serve as a general guide to the order in which treatment should be carried out.

1) Relief of pain.
2) Control of active disease and achievement of stability:
   • OHI, dietary advice, topical fluoride, and initial periodontal therapy;
   • extraction of unsaveable teeth;
   • treatment of large and active carious lesions;
   • consideration of definitive denture design;
   • remaining simple restorations;
   • RCT.
3) Reassessment of success of initial treatment, OH, periodontal condition, and prognosis of teeth.
4) Definitive treatment: crowns, bridgework, and dentures.
5) Maintenance and review.

Practical points

• The priority of items of treatment must be taken into account when formulating a treatment plan, which may lead to deviations from the scheme described above. For example, in an apprehensive patient it would be more appropriate to complete small restorations before dealing with the large ones.

• Explain what the treatment plan involves to the patient and the role they will have to play in controlling their dental disease. Success is dependent upon patient compliance, therefore time spent discussing their expectations, treatment options, time involved, cost implications present and future, and their role in maintenance is never wasted. Equally without such a discussion consent is not by definition informed.

• If need to check a medical history with patient's GMP or refer patient to a specialist, allow sufficient time to elapse before arranging to carry out any treatment that is dependent upon the outcome.

• It is important to bear in mind subsequent items on a treatment plan, e.g. the design of a P/- may influence the choice of material and contour of restorations.

- For complex cases, several short treatment plans, each ending with a reassessment, are more logical and efficient than one long one that keeps changing.
- When formulating a treatment plan group items together into appointments to form a visit plan. Decide how long you will need for each visit.
- Although it is usually advantageous to complete as much work as possible at each visit, in a proportion of patients (or if carried to an extreme, in any patient) this can be counter-productive. If in doubt about how much treatment to do at a visit, discuss this with the patient.
- Regularly reinforce the OH throughout the treatment (e.g. whilst waiting for LA to take).
- Record-keeping is very important. At the end of each visit carefully note what has been done and the materials used (including sizes and shades). Cross that item off the treatment plan and adjust the patient's chart. Note what is to be done next visit: this will save time.
- It is important to recognize your own limitations, and where appropriate refer a patient for advice or treatment.

Stabilization or caries control In patients with multiple carious lesions it may take several weeks/months to complete the permanent restorations necessary to secure OH. In these cases it may be advisable to prevent any symptomless large lesions increasing in size by placing temporary dressings. The cavities should be rendered caries-free at the margins, and temporarily restored with a strong cement, e.g. traditional or resin-modified GI cement.

Dental pain

When a patient attends the surgery and complains of toothache, pain may be arising from a variety of different structures and may be classified as follows:

- Pulpal pain
- Periapical/periradicular pain.
- Non-dental pain.

Dental pain can be very difficult to diagnose, and the clinician must first gather as much information as possible from the history, clinical and radiographic examinations, and other special tests (see Chapter 1).

Pulpal pain

The pulp may be subject to a wide variety of insults, e.g. bacterial, thermal, chemical, traumatic, the effects of which are cumulative and can ultimately lead to inflammation in the pulp (pulpitis) and pain. The dental pulp does not contain any proprioceptive nerve endings, therefore a characteristic of pulpal pain is that the patient is unable to localize the affected tooth. The ability of the pulp to recover from injury depends upon its blood supply, not the nerve supply, which must be borne in mind when vitality (sensibility) testing is carried out (📖 p. 14).[1] It is impossible to reliably achieve an accurate Δ of the state of the pulp on clinical grounds alone; the only 100% accurate method is histological section.

Although numerous classifications of pulpal disease exist, only a limited number of clinical diagnostic situations require identification before effective treatment can be given.

Reversible pulpitis

Symptoms Fleeting sensitivity/pain to hot, cold or sweet with immediate onset. Pain is usually sharp and may be difficult to locate. Quickly subsides after removal of the stimulus.

Signs Exaggerated response to pulp testing. Carious cavity/leaking restoration.

Rx Remove any caries present and place a sedative dressing (e.g. ZOE) or permanent restoration with suitable pulp protection.

Irreversible pulpitis

Symptoms Spontaneous pain which may last several hours, be worse at night, and is often pulsatile in nature. Pain is elicited by hot and cold at first, but in later stages heat is more significant and cold may actually ease symptoms. A characteristic feature is that the pain remains after the removal of the stimulus. Localization of pain may be difficult initially, but as the inflammation spreads to the periapical tissues the tooth will become more sensitive to pressure.

Signs Application of heat (e.g. warm GP) elicits pain. Affected tooth may give no or a reduced response to electric pulp tester. In later stages may become TTP.

---

1 A. H. R. Rowe 1990 *Int Endo J* **23** 77.

Rx Extirpation of the pulp and RCT is the treatment of choice (assuming the tooth is to be saved). If time is short or if anaesthesia proves elusive then removal of the coronal pulp and a Ledermix® dressing can often control the symptoms until the remaining pulp can be extirpated under LA at the next appointment.[1]

Dentine hypersensitivity

This is pain arising from exposed dentine in response to a thermal, tactile, or osmotic stimulus (but not all exposed dentine gives rise to symptoms). It is thought to be due to dentinal fluid movement stimulating pulpal pain receptors. Prevalence is ~1:7 adults with a peak in young adults, then ↓ with age.[2] Δ is by elimination of other possible causes and by evoking symptoms.

Rx Involves ↓ aetiological factors (i.e. OHI, possibly including tooth- brushing technique and intrinsic and extrinsic dental erosion) and by ↓ permeability of dentinal tubules (e.g. by toothpaste containing strontium &/or fluoride; placement of varnishes, dentine desensitizers, dentine adhesive systems, or, if indicated, a restoration).

Cracked tooth syndrome

Symptoms Sharp pain on biting—short duration.

Signs Often relatively few, therefore Δ difficult. Tooth often has a large restoration. Crack may not be apparent at first but transillumination and possibly removal of the restoration may aid visualization. Positive response to vitality (sensibility) testing and pain can normally be elicited by getting the patient to bite with the affected tooth on a cotton-wool roll or a 'tooth slooth'. May be associated with bruxing habit.

Rx An adhesive resin composite restoration may be appropriate in teeth which are minimally restored, but in some cases a cast restoration with full occlusal coverage will be needed. Occasionally RCT may be required.

Periapical/periradicular pain

Progression of irreversible pulpitis ultimately leads to death of the pulp (pulpal necrosis). At this stage the patient may experience relief from pain and thus may not seek attention. If neglected, however, the bacteria and pulpal breakdown products leave the root canal system via the apical foramen or lateral canals and lead to inflammatory changes and possibly pain. Characteristically the patient can precisely identify the affected tooth, as the periodontal ligament, which is well supplied with proprioceptive nerve endings, is inflamed.

1 Scottish Dental Clinical Effectiveness Programme 2007 *Emergency Dental Care.*
2 P. Dowell 1985 *BDJ* **158** 92.

Pulpal necrosis with periapical periodontitis

Symptoms Variable, but patients generally describe a dull ache exacerbated by biting on the tooth.

Signs Usually no response to vitality testing, unless one canal of a multirooted tooth is still vital. The tooth will be TTP. Radiographically the apical PDL may be widened or there may be a periapical radiolucency (granuloma or cyst).

Rx RCT or extraction.

Acute periapical abscess

Symptoms Severe pain which will disturb sleep. Tooth is exquisitely tender to touch.

Signs Affected tooth is usually extruded, mobile, and TTP. May be associated with a localized or diffuse swelling. Vitality (sensibility) testing may be misleading as pus may conduct stimulus to apical tissues. Radiographic changes can range from a widening of the apical PDL space to an obvious radiolucency. It is important to differentiate this condition from a periodontal abscess.

Rx Drain pus and, if indicated, relieve occlusion. Drainage of pus can often be achieved by entering the pulp chamber with a high-speed diamond bur, steadying tooth with a finger to prevent excessive vibration. After drainage has been achieved it is preferable to prepare the canal and place a temporary dressing. Avoid 'open drainage' if possible, but if absolutely necessary for <24h, as after this time further bacterial contamination of the root canal makes subsequent RCT very difficult. If a fluctuant soft tissue swelling is present, this should be incised to achieve drainage. Antibiotics should be prescribed if there is systemic involvement or if the infection is spreading significantly along tissue planes. When the acute symptoms have subsided, RCT must be performed or the tooth extracted.

Chronic periapical abscess

Often symptomless. Possibly associated with persistent sinus. Presentation may be: coincidental finding or acute exacerbation.

Lateral periodontal abscess

Symptoms Similar to periapical abscess with acute pain and tenderness, and often an associated bad taste.

Signs Tooth is usually mobile and TTP, with associated localized or diffuse swelling of the adjacent periodontium. A deep periodontal pocket is usually associated, which will exude pus on probing. Radiographs normally show vertical or horizontal bone loss, and vitality (sensibility) testing is usually positive, unless there is an associated endodontic problem (perio-endo lesion).

Rx Achieve drainage of pus. Irrigate with a chlorhexidine solution. If there is systemic involvement or it is a recurrent problem, prescribe antibiotics (metronidazole or amoxicillin). Debride the pocket once acute symptoms have settled.

Non-dental pain

When no signs of dental or periradicular pathology can be detected then non-dental causes must be considered. Other causes of pain that can present as toothache include:

- TMPDS (📖 p. 446);
- sinusitis (📖 p. 384);
- psychological disorders (atypical odontalgia) (p. 426);
- tumours (📖 pp. 382 and 480).

Isolation and moisture control

Isolation is required to aid visibility, prevent contamination during moisture-sensitive techniques, maintain a relatively aseptic environment, and protect the patient from caustic materials or aspiration of foreign material.

High-volume suction, e.g. an aspirator.

Low-volume suction, e.g. a saliva ejector.

Compressed air This tends to redistribute the moisture to somewhere else (e.g. your eye) rather than remove it. Should be used with care in deep preparations as prolonged use can cause pulpal damage, let alone displace adhesive materials when the solvent is being evaporated prior to curing.

Absorbents
- Cotton-wool rolls. Insert with a rolling action away from the alveolus. Moisten before removal to prevent tearing mucosa.
- Paper pads.
- Carboxymethylcellulose pads (Dry Tips). Very effective if inserted the correct way round with the impermeable plastic against the tooth.

Rubber dam This provides effective isolation and also improves access to operating site. It is indicated where moisture control and airway protection are essential, e.g. RCT (RCT without rubber dam is considered negligent), acid-etch technique. With practice, rubber dam can be applied quickly and often saves time in the long run. The dam must be secured to the teeth; several methods are available:
- Rubber dam clamps. These consist of two metal jaws linked by one or more bows. Commonly used for posterior teeth.
- Floss ligatures.
- Wedges.
- Proprietary rubber bands (Wedjets®) or pieces of dam, worked through contact points.
- By pinching dam between a tight contact point.

Types of dam:
1) Sheet grade, 6-inch square (15cm), which is supported with a frame. Moderate to thicker gauges are preferable.
2) Mask type, which is supported by a paper margin and looped over ears with elastic. Increasingly, latex-free rubber dam is available and arguably should be used routinely.

Placement: Several regimens have been described; the following is popular:
1) Place cotton-wool roll in sulcus beside tooth for treatment.
2) Punch holes, which correspond to tooth size, cleanly in the rubber dam at the centre of each tooth to be included.
3) Try in clamp (with floss tied to it).
4) Fit clamp into appropriate hole, with bridge distally, and using forceps place clamp and dam on to tooth (winged technique). Alternatively, the clamp may be placed first and the dam pulled over (wingless). The latter is especially useful for broken down teeth or poor access.
5) Position dam on other teeth, using floss to ease through contact points.
6) Secure dam anteriorly using one of the methods above.
7) If frame required, position.

8) Put napkin on patient's chin under dam. A saliva ejector will add to the patient's comfort.

If using caustic materials, a rubber dam sealer (e.g. OraSeal®) should be used.

Removal:

1) Take away clamps/ligatures, etc.

2) Stretch dam, carefully cut interdental septa with scissors, and remove.

Protection of the airway Mandatory when fitting crowns, bridges, inlays, and carrying out RCT. Best provided by rubber dam, but if this is not possible a butterfly sponge or gauze can be used.

Gingival retraction ↓ gingival exudate and exposes subgingival preparations prior to impression-taking. Some retraction cords are impregnated with substances such as adrenaline to ↓ bleeding. The cord should be gently placed into the gingival crevice with a cord packing instrument (leaving no tag hanging out) prior to impression-taking and temporization. Braided cords are better than twisted. Bleeding from the gingival margin can be ↓ by applying an astringent. A paste (Expasyl™) which contains aluminium chloride provides for retraction and haemorrhage control. Expasyl™ is useful for preparations finished within or just below the level of the gingival crevice, otherwise retraction cord is more appropriate.

Electrosurgery May be indicated where a margin extends subgingivally and gingival overgrowth is hampering restoration placement or impression-taking. Also for crown-lengthening procedures, although bone removal is required too.

(📖 See p. 102 on crown lengthening).

Principles of tooth preparation

Why restore?
- To restore function.
- To prevent further spread of an active lesion which is not amenable to preventive measures.
- To preserve pulp vitality.
- To restore aesthetics.

However, these reasons need to be evaluated with regard to the patient and the rest of the dentition.

Preparation design With caries prevalence declining, emphasis has changed from extension for prevention, to minimizing removal of tooth tissue. Tooth preparation should be based on the morphology of the carious lesion and the requirements of the restorative material being used.

General principles of tooth preparation
- Gain access to caries.
- Remove all caries at ADJ (to prevent spread laterally).
- Cut away all significantly unsupported enamel.
- There is no need to extend a cavity into self cleansing areas buccally and lingually
- Shape preparation so that remaining tooth tissue and restorative material will be able to withstand functional forces.
- Shape preparation so that restoration will be retained, i.e. slight undercut for amalgam, none required for resin composite or bonded amalgams.
- Check preparation margins are appropriate for the restorative material. Small areas of unsupported enamel may be left if a resin composite restoration is being placed.
- Remove remaining caries.
- Wash and dry preparation.

Helpful hints
- While care must be exercised not to overcut a preparation, do not skimp on access so that caries removal is compromised by poor visibility.
- Mark centric stops with articulating paper prior to tooth preparation and try to preserve if possible, or place the preparation margins past the occlusal contact areas.
- Avoid crossing marginal ridges.
- In removing caries a tactile appreciation of the hardness of dentine is important, therefore use slow-speed instruments or excavators.
- The base of the preparation should not be flattened as this runs the risk of pulp exposure.
- Unless caries dictates, margins should be supragingival.
- All internal line angles should be rounded to ↓ internal stresses.
- Removing caries with a large diameter round bur automatically produces the desired shape.
- In a proximal box, the margin should extend below the contact point because this is where the caries is!

Amalgam[1] (📖 see also p. 608)

- Amalgam is brittle, therefore an amalgam cavo-surface margin of at least 70°, preferably 90°, is required to prevent ditching. Also avoid leaving amalgam overlying cavity margins and overcarving.
- Accepted minimal dimensions for amalgam are 2mm occlusally and 1mm elsewhere.
- In deep preparations, sealers &/or liners are required to seal the dentine and prevent ingress of bacteria.

Resin composite, 📖 p. 610.

Glass ionomer, 📖 p. 618.

- Wear precludes their use in load-bearing situations except for 1° teeth, management of root caries, temporary restorations, and the atraumatic restorative technique.

Gold

- Relies on minimally divergent walls and cement lute for retention.
- A preparation margin of >135° is advisable to give good marginal fit to restoration and to allow burnishing.

It would be foolish to think that experience in tooth preparation can be adequately assimilated from the written text. The purpose of the following pages is to give the reader some practical tips on how to do the procedures considered, as well as to describe recent innovations and techniques.

Nomenclature

Black's classification of cavities is now not widely used. It has been replaced by the following:

Occlusal (Class I)	Cavity in pits and fissures
Proximal (Class II or III)	Cavity in proximal surface(s) of any tooth
Incisal (Class IV)	Proximal in an anterior tooth, but including incisal edge
Cervical (Class V)	Cavity in cervical third of buccal or lingual surface of any tooth.

1 P. B. Robinson 1985 *Dental Update* **12** 357.

Occlusal (Class I)

Amalgam

Amalgam is still the most widely used material for occlusal cavities, probably because it is more forgiving of technique than some of the newer materials. It is now widely accepted, however, that resin composite placed in conjunction with minimal preparation techniques has a role in initial lesion management. If enamel margins are cut to an angle of 90° (or, if cusps steeply inclined, >70°) the resultant preparation will be adequately retentive.

Lining Recently, emphasis has changed, with linings being used to seal the underlying dentine for moderate to deep cavities. Light-cured RMGIs (e.g. Vitrebond™) are now recommended. A preparation sealer (Gluma® Desensitizer) can be used in minimal preparations.

Resin composite

Use of these materials in posterior teeth is increasing as patients request tooth coloured restorations and their concern about amalgam grows. The controversy surrounding posterior resin composites is dealt with on 📖 pp. 230 and 612. A technique which has gained more widespread acceptance is:

Preventive resin restoration Introduced by Simonsen (then by others as the minimal resin composite restoration or sealant restoration!). Preparation is limited to caries removal and the resultant preparation restored using fissure sealant alone if small, or resin composite followed by sealant if larger. Alternatively, GI can be used instead of resin composite. The rationale of this approach is that adjacent fissures are sealed for prevention. It is particularly useful for investigating any suspect areas of a fissure, a technique that is often referred to as an enamel biopsy (obviously coined by an academic). This involves exploring the area with a small bur, and if no caries is found further preparation can be aborted and sealant placed. If carious, a PRR can be carried out. It is often possible to complete preparation of a PRR without LA; however, if the cavity appears larger than originally thought, LA can then be given. If the preparation extends significantly into load-bearing areas, conventional tooth preparation should be carried out and the tooth restored with resin composite or other suitable material.

Technique for medium-sized cavities:

1) Assess whether LA required. If not, ask patient to signal if tooth becomes sensitive.
2) Isolate tooth (preferably with rubber dam).
3) Gain access to caries with a small bur at high speed.
4) Use a small round bur run at slow speed to remove caries. Only remove as much enamel as required for access.
5) Etch preparation margins and occlusal surface. Wash and dry.
6) Apply a dentine adhesive system.
7) Restore preparation with resin composite placed and cured in increments, but don't overfill.
8) Paint sealant over whole of occlusal surface and cure.
9) Check occlusion.

Where possible a related sealant and resin composite should be used to ensure a good bond.

Hints for resin composite restorations

- Use etchant gel in a syringe to aid placement. Many newer adhesive systems do not have a separate etch stage, however, and rely on the use of acidic primers often used in conjunction with bonding resins or as a separate stage, 📖 p. 616 in Chapter 14 on dental materials.
- Additions are generally easy as new resin composite will bond to old.
- Avoid eugenol-containing cements with resin composite restorations.
- Resin composite must be cured incrementally, with increments being no deeper than 2mm.

Proximal (Class II)

▶ Avoid the creation of an overhang at the cervical margin and ensure a good contact point with adjacent tooth with a well-contoured matrix band and wedges.

Amalgam In practice, preparation size is determined by the size of the carious lesion and extension beyond this should be minimal. Proximal preparations comprise a proximal box with vertical grooves. The preparation should only extend occlusally if there is evidence of caries in the occlusal fissures. Retention from occlusal forces is derived from a 2–5° divergence of the walls towards the floor in both parts of the preparation. Amalgam restorations are prone to # at the isthmus in restorations extended occlusally, therefore sufficient depth must be provided in this area. The width of the isthmus should not be overcut (ideally ¼ to ⅕ intercusp width). If the cusps are extensively undermined or missing they should be replaced with a bonded restoration (📖 p. 232). A chisel can be used to plane away unsupported enamel from the margins of the completed preparation to produce a 90° butt joint. In molar teeth with mesial and distal caries it is preferable to try and cut two separate cavities, but often a confluent mesio-occlusal-distal preparation is unavoidable. Increasingly the use of resin composite placed in conjunction with a dentine adhesive system is advocated for the restoration of small to moderate proximal preparations in premolar and molar teeth.

Tunnel preparations A 'tunnel' approach to interproximal caries has been described.[1] Access to the caries is made through either the occlusal or buccal surfaces, leaving the marginal ridge intact. This approach is only suitable for small lesions, as when preparation is completed at least 2mm of marginal ridge must remain. The access cavity may need to be widened buccolingually to complete caries removal. Carisolv™ may have a place here to ensure complete caries removal. A piece of mylar strip wedged into place will act as a matrix. A RMGIC is used to fill the bulk of the preparation and the occlusal access cavity restored with a posterior resin composite. In view of the difficulty of accurately removing all the caries, let alone the incidence of marginal fracture, this technique is rarely used.

Resin composite Posterior resin composites should be used predominately to restore posterior teeth, but the technique is more demanding, taking ~50% longer. In addition, it is difficult to establish adequate contact points and occlusal stops. Polymerization shrinkage can cause cuspal flexure, post-operative pain, and marginal gaps. Direct posterior resin composites are best avoided in the following situations:

- Cusp replacements.
- Poor moisture control.
- Restorations with deep gingival extensions, although a bonded base approach can be adopted.
- Bruxism or heavy occlusion.

1 J. W. McLean 1988 *BDJ* **164** 293.

If a resin composite is to be used then a hybrid material with >75% filler is advisable. Pre-wedging one but not both proximal contacts aids creation of a contact point. Resin composite should be placed, and cured, incrementally. If possible, centric stops should be preserved on sound tooth tissue or the restorative material, but never on the marginal interface of the restoration.[1] Use of indirect composite inlays may combat some of these problems (see next section).

1 R. W. Bryant 1992 *Aust Dent J* **37** 81.

Proximal (Class II)—resin composite and inlays

Resin composite and porcelain inlays These inlay techniques appear to overcome some of the problems associated with direct resin composite restorations. When used in conjunction with an acid-etch technique existing tooth tissue can be reinforced. Curing resin composite outside the mouth with the addition of heat (110° for 5mins) or pressure overcomes polymerization shrinkage and possibly ↑ strength. As the inlays are bonded to the tooth with an adhesive, parallel walls are less important, but undercuts must be removed or blocked out with an RMGI cement (not in the proximal box). In general porcelain inlays offer improved aesthetics, surface finish, and bond in comparison to resin composite inlays; however, placement and adjustment can be more difficult. Ceromers (e.g. belleGlass™) may also be used in similar situations.

Technique: preparation
1) The preparation should have slightly divergent walls, rounded line angles, and a slight bevel of the enamel margins, but not occlusally. For onlays, a minimum 1.5mm reduction of cusps is necessary.
2) Block out any undercuts with RMGIC.
3) Take an impression of the preparation and opposing arch, and if necessary make an inter-occlusal record.
4) Choose shade.
5) Make and place temporary with a proprietary resin-based temporary material (e.g. Fermit, Clip).

Technique: cementation
1) Place rubber dam.
2) Remove temporary and clean tooth.
3) Try-in inlay, and carefully check marginal fit and adjust as necessary. Do not adjust the occlusion at this stage.
4) Polish any adjusted areas.
5) Remove inlay and clean with alcohol. For porcelain only, place layer of silane coupling agent on fitting surface.
6) Etch enamel and dentine (total etch concept). Wash and remove excess moisture, but do not dry.
7) Place dentine-adhesive system to moist surface.
8) Apply dual-cure resin composite luting cement to prep and inlay and carefully seat.
9) Cure for 10sec and then remove any excess resin composite.
10) Complete light-curing (dual-cure resin composite will finish setting chemically under inlay in ~6min).
11) Trim any excess cement (especially interdentally) and polish.
12) Check occlusion and adjust.

Proximal (Class III), incisal (Class IV), cervical (Class V), and root surface caries

Anterior proximal

Resin composite is the most widely used material for anterior proximal restorations.

Access should be gained from either the buccal or lingual aspect, depending on the position of the lesion. As resin composite is adhesive the preparation is just extended sufficiently to remove all peripheral caries. Some unsupported enamel can be retained labially, but the margins should be planed with chisels to remove any grossly weakened tooth structure. Tooth preparation can be almost entirely completed with slow-speed burs and hand instruments. Ideally the margins are bevelled. A slight excess of material should be moulded into the preparation with a mylar strip, wedged cervically. Once the material is set, the excess can be removed. After checking the occlusion the restoration can be polished using one of the proprietary products (e.g. Sof-Lex™ discs, Enhance®) if necessary.

Incisal

The restoration of choice is resin composite, the so-called 'acid-etch tip' (□ p. 100); however, for large incisal cavities in the adult patient, a dentine-bonded crown or porcelain veneer may give better retention and aesthetics.

Cervical

Although cervical cavities are seen less frequently in younger patients, they are an ↑ problem in older age-groups with gingival recession. Resin composite e.g. flowable, compomer, or RMGIC are the preferred materials in this situation. Amalgam should be avoided in this situation due to the possibility of a lichenoid reaction.

Once caries has been removed the occlusal margin should be bevelled. The cervical margin should not be bevelled as it has been shown to ↑ microleakage. The materials are ideally placed incrementally under rubber dam isolation.

Root surface caries

As gingival recession is a prerequisite to root caries, it occurs predominantly in the >40-yr age group. Dentine, which has a critical pH below that of enamel, is thus directly exposed to carious attack. It is sometimes seen secondary to ↓ saliva flow (which reduces buffering capacity and may alter dietary habits) caused by salivary gland disease, drugs, or radiation. Long-term sugar-based medication may also be a factor. Rx requires, first, control of the aetiological factor, and for most patients this involves dietary advice and OHI. Topical fluoride varnishes, high fluoride toothpastes and mouthrinses may aid remineralization and prevent new lesions developing. However, active lesions require restoration, typically with a traditional or RMGIC. See also severe early childhood caries □ p. 90.

Management of the deep carious lesion

Assessment
- Is the tooth restorable and is restoration preferable to extraction?
- Is the tooth symptomless? If not what is the character and duration of the pain?
- Test vitality and percuss the tooth (before LA!).
- Take radiographs to check extent of lesion and if apical pathology.

Management Depends upon a guesstimate of pulpal condition (📖 p. 220).
Irreversible pulpitis/necrotic pulp—Rx: RCT (📖 p. 276) or extraction.
Reversible pulpitis/healthy pulp—aim to maintain pulp vitality by selective removal of carious dentine without pulp exposure. If in doubt Rx as reversible pulpitis. Can always institute RCT later.
There is some evidence that in symptomless teeth with deep carious lesions partial, rather than complete, removal of caries is preferable as it reduces the risk of pulp exposure. It is not known yet whether it is necessary to re-enter and complete excavation at a later date (stepwise excavation of caries)[1]

Rationale Bacteria sealed under a restoration that provides a good peripheral seal are denied substrate, therefore lesion arrests. This allows the pulpodentinal complex to lay down reparative dentine.

Exposure
- If traumatic, small, and uncontaminated, perform direct pulp cap with hard-setting calcium hydroxide or MTA (mineral trioxide aggregate) and restore.
- If carious exposure, and continued pulp vitality is doubtful, RCT will be required. If time short, can dress tooth with Ledermix and a traditional GI cement, and extirpate pulp at next visit.

Pulpotomy
Is removal of coronal part of pulp in order to eliminate damaged or contaminated tissue. It is indicated for teeth with immature apices, as continued vitality of apical pulp will allow root formation to proceed. Once the apex has closed, conventional RCT can be carried out. The pulp is amputated to the cervical constriction, dressed with non-setting or hard-setting calcium hydroxide or MTA and the tooth temporarily restored.

Materials used in the management of pulp vitality
Calcium hydroxide has a pH of 11, which makes it bacteriostatic and promotes the formation of a calcific barrier. When calcium hydroxide comes into contact with the pulp a zone of pulpal necrosis is formed. This is subsequently mineralized with calcium ions from the pulp. It is the material of choice for direct pulp caps, particularly the hard-setting type.

Mineral trioxide aggregate is a very slow setting material. Similar in nature to industrial cement. Very biocompatible.

---

1 D. Rickets 2006 *Cochrane Database Systematic Reviews* Issue 3.

Ledermix is a mixture of triamcinolone acetonide (a steroid) and demethyl chlortetracycline in a water-soluble base. It has anti-inflammatory and bacteriostatic properties, but also suppresses pulpal defences, therefore resulting in the rapid spread of any bacteria not affected by the antibiotic it contains. It is a useful compromise for the management of irreversibly inflamed pulps where anaesthesia may be a problem, or when pulp extirpation has to be delayed.

Survival and failure of restorations

Survival of restorations

The results of Elderton's study into the durability of routine restorations placed in the General Dental Services in Scotland provided both a shock and a stimulus to the profession, as he found that 50% lasted for less than 5yrs.[1] This led to debate over both clinical technique and the profession's readiness to replace restorations. It has been reported that 60% of practitioners' time is spent replacing restorations. It is also interesting to note that those patients who change dentists frequently are more at risk of replacement restorations than those who are loyal to the same GDP.[2] In order to ↑ longevity we need to consider the reasons for the failure of restorations and Δ of secondary caries.

Reasons for failure of restorations

- Incorrect Δ and treatment planning; e.g. pulpal pathology; caries of another surface; extraction of tooth for another reason.
- Poor understanding of the occlusion.
- Incorrect preparation; e.g. caries left at ADJ; incorrect margin preparation; inadequate retention; preparation too shallow; weakened tooth tissue left unprotected.
- Incorrect choice of restorative material; e.g. inadequate strength or resistance to wear for situation.
- Incorrect manipulation of material, e.g. inadequate moisture control; over- or under-contouring.

Before replacing a failed restoration it is important to identify the cause of failure and decide whether this can be dealt with by replacement or repair. When making this decision bear in mind that cavity size is ↑ on average by 0.6mm each time a restoration is removed.[3]

Secondary caries

Unfortunately, placement of a restoration does not confer caries immunity upon a tooth. When caries occurs adjacent to a restoration it is called secondary or recurrent caries. More correctly it is defined as a new lesion which just happens to be adjacent to an existing restoration, and it should be managed in its own right. While secondary caries is an accepted phenomenon, we as a profession have perhaps been a little too ready in the past to diagnose and treat it. Ditched amalgam margins are not a reason for replacement *per se*, and active intervention is only required if caries can definitely be demonstrated as active. Secondary caries is difficult to diagnose, but careful observation (clinically and radiographically) rather than intervention, is now advocated. Intervention is only indicated when the lesion is in dentine, and there is evidence of progression &/or cavitation is present.

To prevent secondary caries it is important not only to educate the patient to reduce their caries rate, but also to examine our restorative technique, to ensure good long term-restorations.

1 R. J. Elderton 1983 *BDJ* **155** 91.
2 J. A. Davies 1984 *BDJ* **157** 322.
3 R. J. Elderton 1979 *Proc Br Paedodont Soc* **9** 25.

Occlusion—1

In a book of this size it is (thankfully) not possible to consider all aspects of occlusion; therefore we will try to concentrate on the practical aspects and leave the more esoteric considerations to other texts. We also suggest that significant occlusal adjustment is rarely indicated and should only be attempted by a specialist.

Definitions

Ideal occlusion Anatomically perfect occlusion—rare.

Functional occlusion An occlusion that is free of interferences to smooth gliding movements of the mandible, with absence of pathology.

Balanced occlusion Balancing contacts in all excursions of the mandible to provide therefore ↑ stability of F/F dentures; not applicable to natural dentition (except rarely in full-mouth reconstruction).

Group function Multiple tooth contacts on working side during lateral excursions, but no contact on non-working side.

Canine-guided occlusion During lateral excursions there is disclusion of all the teeth on the working side except for the canine, and no contacts on non-working side.

Hinge axis The axis of rotation of the condyles during the first few millimetres of mandibular opening.

Terminal hinge axis The axis of rotation of the mandible when the condyles are in their most superior position in the glenoid fossa.

Retruded arc of closure The arc of closure of the mandible with the condyles rotating about the terminal hinge axis.

Intercuspal position (ICP) or centric occlusion Position of maximum interdigitation.

Retruded contact position (RCP) or centric relation Position of the mandible where initial tooth contact occurs on the retruded arc of closure. Occurs when condyles are fully seated in the glenoid fossa. In ~20% of patients RCP and ICP are coincident; the remainder have forward slide from RCP to ICP.

Rest position The habitual postural position of the mandible when the patient is relaxed with the condyles in a neutral position.

Freeway space The difference between the rest and intercuspal positions.

Centric stops The points on the occlusal surface which meet with the opposing tooth in ICP. Normally the cusp tips, marginal ridges and central fossae.

Supporting or functional cusps The cusps that occlude with the centric stops on the opposing tooth. Usually palatal on upper and buccal on lower.

Non-supporting cusps The cusps that do not occlude with the opposing teeth. Usually buccal on upper and lingual on lower.

Deflective contacts Deflect mandible from natural path of closure.

Interferences Contacts that hinder smooth excursive movements of mandible.

Occlusal vertical dimension (OVD) Relationship between maxilla and mandible in ICP, i.e. face height.

Do occlusal factors play a role in temporomandibular disorders?
Well, TMPDS is recognized as being of multifactorial aetiology (📖 p. 446). The evidence would suggest that occlusal interferences usually cause either subclinical or no dysfunction because they lie within the adaptive capacity of the patient's neuromusculature. However, this may be lowered by stress and emotional problems so that in susceptible patients occlusal interferences can result in muscle hyperactivity at certain times. It is important therefore to ensure that iatrogenic interferences are not introduced during restorative procedures.

Occlusion—2

Occlusal examination

Prior to carrying out restorative treatment it is important to examine the patient's occlusion. Occlusal contacts can be identified with a 10μm metal foil (Shimstock) and marked using thin articulating paper (20μm). Important features to look for are:

- Number and distribution of occluding teeth.
- Over-eruption, tilting, rotation, etc.
- Presence or absence of centric stops.
- The RCP and any slide between RCP and ICP.
- Anterior guidance—look for disclusion of posterior teeth on protrusion.
- Lateral excursions—?group function, ?canine guidance. Check for non-working interferences.
- TMJs and muscles of mastication.

The clinical examination can only reveal a limited amount of information and in some circumstances (such as prior to crown and bridgework or in patients with TMPDS) a more detailed occlusal examination is required. This is called an **occlusal analysis** or a **diagnostic mounting**, and is done by mounting study models on a semi-adjustable articulator (see below) to facilitate the examination of the features above.

Occlusal considerations for restorative procedures

In most situations restorations are made to conform to the patient's existing occlusion and the main consideration is to prevent the introduction of iatrogenic occlusal interferences. This approach to treatment is known as the **conformative approach.** In some circumstances the conformative approach is not appropriate and a new occlusal scheme must be planned. This is often the case when extensive crown and bridgework is required, such that the patient's existing occlusion will be effectively destroyed by the preparations. A new occlusion is established, free of interferences and with the patient occluding in retruded contact position, which is the only reproducible position. This approach to treatment is called the **reorganized approach** and further consideration of this line of treatment is beyond the scope of this book.

Generally for simple intracoronal restorations complex methods are not needed, but care must be taken to ensure the correct occlusal scheme is reproduced. Before preparing a tooth it is worthwhile marking the centric stops with articulating paper and trying to preserve them if possible. On completion of the restoration it must be checked in intercuspal position to ensure that it is not high, but also to ensure that it has recreated the centric stops, as if it is out of occlusion then over-eruption will occur (which may produce interferences). The restoration should then be checked in all mandibular excursions to ensure that no interferences have been introduced.

One or two units of extracoronal restorations can again be constructed in a relatively simple manner. This is usually done in the laboratory using hand-held models to reproduce the occlusion. Again, great care must be taken at the try-in stage to check the occlusion as above. Care also required when restoring the most distal tooth in the arch as it is very easy to introduce errors in this situation; it may be more appropriate to use an occlusal record (transfer coping technique—see later) and mount the models on an articulator.

More complex laboratory-made restorations need to be constructed with the models mounted on an articulator. This allows the restorations to be constructed in harmony with the patient's occlusion in all mandibular positions, which should minimize the amount of time spent adjusting the restoration at the try-in stage. Also, if any changes to the patient's occlusion are planned, then they can be made on the articulator in a controlled fashion. An articulator is a device which holds the models in a particular relationship and simulates jaw movements. Numerous types of articulators are available but only certain types are appropriate for use in crown and bridgework, e.g. the Denar mark 2, which is a semi-adjustable articulator. The articulator must accurately reproduce mandibular movements and to do this the casts must be mounted in the correct relationship to the TMJs; this is achieved by taking a facebow record. In a conformative approach casts should be related in ICP for restoration.

Occlusal records

Occlusal records are required to mount the models on an articulator in a particular position. Two positions are commonly used for the mounting, the ICP and the RCP. A wax 'squash bite' has commonly been used to record ICP; however, it is inaccurate as the mandible can be deviated as the teeth 'bite' through the wax. It is far better not to use any record and to mount the models to the position of 'best fit'. After the preparations have been carried out it can be difficult to locate the working model to this position of best fit; in this situation the **transfer coping technique** can be used. In this technique Duralay copings are constructed on the working dies, which are taken to the clinic and seated in place on the preparations; they are then adjusted to ensure they are clear of the occlusion. A further mix of Duralay is applied to the occlusal surface of the coping and the patient asked to close together; this produces an indent of the opposing tooth in the resin and provides a very accurate occlusal registration.

When the models are to be mounted in RCP, this is achieved by recording the position of the mandible on the retruded arc of closure just before tooth contact occurs. This is termed a **pre-centric record** and is generally registered with a relatively hard wax (Moyco® Dental Wax). The record is constructed on the maxillary model and trimmed flush with the buccal surfaces of the teeth. It is then softened and seated on the maxillary teeth and the mandible manipulated onto the retruded arc of closure to indent the wax, without allowing tooth contact to take place. The registration can be refined by using a low viscosity material (e.g. TempBond®) in the wax record.

Alternatively, a proprietary inter-occlusal registration material (e.g. Jet Bite™, Blu-Mousse®) may be used to record the space between prepared teeth and their opponents.

Anterior crowns for vital teeth—1

▶ Defer preparation of any crowns until the patient can attain good OH. Not only will this help to ↑ their motivation, but also healthy gingivae are necessary for correct placement of preparation margins and accurate impressions.

Preliminary treatment

- Check vitality; if non-vital, institute RCT first.
- Take a periapical radiograph to check for apical pathology, health of supporting tissues, and anatomy of pulp.
- Get study models. A trial preparation and diagnostic wax-up on a duplicate model can be helpful (especially for the less confident operator). This helps to anticipate any complications and can also be used for fabrication of a temporary crown.
- Record the shade, so that it can be checked at subsequent visits.
- Examine the occlusion.

Porcelain jacket crown (PJC)

This was previously the first choice for aesthetics in cases where occlusal loading was not a problem. Now being superseded by newer ceramic systems.

All-ceramic crown

Provides better aesthetics and ↑ strength compared with PJC (e.g. In-Ceram®, Empress II®, Procera®, Lava™).

Principles

- Sufficient tooth reduction to permit adequate thickness of crown for strength and aesthetics.
- Reduction should follow tooth contours. **NB** two-plane reduction on labial face of incisor teeth.
- Chamfer preparation: 1.0mm labial (just into gingival crevice) and palatal (supragingival).
- 5° taper of opposing walls for retention.

Preparation

Check shade in natural and artificial light with help of dental nurse and patient.

Interproximal Use a long, tapered chamfer bur. Walls should have 5° taper and converge lingually.

Labial With the same bur, first place three depth grooves and remove intervening tooth tissue. Extend a maximum of 0.5mm subgingivally.

Lingual If possible carry out under direct vision. Continue interproximal shoulder round to form cingulum wall, supra-gingivally. Remainder of pala-tal surface should be prepared with a flame-shaped bur to give 0.8–1.0mm clearance from opposing teeth.

Incisal A reduction of 1.5–2mm is required.

Finishing Finishing burs should be used to round off line angles.

Fabricate temporary crown (📖 p. 270) next, as if time runs out impressions can be deferred, but a temporary crown cannot.

Impressions (📖 p. 628) Record preparation in elastomeric material. Opposing arch can be recorded in alginate (cheaper), inter-occlusal record, and facebow if required. Fit temporary and arrange next appointment.

Fitting crown Protect airway. Remove temporary crown. Check marginal fit, contact points, and occlusion. If any adjustments are required polish with porcelain polishing wheels. Make sure patient is happy before you cement crown.

Anterior crowns for vital teeth—2

Porcelain fused to metal (PFM) crown

↑ strength, but ↑ labial reduction (**NB**, some ceramic crowns can be more destructive than PFMs) and ↓ aesthetics. Preparation requires 0.5mm reduction of lingual surface with chamfered margin and labial reduction of 1.2–1.5mm, with shoulder. Transition from shoulder to chamfer is on proximal surface. The junction between porcelain and metal must not be in an area of contact with the opposing teeth. Ideally, all occlusal surfaces in contact with opposing teeth should be finished in metal.

Common problems with anterior crowns

- *Preparation likely to expose pulp* Consider veneer as interim measure.
- *Completed crown does not seat* Check: (i) no temporary cement left on preparation; (ii) approximal contacts with floss, and if too tight, adjust; (iii) ? distorted impression; check no undercuts on preparation and repeat impressions; (iv) die over-trimmed leading to over-extension of margin, cut-back crown margin.
- *Core material showing through crown* Need to reduce preparation so that sufficient bulk of enamel and dentine porcelain can be built up over core, and remake.
- *Colour not right* If technician handy can see if surface stains will give sufficient improvement. If not, re-choose shade and remake.

Removing old crowns

- Protect airway
- A crown-removing instrument can be used to try and remove a crown without destroying it.
- If crown is to be replaced: cut a longitudinal groove in labial surface of crown. Insert a flat plastic and twist.

Anterior post and core crowns

In root-filled anterior teeth it may be necessary to insert a post and core prior to the placement of a crown. Post and cores provide support and retention; however, as the placement of a post makes further orthograde endodontics difficult, it is important to check first that the root-filling and apical condition are satisfactory. If in doubt, repeat RCT.

Preliminary preparation   The first step is to prepare the crown of the tooth to receive the appropriate coronal restoration. The appropriate reductions and margin preparations are carried out with the intention of retaining as much coronal dentine as possible. Grossly weakened tooth substance is removed, but the root face should *not* be flattened off. The retention of a core of tooth substance is important as it effectively ↑ the length of the subsequent post; obviously in some cases this will not be possible, e.g. if the tooth has fractured at gingival level. The coronal GP is removed with a heated instrument or Gates–Glidden bur, taking care not to disturb apical seal. The root canal is then prepared according to the particular technique being used. As a general guide the post should be at least equal to the anticipated crown height, but a minimum of 4mm of well-condensed GP should be left. A periodontal probe or silicone stop is helpful to check prepared canal length.

Types of post and core system

Many different types of post system are available and they can be classified in numerous ways:

Prefabricated or custom-made   Prefabricated posts obviously have the advantage of being cheap and quick, however, they lack versatility and many of the systems require all coronal dentine to be removed. Custom-made techniques are preferred as they are more versatile, but they are also more expensive and require an additional laboratory stage.

Parallel-sided or tapered   Parallel-sided posts are generally preferred to tapered as they provide greater retention and do not generate as much stress within the root canal. Tapered posts, however, are less likely to perforate in the apical region and are better for small tapered roots, e.g. lateral incisors.

Threaded, smooth, or serrated   Threaded posts provide greater retention than smooth-sided; however, they will ↑ stress within the root canal and are therefore C/I. Serrated posts do not concentrate stress but simply ↑ the surface area for retention. Other design features include antirotational components and cementation vents.

Examples

Custom-made   The cast post and core is a popular choice. First of all the root canal is prepared using parallel-sided twist drills, and an antirotation groove is placed in the coronal dentine. The post and core can then be constructed either by a **direct technique** or by an **indirect technique**. In the direct technique a pattern is fabricated in the mouth using either inlay wax or a burn out resin (e.g. Duralay) which is then sent to the laboratory for casting. For the indirect technique, which is more widely used, an impression is taken using a matched plastic impression post placed in the prepared post hole. When using this technique it is generally inadvisable to have the post and subsequent crown constructed on the same impression.

Preformed These are available in various different forms:

        Parallel, serrated—e.g. ParaPost®.

        Parallel, threaded—e.g. Radix®, Kurer™.

Tapered, threaded—e.g. Dentatus screw. These are the poorest design in terms of stress production and, in the authors' opinion, should not be used. If they are used in small tapered roots they should be cemented 'passively'.

Some of these systems have a prefabricated core on the post whilst with others it must be built up around the neck using resin composite. For the majority of crowns choice is one of personal preference. However, no one system will be versatile enough to cover every eventuality, so it is wise to be familiar with more than one method. Tooth-coloured posts based on ceramic or fibre-reinforced resins (LightPosts™, ParaPosts®, FibreWhite™, and Snowposts®) are increasingly available and the results are promising.

Anterior post and core crowns— practical tips

Some problems and possible solutions

- *Subgingival tooth loss* Either extrude tooth orthodontically or use cast post and core method, extending post into defect in the form of a diaphragm.
- *Insufficient space for separate core and PJC* Construct post crown in one piece with porcelain bonded to labial face.
- *Extensive tooth loss and calcified canal* (e.g. dentinogenesis imperfecta, severe toothwear) Use dentine pins (plus dentine adhesive system) to retain pinned resin composite core for porcelain bonded crown or consider crown lengthening surgery.
- *Perforation of root by post* Apical ⅔—if the post can be removed it is worth trying to encourage the laying down of a calcific barrier by dressing with calcium hydroxide. If successful re-prepare post hole to correct alignment. Alternatively, need surgical approach to cut back excess post and seal perforation with GI or MTA. Coronal ⅓— incorporate perforation into diaphragm preparation and make new cast post and core. Sealing the perforation from an orthograde approach with use of magnification and illumination and MTA is also a useful approach.
- *Loss of post* Check: (i) ? Length adequate. If not, remake with ↑ length. (ii) ? Loose fit or too much taper. Can try sandblasting post and re-cementing with adhesive cement, e.g. Panavia 21. Alternatively, correct and remake. (iii) ? Perforation. Take radiographs in parallax to check, and see above. (iv) ? Root #. Extract.
- *Apical pathology* If post and core, crown and endodontics satisfactory, arrange periradicular surgery. If not, remove and carry out revision endodontic therapy and place new post and crown.

Causes of failure in post and core crowns A survey of failed posts showed that most failed within 1yr, but that a post crown that has survived satisfactorily for 3yrs has a good chance of lasting for 10yrs. Common causes of failure were caries, root #, and mechanical failure of the post.[1]

Removing old posts and cores Unretentive posts may be removed by grasping with Spencer–Wells forceps and twisting. Post removers are available (but C/I for threaded posts) that work by drawing out post using root face as anchorage, e.g. the Eggler post remover. Some proprietary kits, e.g. Masseran, can be used to cut a channel around the post to facilitate removal. In some cases an ultrasonic scaler tip can be used to vibrate the post loose, but heat generation can be a problem.

1 R. Lewis 1988 *BDJ* **165** 95.

Veneers

Indications Mild discoloration (can ↑ success by bleaching first), hypoplasia, fractured teeth, toothwear lesions, closing space, or modifying shape (within limits). Veneers are particularly useful in adolescents, where more extensive tooth preparation may risk exposure.

Contraindications Large existing restorations, severe discoloration, insufficient tooth substance to bond restoration to, and parafunction. Overlapping teeth, pencil-chewing, or nail-biting are relative C/I.

Types

Acrylic laminate veneers No longer used.

Resin composite Useful for the treatment of adolescent patients. Can be made directly or, more commonly, indirectly. Problems are shrinkage, staining, and wear. Average life-span ~4yrs.[1]

Porcelain Better performance and aesthetics than resin composite and long-term follow-up now available.[2] In addition, porcelain is less plaque retentive. They are made indirectly in the laboratory and roughened on their fitting surface by etching or sandblasting. This surface is treated with a silane coupling agent prior to bonding to the etched tooth enamel with resin composite luting cement.

Technique for porcelain veneers

Tooth preparation The veneers are usually 0.5–0.7mm thick, therefore unless deliberate overbuilding is required, the tooth needs to be reduced labially. To guide reduction depth cuts of 0.5mm are advisable. A definite chamfered finishing line will make the technician's job considerably easier and this should be established first. If the tooth is discoloured the margin should be sub-gingival (but still in enamel), otherwise keep slightly supragingival. The finishing line is extended into the embrasures, but kept short of the contact points. Incisally, the veneer can be finished to a chamfer at the incisal edge or wrapped over onto the palatal surface (see Figure 6.1).

An impression of the preparation is taken using an elastomeric impression material in a stock tray and the shade taken with a porcelain shadeguide. Temporary coverage is not usually required (see p. 270).

Try-in Careful handling is necessary so as not to contaminate the fitting surface of the veneer. Do not check the fit of the veneer on the stone cast. The prepared tooth should be cleaned and isolated and then the veneer tried in wet (to ↑ translucency). Minor adjustments are best deferred until after cementation to ↓ risk of #. The effect of different shades of resin composite &/or opaquers and tints can be tried prior to etching to get the best colour match. If several veneers are to be fitted, check them individually and then together to work out the order of placement.

---

1 J. S. Clyde 1988 *BDJ* **164** 9.
2 F. J. Shaini 1997 *J Oral Rehabil* **27** 553.

Placement The fitting surface of the veneer is cleaned with alcohol, dried, and then coated with a thin layer of silane coupling agent followed by bonding resin. The tooth is re-isolated and cellulose acetate strips used to separate from adjacent teeth. After etching, washing, and flash drying, a dentine adhesive system is used. Numerous cementation systems are available, e.g. Calibra®, Nexus™, Variolink®. The resin composite luting cement is placed thinly on the fitting surface of the veneer and the veneer carefully positioned. Excess luting cement should be removed with a brush dipped in bonding resin before curing. Adjustments are made with flame-shaped diamond or multi-blade tungsten carbide bur before polishing. The patient should be instructed in the use of floss.

Porcelain slips are veneered corners or edges used to restore # incisors or close spaces by building out the tooth mesially or distally. Now rarely used as direct placement of resin composite is preferred.

Incisal edge
chamfer

Wrap around
incisal edge

Fig. 6.1 Porcelain veneer preparations.

Dentine bonded crowns

These are full coverage ceramic restorations which are bonded to the underlying dentine. The bond is formed between a dentine bonding agent, composite resin luting material and a ceramic fitting surface which has been made micromechanically retentive by etching. The labial preparation is minimal, but incisal reduction is the same as for other porcelain crowns. They are useful for tooth wear cases or where preparation taper is large or crown height poor. Chair-side fitting is more time consuming than for conventional crowns.

Posterior crowns

Posterior crowns are indicated as bridge abutments; to restore endodontically treated teeth; for repair of tooth substance lost due to caries, wear, or #. Tooth loss due to these causes should first be restored using a suitable plastic restorative material. Prior to preparation replace any doubtful restorations, check vitality and take a pre-operative radiograph.

Full veneer gold crown

Principles

- Remove enough tooth substance to allow adequate thickness of gold, i.e. 1.5mm on functional cusp, 1mm elsewhere, following original tooth contours.
- Wide bevel on the functional cusp (normally buccal—lowers, palatal—upper) for structural durability.
- Convergence of opposing walls <10°.
- Height of axial walls as great as possible (without compromising occlusal reduction).
- Chamfer finishing line.
- Where possible, margins should be supragingival and on sound tooth substance.

Preparation

Occlusal Using a short diamond fissure bur reduce the cusp height, maintaining the original anatomy.

Bucco-lingual With a torpedo-shaped bur eliminate undercuts, retaining 5° taper in cervical ⅔, but usually remaining ⅓ will converge occlusally.

Approximal Using a fine tapered diamond bur within the confines of the tooth, eliminate undercuts at an angle of 5°.

Finishing Round axial line angles and cusps. Check no undercuts and smooth preparation with fine diamonds.

Impressions, 📖 p. 628, and temporary coverage, 📖 p. 270.

Porcelain fused to metal crown

Used where need a combination of strength and aesthetics. Preparation is similar to the full veneer gold crown except that where porcelain coverage is required more tooth substance must be removed. The amount of porcelain coverage must be decided before the preparation is commenced, and the patient consulted at this stage to make sure that they are happy.

Occlusal reduction If it is acceptable to the patient, it is better to provide an all-metal occlusal surface, as less tooth substance needs to be removed. If not and an all-porcelain occlusal surface is required, 2mm will need to be removed from the supporting cusps and 1.5mm from the non-supporting cusps, which will compromise retention in teeth with short clinical crowns and vitality.[1] Porcelain occlusals can also introduce occlusal interferences and wear of the opposing teeth if unglazed.

1 W. P. Saunders 1988 *BDJ* **185** 137.

Buccal reduction 1.2–1.5mm should be removed to provide enough room for the metal and porcelain.

Margins If it is acceptable to the patient, it is better to produce a metal to tooth margin, which will necessitate a narrow collar of metal around the gingival margin. In this case, the finishing line prepared should be a deep chamfer or a bevelled shoulder. If the patient insists on a porcelain to tooth margin then a 1.2–1.5mm shoulder must be produced. Where no porcelain coverage is needed a chamfer finishing line is produced, as for the full veneer gold crown.

Crowning root-filled posterior teeth

Single-rooted posterior teeth can be treated as anterior teeth (📖 p. 246). In multirooted teeth the major problem is the divergence of the root canals. The two most commonly used approaches are:

Direct method Pre-formed posts are cemented into one or more canals. Amalgam may also be packed into the coronal aspect of the root canals (Amalcore technique) and an amalgam core built up, which is the preferred technique. RMGIC or resin composite may also be used. These materials have the advantage that the preparation can be completed at the same visit. A dentine adhesive system should be used with resin composite to enhance retention.

Indirect method A sprue is placed in the least divergent canal and a lubricated post (e.g. SS wire) positioned in the more divergent. A wax pattern (or Duralay) is then built up to form a core. The lubricated post is removed before the pattern is sent to the lab for casting. The cast post (for the least divergent canal) and core is cemented in position, then either Wiptam or SS wire is cemented through the hole in the casting into the more divergent canal.

With either technique a gold shell or porcelain-bonded crown can be used for the final restoration.

All ceramic crowns

These new systems (e.g. Inceram, Empress I and II, Procera, Techceram) are built on high-strength alumina cores and may be used for posterior crowns. Few long-term clinical studies have been completed; although 5-yr data for Procera® is good.[1] Zirconia all ceramic restorations have been introduced recently and appear promising.

Problems with post and core crowns in multi-rooted teeth

- Short or very curved canals: use a sandblasted metal post in conjunction with a metal adhesive system, e.g. Panavia™ 21.
- Subgingival tooth loss: use pre-formed post(s) with amalgam core which is well-condensed into region of defect. Some corrosion between the dissimilar metals may be preferable to extending preparation and impressions below level of amalgam.

---

1 P. A. Brunton 1999 *BDJ* **186** 430.

Bridges

Definitions

Bridge (fixed partial denture) A prosthetic appliance that is permanently attached to remaining teeth and replaces a missing tooth or teeth.

Abutment A tooth which provides attachment and support for a bridge.

Retainer The component that is cemented to the abutments to provide retention for the prosthesis.

Pontic The artificial tooth that is suspended from the abutments.

Connector The component that joins the pontic to the retainer. May be rigid or non-rigid.

Saddle The area of edentulous ridge over which the pontic will lie.

Units Number of units = number of pontics + number of retainers.

Retention Prevents removal of the restoration along the path of insertion or long axis of the preparation.

Support The ability of the abutment teeth to bear the occlusal load on the restoration.

Resistance Prevents dislodgement of the restoration by forces directed in an apical or oblique direction and prevents movement of the restoration under occlusal forces.

Types of bridge

Fixed–fixed The pontic is anchored to the retainers with rigid connectors at either end of the edentulous span. Both abutments provide retention and support. Both preparations must have a single line of draw.

Fixed–movable The pontic is anchored rigidly to the major retainer at one end of the span and via a movable joint to the minor retainer at the other end (Figure 6.2). The major abutment provides retention and support whilst the minor abutment provides support only. This design allows some independent movement of the minor abutment and has the advantage that the preparations need not be parallel.

Direct–cantilever Pontic is anchored at one end of the edentulous span only.

Spring cantilever A tooth-retained, mucosal-supported bridge. The retainer and pontic are remote from each other and connected by a metal bar which runs along the palate. Usually an upper incisor is replaced from the premolars or a molar. It is useful where there is an anterior diastema or if the posterior teeth are heavily restored; however, they are often poorly tolerated. These are rarely used now.

Resin-bonded Retained by resin composite (📖 p. 266).

Compound/hybrid Combination of more than one of above types.

Removable Can be removed by dentist for maintenance.

Types of retainers
- Full coverage crown.
- Three-quarter crown.
- Post-retained crown.
- Onlay.
- Inlay.

All of the above restorations have been used as retainers in conventional bridgework. They are listed in order from most retentive to least retentive. Wherever possible one of the first two should be used, as the failure rate of the last three is much higher. Post crowns should be avoided if possible, and onlays or inlays should only ever be used as minor retainers in fixed–movable bridges.

Selection of abutment teeth
When selecting abutment teeth general factors must be taken into account, such as caries status and existing restorations, but there are two other considerations which specifically relate to bridgework. These are **retention** and **support**.

Assessment of retention
The factors that affect the amount of retention offered by a potential abutment tooth are the clinical crown height and the available surface area. Obviously, the larger teeth offer more retention and should be chosen in preference to the smaller ones. The teeth of both arches are listed below in order of the amount of retention offered (if a full coverage restoration is used).

	Greatest	→	→	→	→	→	Poorest
Maxilla	6	7	4	5	3	1	2
Mandible	6	7	5	4	3	2	1

Assessment of support
Three factors are important:

Crown–root ratio Ideally should be 2:3 but 1:1 is acceptable. As bone is lost so the lever effect on the supporting tissues is ↑.

Root configuration Widely splayed roots provide more support than fused ones.

Periodontal surface area The more of the root that is attached to the bone via the PDL the greater the support offered. At one time great significance was applied to this factor and it formed the basis of Ante's law (1926) which states that '*the combined periodontal area of the abutment teeth must be at least as great as that of the teeth being replaced*', Ante's law has no scientific basis and no longer has a place in contemporary bridgework design. It does not take into account that we are dealing with a biological system—as the load is ↑ on the abutment teeth a biofeedback mechanism operates to cause a reduction in this load.

The teeth of both arches are listed below in order of the amount of support offered, assuming that the periodontal tissues are intact.

	Greatest	→	→	→	→	→	Poorest
Maxilla	6	7	3	4	5	1	2
Mandible	6	7	3	5	4	2	1

Taper and parallelism

- Opposing walls of abutments should have 5° taper.
- For most designs abutments should be prepared with a common line of draw.
- Checking parallelism: direct vision, with one eye; survey mirror with parallel lines inscribed.
- Management of tilted abutments, p. 261.

Types of pontic

Ridge lap As name suggests, this type of pontic should make (minimal) contact with buccal aspect of ridge. Gives good aesthetics and is the most popular type.

Hygienic Does not contact saddle, therefore easy to clean. Unaesthetic, therefore limited to molar replacement.

Bullet Makes point contact with tip of ridge.

Saddle Extends over ridge buccally and lingually, therefore difficult to clean. Should not be used.

Fig. 6.2 Fixed movable bridge replacing the lower left first permanent molar.

Bridges—treatment planning and design

Treatment planning

First consider whether benefits of replacing missing teeth (improved aesthetics, occlusal stability, mastication, and speech) outweigh disadvantages (↑ oral stagnation, tooth preparation, cost). Do not forget to consider implants or shortened dental arch therapy. If replacement is indicated ? fixed or removable prosthesis. A number of factors affect this decision:

General	Local
Patient's motivation/condition	OH and periodontal health
Age	Number of missing teeth
Health	Position of missing teeth
Occupation	Occlusion
Cost	Condition of abutments
	Length of span
	Degree of resorption

These factors need to be favourable if expensive and complex bridgework is required. Removable prostheses are indicated if general or local factors are less than ideal (📖 p. 294). Remember that removable prostheses can be more harmful than fixed partial dentures.[1]

Designing bridges

- Assess prognosis of all teeth in vicinity to reduce risk of another tooth requiring extraction in near future.
- Assess possible abutment teeth (check restorations, vitality, periodontal condition, mobility, and take periapical radiographs).
- Select design of retainers, e.g. full or partial crown. Full coverage is to be preferred.
- Consider pontics and connectors.
- With this information compile a list of possible designs for bridge.
- Consideration of the advantages and disadvantages of each design combined perhaps with a diagnostic wax-up should help to narrow down the choice. Where possible try the least destructive alternative first.

Specific design problems

Periodontally involved abutments First control periodontal disease. Then ? bridge indicated. Fixed–fixed type of design preferable to splint teeth together. Consider fibre-reinforced resin composite fixed partial dentures for this specific indication.

---

1 E. Budtz-Jorgensen 1990 *J Prosthet Dent* **64** 42.

Pier abutments This is the central abutment in a complex bridge that supports pontics on either side, which are in turn anchored to the terminal abutments. In this situation the pier abutment can act as a fulcrum and when one part of the bridge is loaded the retainer at the other end experiences an unseating force which can lead to cementation failure. To overcome this a stress-breaking element must be introduced, e.g. fixed–movable joint, or avoid pier abutments by simplifying the design.

Tilted abutments This occurs most commonly following loss of a molar. There are several approaches:
- Orthodontic treatment to upright abutments.
- Two-part bridge, e.g. fixed–movable.
- Telescopic crowns—placement of individual gold shell crowns on abutments, over which telescopic sleeves of bridge fit.
- Partial veneer preparations in which pins or slots are prepared to compensate for slight malalignment of abutments (least satisfactory).
- Precision attachments—a precision screw and screw tube can be incorporated into a two-part bridge. After cementation the screw is inserted, which effectively converts the bridge to a fixed–fixed design.

Canines The canine is often the keystone of the arch, and a very difficult tooth to replace. The adjacent teeth are poor in terms of the amount of retention and support that they offer and the canine is often subject to enormous stresses in lateral excursion (in a canine-guided occlusion). If a canine is to be replaced with a bridge the occlusal scheme should be designed to provide group function in lateral excursion—never canine guidance.

Bridges—practical stages

1) Take a **history**—Why is a bridge necessary? When and why was tooth lost? Remember the medical history, dental history and social history.

2) Carry out a **clinical examination**—EO look for signs of TMPDS. IO look at the general condition of the mouth, the length of edentulous span, the condition and position of the potential abutment teeth and periodontium. Carefully examine the occlusion and try to formulate some initial ideas on possible bridge designs.

3) Special tests—Radiographs of the potential abutments are mandatory along with vitality (sensibility) tests, accepting their limitations.

4) Diagnostic mounting—Take accurate impressions of both arches, a facebow record and have the models mounted on a semi-adjustable articulator. The mounting can be carried out either in ICP (best fit) or in RCP, for which a precentric record will be necessary. If a reorganized approach to reconstruction is being considered, or if the clinical examination has revealed significant occlusal interferences, an RCP mounting should be performed. Carefully examine the occlusion and consider what occlusal consequences the proposed restoration will have.

5) Diagnostic waxing—In effect, this is a mock-up of the final restoration on the mounted models. Wax can be added to the teeth to simulate the effect that the restoration will have on the final occlusion and aesthetic result. In the anterior part of the mouth a denture tooth can be used. In addition to assessing aesthetics and occlusion the diagnostic wax-up can serve as a template from which the temporary bridge can be constructed. An impression is taken of the wax-up in a silicone putty and saved for later. At this stage the design of the prosthesis must be finalized.

6) Preparations—Before the preparations are carried out any suspect restorations in the abutment teeth are replaced. Preparations are carried out in accordance with basic principles (📖 p. 226) and care is taken to ensure that a single path of insertion is established. When checking for parallelism one eye should be kept closed and the use of a large mouth mirror is very helpful. Custom-made paralleling devices can be used but they are very cumbersome.

7) Temporary bridge—This is normally constructed using the matrix which has been formed from the diagnostic wax-up; in this way the temporary bridge should reproduce the aesthetics and occlusion of the final bridge (if the wax-up was done properly!). The matrix is filled with one of the proprietary temporary crown and bridge resins (e.g. Protemp) and seated over the preparations. After it has set it is removed, trimmed, polished, and cemented with a temporary cement (e.g. Temp bond).

8) Impressions—An impression is taken using an elastomeric material. Ideally all of the preparations should be captured on one impression, but this can be very difficult if multiple preparations are involved. If difficulties are encountered in this respect they can often be overcome by using the transfer coping technique. In this technique acrylic (Duralay) copings are made on dies of the preparations for which a successful impression has been achieved. These are then taken to the mouth and seated on the appropriate tooth, and the impression repeated to capture the other preparations. On removal, the coping will be removed in the impression and the dies can be reseated in the copings and a new model poured around them.

9) Occlusal registration—Under most circumstances the models will be mounted in ICP in the position of best fit, and therefore an occlusal registration will not be necessary. Where numerous preparations have been carried out and it is difficult to locate this position, some form of inter-occlusal record will be necessary. A popular technique involves the use of transfer copings, and is described in the section on occlusion (📖 p. 240).

10) Metal work try-in—If a porcelain fused to metal bridge is being constructed it is advisable to try in the metal work before the porcelain is added. At this stage the fit of the framework can be evaluated and the occlusion adjusted. On occasions it will be found that one retainer seats fully whilst the other does not. This can occur if there has been some minor movement of the abutments since the impression was taken. If this is the case the bridge should be sectioned, and hopefully both retainers will then seat. The two parts are then secured in their new position with acrylic resin (Duralay™) and sent back to the lab for soldering.

11) Trial cementation—The finished bridge is tried in and any necessary adjustments made. The bridge should then be temporarily cemented (with modified Temp Bond®) for a period of a month or so. The advantage of a trial cementation period is that if any further adjustments are necessary they can be carried out outside the mouth and the restoration repolished and reglazed. The patient is instructed in how to clean the bridge (use of Super Floss®).

12) Permanent cementation—After the period of trial cementation the bridge is re-evaluated and the patient asked if they are happy with it. If all is well the bridge is removed and cemented with a permanent cement (usually traditional or RMGIC).

13) Follow-up—Arrangements are made to recall the patient to check that the bridge is still functioning satisfactorily.

Bridge failures

Most common reasons

- Loss of retention.
- Mechanical failure, e.g. # of casting.
- Problems with abutment teeth, e.g. secondary caries, periodontal disease, loss of vitality.

Management of failures

Depending upon type and extent of problem:
- Keep under review.
- Adjust or repair *in situ*.
- Replace.

Replacement

Before replacement of a bridge is embarked upon, a careful analysis of the reasons for failure is necessary. Minor problems in an otherwise satisfactory bridge should be repaired if at all possible. Fractured porcelain can be repaired with one of the specialized repair kits available (e.g. CoJet™). Secondary caries or marginal deficiencies, if small, can be restored with traditional GI cement.

A survey of bridges placed by GDPs in Sweden found that 93.3% were still in service after 10yrs.[1] The most common reason for failure was loss of vitality. This is not necessarily an indication for removal of the bridge because RCT can often be carried out through the retainer of the abutment.

Removing old bridges

To remove intact, try a sharp tap at cervical margin with a chisel or preferably a slide hammer. Orthodontic band-removing pliers can also be used but these require a small hole to be cut in the occlusal surface. If only one retainer is loose, support bridge in position while trying to remove it so that it does not bind.

Retainers can be cut through (📖 p. 244), but this will destroy bridge.

---

1 S. Karlsson 1986 *J Oral Rehab* **13** 423.

Resin-bonded bridges

This technique involves bonding a cast metal framework, carrying the pontic tooth, to abutment teeth using an adhesive resin. This type of bridge is almost exclusively used for cantilever adhesive bridgework, i.e. one abutment and one pontic (Figure 6.3). Fixed–fixed designs have been problematic, with one retainer debonding being a common clinical finding. The resin bonds to the abutment tooth using the acid-etch technique and to the metal framework by either mechanical or chemical means.

Classification by:

1) Position: anterior or
            posterior.

2) Retention: Macromechanical: (a) perforated (Rochette);
                          (b) mesh (Klettobond);
                          (c) particular (Crystalbond).
            Micromechanical: (a) electrolytically etched (Maryland);
                          (b) chemically etched.
            Chemical: (a) sandblasted;
                          (b) tin-plated.

Chemical retention to a sandblasted metal surface is now used virtually exclusively. A dual-affinity cement (Panavia 21) is used, which chemically bonds to both enamel and non-precious alloys.

Indications	Advantages
Short span	Cheaper than conventional bridge
Sound abutment teeth	Minimal tooth reduction
Favourable occlusion	No LA required
	Disadvantages
	Tendency to debond especially if tooth preparation is poor
	Metal may show through abutments

Treatment planning as for conventional bridgework. If orthodontic treatment is needed to localize space or upright adjacent teeth, it is advisable to retain with a removable retainer for at least 3 months prior to bridge placement.

Tooth preparation is required to:
- Give a single path of insertion. Provide near parallel guiding planes eliminating undercuts, which allows coverage of maximal surface area for bonding.
- Provide space in occlusion to accommodate bridge. Need at least 0.5mm for wings.
- ↑ retention, e.g. using a wrap-around design (covering >180° of tooth circumference) to resist lateral displacement.
- Mesial and distal grooves enhance resistance form.
- To prevent gingival displacement. A minimal chamfer is recommended.
- Provide axial loading of the abutments—prepare cingulum or occlusal rests.

NB Tooth preparation should usually be confined to enamel, and the framework should be designed with maximal coverage (to ↑ surface area available for bonding).

Technique (chemical method using Panavia™ 21) Following tooth preparation an elastomeric impression of the abutment teeth is taken plus an alginate impression of the opposing arch. At the try-in stage the bridge should be assessed for fit, aesthetics, occlusion, etc., and then the fitting surface thoroughly cleaned with alcohol. Contamination of the fitting surface with saliva must be avoided and cementation is best done under rubber dam. Following etching and washing of the abutment(s), and placement of a dentine adhesive system, the wings of the bridge are coated with Panavia™ 21 and the bridge seated into place and held firmly until set. Use of acetate strips and Superfloss at this stage will clear most of the excess cement and prevent it adhering to the adjacent teeth. The cement must then be covered with a substance known as OxyGuard®, which prevents O_2 inhibition of the surface layer. After 5min or so the rubber dam is removed and any excess cement removed.

Problems
- Dentine exposed during preparation: Use a dentine adhesive system.
- Metal shining through abutments: Cut wings away incisally before cementation or use a more opaque cement. May have to consider conventional bridge or placing veneer on labial surface.
- Debonds: If one flange only, can usually detach other by a sharp tap with a chisel or by using ultrasonic scaler tips. If persistent problem, consider conventional bridge. The trend is for these bridges to be used for cantilevered bridgework and it is not usual for fixed–fixed adhesive bridgework to be prescribed due to problems with unilateral debonding.
- Caries occurring under debonded wings: Remove bridge and repair.

Fig. 6.3 Adhesive cantilever bridgework replacing missing upper canines.

Attrition, abrasion, and erosion

As these rarely occur individually, the term 'toothwear' is preferred. Also called 'non-carious tooth tissue loss' or 'tooth surface loss', but this is often an understatement!

Some toothwear during life is inevitable, but where it has resulted in an unsatisfactory appearance, sensitivity, loss of vitality or mechanical problems, the condition warrants investigation and treatment.

Abrasion is physical wear of a tooth caused by an external agent. Classically, toothbrushes are blamed for the characteristic cervical notches, but it is now believed that other factors may also be operating.[1] Abfraction lesions are now typically thought to be due to flexure of teeth under excursive occlusal loading, possibly coupled with some form of stress corrosion.

Attrition is physical wear caused by movement of one tooth against another. It affects interproximal and occlusal surfaces. ↑ in more abrasive diets and in bruxism. It is often assumed that attrition is greater in patients with reduced posterior support, but no evidence exists to support this.[2] Bruxism ↓ with ↑ age.

Erosion is loss of tooth substance from non-bacterial chemical attack. The incidence of erosion appears to be ↑, but this may be the result of an ↑ awareness of the problem. As the presence of acid results only in demineralization, for loss of tooth substance to occur erosion must act in conjunction with attrition, abrasion, or both. Erosion will be enhanced if the buffering capacity of the saliva is ↓, e.g. in dehydration secondary to alcoholism. Classically, one sees smooth plaque-free surfaces with proud restorations whether the acid is industrial (rare), dietary, or gastrointestinal in origin. The latter may be caused either by gastric reflux, which can be asymptomatic, vomiting (e.g. bulimia, 🕮 p. 517, or pregnancy). Such conditions warrant referral.

Diagnosis From the history, clinical picture and special investigations. As toothwear may be due to a factor which no longer operates, it may be necessary (tactfully) to delve into the patient's past. In a proportion of cases, the aetiology will remain obscure and this will complicate prevention. It is important to establish whether the toothwear is ongoing. If teeth are sensitive, probably yes; however, sequential study models will provide definitive evidence.

Toothwear indices are only of value if reproducible, i.e. used regularly. If interested, see paper by Smith.[3]

1 B. G. N. Smith 1989 *Dental Update* **16** 204.
2 A. F. Kayser 1985 *Community Dental Health* **2** 285.
3 B. G. N. Smith 1984 *BDJ* **156** 435.

Management[1]

- Prevention requires an understanding of the aetiology. However, an explanation of possible exacerbating factors to the patient may help to limit loss even if the exact aetiology is unknown.
- For patients where parafunction is thought to be a contributory factor a splint may be provided for night wear. Hypnotherapy may also be useful.
- Referral to a physician (gastrointestinal problems), psychiatrist (bulimic patient), or restorative specialist (complicated restorative problem).
- Monitoring. Take study models, silicone indices and photos to allow rate of wear to be monitored. Intervention is indicated in cases with an unsatisfactory appearance, sensitivity, or functional problems.
- GI or resin composite restorations may help improve appearance and ↓ sensitivity
- If toothwear is excessive it may not be possible to provide an aesthetic result without ↑ OVD. This can be achieved by direct composite restorations or by indirect restorations. These may be full coverage crowns or bonded onlays. In some cases surgical crown lengthening may be required. If there is sufficient freeway space direct composite resin or dentine bonded crowns may be used to restore the dentition.
- Overdentures may be indicated in cases of excessive toothwear, but are aesthetically less satisfactory.

1 E. A. M. Kidd 1993 *Dental Update* 20 174.

Temporary restorations

Indications
- Protection of pulp and palliation of pulpal pain.
- Restoration of function.
- Stabilization of active caries prior to permanent restoration.
- Aesthetics.
- Maintenance of position of prepared and adjacent teeth.
- To prevent over-eruption of opposing teeth.
- To prevent gingival overgrowth.

Temporary dressings Choice of material depends upon the main purpose of the dressing, i.e. therapeutic or structural, but the dressing must also be capable of promoting a good seal and being readily removed. For palliation of pulpal pain ZOE is indicated. For caries control, a calcium hydroxide liner and traditional GI cement. If the remaining tooth tissue requires support this can be gained using a copper ring or an orthodontic band. The interim seal during RCT is very important, a relatively strong material which prevents microleakage (e.g. GI) should be used.

Temporary crowns Three main types:

Pre-formed: (i) Polycarbonate crown (e.g. Directa), which is trimmed to correct shape and customized by lining with a bis-acryl material (e.g. Protemp™). **NB** roughen the inside of the crown to facilitate retention. (ii) Soft metal alloy crowns (e.g. Ion).

Laboratory made: Advisable if preparing multiple crowns or if temporary crown needs to last for several months while other aspects of treatment are completed. Preferred method for temporary bridges.

Chair-side: This is a versatile technique. Crowns are custom-made using an alginate impression of the tooth taken prior to preparation as a mould. When the preparation is completed, any undercuts should be blocked out with carding wax to prevent the temporary crown material locking in the mouth. The material for the crown is then syringed into the impression around the preparation and re-seated in the mouth. When the initial set has been reached the impression is removed and the temporary left to finish curing before being polished. Suitable materials are Protemp® (a bis-acryl resin) and Trim™ (poly-n-butyl methacrylate). Care must be taken when using the latter due to high exotherm on curing. An alternative technique is to make a duplicate model of the diagnostic waxing. This approach is useful for multiple crowns or where changes are being made to occlusion/aesthetics. Applicable to both anterior and posterior crowns.

If preparing several adjacent teeth, consider linking temporary crowns to aid retention.

Temporary post and core crowns Some systems (e.g. ParaPost®) come complete with temporary posts, otherwise they can be made at the chairside with a suitably sized piece of wire. The length of the post should be adjusted so that it protrudes 2–3mm out of the canal without interfering with the occlusion. A one-piece temporary post and crown is made either by the chair-side method described above or with a polycarbonate crownformer and acrylic.

Temporary bridges The best type is made in the laboratory in acrylic and re-lined at the chair-side. Alternatively, make a chair-side bridge using the diagnostic waxing.

Veneers Temporary coverage is usually not necessary, but if the patient complains of sensitivity tack a temporary composite veneer to the prepared surface by etching two small areas of enamel.

Temporary inlays A light-cured temporary material (e.g. Fermit, Clip) is useful.

Temporary cements The preferred material is Temp bond or similar. Fears about eugenol-containing cements and subsequent use of resin composite materials are unfounded as the etching stage removes residual eugenol from the dentinal tubules.

Pinned restorations

Extensive loss of the crown of a tooth leads to problems with retention of subsequent restorations. In posterior (and occasionally anterior) teeth these can be alleviated by the use of dentine pins although their use is ↓. Pin retention may also be necessary to support the cores of full coverage crowns. Pins ↓ the compressive and tensile strength of amalgam and therefore should not be over-prescribed. A rule of thumb is one pin per missing cusp. Now virtually all pins used are of the self-threading variety, where the pin is carried to the prepared channel in a handpiece. They are usually self-shearing when the correct depth (usually 2mm) is reached. Pins have largely been replaced by bonding of amalgam coupled with the use of auxiliary forms of retention such as boxes and slots, circumferential grooves, and the use of Amalcores in the treatment of non-vital teeth. Retention can be ranked: self-threading >> friction lock > cemented.

▶ Care is required to avoid perforation into the pulp or PDL.

Technique **(self-shearing threaded pin system)**
1) Complete tooth preparation and place lining.
2) Choose pin site: 1mm away from amelo-dentinal junction and pulp and clear of bi- or trifurcation areas. A radiograph may be helpful.
3) Use a small round bur to indent chosen site.
4) Pin channel is then cut parallel to root surface and bur removed whilst still running, then reintroduced to full depth and removed.
5) Line up pin with channel and insert. Pins usually shear off when base of channel is reached. If not, move handpiece to and fro until it does.
6) Check occlusion and if necessary bend pin inwards. An old chisel with a groove cut in it is a suitable instrument.
7) Fit matrix band or copper ring and condense amalgam (or resin composite).

Problems and their management
- Pin perforates into pulp: isolate to prevent contamination with saliva; place hard-setting calcium hydroxide and seal with RMGIC (e.g. Vitrebond). Monitor vitality of pulp.
- Pin perforates into PDL: can monitor; extend preparation margin to include defect and carefully re-site pin (!); or try to smooth off if accessible in gingival crevice.

Pin retention in anterior teeth Following the introduction of the acid-etch technique pins are rarely required in anterior teeth. Pins used to retain resin composite restorations may show through, detracting from the aesthetics, and are rarely indicated. Gold veneer pinledge preparations are occasionally used as bridge abutments. They rely on pins (which are an integral part of the gold casting) for retention and avoid proximal involvement necessary for ¾ crown.

Bleaching

Bleaching provides a conservative solution for mild to moderately discoloured vital or root-filled teeth. Take photos as a pre-operative record or alternatively note shade of tooth, using a porcelain shade-guide.

Vital bleaching

Two methods have been described.

In-surgery or in-office bleaching This uses carbamide or hydrogen peroxide (30–35%) as the bleaching agent. It is caustic, therefore protective eyewear and care is required. Dental curing lights are commonly used to activate the bleaching agent.[1] It is likely, however, that no activation is required.

Home bleaching A gel of 10–15% carbamide peroxide in a soft splint has also been advocated for 'home bleaching'. This is worn for a few hours, typically 8h each day for several weeks, usually two, and is the preferred technique.

'In-office' bleaching technique

1) Apply Orabase™ to gingivae prior to placing rubber dam over teeth to be treated.
2) Polish teeth with pumice.
3) Etch enamel, wash, and dry, although the need to etch has been questioned.
4) Apply the bleaching agent according to the manufacturer's instructions.
5) Wash teeth with copious amounts of water.
6) Remove rubber dam and polish teeth.
7) Advise patient to avoid tea, coffee, red wine, cigarettes, etc., for 1 week and that some sensitivity may occur.
8) Can repeat as required.

Home bleaching technique

1) Take an alginate impression.
2) Ask the laboratory to make a bleaching splint.
3) Fit the splint, dispense the carbamide peroxide (10%), and give instructions.
4) Advise 6–8h treatment per day.
5) Review weekly.

Non-vital bleaching

This provides a conservative alternative to a post-retained crown for the discoloured root-filled tooth. However, it usually only achieves an improvement in shade. There is a tendency for the discoloration to recur over time, therefore warn the patient and over-bleach. Interestingly, it has been shown that the degree and duration of discoloration and the age of the patient do not affect the prognosis for a successful result.[1]

1 R. A. Howell 1980 *BDJ* **148** 159.

Walking bleach technique

1) Place Orabase™ around gingivae of tooth to be treated and isolate with rubber dam.
2) Open access cavity and remove root filling to 2mm below gingival margin (a period probe is a useful guide).
3) Place thin layer of GI cement over root filling to prevent root resorption.
4) Remove any stained dentine within pulp chamber.
5) Clean access cavity with etchant on a pledget of cotton wool and then repeat with alcohol. Wash and dry.
6) Place 35% carbamide peroxide.
7) Seal with a pledget of cotton wool and GI.
8) Review patient after 1–2 weeks and repeat (up to two times) if necessary.
9) Seal access cavity permanently with a light shade of resin composite.
10) Alternatively, after sealing and cleaning access cavity, place 10% carbamide peroxide into pulp chamber and ask patient to change the material regularly through the open access cavity over a 24-h period combined with wearing a tray for simultaneous external bleaching of the tooth (inside/outside bleaching). The tooth is sealed coronally when the patient returns.

Thermocatalytic techniques, where the hydrogen peroxide is heated within the pulp chamber, should no longer be used, as they are associated with the development of cervical resorption lesions.

Root canal treatment

RCT involves the removal of pulpal remnants and cleaning and obturation of the resultant space, in order to prevent or manage microbial proliferation within the root canal system and apical periodontitis.[1]

Indications

- Pulp irreversibly damaged or necrotic &/or evidence of apical periodontitis.
- Elective devitalization prior to further restorative treatment e.g. overdenture.

Contraindications

- Non-functional or non-restorable teeth.
- Insufficient periodontal support.

Preparation for treatment

Pre-operative radiograph Must show the full length of the root(s) and 2–3mm of the periapical region.

Local anaesthesia Should be given at this stage if required

Preparation of tooth Before starting RCT all caries must be removed from the tooth and an interim restoration placed so that it can withstand placement of rubber dam, ingress of bacteria from the mouth is prevented and a stable reference point for measurement of working length is provided. Occlusion may be adjusted to protect the tooth against fracture if necessary.

Isolation Rubber dam use is mandatory to maintain an aseptic environment, protect the patient from toxic materials and prevent inhalation or ingestion of small root canal instruments. Seal may be optimized with use of OraSeal®/OpalDam®.

Access Should be designed to remove the roof of the pulp chamber so that the chamber can be cleaned and the canal orifices clearly seen and should reduce the curvature required to negotiate the apical ⅓ of the canals. This should be balanced with conservation of as much sound tooth tissue as possible (Figure 6.4). The access cavity in anterior teeth should be midway between incisal edge and the cingulum, and in posterior teeth will vary according to the anatomy of the pulp chamber. Lining up a bur with the pre-operative radiograph will help to gauge the depth of preparation. The turbine handpiece should be used to gain initial access, reverting to slow speed for removal of the roof of the pulp chamber and subsequent preparation. When completed the access cavity should have a smooth funnel shape. Proprietary access cavity burs are available. Magnification and additional illumination are helpful.

1 European Society of Endodontology 2006 *Int Endo J* **39** 921.

Extirpation of the pulp Achieved using a barbed broach or fine files. Often the pulp remnants are necrotic and copious irrigation is required for complete removal.

Working length[1] Definable as the distance from a fixed reference position on the crown of the tooth to the apical constriction of the root canal. Remember that the apical constriction is normally 0.5–2mm short of the radiographic apex of the tooth. There are two methods of establishing the working length: (i) involves the use of radiography; a file fitted with a silicone stop and of sufficient size that its tip can be clearly seen on a paralleling radiograph is inserted into the canal prior to taking the radiograph; (ii) uses an electronic device known as an apex locator. This works by measuring electrical impedance with an electrode in the root canal; when the electrode reaches the apical foramen it emits an audible or visible signal.

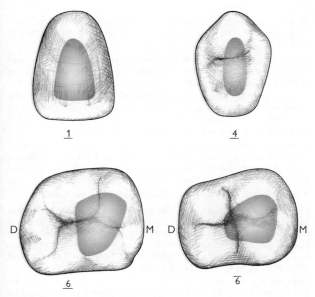

Fig. 6.4 Access cavity preparations.

1 C. J. R. Stock 1994 *BDJ* **176** 329.

Root canal therapy—instruments

It is helpful to make up RCT kits containing the commonly used instruments, e.g. front surface mirror, double ended endodontic explorer, endo-locking tweezers, long-shanked excavator, flat plastic, root-canal spreaders and condensers, and a metal ruler. The whole kit can then be sterilized.

Stainless steel instruments

Broaches These are either smooth for exploring or barbed for pulp extirpation.

K-type-files These are usually used in a watchwinding action[1] or with balanced force which involves using blunt-tipped files and rotating clockwise to bind the flutes into the dentine and then rotating anticlockwise whilst applying an apically directed force to remove dentine. It requires practice to master but is particularly useful when preparing the apical part of severely curved canals.

Hedstroem file Made by machining a continuous groove into a metal blank. More aggressive than K-file. Must never be used with a rotary action as liable to #.

Nickel Titanium instruments (NiTi) Files have traditionally been made from steel, but newer varieties made of NiTi are gaining popularity as they are much more flexible.

Greater taper (GT) Hand files made from NiTi. Unlike standard instruments which have a taper of 0.02, they have a range of tapers (0.06–0.12) with matched GP cones. The flutes of the instruments are machined in reverse so are used in a reverse balanced force method.

Hand Protaper files Have a variable taper over the length of the instrument (like the Eiffel tower!). They are used by hand in either continuous rotations or watchwinding movements. Their sequence of use is the same as for the rotary Protaper series.

Rotary NiTi files There are many different systems on the market.

There are concerns about the ability to effectively clean and decontaminate files after contact with pulpal tissue. It is unclear whether vCJD prions could be transmitted by such instruments. No evidence has yet linked vCJD transmission with endodontic treatment but single use of endodontic files is advised by the Chief Dental Officer due to the theoretical risk of transmission from neural pulpal tissues as in animal models.

Ultrasonic instrumentation
Can be used for shaping but less effective than other methods. Useful for using with irrigation for effective canal cleaning, for assisting with loosening of posts/crowns prior to removal, removing fractured instruments, identifying canal orifices and for apical surgery.

---

1 W. P. Saunders 1997 *Dental Update* **24** 241.

Spiral root fillers May be used to deposit paste materials within the canal, but are liable to #, therefore the inexperienced operator should use them by hand. A preferred alternative is to coat a file with the paste and spin it by hand in an anticlockwise direction to deposit the paste in the canal.

Gates–Glidden burs These are bud-shaped with a blunt end and are used, at slow speed, for preparing the coronal ⅔ of the canal. An 'Orifice opener' works in the same fashion.

Silicone stops These indicate the working length on RCT instruments. Some have a notch to indicate the direction of a curvature.

Finger spreaders These are used to condense the cones of GP during canal obturation. They may be sized to match the GP accessory cones.

Other equipment Sterile cotton-wool pledgets and paper points will be required for drying canals, and a syringe and endodontic needle (gauge 27 or 28) for irrigating them.

The root canal system

The root canal system is complex and radiographically can only be viewed in 2 dimensions. The apical foramina are usually sited 0.5–0.7mm away from the anatomical and radiographic apex. The apical constriction usually occurs 0.5–0.7mm short of the foramina. These distances ↑ with age due to deposition of secondary cementum. Root-filling to the constriction provides a natural stop to instrumentation, thus the working length should be established 1–2mm from the radiographic apex.

Average working lengths (in mm):

	1	2	3	4/5	6	7
Maxilla	21	20	25	19	19	18.5
Mandible	19	19.5	24	20	19.5	18.5

Most canals are flattened mesio-distally, but become more rounded in the apical ⅓. Lateral canals are branches of the main canal and occur in 17–30% of teeth.

NB:

Maxillary

4   74% have >1 canal with >1 foramina.
5   75% have 1 canal with 1 foramen.
6,7 Assume these teeth have 4 canals (2MB; 1P; 1DB) until second MB canal cannot be found.

Mandibular

1,2 >40% have 2 canals, but separate foramina are seen in only 1%.
4,5 May have 2 canals, but these usually rejoin to give 1 foramina.
6,7 Generally have 3 canals (MB; ML; D), but ⅓ have 4 canals (2 in D root).

Some endodontists are using a technique involving maintenance of apical patency, but at present there is little research evidence to support this approach.

Canal preparation

Aims of RCT are elimination of microorganisms and remaining pulp tissue from the root canal system and prevention of reinfection

Aims of chemomechanical preparation. These are twofold, and generally described as *shaping* and *cleaning*

Shaping Aims To produce the ideal shape for effective penetration of irrigant and the reception of the root filling material.

Shaping objectives

Shape
The prepared canal should be a continuously tapering funnel from crown to apex and should maintain the original anatomy. The apical constriction and original canal length should be maintained.

Length
The termination point of the preparation has been controversial. In teeth with vital inflamed pulp bacteria are not present in the apical region of the canal and several authors recommend terminating instrumentation 2–3mm short of the radiographic apex in order to leave a clinically normal apical pulp stump.[1] In teeth with necrotic infected pulp, bacteria may penetrate to the most apical part of the root canal. Therefore length of instrumentation should be the entire root canal.

Apical width
The apical width is gauged with hand files once working length is reached.

Cleaning aims To remove bacteria and organic debris from the root canal. Mechanical preparation alone does not reduce bacterial numbers sufficiently. Antibacterial irrigation is also required.

Cleaning objectives
Flush out debris and eliminate microorganisms, lubricate root canal instruments and dissolve organic debris. The irrigant solution should have broad antimicrobial spectrum and should be active against endodontic pathogens biofilms. They should dissolve pulp remnants and smear layer with no irritant effect on the periradicular tissues. Solution can be delivered gently with a syringe or with ultrasonic or sonic systems. Sodium hypochlorite is an effective irrigant as it is bacteriocidal agent and dissolves organic debris. There is some controversy over the appropriate concentration. It is usually used at 2.5%. It is caustic and should not be extruded beyond the apex. Frequent exchange of fluid and flooding of the root canal system is important as it reduces torque and promotes disinfection. Instrumentation of the root canal wall produces a smear layer.

1 M. K. Wu *Oral Surg Oral Med Oral Pathol Oral Radiol Endod* 2000 **89** 99.

EDTA is a chelating agent which dissolves the inorganic component of the smear layer which sodium hypochlorite cannot do. EDTA solution can be used after instrumentation is complete followed by a final rinse of sodium hypochlorite.

Paste or gel type chelators can be useful for negotiating canal blockages but are not recommended for use with rotary instruments as they can increase torque for some instruments.

Root canal preparation

Current thinking favours the development of shape in a crown-down manner. Preparation of the coronal part of the canal is done first with larger instruments and then working down the root canal with progressively smaller instruments. This principle is adhered to whether hand or rotary techniques are used. The advantages of this are[1]

- Effectively, ↓ the curvature in the coronal part of the root canal, allowing straighter access for files to the apical region. It therefore reduces the likelihood of apical transportation (zipping).
- It allows improved access for the flow of irrigant solution within the canal.
- It reduces the likelihood of apical extrusion of infected material as most of the canal debris is removed before apical instrumentation takes place. This is particularly important because the majority of bacteria in an infected root canal are located in the coronal region.

Can be achieved by using hand or rotary instruments. In either case adequate access is required and the choice of technique, instrument and final preparation size have to be decided for each root canal system. (Figure 6.5.)

Sequence of canal preparation

Following coronal access preparation the root canal orifices are identified. The sequence for canal preparation is as follows:

Preparation of coronal two-thirds of root canal. This can be straightforward in large straight canals but in small curved canals may require coronal pre-enlargement with standard hand files prior to producing straight line radicular access with Gates–Glidden burs or orifice shapers.

Working length determination

Apical third preparation. Preparation to the working length and apical width is now achieved.

Canal patency must be maintained at all times during preparation. This is helped by copious irrigation and frequent recapitulation with small files.

1 M. A. al Omari 1995 *J Endod* **21** 154.

Rotary instrumentation (e.g. ProFile, Rotary GT, Protaper) Rotary instruments are made with nickel titanium, a highly flexible alloy. They are made in a range of tapers (0.02 to 0.12) and tip sizes. There are many different systems on the market and any chosen technique must be carefully learned and practiced. Rotary files are vulnerable to flexural and torsional fracture. They should be used with care in very (especially coronally) curved canals. They are not designed for initial negotiation of canals or for bypassing ledges. Initial hand preparation to a no. 20 ISO instrument and production of a glide pathway is always required. Frequent irrigation is important and recapitulation with a small hand file between each rotary file use helps maintain a glide path. A light touch and slow speed is essential. Apical preparation should be completed by hand.

Common errors in canal preparation
- *Incomplete debridement*: working length short, missed canals.
- *Lateral perforation*: often occurs as a result of poor access.
- *Apical perforation*: makes filling difficult.
- *Ledge formation*: can be very difficult to bypass.
- *Apical transportation (zipping)*: A file will tend to straighten out when used in a curved canal and straightening can transport the apical part of the preparation away from the curvature. The use of flexible files reduces the likelihood of this happening.
- *Elbow formation*: When apical zipping happens, a narrowing often occurs coronal to this in the canal such that the canal is hourglass in shape. This narrowing is termed an elbow.
- *Strip perforation*: A perforation occurring in the inner or furcal wall of a curved root canal, usually towards the coronal end.

Anticurvature filing This was developed to minimize the possibility of creating a 'strip' perforation on the inner walls of curved root canals. It is used in conjunction with other techniques or preparation, and the essential principle is the direction of most force away from the curvature. Filing ratio 3:1 Outer wall: Inner wall.

NiTi rotary instruments reduce creation of blocks, ledges, transportations and perforations by remaining centred within the natural path of the canal.

Inter appointment medication
The objective of medicament placement is to prevent growth and multiplication of microorganisms between visits. Materials used are non-setting calcium hydroxide or iodine-containing pastes.

NB It is essential to place an effective temporary restoration to prevent contamination of the canal system between visits.

Pre-operative   Orifice enlargement

Completed canal

Fig. 6.5 Access cavity preparations.

Canal obturation

Objectives

To provide a three-dimensional hermetic seal to the root canal that will prevent the ingress of bacteria or tissue fluids which might act as a culture medium for any bacteria that remain in the root canal system. In the past, the critical factor was considered to be the achievement of an apical seal, but now it is realized that coronal seal is also important. For this reason the whole of the root canal must be filled, and techniques that only seal the apical region (e.g. silver points) have fallen from favour.

Timing

Root canal filling should be undertaken after completion of root canal preparation and when the infection is considered eliminated and the canal can be dried. There is no evidence to suggest that RCT is more effective, in terms of radiological success between single and multiple visit RCT. Patients undergoing single visit RCT may experience a slightly higher frequency of swelling and are significantly more likely to take painkillers.[1]

Materials[2]

Core materials

- Gutta percha: a form of latex derived from tropical trees.
- Resin based core materials: Resilon a polyester core material.

Both types are supplied as master/accessory points for placement with lateral condensation and as pellets for thermoplastic, vertical condensation techniques.

Sealers

A wide variety is available

- Zinc oxide eugenol bases sealers (e.g. Tubliseal™)
- Calcium hydroxide-based materials (e.g. Sealapex™)
- Resin-based sealers (e.g. AH Plus®), RealSeal® for use with Resilon®
- Silicone-based sealers e.g. RoekoSeal®
- Gutta flow is a material based on Roeko Seal with powdered GP added

Techniques

Numerous techniques have been described; all of those mentioned here use GP.

Cold lateral compaction

This is a commonly taught method of obturation and is the gold standard by which others are judged. The technique involves placement of a master point chosen to fit the apical section of the canal. Obturation of the

---

1 L. Figini, *Cochrane Database of Systematic Reviews* 2007 Issue 4.

2 J. Whitworth 2005 *Endod Top* **12** 2.

remainder is achieved by compaction of smaller accessory points. The steps involved are:

1) Select a GP master point to correspond with the master apical file instrument. This should fit the apical region snugly at the working length so that on removal a degree of resistance or 'tug-back' is felt. If there is no tug-back select a larger point or cut 1mm at a time off the tip of the point until a good fit is obtained. The point should be notched at the correct working length to guide its placement to the apical constriction.

2) Take a radiograph to confirm that the point is in correct position if you are in any doubt.

3) Coat walls of canal with sealer using a small file.

4) Insert the master point, covered in cement.

5) Condense the GP laterally for 20sec with a finger spreader set to within 1mm of working length to provide space into which an accessory point can be inserted. Repeat until the canal is full.

6) Excess GP is cut off with a hot instrument 1mm below the amelocemental-junction and the remainder packed vertically into the canal with a cold plugger.

Warm Gutta Percha techniques

Warm lateral condensation As above, but uses a warm spreader after the initial cold lateral condensation. Special heat carriers can be used with a flame or a special electronically heated device (Touch and heat).

Vertical condensation In this technique the GP is warmed using a heated instrument and then packed vertically. A good apical stop is necessary to prevent apical extrusion of the filling, but with practice a very dense root filling can result. Time consuming. The System B heat carrier has simplified this technique.

Thermomechanical compaction This involves a reverse turning (e.g. McSpadden compactor or GP condenser) instrument which, like an inverted Hedstroem file, softens the GP, forcing it ahead of, and lateral to the compactor shaft. This is a very effective technique, particularly if used in conjunction with lateral condensation in the apical region, but requires much practice to perfect.

Thermoplasticized injectable GP (e.g. Obtura, Ultrafil) These commercial machines extrude heated GP (70–160°C) into the canal. It is difficult to control the apical extent of the root filling, and some contraction of the GP occurs on cooling. Useful for irregular canal defects, e.g. following internal root resorption. Can be used for backfill in combination with System B.

Coated carriers (e.g. Thermafil) These are cores of metal or plastic coated with GP. They are heated in an oven and then simply pushed into the root canal to the correct length after size verification and sealer placement. The core is then severed with a bur. A dense filling results, but again apical control is poor and extrusions common. They are expensive and difficult to remove.

Once the filling is in place the tooth will need to be permanently restored, provided the follow-up radiograph is satisfactory. Fillings that appear inadequate radiographically may be reviewed regularly, or replaced, depending upon the clinical circumstances.

Coronal seal

After completing obturation a good coronal seal must be achieved by place-ment of resin modified glass ionomer on the pulp chamber floor and canal orifices and placement of a definitive restoration. This is now recognized as very important for success in endodontics. Too often good endodontic therapy is jeopardized by a poor restoration that does not provide a good coronal seal.[1]

Follow-up

The tooth should be reviewed clinically and radiographically for 1yr. Suc-cess is indicated by absence of pain, swelling or sinus and the presence of a normal periodontal space. If radiographic assessment shows no change in the size of the lesion or incomplete healing then it should be followed up for 4yrs. If not completely healed by then it is judged a failure.

Failure of endodontic treatment

May present as pain, swelling, discharge, or radiographically as an enlarge-ment of a periapical radiolucency. Following effective RCT most radiolu-cent periapical lesions show signs of resolution within 2yrs.

Failure may be the result of untreated/missed canals, incomplete cleaning of the canals, loss of coronal seal, root fracture, iatrogenic damage. Managed by root canal retreatment, periradicular surgery or extraction.

Cleaning and shaping of the root canal is the single most important factor in preventing and treating endodontic diseases. There is no evidence that any particular root canal filling technique is superior in terms of promoting healing.

1 H. A. Ray *Int Endod J* **28** 12.

Root canal therapy—materials

Irrigants These are required to flush out debris and lubricate instruments. Dilute sodium hypochlorite is generally considered to be the best irrigant as it is bacteriocidal and dissolves organic debris. The normal concentration is 2.5% available chlorine. Chelating agents which soften dentine by their demineralizing action are particularly helpful when trying to negotiate sclerosed or blocked canals (e.g. EDTA paste, File-Eze®, RC Prep™).

Canal medication Some would advocate the routine use of non-setting calcium hydroxide paste (Hypocal™, Ultracal®) as an inter-appointment medicament. It can be very effective in treating an infected canal where there is a persistent inflammatory exudate from the periapical tissues.
- *Antibiotic/steroid paste* (Ledermix) is useful if you are unable to achieve anaesthesia of a hyperaemic pulp. Dressing with Ledermix® ↓ inflammation and may allow pulp extirpation under LA next visit.
- *Iodine-containing pastes* are useful in retreatment cases as certain organisms are resistant to calcium hydroxide.

Filling materials GP, a form of latex extracted from tropical trees, comes the nearest to meeting the requirements of an ideal filling material. It is supplied in cones which come in two forms: *master cones*, sized according to ISO standards; *accessory cones*, sized to match the finger spreaders.

Sealers A wide variety is available. The calcium hydroxide materials (e.g. Sealapex™) or the eugenol-based sealers (e.g. Tubliseal™) are perhaps the safest choice Other sealers based on resin (AH Plus®) and GI (Ketac™ Endo) are available.

Calcium hydroxide Has a wide range of applications in endodontics due to its antibacterial properties and an ability to promote the formation of a calcific barrier. The former is thought to be due to a high pH and also to the absorption of carbon dioxide, upon which the metabolic activities of many root-canal pathogens depend. It is also proteolytic. Indications for the use of calcium hydroxide include:
- To promote apical closure in immature teeth.
- In the management of perforations.
- In the treatment of resorption.
- As a temporary dressing for canals where filling has to be delayed. In the management of recurrent infections during RCT.

Some endodontic problems and their management

Acute periapical abscess Relief of symptoms requires drainage of the abscess and where possible this should be obtained through the tooth under rubber dam. Open the pulp with a diamond bur in a turbine handpiece whilst supporting the tooth to ↓ vibration. Regional anaesthesia and occasionally sedation may be required. Once opened the canal is irrigated with sodium hypochlorite and, if at all possible, resealed. It may be necessary to see the patient again in 24h, but this is more labour-saving long term than leaving the tooth on open drainage. Relieve any traumatic occlusion.

If a fluctuant abscess is associated with the tooth this should be incised. If drainage can be obtained through the tooth and there is no evidence of a cellulitis then antibiotics are not required (p. 370).

Pain following instrumentation This is usually due to instruments or irrigants, or to debris being forced into the apical tissues. Placement of a small amount of Ledermix in the canal may provide symptomatic relief, but care is required not to breach the apex. Occasionally, an acute flare-up of a previously asymptomatic tooth occurs following initial instrumentation—this is called a phoenix abscess. Loss of face is saved by warning patients that this can happen. Affected teeth should be opened and irrigated and if possible resealed. This may need to be repeated after 24–48h.

Sclerosed canals As the incidence of pulp necrosis following canal obliteration is only 13–16%, elective RCT is not warranted.[1] However, where pulp death has occurred finding the canal orifice may be difficult.

If careful exploration with a small file is unsuccessful, investigation of the expected position of the canal entrance with a small round bur or ultrasonic tips may help. Once the canal is found, a No. 8 or 10 file should be used to try and negotiate it, using EDTA-containing File-Eze®, Glyde™ or RC Prep™ as a lubricant, and the canal prepared and filled conventionally. Success rates of 80% have been reported for canals that were hairline or undetectable on radiographs.[1] Occasionally, a total blockage of the canal is encountered, in which case the filling is placed to this level &/or periradicular surgery done.

Pulp stones in the pulp chamber can usually be flicked out. If they occur in the canal use EDTA and a small file to try and dislodge them.

Fractured instruments Sometimes it is possible to get hold of the fractured portion with a pair of fine mosquitos. If not, insertion of a fine file beside the instrument may dislodge it or ultrasonic tips may be used to dislodge; should this be unsuccessful a Masseran kit (p. 248) may be required. Should the fractured piece be lodged in the apical portion of the canal it may be better to fill the canal below it and keep it under observation, resorting to periradicular surgery as a last-ditch solution.

---

1 J. O. Andreasen 1994 *Text book and Colour Atlas of Traumatic Injuries to the Teeth*, Munksgaard.

Immature teeth with incomplete roots, 📖 p. 110.

Removing old root-fillings   If a single-point technique or a root-filling paste has been used removal is straightforward. If a well-condensed GP filling is present this may be softened, using a heated probe to gain purchase for a fine file to be inserted. Rotary NiTi instruments can be helpful. Use of chloroform or oil of cajeput may aid softening and removal. Apical silver points or amalgam may require apical surgery to achieve a satisfactory apical seal if pathology is present.

Perforations   can be iatrogenic or caused by resorption (📖 p. 110). In the latter case, dressing with non-setting calcium hydroxide may help to arrest the resorption and promote formation of a calcific barrier. Increasingly MTA is being used for the repair of perforations and in surgical endodontics as a retrograde filling material with excellent results.[1] Management of traumatic perforations depends upon their size and position:
- *Pulp chamber floor* If small, can cover with calcium hydroxide and fill with GP or GI, but if large, hemisection or extraction may be necessary. MTA can also be used but is expensive.
- *Lateral perforation* If this occurs near the gingival margin it can be incorporated in the final restoration of the crown, e.g. a diaphragm post and core crown. If in the middle ⅓, the remainder of the canal may be cleaned by passing instruments down the side of the wall opposite the perforation. Then the canal can be filled with GP, using a lateral compaction technique to try and occlude the perforation as well. Larger perforations may require a surgical approach and in multirooted teeth hemisection or extraction may be unavoidable.
- *Apical ⅓* It is usually worth trying a vertical compaction technique to attempt to fill both the perforation and the remainder of the canal. If this is unsuccessful periradicular surgery will be required.

Ledge formation If this occurs, return to a small file curved at the apex to the working length and use this to try and file away the ledge, using EDTA or RC Prep™ as lubricants.

Perio-endo lesions, 📖 p. 194.

---

1 M. Torabinejad 1999 *J. Endod* **25** 197.

Four-handed dentistry

Working in a seated position is now the norm for all dentists. This has resulted in the dental nurse taking a more active role by working closely with the dentist. The development of four-handed dentistry is credited to Ellis Paul.[1]

Advantages and disadvantages
- ↑ comfort for dentist and nurse
- ↑ efficiency
- ↑ patient comfort
- ↑ operator visibility
- ↓ backache
- ↑ professional satisfaction for the dentist and dental nurse

Seating the patient Except for the old, infirm or pregnant patient, a totally supine position is preferable. Remember to warn the patient that you are about to whisk them backwards.

Seating the dentist The aim is a relaxed, undistorted, and comfortable posture, with good vision of the teeth to be treated. Adjust the dentist's stool so that the top of their thighs slope at 15° to the floor. Position the dental chair so that, with the operator's back straight, the patient's mouth is at the dentist's focal distance (mid-sternal level). Forearms should slope upwards to this point. The operator's location is between 10 and 11 o'clock relative to the patient's head. Ensure the patient's head is at the top of the headrest.

Seating the dental nurse The dental nurse must also be seated comfortably with a straight back, with their eye level 10cm higher than the dentist's for maximum vision. The dental nurse's normal working environment is at between 2 and 3 o'clock, within easy reach of the instruments and equipment to be used.

Role of the dental nurse
- Receive, seat, and look after the patient.
- Place bib and protective glasses on patient.
- Position dental light.
- Retract patient's lips and protect their soft tissues.
- Aspirate fluids—hold aspirator in right hand.
- Hold 3-in-1 syringe in left hand whilst aspirating.
- Pass instruments to the operator.

Instrument transfer The transfer zone is just in front of, and slightly below the patient's mouth, not over their eyes. There are several techniques which enable the dental nurse to pass and receive instruments effectively from the dentist. All require practice. Each dental team needs to choose, adapt, practise, and perfect a system that safely achieves instrument transfer.[2]

---

1 J. E. Paul 1991 *Team Dentistry*, Dunitz.
2 J. E. Paul 1997 *Fact File: Occupational Back Pain*, BDA.

Prosthetics and gerodontology

Contents

Relevant pages in other chapters Bridges—treatment planning and design, 📖 p. 260; occlusion, 📖 p. 238; acrylic and other denture materials, 📖 p. 640; casting alloys, 📖 p. 630; impression materials, 📖 p. 626.

Principal sources and further reading M. R. Y. Dyer 1989 *Notes on Prosthetic Dentistry*, Wright. J. C. Davenport 1988 *A Colour Atlas of Removable Partial Dentures*, Wolfe. J. F. McCord 2002 *Missing Teeth: A Guide to Treatment Options*, Churchill Livingstone. D. W. Bartlett 2004 *Clinical Problem Solving in Prosthodontics*, Churchill Livingstone.

Treatment planning

Reasons for prosthetic replacement of missing teeth
- Restore aesthetics.
- ↑ masticatory efficiency.
- Improve speech.
- Preserve or improve health of the oral cavity by preventing unwanted tooth movements.
- Improve distribution of occlusal loads.
- Space maintenance.
- Prepare patient for complete dentures.

Disadvantages of prosthetic replacement
- ↑ plaque accumulation/changes in composition.
- Damage to soft tissues and remaining teeth, exacerbated by poor denture design and/or lack of patient care.

Treatment options for the partially dentate mouth
- No replacement of missing teeth. If the benefits of a prosthesis do not outweigh the disadvantages, then replacement is C/I. An occlusion with first premolar to first premolar present in each jaw (shortened dental arch) is usually functionally adequate. Poorly controlled epilepsy is a C/I to dentures.
- Bridges (📖 p. 260) are preferable for short bounded spans in well-motivated patients.
- Removable partial dentures. Indicated for patients with satisfactory OH and whose remaining teeth have an adequate prognosis, or as a training/interim appliance prior to F/F.
- Complete immediate dentures. These are indicated for patients who have already mastered wearing a partial denture and whose remaining teeth have a poor prognosis.
- Extraction of the remaining teeth and provision of a denture after healing has occurred. Avoid if possible as considerable guesswork is involved in the subsequent denture and the chances of the patient coping successfully are ↓.
- In the older, partially dentate patient it is important to assess whether the patient is likely to retain some functional teeth for the remainder of their life-span. If this is improbable, some advocate providing F/F dentures while the patient is still young enough to adapt.

Treatment planning for partial dentures
NB It is important to enquire about previous denture history (just because a patient is not wearing a denture does not mean that they have not had one) and assess the reasons for failure or success. If a patient produces an extensive collection of unsuccessful dentures, unless there is an obvious and easily remedied fault, it is probably wiser to assume that you are unlikely to succeed where so many have failed and refer the patient for a specialist opinion.
- Relief of pain and any emergency treatment.
- History and exam, including a thorough clinical and radiographic assessment of remaining teeth and edentulous areas.

- Unless immediate dentures planned, extract any teeth with poor prognosis.
- OH and periodontal treatment.
- Preliminary design of partial denture.
- Carry out restorative treatment required.
- Modify design if necessary and commence prosthetic treatment (📖 p. 304).

Treatment planning for complete dentures

- Relief of pain and any emergency treatment, including temporary modification of existing dentures, if indicated.
- History and exam.
- Investigation and treatment of any systemic problems.
- Removal of pathological abnormalities (e.g. retained roots), and pre-prosthetic surgery, if required.
- ? rebase (📖 p. 318), copy (📖 p. 326), or construct new dentures (📖 p. 308).

▶ Discussing with the patient the limitations of dentures prior to their construction is more likely to be viewed as explanation, whereas leaving it until after fitting the dentures will be seen as making excuses!

Principles of removable partial dentures

Definitions

Saddle That part of a denture which rests on and covers the edentulous areas and carries the artificial teeth and gumwork.

Connector (major and minor) Joins together component parts of a denture.

Support Resistance to vertical forces directed towards mucosa.

Retainers Components which resist displacement of denture.

Indirect retention Resistance to rotation about clasp axis by acting on the opposite side to the displacing force.

Fulcrum axis Axis around which a tooth- and mucosa-borne denture tends to rock when saddles are loaded.

Bracing Resistance to lateral movement.

Guide planes Two or more parallel surfaces on abutment teeth used to limit path of insertion, and improve retention and stability.

Survey line Indicates the maximum bulbosity of a tooth in the plane of the path of withdrawal.

Free-end saddle An edentulous area posterior to the natural teeth.

Stress-breaker A device allowing movement between saddle and the retaining unit of partial denture.

Gum-stripper A tissue-borne partial denture which can 'sink'.

Dysjunct denture Has complete separation between tooth- and mucosa-borne parts.

Swinglock denture[1] Has a labial retaining bar or flange which is hinged at one side of the mouth and locks at the other.

Sectional denture Made in two or more sections which are then fixed together with screws or other devices.

Classification

Kennedy Describes the pattern of tooth loss (Figure 7.1):
 I Bilateral free-end saddles.
 II Unilateral free-end saddle.
 III Unilateral bounded saddle.
 IV Anterior bounded saddle, only.

Any additional saddles are referred to as modifications (except Class IV), e.g. Class I modification 1 has bilateral free-end saddles and an anterior saddle.

---

1 M. Chan 1998 *Dental Update* **25**, 80.

Craddock Describes the denture type:
1) Tooth-borne.
2) Mucosa-borne.
3) Mucosa- and tooth-borne.

Acrylic versus metal dentures

Approximately 75% of the dentures provided in the UK have an acrylic connector and base. Although metal bases are generally preferred because the greater strength of metal permits a more hygienic design, an acrylic base is indicated for:

- Temporary replacement, e.g. following trauma or in children.
- Where there is inadequate support from the remaining teeth for a tooth-borne denture.
- When additions to the denture are likely in the near future.

However, where financial constraints C/I a metal base, attention to the following may avoid the production of a gum-stripper:

- Wide mucosal coverage to provide maximum support.
- Keep base clear of the gingival margins wherever possible.
- No interdental extensions of acrylic.
- Point contact and wide embrasures between natural and artificial teeth.
- Labial flanges for extra retention and bracing.
- Additional support from wrought SS rests.

Kennedy Class I

Kennedy Class II

Kennedy Class III

Kennedy Class IV

Fig. 7.1 Kennedy classification.

Components of removable partial dentures

Saddles can be made entirely of acrylic or have a sub-framework of metal overlaid by acrylic.

Rests are an extension of the denture onto a tooth to provide support &/or prevent over-eruption. Occlusal rests are used on posterior teeth (usually over either the mesial or distal marginal ridge and fossa) and cingulum rests on anterior teeth. Rests may be wrought or cast; the latter is preferred for strength and fit.

Clasps provide direct retention by engaging the undercut portion of a tooth (Figures 7.2 and 7.3). The action of a clasp must be resisted either by a non-retentive clasp arm above the maximum bulbosity of the tooth or by a reciprocal connector. Clasps can be classified by their position (occlusally approaching or gingivally approaching) or by their construction and material.

Cast (cobalt chrome) clasps are stiff, easily distorted and liable to #. However, provided they are limited to undercuts of 0.25mm, the advantage of being able to cast them as an integral part of a denture framework offsets these drawbacks.

Wrought clasps are usually attached by insertion into the acrylic of a saddle. SS is the most commonly used alloy, but gold clasps are more flexible and easily adjusted (and distorted).

The stiffer the wire the smaller the undercut that can be engaged. This can be offset by reducing the diameter of the wire to ↑ flexibility (but ↑ the likelihood of #) or by increasing the length of the clasp arm (e.g. gingivally approaching clasp). Cast cobalt chrome can be too stiff for occlusally approaching clasps on premolar teeth. The actual design used depends upon:

- Depth of undercut: 0.25mm—cast cobalt chrome; 0.5mm—SS wire; <0.75mm—wrought gold.
- Position of undercut on tooth and relative to saddle, e.g.:
  - High survey line: gingivally approaching clasp or modify tooth shape by grinding.
  - Diagonal survey line, (a) sloping down from saddle: gingivally or occlusally approaching (ring or recurved) clasp; (b) sloping up from saddle: gingivally or occlusally (circumferential) approaching clasp.
  - Medium survey line: as above.
  - Low survey line: modify tooth shape, e.g. with resin composite.
- Position of tooth. Gingivally approaching clasps are less conspicuous and are therefore preferred for anterior teeth.
- Occlusion: adequate inter-occlusal space should be present or created for a clasp arm to cross a contact point between two natural teeth, to prevent occlusal disruption.
- Shape of sulcus: fraenal attachments and alveolar undercuts may prevent use of gingivally approaching clasps.
- Periodontal health: reduced periodontal support requires more flexible clasps to avoid overload.
- Material of denture base. Cast clasp arms are easily cast as part of the framework but for acrylic dentures wrought clasps are more usual.

Connectors

In addition to joining parts of the denture together, the connector can also contribute to support and retention.

P/– connectors

	Patient tolerance	Indirect retention	Support	Comments
Ant. Bar	–	+	–	useful for Kennedy IV
Mid. Bar	+	–	++	C/l torus
Post. Bar	++	+	–	need mucocompression
Ring	–	++	+	
Plate	+	++	++	less hygienic
Horseshoe	+	+	++	useful for multiple saddles

–/P connectors

- Lingual bar should only be used if there is >7mm between floor of mouth and gingival margin to give 3mm clearance from gingivae. Does not contribute to indirect retention. Usually cast. C/l if incisors are retroclined. If insufficient space can use sublingual bar.
- Sublingual bar lies horizontally in anterior lingual sulcus, but opinions differ as to patient tolerance. More rigid than lingual bar.
- Lingual plate is well tolerated and provides good support, bracing, and indirect retention if used in conjunction with rests but covers gingival margins. Can be made of cast metal or acrylic.
- Continuous clasp is really a bar which runs along the cingulae of the lower anterior teeth and is usually used in conjunction with a lingual bar. Poorly tolerated.
- Dental bar is similar to continuous clasp, but of ↑ cross-sectional area and without lingual bar. Useful for teeth with long clinical crowns. Provides support and indirect retention. May not be well tolerated.
- Buccal/labial bar is indicated when the lower incisors are retroclined.

Figures 7.2 and 7.3 show the two most commonly used types of clasp.

Fig. 7.2 Occlusally approaching three-arm clasp.

One arm is the bracing reciprocal arm
One arm is the retentive component
One arm is the occlusal rest

Fig. 7.3 Gingivally approaching T clasp.

Removable partial denture design

P/P design is carried out after assessment of the patient and with reference to any previous dentures (Figure 7.4). A set of accurately articulated study models is essential.

Surveying

Objectives:
- Establish path of insertion.
- Define those undercuts which may be used to retain denture.
- Define those undercuts which require blocking out prior to finish.

If the path of insertion is at 90° to the occlusal plane insertion of the denture will be straightforward; however, where the teeth are tilted or few undercuts exist, an angled path of insertion may be advantageous. Which provides more resistance to displacement during function is controversial.

A survey line can then be marked on the teeth to indicate their maximum bulbosity in the plane of the path of withdrawal. This is done using a dental surveyor.

Design

1. Outline saddles Usually straightforward. If <½ tooth width or if in doubt of the need to replace a missing tooth, omit.

2. Plan support Support can be tooth only, mucosa only, or both. Tooth-borne support (occlusal and cingulum rests) should be used wherever possible, as teeth are better able to withstand occlusal loading and support will not be compromised following resorption. Tooth and mucosa support are inevitable with large or free-end saddles and where plate designs are used. Tissue-only support should be utilized when no suitable teeth are available, and is less damaging in the upper than the lower arch, because of the palatal vault.

Need to assess the role of the denture, length of the saddles, the amount of support required (? denture opposed by natural or artificial teeth), and the potential of remaining teeth to provide support (root area in bone), before a final decision is made.

3. Obtain retention Retention can be:
Direct e.g. clasps, guide planes, soft tissue undercuts, or precision attachments. Of these, clasps are the most commonly used. The best arrangement is to use three clasps as far away from each other as possible. Guide planes help to establish a precise path of insertion and withdrawal. Need be only 2–3mm in length, reducing reliance on clasps.
Indirect This is derived by placing components so as to resist 'rocking' of the denture around direct retainers, e.g. by the position of clasps and rests and the type of connector. Particularly important with free-end and large anterior saddles.

4. Assess bracing required Bracing is provided by the connector, maximum saddle extension, and the reciprocal arms of clasps. Elimination of occlusal interferences ↓ need for bracing.

5. Choose connector After consideration of above. Is there space in the occlusion to accommodate the chosen connector? Where possible the connector should be cut away from the gingival margins.

6. Reassess ?as simple as possible ?aesthetic.

Instructions to technician Should include written details and diagram. Where some confusion may arise over the precise position of a component it may be helpful to mark this directly on the cast. Computer aided design programs are now available.

Some design problems

The lower bilateral free-end saddle (Class I) This presents a particular problem because of a lack of tooth support and retention distally, small saddle area compared to force applied, and distal leverage on abutment tooth in function (which ↑ with resorption). Possible solutions include:

- Maximize indirect retention by placing rests and clasps on mesial aspect of the abutment tooth and using lingual plate design.
- Using a muco-compressive impression of saddle area to ↓ displacement in function. The altered cast technique.
- Use fewer, smaller teeth and maximize base extension.
- RPI system for distal abutment teeth. Mesial **R**est, distal guiding **P**late and mid-buccal **I** bar. During function the saddle moves tissue-ward and rotates around the mesial rest. The plate and I bar are constructed in such a way as to disengage from the tooth and avoid potentially harmful loading.
- Stress-breaker design (advantages more theoretical than practical).
- Use precision attachments (beware of overloading abutments).

Class IV Can sometimes avoid unsightly clasps anteriorly by the use of:
- A flange engaging a labial alveolar undercut.
- A rotational path of insertion[1] utilizing rigid minor connectors that are rotated into proximal undercuts anteriorly.
- Inter-proximal undercuts, which may allow minimal display of clasps—'hidden clasps'.
- An acrylic spoon denture held in place by the tongue.

Multiple bounded saddles A horseshoe design, which utilizes guide planes for retention, may be indicated.

Fig. 7.4 Sectional partial denture.

1 Chow *et al.* 1988 *BDJ* **164** 180.

Clinical stages for removable partial dentures

1. Assessment and treatment plan, 📖 p. 294.

2. Take first impressions These are usually taken using alginate in a stock tray. For free-end saddles modify the tray first with compound or silicone putty.

3. Record occlusion If ICP is obvious the occlusion can be recorded conventionally (📖 p. 240) at the same visit as first impressions. If ICP is not obvious, wax record blocks will be required and a separate visit. Where there are no teeth in occlusal contact, the steps involved are the same as for recording the occlusion for F/F (📖 p. 312). If there is an occlusal stop, but insufficient standing teeth to produce a stable relationship of the casts, the procedure is as follows:

- Determine the OVD and mark the position of two index teeth with pencil.
- Define the occlusal plane using the record block on which this is easiest, e.g. tooth to tooth, tooth to retromolar pad.
- Check the record blocks in the mouth, using the mark on the index teeth as a guide, and adjust blocks if necessary.
- Record occlusion with bite-recording paste.
- Check the relationship of the index teeth on the articulated casts corresponds to that in the mouth.

4. Mounted casts are surveyed and denture designed, 📖 p. 202.

5. Tooth preparation may be required to:
- Accommodate rest seats. Rests need to be >1mm for strength, therefore if insufficient room in occlusion to accommodate this bulk, tooth reduction is required.
- Establish guide planes.
- Modify unfavourable survey line, e.g. ↓ bulbosity.
- Increase retention, e.g. by the addition of resin composite to create undercuts.

6. Record second impressions using a special tray. Alginate is the most commonly used material, but elastomers are preferable for deep undercuts. It is helpful to have a wax try-in before the framework is made. This enables you to confirm tooth position so that the retentive elements for the acrylic are placed appropriately.

7. Try-in of framework
- Check extension, adaptation, and position of clasp, and rests. If casting does not fit, use of correcting fluid may reveal which areas to relieve.
- Check upper and lower separately for OVD and occlusion, and then together.
- Major faults: repeat second impressions.
- Minor faults: adjust at finish.
- Re-record occlusion, if required.
- Select tooth mould and shade.
- Altered cast technique, if required.

8. Try-in of waxed denture
- Check position of denture teeth.
- Check flange extensions/thickness.
- Check OVD and occlusion.
- Check aesthetics with patient and only proceed when patient is satisfied.
- Prescribe post-dam relief areas and management of undercuts.

9. Finish Once any fitting surface roughness is eliminated, the dentures are tried in separately, adjusting undercuts and contacts as required. The extension, occlusion, and articulation are then adjusted if necessary. Give the patient written and verbal instructions, and a further appointment.

Rebasing P/P

Acrylic mucosa-borne dentures can be rebased at the chair-side with self-cure materials, but difficulty may be experienced in removing the denture in the presence of undercuts, and the materials are generally inferior to the original denture base. Alternatively, P/P can be rebased in the laboratory by means of a technique similar to that used for F/F (p. 318). Alternatively, make a new denture. For cast metal dentures an impression can be recorded of saddle area using an elastomer or ZOE, whilst holding denture by the framework. In all cases care must be taken to avoid the introduction of occlusal errors, e.g. ↑ OVD.

Immediate complete dentures

When the remaining teeth have a poor prognosis management depends upon whether the patient is already a partial denture wearer or not.

Rx alternatives for patients with no previous denture experience

- Extract remaining teeth, wait 6 months for resorption to slow, and then construct F/F dentures. A recipe for disaster!
- Extract majority of posterior teeth leaving sufficient only to maintain OVD and occlusal relationship, and then make immediate complete dentures when resorption has slowed.
- Provide partial denture and allow patient to adapt before progressing to an immediate complete denture. The best solution.

Rx alternatives for partial denture wearer

- A 'creeping partial denture' to which teeth are added as required. This allows a gradual progression towards edentulousness and is preferable for the elderly patient.
- Immediate complete denture. This has the advantage that the form and position of the natural teeth can be copied and is said to promote better healing and reduce resorption, but frequent adjustments and early replacement are necessary.
- Overdenture (📖 p. 328); may retain alveolar bone.

Types of immediate complete denture

- *Flanged* Either full or part (extended 1mm beyond maximum bulbosity of ridge).
- *Open face* No flange, artificial teeth sit over (or just into) the socket of natural predecessor.

Flanged dentures are preferable as they afford better retention and make subsequent rebasing easier. However, where a deep labial undercut exists into which it would be impossible to extend a flange, the choice is either surgical reduction or an open-face denture. Most patients choose the latter.

Clinical procedures

1) *Assessment* Warn the patient about the effects of resorption and the need for early rebasing/replacement.
2) *Primary impressions* (as for P/P, 📖 p. 304).
3) *Secondary impressions* in alginate or silicone.
4) *Recording occlusion.* Where there are sufficient posterior teeth remaining a wax wafer should suffice, and this can be taken at the same visit as impressions are recorded. Otherwise, record blocks will be required.
5) *Try-in* This will be limited to those teeth that are already missing. Check fit, extension, and stability, etc. In addition, need to prescribe:
   - type of flange required;
   - any proposed changes in position of anterior artificial teeth compared to natural teeth.
6) *Extraction* of remaining teeth as atraumatically as possible.

7) *Finish* Repeated removal and insertion of the denture should be avoided, therefore adjustments should be limited to making the patient comfortable. They should be instructed not to remove the denture before the review appointment in 24h.

- *Review* The fitting and occlusal surfaces are adjusted as required. If dentures are unretentive they will require temporary reline (see below).
- *Recall* Regular inspection of immediate dentures is important as rapid bone resorption means that they will require rebasing early. However, this should be deferred, if feasible, for at least 3 months after the extractions. A possible regimen is 1 week, 1 month, 3 months, 6 months, and then yearly.

Laboratory procedures These are similar to F/F except that the plaster teeth are removed and the cast trimmed, before final processing.

Surgical procedures, 📖 pp. 345 and 388.

Problems

- *Denture unretentive* Use a temporary reline material (replaced regularly) to tide patient over initial 3 months and then reline with heat-cure acrylic.
- *Gross occlusal error* Adjust occlusal surface of one denture until even contact attained. This denture can then be replaced after initial resorption has occurred.

Principles of complete dentures

Patient assessment

This should include:
- Previous dental history: including the age of the patient, when they became edentulous, number and degree of success of previous dentures, and their opinion of present F/F.
- PMH: Medical factors can impact upon availability for treatment and ability to cope with dentures. Some drugs may reduce salivary flow.
- Social history: other considerations may affect treatment e.g. transport arrangements.
- EO examination of skeletal pattern and biological age.
- IO examination for signs of any pathology, and an assessment of ridge form, compressibility of mucosa, tongue size, tonicity of the lips, and the volume and viscosity of saliva.
- An evaluation of their present F/F. What to copy and what to correct.
- Personality.

Retention

The resistance of a denture to displacement. Dependent upon: (i) peripheral seal; (ii) contact area between denture and tissues; (iii) close fit; (iv) viscosity/volume of saliva. Neuromuscular control has more to do with stability than retention.

Stability

The ability of denture to resist displacing forces during function. Influenced by forces acting on polished and occlusal surfaces, as well as the form of the supporting tissues.

Neutral zone

The area where the muscular displacing forces are in balance.

Ways to optimize retention and stability

- Maximum extension of denture base (as far as the surrounding musculature will allow). The upper denture should extend distally over the tuberosities and onto the compressible tissue just anterior to the vibrating line on the palate. The lower denture should extend the full depth and width of the lingual pouch, and halfway across the retromolar pad. **NB** Over-extension will result in a denture that is easily displaced in function.
- As close an adaptation of denture base to mucosa as possible, to maximize the surface tension effects of saliva.
- Placement of the teeth in the neutral zone. More important in -/F. The better retention of F/- often allows some latitude in this respect.
- Correct shape of the polished surfaces so that muscle action tends to re-seat the denture.
- A good border seal. This is achieved by ensuring that the flanges fill the entire sulcus width and by placing a post-dam on compressible tissue.
- Balanced occlusion free from interfering contacts.

Common denture faults

These are, in order of decreasing prevalence:[1]

- Lack of freeway space.
- Failure to reproduce closely enough the features of previous successful dentures.
- Occlusal errors.
- Incorrect adaptation and extension.

1 R. Yemm 1985 *BDJ* **159** 304.

Impressions for complete dentures

▶ Tissues must be healthy before final impressions are recorded. If necessary use tissue conditioner in present F/F (📖 p. 318).

Classically, two sets of impressions are recorded of the edentulous mouth. The purpose of the first is to record sufficient information for a special tray to be made in which to record the second or master impression.

Preliminary impressions

These are recorded using an (edentulous) stock tray and alginate, elastomer (both preferable for undercut or flabby ridges) or impression compound. A line should be marked on the impression to indicate to the technician the desired extension of the special tray. In the upper, the posterior limit should be the hamular notches and the vibrating line, and in the lower the retromolar pads.

Special trays can be made in self-cure or light-cure acrylic. The space left for the impression depends upon the material to be used: ZOE = 0.5mm; elastomer = 0.5–1.5mm (depending on viscosity); alginate = 3mm. For trays with >1mm space use greenstick stops clinically to aid positioning.

Master impressions

These aim to record the maximum denture-bearing area, and to develop an effective border seal, the functional width and depth of the sulcus. The special tray should be modified by reducing any over-extension and the peripheries adapted by the addition of greenstick tracing compound. It is important that the trays are not perforated and that you can demonstrate a peripheral seal with the upper tray before you take your impression. Gently manipulate the patient's soft tissues and ask them to slightly protrude their tongue to imitate functional movements.

Muco-compressive versus muco-static A muco-compressive impression technique is sometimes advocated to give a wider distribution of loading during function and to compensate for the differing compressibility of the denture-bearing area, thus preventing # due to flexion. ZOE or composition is used. However, dentures made by this method are less well retained at rest, which is the greater proportion of time. Alginate is said to be more muco-static. Tissue adaptation following a period of use probably reduces the clinical difference between the two techniques.

Special techniques

Neutral zone impression technique This is used for recording the neutral zone in patients with limited natural retention for -/F.
- Record second impressions and occlusion.
- A fully extended acrylic baseplate is made on the lower cast, with wire loops added which do not extend above occlusal plane.
- The upper trial denture or record block is inserted.
- Tissue conditioner is placed on the baseplate and around loops, and inserted.
- Ask patient to swallow, purse lips and say 'Ooh' and 'Eee'.
- The impression is removed and trimmed down until it can be fitted onto the articulator to replace the lower occlusal rim.

- A mould of the impression is made into which wax is poured.
- The wax is cut away so that each denture tooth can be positioned within the zone recorded to make the trial denture. The polished surfaces should replicate the impression.

Flabby (displaceable) ridge Classically occurs under a F/- opposed by natural lower teeth. If mild, then an impression recorded with alginate or elastomer in a tray perforated over the flabby area may suffice. For more severe cases a two-stage technique is required, using a special tray with a window cut out over the flabby tissue. First, an impression is recorded in the tray with ZOE and the paste trimmed away from the flabby area. This is then re-seated and low-viscosity elastomer or impression plaster placed into the window to complete the impression. **NB** Combination type cases should have the dentures constructed on a semi-adjustable articulator to minimize occlusal displacing forces.

Functional impression Tissue conditioner is placed inside the patient's existing denture. After several days of wear a functional impression is produced.

Common impression problems and faults

- A feather edge indicates under-extension. This can be corrected by the addition of greenstick to the tray and repeating.
- Tray border shows through impression material. Reduce tray in the area of over-extension and repeat the impression.
- Air blows. If small, can be filled in with a little soft wax. If large, retake the impression.
- Tray not centred. Often partially due to using too much material so that it is difficult to see what is where. Remember to line up the tray handle with the patient's nose (except for ex-boxers).
- Retching. A calm and confident manner is necessary for successful impressions. Gain the patient's confidence by attempting the lower first and use a fast-setting, viscous material. Distraction techniques may help, e.g. wriggling the toes on the left foot and the fingers of the right hand at the same time (the patient, not the operator!).
- Patient with dry mouth: ZOE is C/I; use elastomer instead.
- Areas where tray shows through in otherwise good impression. Can be overcome by prescribing a tin-foil relief when dentures being processed.

Recording the occlusion for complete dentures

When recording the occlusion with wax rims mounted on rigid acrylic or shellac bases the aim is to provide the technician with information for constructing trial dentures.

As head posture can affect FWS, position the patient so that the Frankfort plane is horizontal. A heated wax trimmer and a heat source are required to adjust the rims.

1) Check fit of bases. If poor, can either repeat second impressions, or take a ZOE or low viscosity elastomer impression with the base and proceed.
2) Adjust upper rim to give adequate lip support.
3) Trim occlusal plane of upper rim.

Position of the occlusal plane This should be placed so that approx 1–2mm (↓ with age) of tooth are visible below the patient's upper lip at rest. The occlusal plane should lie midway between the ridges parallel to the inter-pupillary and the alatragal lines. At rest the tongue should rise just above the lower occlusal plane posteriorly. Centre lines, canine lines and smile line should be marked

4) Trim lower record block to obtain correct lip support and bucco-lingual position of posterior teeth.
5) Adjust lower rim so that it meets upper evenly in RCP, with 2–4mm of FWS.

Vertical dimension The FWS is the space between the occlusal surfaces of the teeth when the mandible is in the rest position. In the majority of patients it is 2–4mm. The OVD for an edentulous patient can therefore be determined by measuring their resting face height and subtracting a FWS. Resting face height is assessed using:

- A Willis gauge, to measure the distance between the base of nose and the underside of the chin. Is only accurate to ± 1mm.
- Spring dividers, to measure the distance between a dot placed on both the chin and the tip of the patient's nose. This method is less popular with patients and is C/I for bearded gentlemen (or ladies!).
- The patient's appearance and speech.

6) Mark the centre lines
7) Locate rims in RCP e.g. with bite-recording paste

Horizontal jaw relationship Record the more reproducible RCP. In the natural dentition, ICP is approx 1mm forward of RCP, some prosthetists advise adjusting the finished dentures to allow the patient to slide comfortably between the two positions.

8) Prescribe mould and shade of artificial teeth for try-in
9) Consider using a facebow registration to mount the maxillary cast on the articulator

Position of the anterior and posterior teeth, Ideally, the artificial teeth should lie in the space occupied by the natural dentition. The extent to which it is possible to compensate for a Class II or III malocclusion depends upon the retention afforded by the ridges. In the natural dentition the upper incisors lie approx 10mm anterior to the posterior border of the incisive papilla.

With resorption this comes to lie on the ridge crest, therefore the artificial teeth should be placed labial and buccal to the ridge, to give adequate lip support and a naso-labial angle of approx 90°.

Posterior teeth should be narrow to ↑ masticatory efficiency. Low cusped teeth are preferred, but cuspless teeth are useful for patients with poor natural retention or a 'wandering' ICP. When considering the colour, mould, and arrangement of the anterior teeth, the patient's age, facial appearance, and most importantly their opinion, must be taken into account. If you disagree about the suitability of their choice, document it.

Type of articulator to be used for setting-up the teeth Most textbooks advocate semi-adjustable or average value articulators for F/F dentures. However, most dentures are made on simple hinge articulators to the satisfaction of the majority of patients, probably because they are able to adapt to the occlusion that results. An average value type will give some degree of balanced articulation which can then be refined in the mouth and will help avoid the introduction of occlusal interferences, and is the preferred method.

Common pitfalls

- Inaccuracies caused by poorly fitting bases.
- Rims contacting prematurely posteriorly and flipping-up anteriorly, or vice versa.
- Failure to provide adequate FWS. This is less likely to occur if the rest position is recorded with only one denture or rim in position.
- Attempting to correct too much when replacing old worn dentures and exceeding the adaptive capacity of the patient.

Trial insertion of complete dentures

Trial dentures are constructed by setting-up the prescribed teeth in wax on acrylic or shellac bases. Both the dentist and patient must be satisfied before the dentures are processed in acrylic.

Clinical procedures

Check the trial dentures

- On and off the articulator. Comparison with the patient's existing dentures is helpful to see if the features to be copied or modified have been successfully incorporated.
- Singly in the mouth. To check extension, stability, and the position of the teeth relative to the soft tissues.
- Together in mouth. Examine vertical dimension, occlusion, aesthetics, and phonetics ('S' sound will be affected by an ↑ or ↓ FWS).

Seek the patient's opinion Some advocate getting patients to sign an acceptance slip before going to finish.

Prepare post-dam This should be placed just anterior to the vibrating line on the palate, which can be assessed by asking patient to say 'Aah'. The degree of compressibility of the tissues is assessed and the depth of the post-dam cut accordingly (usually ~1mm). The post-dam is recorded by marking the master impression with indelible pen and prepared on the upper cast with a wax knife in the shape of a Cupid's bow.

Complete prescription to the technician This should include:
- Any changes in posterior tooth position or anterior tooth arrangement.
- For fibrous undercuts >4mm and bony undercuts >2mm, decide whether they are to be plastered out or the flange thickened for adjustment at finish.
- Tin-foiling for relief of hard or nodular areas, if required.
- Gingival colour and contour.
- Denture base material. This is usually heat-cure acrylic; however, metal bases are indicated for patients with a history of fractured dentures.
- Identification marker, which is preferably legible.

Common problems and possible solutions

- Over-extension of flanges. Reduce.
- Under-extension of flanges. Try a temporary wax addition to flange first, to check effect of extending it. If this is satisfactory a new impression is required.
- Teeth outwith neutral zone. Remove offending teeth and replace with wax which can be trimmed until correct.
- Incorrect OVD. If too small, can increase by adding wax to the occlusal surfaces of teeth, but if too large, will need to replace lower teeth with wax and re-record OVD.
- Occlusal discrepancy or anterior open bite or posterior open bite. Replace lower posterior teeth with wax and re-record OVD.
- Too little of upper anterior teeth visible. Reset anterior teeth to correct position and ask lab to adjust occlusal plane accordingly.

- Too much of upper anterior teeth showing. The effect of reducing the length of the incisors can be judged by colouring incisal region with a black wax pencil and then indicating desired change in position to lab.
- Inadequate lip support. An increase in support can be assessed by adding wax to the labial aspect of the upper try-in.

A new try-in will be required if large errors are being corrected or if any doubt still exists about the occlusion.

Fitting complete dentures

Some adjustment of completed dentures is inevitable following processing. On average, a 0.5-mm increase in height occurs and a slight shift in tooth contact posteriorly. The main steps are:

Adjustment of fitting surface First, smooth any roughness and if necessary gradually reduce the bulk of the flanges in areas of undercut until the denture can be easily inserted without compromising retention.

Check occlusion The vertical dimension of the dentures is maintained by contact between the upper palatal and lower buccal cusps, therefore adjustment of these should be avoided if possible.

- Get patient to occlude and check contact with articulating paper. If contact uneven, or heavy contacts seen, adjust the fossae.
- For cusped teeth only, place articulating paper between occlusal surfaces and ask patient to make small lateral movements and adjust Buccal Upper and Lower Lingual (BULL rule) cusps only to remove any interferences.
- Remove any interferences to protrusive movements.
- Balancing contacts are desirable, but not essential unless they can be established easily by minor adjustments to working side contacts. Some authorities suggest providing even occlusal contact only at the time of fitting, allowing the patient to adapt to their new dentures before trying to achieve balanced articulation.

Advice to the patient Verbal and written instructions should be given.

- Most patients take some time to adapt to their new dentures. During this time a softer diet is advisable.
- If pain is experienced the patient should try to continue wearing their dentures and return for adjustment as soon as possible so that affected areas can easily be seen. If this is not possible they should stop wearing the dentures until 24h prior to the next visit.
- Although patients should be encouraged not to wear their dentures at night, adaptation may be speeded up if they are worn full-time for the first 1–2 weeks.
- When the dentures are not being worn they should be stored in water to prevent them drying out and warping. Plastic denture boxes are cheap, and safer than a glass of water at the bedside.
- Cleaning, 📖 p. 320.

Review The patient should be seen 1–2 weeks after fitting to ease the dentures and adjust the occlusion. Localization of the cause of any irritation due to a flaw on the fitting surface can be helped by:

- Pressure relief cream which is painted onto the fitting surface of the denture.
- Indelible pencil, or denture fixative powder mixed with zinc oxide, which is applied carefully to area thought to be responsible and the denture inserted. On removal the mark will have been transferred to the adjacent mucosa and should correspond with the damaged area.

- If there is no obvious cause relating to the fitting surface remember that occlusal faults can cause displacement and mucosal trauma, and an excessive OVD is a common cause of generalized soreness under -/F (📖 p. 322).

Stress the importance of regular review of all patients with dentures.

Denture maintenance

▶ Review patients with F/F annually. Regular maintenance will help prevent damage due to ill-fitting dentures and will ↑ the likelihood of early detection of oral pathology.

Problems caused by lack of aftercare of F/F As a result of resorption all dentures become progressively ill-fitting, leading to loss of retention and stability. Movement of dentures in function may result in:

- Resorption.
- Predisposition to candidal infection.
- Denture irritation hyperplasia, 📖 p. 388.
- Inflammatory papillary hyperplasia of the palate.

All of these are exacerbated by wear of the occlusal surfaces.

Rebasing

The terms 'rebasing' and 'relining' are commonly used interchangeably. Strictly speaking relining is replacement of the fitting surface (e.g. with a temporary material) and rebasing is replacement of most or all of the denture base.

Rebasing is indicated where the only feature of F/F that requires improvement is the fitting surface; otherwise consider replacement F/F using copy method. For rebasing the material of choice is heat-cure acrylic (📖 p. 642), but this necessitates the patient being without their dentures while the addition is being made. Self-cure acrylic applied at the chair-side appears attractive, but its properties are inferior. For a heat-cure rebase, a wash impression (ZOE or low viscosity elastomer) must be recorded inside the denture.

Technique To avoid an ↑ in OVD, record the impression for one denture at a time.

- Check occlusion and adjust if required. Note OVD.
- Remove undercuts from fitting surface.
- Correct extension and place post-dam in greenstick.
- Apply impression material and insert in mouth. Get patient to close into contact with opposing denture. Check OVD and occlusion.
- Remove and examine impression; if unsatisfactory (or if in doubt) repeat.

An alternative method for inflamed tissues is to record a functional impression (📖 p. 311) over several days with a tissue conditioner, in which case the resulting impression needs to be cast immediately.

Tissue conditioners

These are resilient materials which give a more even distribution of loading and thus promote tissue recovery. They are particularly useful where ill-fitting dentures have caused trauma, as it is important to allow the tissues to recover before impressions for replacement dentures or a rebase are taken.

Technique Relieve any areas of pressure on the fitting surface and reduce any over-extension. A minimum thickness of 2mm is required and the material should not be left for >1 week. Repeated applications may be necessary.

Soft linings are indicated for

- Older patients with a thin atrophic mucosa. Usually for -/F.
- Following prosthetic surgery.
- To utilize soft tissue undercuts for ↑ retention, e.g. following hemimaxillectomy, clefts.

It is wise to make a new denture first in acrylic and adjust the occlusion, before placing soft lining. A minimum thickness of 2mm is required, which may significantly weaken a lower denture necessitating placement of a metal strengthener on the lingual aspect. No material is ideal and soft linings are best avoided (□ p. 642).

Cleaning dentures

When new dentures are fitted the importance of regular, thorough cleaning, especially of fitting surfaces with soap, water, and a brush to prevent the build-up of plaque, stain, and calculus should be emphasized. Unfortunately, few patients are sufficiently diligent, due in part to being conditioned by advertising, to expect to use a denture cleaner.

Advise patients to clean their dentures over a basin of water to act as a safety net.

Formulation	Active ingredients	Problems
Powder	Abrasives, e.g. calcium carbonate	Abrasion
Paste	Abrasives + eugenol	Abrasion + crazing
(Dentu-creme)	Abrasive + phenol oil	Abrasion + sensitivity
Hypochlorite (Dentural)	Sodium hypochlorite	Can corrode metal
Effervescent (Steradent)	Dissolves to give alkaline peroxide solution	Doubts about effectiveness
Dilute acids (Denclen)	3–5% hydrochloric acid or 5–10% phosphoric acid	Can corrode metal
Enzymatic	Proteolytic enzymes	Not widely available

Practical tips

Hypochlorite solutions are effective for acrylic dentures when used overnight, but if used with hot water are liable to cause bleaching, therefore warn patient.[1] The peroxide cleaners are popular but are ineffective if used for only 15–30min as the manufacturers advise.

	Avoid	Use
Viscogel®	Acids, alkaline peroxide	Hypochlorite
Molloplast®	Acids, alkaline peroxide	Hypochlorite
Coe-Comfort™	Hypochlorite, alkaline peroxide	Soap + water
Metal denture	Hypochlorite	Alkaline peroxide
Any denture	Household bleach	

1 C. A. Crawford 1986 *J Dent* **14** 258.

Denture problems and complaints

The most common complaints are of pain &/or looseness, which can be due to denture errors or patient factors. The latter should be foreseen and the patient warned in advance of the limitations of dentures. The wise prosthetist will tend to overestimate the difficulty of providing successful dentures. Unless the cause is immediately obvious, e.g. a flaw on the fitting surface, a systematic examination of the fitting, and polished and occlusal surfaces (including the jaw relationship) should be carried out.

Pain This can be due to a variety of causes, including roughness of the fitting surface, errors in the occlusion, lack of FWS, a bruxing habit, a retained root, or other pathology. Forward or lateral displacement of a denture due to a premature contact can lead to inflammation of the ridge on the lingual or lateral aspect, respectively. With continued resorption bony ridges become prominent and the mental foramina exposed, which can lead to localized areas of specific pain.

Pain from an individual tooth on P/P

- Excessive load &/or traumatic occlusion.
- Leverage due to unstable denture.
- Clasp arm too tight.
- Inadequate lining under amalgam restoration failing to insulate against a galvanic couple with metal denture.

Looseness This more commonly affects the lower than the upper denture.

Denture faults	Patient factors
Incorrect peripheral extension	Inadequate volume of saliva
Teeth not in neutral zone	Poor ridge form
Unbalanced articulation	↓ adaptive skills, e.g. elderly patient
Polished surfaces unsatisfactory	

Burning mouth This can be due to: (i) local causes: e.g. ↑ OVD or sensitivity to acrylic monomer, or be unrelated to the denture (e.g. irritant mouth washes, candidiasis); (ii) systemic causes: e.g. the menopause, deficiency states, cancerophobia, xerostomia.

Speech

Patient's complaint	Possible cause
Difficulty with f, v.	Incisors too far palatally
Difficulty with d, s, t	Alteration of palatal contour
	Incorrect overjet and overbite
s becomes th	Incisors too far palatally
	Palate too thick
Whistling	Palate vault too high behind incisors
Clicking teeth	OVD
	Lack of retention

Cheek biting Check first that teeth are in neutral zone. If satisfactory, ↓ buccal 'overjet', i.e. reduce buccal surface of lower molars (provided normal bucco-lingual relationship).

Retching

- Map out extent of sensitive area on palate using a ball-ended instrument and firm pressure, and check extension of denture.
- Palateless dentures may be a solution, but their retention is poor.
- Training dentures. These can take the form of a simple palate to which teeth are added incrementally, starting with the incisors.
- Hypnosis.
- Implants (📖 p. 330) and a fixed prosthesis.

The grossly resorbed lower ridge Resorption is progressive with time, which is a good argument for avoiding rendering young patients edentulous. The mandible resorbs more quickly than the maxilla, which exacerbates the problem of retention for -/F. Management is dependent upon the severity of the problem and the patient's biological age.

- Minimizing destabilizing forces upon the lower denture, e.g.
  (1) maximum extension of denture base; (2) ↓ number and width of teeth; (3) ↑ FWS; (4) lowering occlusal plane.
- Neutral zone impression technique (📖 p. 310).
- Surgery (📖 p. 388).
- Implants (📖 p. 330).

Recurrent fracture Apart from carelessness, this is usually caused by occlusal faults or fatigue of the acrylic due to continual stressing by small forces. Flexing of the denture can occur with flabby ridges, palatal tori, and following resorption. Notching of a denture, e.g. relief for a prominent frenum, can also predispose to #. Treatment depends upon the aetiology, but in some cases provision of a metal plate or a cast-metal strengthener may be necessary.

Candida and dentures

Candida is a common oral commensal. It becomes pathogenic if the environment favours its proliferation (e.g. dentures, ↑ carbohydrate intake, antibiotic alteration of the bacterial flora) or the host's defences are compromised, 🕮 p. 400.

Denture stomatitis

Also known as denture sore mouth, a misnomer because the condition is usually symptomless. Classically, seen as redness of the palate under a F/- denture, with petechial and whitish areas. 90% of cases due to *Candida albicans*, 9% to other candida, and <1% to other organisms, e.g. *Klebsiella* spp.

Incidence A common condition, having been reported in 30–60% of patients wearing F/F. It affects F more commonly than M, in a ratio of 4:1, and usually affects the upper denture-bearing area only.

Aetiology is still not completely understood.
- Infection with *Candida* spp.
- Poor denture hygiene.
- Night-time wear of dentures.
- Trauma is often cited as a contributing factor to denture stomatitis, BUT
  - it occurs more commonly under F/- than -/F;
  - it can affect patients wearing F/- only;
  - it is also found under well-fitting orthodontic appliances.
- Systemic factors can predispose to candida infection, e.g. iron and vitamin deficiency, steroids, drugs which cause xerostomia, and endocrine abnormalities.
- A high sugar intake provides substrate for candida to multiply.

Management
- Patients should be encouraged to remove their dentures at night.
- They should cleanse denture thoroughly e.g. brushing fitting surface and soaking in hypochlorite cleanser.
- New dentures may be required if these measures fail despite good compliance. The denture can act as a reservoir for candida.
- Reduce sugar intake.
- Miconazole gel can be added to the fitting surface of the denture before insertion or nystatin pastille (1 pastille qds) can be allowed to dissolve slowly in the mouth but they are less effective at resolving stomatitis.
- If suspect systemic factors exacerbating condition, refer to GMP.
- Coexisting papillary hyperplasia of palate may need surgical reduction.
- Systemic fluconazole may be used in some cases

Angular cheilitis, 🕮 p. 400.

Denture copying

Successful function with complete dentures depends to a marked degree upon the patient's ability to control them. This ability is learnt during a period of denture use. When replacement dentures become necessary, it is helpful if the new appliances require as little adaptation as possible to the existing skills. This is generally considered to be particularly important for the older patient. Not only may skills have been developed over a long period, but also the ability to relearn may be diminished. So-called denture copying techniques provide a more reliable method for provision of replacements.

Treatment planning

Before undertaking treatment it is essential to decide which features of the previous dentures are satisfactory, and which require modification, and by how much. Consider:

- Fitting surface—if this is the only feature that requires improvement, then rebasing is a possibility.
- Polished surface shapes.
- Occlusal surface; jaw relationship; OVD. The effect of an increase in OVD can be assessed by self-cure addition to the existing dentures (occlusal pivots), but remember that this irreversibly alters them.
- Anterior tooth size, arrangement, relation to lips.
- Posterior tooth mould and arch width (relation to tongue and cheeks).

Copying complete dentures

A number of techniques have been described. They vary in the materials used, and these in turn affect the acceptability of laboratory work, and the clinical freedom to incorporate 'corrections'. In general, copies of the old appliances are used as substitutes for record blocks, and as special trays. Typical method:[1]

1. Clinic

- Correct under-extension with greenstick tracing compound.
- Record impressions with silicone putty of polished surface and teeth, using large disposable tray. Complete mould with second mix of putty to record fit surface (use a separating medium—Vaseline or, better, emulsion hand cream).
- Open mould, clean dentures, and return to patient.
- Send putty moulds to laboratory.

2. Laboratory

- Fabricate self-cure acrylic baseplates on the silicone model of the fit surface.
- Pour wax into remaining space.
- After cooling remove completed copy, cut off sprues, and polish.

---

1 R. Yemm 1991 *Int Dent J* **41** 233.

3. Clinic

- Employ the copies ('replica record blocks') to record required changes in denture shapes (see treatment planning), by adding or removing wax. Record working impressions in low viscosity silicone *with adhesive* to aid retention on base.
- Record jaw relationship with 'bite recording paste'.
- Select shade/moulds for new teeth.

4. Laboratory

- Cast impressions and articulate.
- Set-up, cutting away modified replica rims to substitute new teeth (rather like setting up an immediate denture!).
- Wax-up, including borders defined by working impressions.

5. Clinic

- Try-in stage.

6. Laboratory

- Finishing stages as normal.

7. Clinic

- Normal insertion stage (and subsequent review).

Other methods use alternative materials (e.g. alginate for impressions of existing dentures, wax, and shellac to form the copy dentures). Choice will depend on acceptability to both clinic and laboratory. In no instance, however, is an all-wax copy regarded as being acceptable, since rigidity is inadequate for use as an impression tray.

Copying partial dentures for immediate dentures[1]

In patients with successful P/P, for whom extraction of the remaining teeth is planned, the transition to complete dentures can be facilitated by using a copy technique.

Clinic 1 Correct under-extended flanges with greenstick and then take impressions of the dentures with putty in stock trays (see F/F technique). Record an alginate impression of the opposing arch, if no denture is planned for that arch.

Lab 1 Wax/shellac or acrylic replica of partial denture is constructed.

Clinic 2 Use the replica denture to develop the prescription and then record a wash impression inside the base with a light-bodied silicone. Record the occlusion using bite registration paste. Finally, take an overall impression in a stock tray with the modified replica denture *in situ*.

Lab 2 The impression is cast and used as a base for articulating the wax replica with the cast of the opposing arch. The teeth prescribed are then set up, and the wash impression retained in the replica, for the try-in. Try-in and Finish as for complete immediate dentures, 📖 p. 306.

1 J. R. Drummond 1983 *BDJ* **155** 297.

Overdentures

An overdenture (OD) derives support from one or more abutment teeth by completely enclosing them beneath its fitting surface. It can be a partial or complete denture.

Advantages

- Alveolar bone preservation around the retained tooth.
- Improved retention, stability, and support.
- Preservation of proprioception via PDL.
- Improved crown to root ratio, which ↓ damaging lateral forces.
- ↑ masticatory force.
- Additional retention possible using attachments.
- Aids transition from P/P to F/F.

Disadvantages

- RCT probably required.
- To avoid excessive bulk in region of retained tooth (which may compromise aesthetics) denture base may need to be thinned, which ↑ likelihood of #.
- ↑ maintenance for both patient and dentist.
- Roots may be prone to caries.

Indications

- Motivated patient with good oral hygiene.
- Because of ↓ retention and stability of -/F and ↑ rate of mandibular resorption, ODs are particularly useful for -/F or free-end saddle.
- Cleft lip and palate.
- Hypodontia.
- Severe toothwear.

Choosing abutment teeth

- Ideally: bilateral, symmetrical with a minimum of one tooth space between them.
- Order of preference: canines, molars, premolars, incisors.
- Healthy attached gingiva, adequate periodontal support (>½ root in bone), and no or limited mobility.
- Is RCT required and if so is it feasible?

Preparation of abutment teeth

Alternatives include:

- Removal of undercuts only.
- Preparation of crown for thimble/telescopic gold coping.
- RCT, tooth cut to dome shape, and access cavity restored with amalgam or an adhesive restoration.
- RCT and gold coping over root face.
- RCT and precision attachment.

Precision attachments[1] are useful for ↑ retention of dentures or bridges, especially in cases with tissue loss (e.g. trauma or CLP), but they ↑ loading on abutment teeth, and are expensive and difficult to rebase and repair. Usually of two parts, which are matched to fit together. One part is attached to the abutment tooth and the other to the denture. A variety of attachments are available, including stud/anchor (e.g. Rotherman eccentric clip), bar (e.g. Dolder), and magnets.

Since precision attachments require the highest technical skill and are highly dependent on patient and professional maintenance, it is wise to first use a basic OD and then reassess the need for additional retention. Hybrid dentures are partial dentures that utilize precision attachments (either intra- or extracoronal) on the abutment teeth for retention. Implants which are inserted in edentulous areas can be used with precision attachments to increase retention.

Clinical procedures

- Assessment (clinical examination, study models, radiographs, etc.).
- RCT if required.

If abutment preparation is limited to crown reduction:

- The steps involved are as for immediate dentures, with the abutment teeth reduced less on cast than is planned clinically. At the visit during which the final dentures are to be fitted, the abutment teeth are prepared and the dentures relined with self-cure acrylic to improve their adaptation.

If precision attachments or copings to be used:

- The teeth are prepared and an impression of the abutments, including post holes, taken. In the lab, dies are prepared and transfer copings (usually metal) made. The transfer copings are tried on the abutments, and if satisfactory an overall impression is recorded to accurately locate the copings to the remainder of the denture-bearing area. Alternatively, a two-stage technique using a special tray with windows cut out over abutments can be used.
- Regular review (6-monthly) and maintenance is necessary for success.

Problems

The most important are:

- Caries of abutment teeth, therefore need good oral and denture hygiene and topical fluoride, e.g. toothpaste, applied to the fitting surface of the denture. Patients should be encouraged to remove their denture at night.
- Periodontal breakdown.

1 H. W. Preiskel 1984 *Precision Attachments in Prosthodontics*, Quintessence.

Implantology

Implantology is based on the principle of osseointegration i.e. a direct functional and structural connection between a load carrying titanium implant with bone with no intervening connective tissue.

This concept has revolutionized tooth replacement in recent years (Figure 7.5). Successful osseointegration depends on meticulous planning. There is little point in a successfully integrated implant in the wrong place!

Preparation for implants

There are two aspects to treatment planning:

Assessment of suitability for implant placement

Achieved by thorough history, clinical examination of hard and soft tissue availability, periodontal health, dentition, occlusion, available interdental and interocclusal space and mouth opening ability. Smoking and untreated periodontal disease are risk factors for implant placement. Poorly controlled diabetes, immunosuppression, scleroderma, use of bisphosphonates are possible contra-indications to implant placement. Radiographic examination looks at the quality and quantity of bone and adjacent anatomical structures (e.g. ID canal/maxillary sinus), and any bony pathology. All prosthetic options (i.e. no treatment, removable partial denture, fixed bridge or implant) are considered.

Planning of implant position if implant indicated

This uses the 'top down' approach. This means deciding on tooth position first using wax-ups on mounted study models. If there is insufficient bone available in the right place then either bone augmentation is required or other prosthetic options need to be considered.

Bone augmentation may be achieved by onlay grafting, ridge expansion, sinus elevation or distraction osteogenesis. The material used may be autogenous bone or allografts, xenografts (e.g. Bio-Oss®) or alloplastic materials. Barrier membranes (e.g. Bio-Gide®) may be used to support the graft material. Bone morphogenetic proteins may be used as bioactive mediators.[1]

The wax up is used to produce a radiographic stent which is used to help plan the appropriate size and position of implant. A surgical stent is also made to help guide implant placement. Digital implant planning systems (e.g. Simplant) are now available. These allow for 3-dimensional planning and the production of surgical guides.

Placement

Careful technique is required to avoid overheating bone resulting in bone necrosis. There are many implant systems available. Some use a two-stage technique where the implant is buried while it integrates and has to be exposed at a later date. Others are transmucosal while they integrate.

1 M. Esposito 2008 *Cochrane Database Systematic Reviews* Issue 3.

Integration times

Traditionally the time from placement to integration and loading has been accepted as 3 months in the mandible and 4–6 months in the maxilla. There is now some evidence that, in certain circumstances, implants may be loaded earlier than this.[1]

Abutment connection

Once integrated (and, if necessary, exposed) an abutment is connected to the implant. This allows the prosthetic superstructure to be manufactured and connected via the abutment to the implant.

Implant superstructures may be single tooth crown, implant retained bridge or implant retained overdentures.

Follow-up and maintenance

Implant retained restorations need to be carefully maintained by the patient. The implant needs to be followed up long term clinically and radiographically by the clinician. Implant failure may be early or late. Early failure may be due to inadequate site preparation, overheating of bone, infection, premature loading or lack of primary stability. Late failure may be due to overloading or infection (peri-implantitis). Literature shows maintenance of restorations will be an ongoing problem for the implant patient, e.g. #screws, clips, porcelain, acrylic.

Fig. 7.5 Implant placed to replace the upper right central incisor.

1 M. Esposito 2007 *Cochrane Database Systematic Reviews* Issue 2.

Gerodontology

(or Gerodontics or Gerontology)

Definition Dentistry for the elderly. For those who have not reached pensionable age, the elderly is anyone over 65yrs. Others suggest that it is >75yrs of age. Rather than arbitrary cut-offs, biological age should be considered.

Epidemiology Two factors are mainly responsible for the increasing relevance of dentistry for the elderly: an increase in the proportion of the elderly in the population and the improvements in dental health that have resulted in more people keeping their natural teeth for longer. The proportion of edentulous adults in the UK fell from 30% in 1978 to 13% in 1998.[1]

Problems The major overall problems are:
- Age changes, both physiological and pathological.
- Disease and drug therapy (Chapter 11).
- Delivery of care.

Restorative problems include:
- Reduced adaptive capacity; therefore if teeth are unlikely to last a lifetime, the transition to at least partial dentures should be made whilst the patient is able to learn the new skills necessary.
- Age changes in the denture-bearing areas, including bone resorption and mucosal atrophy.
- Root caries, which can occur following exposure of root surfaces by gingival recession, in association with changes in diet, ↓ self-care, and ↓ salivary flow. Details of management are given 🕮 p. 25. Prevention of root caries in susceptible patients is possible using either a topical fluoride mouthrinse, high fluoride toothpaste or fluoride-containing artificial saliva, e.g. Luborant or Saliva Orthana.
- Toothwear (🕮 p. 268) is especially prevalent when partial tooth loss has occurred.
- Pulpal changes, including sclerosis (🕮 p. 290) and ↓ repair capacity.
- Reduced manual dexterity, making OH procedures difficult. Epidemiological studies of the periodontal needs of the elderly population are still sparse and some trends may be masked by a high rate of edentulousness. The available evidence suggests that, although older patients develop plaque more quickly, the need for periodontal treatment ↑ up to middle age, and thereafter the majority can be maintained by regular non-surgical management.

1 M. Kelly et al. 2000 Adult Dental Health Survey: Oral Health in the United Kingdom 1998, HMSO.

Age changes

Age changes are defined as an alteration in the form or function of a tissue or organ as a result of biological activity associated with a minor disturbance of normal cellular turnover.

In general

↓ microcirculation, ↓ cellular reproduction, ↓ tissue repair, ↓ metabolic rate, ↑ fibrosis. Degeneration of elastic and nervous tissue. These result in reduced function of most body systems.

Oral

Oral soft tissues A ↓ in the thickness of the epithelium, mucosa, and submucosa is seen. Taste bud function ↓. With age, an ↑ occurs in the number and size of Fordyce's spots (sebaceous glands), lingual varices, and foliate papillae. Recent evidence suggests that stimulated salivary flow rate does not fall purely as a result of age. However, medications or systemic disease can affect salivary output.

Dental hard tissues Enamel becomes less permeable with age. Clinically, older teeth appear more brittle, but there is no significant difference between the elastic modulus of dentine in old or young teeth. The rate of secondary dentine formation reduces with age, but still continues. Occlusion of the dentine tubules with calcified material spreads crownwards with age.

Toothwear is an age-related phenomenon and can be regarded as physiological in many cases. However, excessive and pathological wear can be caused by parafunction, abrasion, erosion (dietary, gastric, or environmental), or a combination of these factors (p. 268).

Dental pulp ↑ fibrosis and ↓ vascularity mean that the defensive capacities of the pulp ↓ with ↑ age, therefore pulp capping is less likely to succeed. Also ↑ secondary dentine and ↑ pulp calcification.

Periodontium ↑ fibrosis, ↓ cellularity, ↓ vascularity, and ↓ cell turnover are found with ↑ age. Whether gingival recession is pathological or physiological (developmental) is still hotly debated.

Systemic

Immune system A ↓ in cell-mediated response and ↓ in number of circulating lymphocytes leads to an ↑ incidence of autoimmune disease as well as a ↓ in the older patient's defence against infection. Also an ↑ in neoplasia is seen. Steroid treatment for autoimmune disease may complicate dental treatment.

Nervous system Ageing involves both a physiological decline in function and dysfunction associated with age-related disease (e.g. strokes, parkinsonism, trigeminal neuralgia). A ↓ in acuity compounds the problem.

Cardiovascular Hypertension and ischaemic heart disease worsen with age. Anaemia is more common in the elderly. In general, the greatest problems arise when a GA is required, or the practice is on the second floor.

Pulmonary system Lung capacity ↓ with age and chronic obstructive airways disease ↑ in prevalence.

Endocrine system Diabetes is more common.

Muscles ↓ bulk, slower contractions, and less precision of control occur.

Nutrition Poverty, impaired mobility, ↓ taste acuity, and ↓ masticatory function can result in nutritional deficiencies in the elderly. These can manifest as changes in the oral mucosa.

Mucosal disease, which is more common with increasing age

- Oral cancer, 📖 p. 416.
- Lichen planus, 📖 p. 430.
- Herpes zoster is more common with ↑ age due to a ↓ in T-cell function. Neuralgia occurs more frequently after an attack in the elderly.
- Benign mucous membrane pemphigoid, 📖 p. 408.
- Pemphigus, 📖 p. 406.
- Candida is seen more frequently in the older age groups due to an ↑ proportion of denture wearers and ↑ immune deficiencies.

This list is obviously not exhaustive.

Dental care for the elderly

The basis for delivery of care to the older patient has been, and is likely to continue to be, via the GDP.

General management problems

Medical and drug history (Chapter 11) It is wise to check any complicated medical problems with the patient's GMP or physician. Unfortunately, many doctors are only familiar with the dental treatment they have personally received, therefore give details of what is proposed.

Communication with the elderly may sometimes require patience and understanding. Older patients may try to cover up deafness, poor eyesight, and lack of comprehension, so it is better to err on the side of over-stressing an important point or instruction, but avoid sounding patronizing. It is often helpful to enlist the assistance of a relative or friend of the older patient.

Oral hygiene may be compromised by arthritis &/or a stroke. Advise an electric toothbrush or modifying the handle of an ordinary toothbrush to make it easier to grip, e.g. with elastoplast or bicycle handlebar grips. Alternatively, self-cure acrylic can be used to make a custom grip for a toothbrush.

Delivery of care

Dental practice Consideration should be given to:
- Access for a wheelchair or Zimmer frame. Dental practices are required to provide reasonable adjustments to ensure treatment is accessible.
- Timing of appointments; e.g. for a diabetic patient these need to be arranged around meals and drug regimens, and early morning visits are probably C/I for arthritic patients as it may take them a couple of hours to 'get going'.
- Positioning of the patient. Some elderly patients are unhappy to be recumbent in the dental chair. In addition, this position is C/I for those with cardiovascular or pulmonary disease. Adjust dental chair gradually as rapid movement from a flat to upright position can result in postural hypotension.

Domiciliary care An estimated 12–14% of the elderly population is bedridden or housebound to such a degree that they cannot visit their GMP or GDP. Unfortunately, although the dental needs of this group are high the uptake of dental care is low, due to the low priority placed on such care and the difficulty experienced in obtaining it. Hygienists can now make domiciliary visits.
- *Site* The kitchen is probably the most suitable room, with access to water and heat. However, it is wise to defer to the patient should they prefer another location for the improvised surgery. Care must be taken to protect the floor and work surfaces from any spillages.
- *Seating* Where possible the patient should be seated in their wheelchair, or a straight-backed chair placed against a wall with a cushion for additional head support. When a patient is bedridden there

is no choice, but the dentist(s) should take frequent rests from bending over, to prevent back strain.
- *Equipment* The expenditure on this will be determined by the volume of such work undertaken. Portable dental units are available, but costly. However, the outlay could be shared by several practices or PCT. A Mothercare or fishing-tackle box is useful for holding small items.
- *After-care* This is particularly important. It is the dentist's responsibility to ensure that the relatives or carers appreciate the need for good oral and denture care and how to carry it out. In the bedridden, chlorhexidine can be applied to the teeth with cotton swabs.

▶ Take a chaperone.

Key points
- Can treatment be carried out successfully?
- Consider maintenance required by any proposed treatment. Elaborate procedures which fail may leave the patient worse off.
- The objective is to maintain optimum oral function. Sometimes retention of a few teeth can be disadvantageous.
- Medical crises (e.g. a period in hospital) can result in a very rapid change in a previously stable oral state, e.g. rapid caries attack, loss of denture-wearing skill through lack of use.
- Avoid sudden changes in occlusion. The shape/form of dentures should not be changed anteriorly. During restorative work refrain from introducing significant occlusal change. If necessary to extract teeth, do so a few at a time, with additions to existing dentures.

Some clinical techniques of particular value in elderly
- Adhesive restorations, e.g. GI for root caries.
- Acid-etch bridgework is less destructive to abutments and is therefore more fail-safe.
- Gradual tooth loss, with additions to existing P/P, is less demanding of a ↓ adaptive capacity.
- Replacement dentures should be made with careful regard to existing appliances. Use of copying techniques again ↓ amount of adaptation required.
- If recording the occlusion proves difficult, use cuspless teeth.
- Mark dentures with the patient's name.

Oral surgery

Contents

Principal sources and further reading D. Mitchell 2006 *An Introduction to Oral and Maxillofacial Surgery*, OUP. L. Peterson 2004 *Contemporary Oral and Maxillofacial Surgery*, Mosby. J. Pedlar and J. Frame 2001 *Oral and Maxillofacial Surgery: An Objective Based Textbook*, Churchill Livingstone. *Additional background Pathology*: J. Soames and J. Southam 2004 Oral Pathology, 3rd edn, OUP. Third molars: NICE 2000 *Guidance on Removal of Wisdom Teeth*. A. MacGregor 1985 *The Impacted Lower Wisdom Tooth*, OUP.

Principles of surgery of the mouth

The mouth is a remarkably forgiving environment in which to operate, because of its excellent blood supply and the properties of saliva. It is compromised less than could be expected by its teeming hordes of commensal organisms. This does not, however, constitute *carte blanche* for ignoring the basic principles of surgery, although these can and should be modified to suit the nature and the site of the surgery.

Asepsis and antisepsis, 📖 p. 342.

Analgesia Thankfully, nowadays all patients should expect and receive painless surgery, both perioperatively and post-operatively. Analgesia and anaesthesia, Chapter 13.

Anatomy and pathology are the interdependent building blocks of surgery. Know the anatomy and you can understand or even devise the operation. Know the pathology and you know why you are doing it, what can be sacrificed, and what must be preserved.

Access For all minor and certain major oral surgical procedures, access is through the mouth via intra-oral incisions. Extra-oral surgery, Chapter 10.

Incisions for dento-alveolar surgery are full thickness, i.e. mucoperiosteal flaps; for mucosal and periodontal surgery split thickness flaps are raised (📖 pp. 204 and 212). For mucoperiosteal flaps, although the base does *not have* to be longer than its length, this design improves the blood supply to the flap and should be used where this is a concern. Improved access via a large flap, allowing minimally traumatic surgery, virtually always outweighs the trauma of additional periosteal stripping.

Always plan the incision mindful of local structures. *One cut*, at right angles, through mucoperiosteum to bone, is the aim. Do not split interdental papillae. Try to cut in the depth of the gingival sulcus. Raise the flap cleanly, working subperiosteally with a blunt instrument, moving from easily elevated areas to the more difficult (📖 p. 344).

Retraction of the raised flap should be gentle and precise. It is the assistant's duty to prevent trauma to the tissues by sharp edges, overheated drills, or bullish surgeons.

Bone removal by drills must be accompanied by sterile irrigation to prevent heat necrosis of bone, damage to soft tissues, and clogging of the bur. When using chisels to remove bone remember the natural lines of cleavage of the jaws and make stop cuts (chisel technique, 📖 p. 362).

Removal of the tooth/root is carried out using controlled force.

Debridement is removal from the wound of debris generated by both the pathology and the operation. It is as important as any other part of the operation. Subperiosteal bone dust is a common cause of pain and delayed wound healing.

Haemostasis and wound closure are covered on 📖 p. 350.

Post-operative oedema is, to some degree, inevitable; it is minimized by gentle efficient surgery, which is more important than such measures as ice packs and peri- or post-operative steroids, although these can help.

Asepsis and antisepsis

Asepsis is the avoidance of pathogenic microorganisms. In practical terms, 'aseptic technique' is one which aims to exclude all microorganisms. Surgical technique is aseptic in the use of sterile instruments, clothing, and the 'no touch' technique.

Antisepsis is an agent or the application of an agent which inhibits the growth of microorganisms while in contact with them. Scrubbing up and preparation of operative sites are examples of antisepsis.

Disinfection is the inhibition or destruction of pathogens, whereas **sterilization** is the destruction or removal of **all** forms of life. Pre-packaged sterile supplies and the use of an autoclave (121°C for 15min or 134°C for 3min) for resterilizable equipment are the only really acceptable techniques in dentistry. Disinfection using gluteraldehyde or hypochlorite is second choice, for use where true sterilization is not feasible. There are strict restrictions on the use of gluteraldehyde which limit its usefulness outside hospitals. It is not possible to render the mouth aseptic and it is fruitless to try; there are, however, three basic techniques which are of value:

Avoid introducing infection This is achieved by *always* using sterilized instruments, and wearing gloves.

Avoid being infected yourself by the operative site Wear gloves, face, and eye protection.

Reduce the contaminating load to the site By pre-extraction cleaning of teeth, use of chlorhexidine mouthrinse, and prophylactic antimicrobials, when appropriate. There is no evidence base, but it is commonsense.

Cross-infection and its control

Much attention has been focused on this problem in recent years, first with hepatitis B and its related agents, then with HIV, and now with prions. Although screening is possible in some instances, this is of little real value since the majority of individuals with communicable viral particles *are asymptomatic* and hence not identifiable. Therefore safe practice mandates the use of sound cross-infection control as part of everyday practice on *all* patients.

Aerosols are easily created and are a potential source of cross-infection. Minimize wherever possible by high vacuum suction. Wear glasses and a mask if exposure to an aerosol cannot be avoided. Masks are routine in theatre, although of unproven value in preventing wound infection.

Cleaning and sterilizing Use disposable equipment when possible and **never** reuse. Clean instruments prior to sterilization. Use disposable or easily disinfected work surfaces. This book cover can be wiped down!

Gloves should be worn routinely. Sterile gloves for surgery.

Immunization against Hep B is available. Get it and get all staff with clinical contact to do likewise.

Waste disposal It is everyone's responsibility to ensure sharps are carefully placed in rigid, well-marked containers and disposed of by an appropriate service. Dealing with potentially contaminated impressions and appliances, 📖 p. 629. Treatment of the known high-risk patient, 📖 p. 718.

Needlestick injuries If this happens to you, rinse wound under running water and record date and patient details. In hospital, follow local policy; in practice, contact local public health laboratory. DH guidance in the UK recommends universal source testing for Hep B, C, and HIV after an appropriate risk assessment. Antiretroviral 'prophylaxis' post contamination with HIV can help reduce risk of developing HIV-positive status.

Forceps, elevators, and other instruments

Extraction forceps come in numerous shapes and sizes. The choice of forcep is largely down to individual preference or, more frequently, availability. 'Universal' forceps are straight-bladed upper or lower forceps used to grip the roots of teeth to allow a controlled extracting force. 'Eagle beak' forceps are upper and lower molar forceps which engage the bifurcation of molar teeth allowing a buccally directed extraction force. 'Cowhorns' are designed to penetrate the molar bifurcation either to be used in a figure of eight loosening pattern or to split the roots. Most forceps come with a deciduous tooth equivalent.

Elevators used to dilate sockets to facilitate extraction or to remove dental hard tissue by themselves. These are the instruments which should **always** be used to remove impacted teeth. They should be used with gentle (finger pressure) forces. The commonly used patterns are Couplands No. 1, 2, and 3, Cryers right and left, and Warwick–James right, left, and straight.

Scalpel A Bard–Parker handle with a No. 15 blade is the usual.

Periosteal elevators A number are available; the Howarths, originally designed as a nasal rasparatory, is a favourite. McDonalds and 'No 9' are others.

Retractors Tongue, cheek, and flap retractors are needed and are legion in number; Dyson's tongue retractor, Kilner's cheek retractor, Bowdler–Henry's rake retractor, and the Minnesota flap retractor are favourites. Lack's is an all-purpose retractor (really a bent bit of metal)!

Chisels versus burs Depends upon your training. Generally, burs (No. 8 round T-C for bone removal, medium taper fissure TC for tooth division) are kinder on the conscious patient and the best bet for the inexperienced. Chisels are more appropriate in theatre and are particularly useful (3mm and 5mm TC tipped) for disto-angular third molars and upper third molars.

Curettes The Mitchells (no relation) trimmer is probably the most valuable instrument in this category.

Needle holders and sutures vary more than any of the above, depending on your location. The usual suture size for IO work is 4/0; the material may be non-absorbable (silk) or absorbable (Dexon®, Vicryl®). It is difficult to justify the continued use of any non-absorbable IO suture for routine use.

Scissors Remember to keep dissecting scissors, e.g. McIndoe's, separate from suture-cutting scissors, and keep both sets sharp.

Dissecting forceps are designed to hold soft tissue without damaging it; Gillies dissectors are popular. College tweezers are *not* dissecting forceps and are used to lift up sutures prior to removing them.

Aspirator Sterile/disposable suction tip small enough to get into the defect.

The extraction of teeth

The extraction of teeth must be viewed as a minor surgical procedure; therefore the medical history will be pertinent, e.g. bleeding diathesis, etc. More common and specific considerations are the sex, age, and build of the patient. NICE guidelines currently state that patients at risk of bacterial endocarditis do **not** require antibiotic cover. Extractions in children are technically simple; it is the child who is most likely to be a problem, whereas stoical old men who may not bat an eye at the procedure often have teeth aptly described as 'glass in concrete'. Malpositioned teeth present problems of access and isolated teeth, especially upper second molars, tend to be ankylosed. Heavily restored and root-filled teeth can be very brittle. In all these cases a pre-extraction X-ray can help.

Extraction of teeth begins with *positioning* After LA has taken, the patient is positioned supine at the height of the operator's elbow for upper teeth, and sitting with the operator behind for (right-handed dentists) lower extractions on the right and in front for lower extractions on the left. The position is reversed for left-handers, but unfortunately the world seems biased against this group, and many dental chair systems seem to preclude comfortable positioning for them.

Common technique   The socket is dilated either using an elevator between the bone of the socket wall and the tooth or by driving the forceps blades into the socket. The blades of the forceps are applied to the buccal and palatal/lingual aspects of the tooth and pushed either along the root of the tooth or, in certain molar extractions, into the bifurcation. The tooth is then gripped in the forceps and, maintaining a consistent and quite substantial vertical force, the tooth is moved depending on its anatomy:

1, 2, 3 have conical roots—rotate then pull.

4, 5 have either two fine roots or a flattened root—move buccopalatally until you feel them 'give', then pull down and buccally.

6,7 have three large divergent roots—these are moved buccally while maintaining upward pressure, but frequently need a variety of rocking movements before they are sufficiently disengaged to complete extraction.

1,2,3 can usually be removed with a simple buccal movement, but sometimes need to be rocked or even rotated.

4,5 are rotated and lifted out.

6,7 are two-rooted and can usually be removed by a controlled buccal movement. Remember to support the patient's jaw.

Deciduous teeth are extracted using the same principles, but while permanent molars can be removed using forceps which engage the bifurcation, these should not be used on deciduous teeth.

Third molars (📖 pp. 358–362).

As with all operative techniques in dentistry, the doing is worth a thousand words. To become competent there are three golden rules: practice, practice, and practice.

Complications of extracting teeth

Access Small mouths present an obvious, but usually manageable problem. Crowded or malpositioned teeth may need trans-alveolar approach. Trismus, if due to infection, e.g. submasseteric abscess, should be managed in hospital where facilities for external drainage and airway protection are available.

Pain Has the LA worked? Try further LA as regional block, infiltration, or intraligamentary injection. Is it pain or pressure? If pressure, reassure and proceed. If pain and other signs of adequate LA are present, then acute infection is the most likely culprit. Can the extraction wait by using delaying tactics such as draining an abscess? The vast majority can and very few adult extractions really justify a GA.

Inability to move the tooth Don't worry; it happens to us all. Have you got an X-ray? If not, get one and look for: bulbous or diverging roots, very long roots, ankylosis, or sclerotic bone. Do not press on regardless; it will work sometimes but shows lack of consideration and will cost you in time and goodwill in the long run. Most 'solid' teeth have an easily identifiable cause, e.g. diverging roots, and raising a flap and using a trans-alveolar procedure (📖 p. 354) will quickly and easily remedy this.

Breaking the tooth is a common occurrence and may even assist extraction if, e.g. the roots of a molar are separated. More often, unfortunately, the crown #, leaving a portion of root(s) *in situ*. It is quite acceptable to leave small (<3mm) pieces of deeply buried apex, but provide antibiotics, tell the patient, and review. Larger pieces of root must be removed as they have a high incidence of infective sequelae (📖 p. 370).

# of alveolar &/or basal bone Breaking the alveolar bone is relatively common. If # only involves the alveolus containing the extracted tooth, remove any pieces of bone not attached to periosteum and close the wound. Rarely, the alveolus carrying other teeth will be involved, in which case remove tooth by a trans-alveolar procedure and splint remaining teeth (📖 p. 106). Basal bone # is rare; ensure analgesia (LA &/or systemic analgesics) and arrange reduction and fixation (📖 p. 464).

Loss of the tooth Stop and look; in the mouth, is it under the mucoperiosteum or in a tissue space: these can usually be milked out. Look in the suction apparatus. Is it in the antrum (📖 p. 384), through the lingual cortex or even the ID canal? Has it been swallowed or inhaled? Chest X-ray is mandatory if not found.

Damage to other teeth/tissues and extraction of the wrong tooth Prevent by confirming with the patient the teeth to be removed and making careful notes. Plan the operation; do not use inappropriate instruments or ones which you don't know how to use. If the wrong tooth is extracted, replant if feasible and proceed to remove the correct tooth. Tell the patient and make careful notes.

Dislocated jaw Reduce (📖 p. 468); **bleeding** (📖 p. 350); **pain, swelling**, and **trismus** are common sequelae, and discussed on 📖 p. 362.

Bisphosphonate Related Osteonecrosis (BRON) (📖 p. 581); the principle is not to carry out any surgery which requires osteoclast activity for healing on someone taking these drugs. If this is inevitable, explain relative risks to patient and take recommended precautions (📖 p. 352).

Post-operative bleeding

Bleeding disorders are covered on 🕮 p. 492.
Principles of management of post-operative bleeding.
- Support the patient. If hypotensive and tachycardic, establish IV access and replace lost blood volume.
- Diagnose each cause, nature, and site of blood loss.
- Control the bleeding point.

Classically, post-op bleeding is described as: immediate (primary), reactionary, and secondary.

Immediate When true haemostasis has not been achieved at completion of surgery.

Reactionary Occurs within 48h of surgery and is due to both general and local rise in BP opening up small divided vessels which were not bleeding at completion of surgery.

Secondary Occurs ~7 days post-op and is usually due to infection destroying clot or ulcerating local vessels. In practice, bleeding following removal of teeth is common and usually simple to diagnose. The patients are seldom shocked or hypotensive but are often very anxious and nauseated by the taste, smell, and sight of blood, and by blood in the stomach, which is irritant. Bleeding usually comes from one or all of three sources: (i) gingival capillaries; (ii) vessels in the bone of the socket; and (iii) a large vessel under a flap or in bone, such as the inferior alveolar artery. The first two are by far the more common.

Management

Reassure the patient they won't bleed to death. Remove accompanying entourage and get the patient to an area with reasonable facilities. Take a drug history (anticoagulants?). *Wear gloves and apron*: patients often vomit. (If patient has to wait to be seen they should bite firmly on a clean handkerchief or gauze, rolled to fit the area the bleeding seems to be coming from). In good light, with suction, clean the patient's face and mouth, remove any lumps of clot, and identify the source of bleeding. Is it from under a flap? If from a socket, squeeze the gingivae to the outer walls of the socket between finger and thumb; if bleeding stops it is from a gingival vessel. In these cases, LA and suturing are needed. If bleeding continues it is from vessels in bone, which need some form of pack.

Technique

Give LA if needed, and have assistance with suction. If flap involved remove old sutures, evacuate clot, identify bleeding point, and place a tight suture around it. Bleeding should be much ↓; if not, repeat until it is, then close wound and have the patient bite on a swab for at least 15min. If it is a gingival bleed a tight interrupted or mattress suture will compress the capillaries, again followed by a swab to bite on. If bleeding is from the depths of the socket, the clot may need to be removed and replaced by a pack or supported by a resorbable mesh (oxidized cellulose) &/or agents such as tranexamic acid, adrenaline, or epsilon aminocaproic acid soaked into the mesh. If removing clot and packing the socket, remember this will delay healing and predispose to infection, so use BIPP or Whitehead's varnish packs. If all else fails, all the above measures plus a pressure pack, analgesia, a sedative antiemetic, and a night in a hospital bed will do the trick. Patients requiring this degree of treatment should be investigated haematologically and for liver disease.

Suturing

Every dentist should master the basic skills of suturing.

Materials Most sutures are suture material fused to a needle, although threaded reusable needles are used in some countries. Needles may be round-bodied, cutting or reverse cutting. Straight, curved, or J-shaped. Almost all IO work is done with a 16–22mm curved cutting or reverse cutting needle held in a needle holder. Suture material may be resorbable (Dexon®, Vicryl®, or Monocryl®) or non-resorbable (silk, nylon, prolene, or Novafil®). Monofilament suture (e.g. nylon) causes less tissue response than braided (e.g. silk).

Skin is best closed with nylon, prolene, or Novafil®. *Mucosa* and *deep tissues* best closed with an absorbable. *Vessels* are tied off using resorbables, except major veins and arteries, which are transfixed and tied with silk. BSS can be used for skin but must be removed *early*. Suture strength is described as 0 (thickest) to 4/0 (commonest in IO use) to 11/0 (thinnest for microvascular work).

Types of stitch are shown in Figure 8.1.

Suture technique Closure of a wound or incision should, whenever possible, be without tension, by closing deep layers and over supporting tissue. Hold the needle in the needle holder ~⅔ of the way from its tip. Suture from free to fixed tissue taking a bite of 2–3mm on both sides. Leave the sutured wound edges slightly everted in apposition. Except when swaging tissue to bone, e.g. when arresting haemorrhage or when tying vessels, do not overtighten the suture as wound margins become swollen, and you need to allow for this.

Knot tying The two most useful are the square (reef) knot and the surgeon's knot (see diagram).

Instrument tying is easy to learn from a book but needs considerable practice to perfect. The knot is started by passing the suture once (square knot) or twice (surgeon's knot) around the tip of the needle holders; the knot is tightened and then locked by passing the suture around the needle holder in the opposite direction once. It is possible to control the suture tension by completing the knot in three loops instead of two.

Hand tying is invaluable for those wishing to develop surgical expertise or involved in major maxillofacial surgery. It takes a substantial amount of time and practice and is impossible to learn from a book. Get a sympathetic senior to demonstrate.

Suture removal is not someone else's job to be casually forgotten about. Do the stitches need to be removed? In inaccessible sites, difficult patients, or areas in which scar quality is less important, a resorbable suture should be used. An alternative is tissue glue, e.g. Dermabond®, Indermil®. Facial skin sutures should be removed at 4–6 days. When removing sutures use sharp scissors (avoid 'stitch cutters' if you can), lifting up and cutting a bit of suture that has been in the tissue, thus avoiding dragging bacteria through the incision on removal.

Fig. 8.1 A Reef knot. B Surgeon's knot.

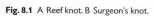

1 Simple interrupted suture.
2 Horizontal mattress suture.
3 Vertical mattress suture.
4 Continuous subcuticular suture.

Dento-alveolar surgery: bisphosphonates

These drugs are mentioned in 📖 p. 581. They constitute a wide group of agents which act primarily by inhibiting osteoclast function which helps prevent fractures in osteoporosis, stabilizes Paget's disease, relieves bone pain and fractures in bone metastases in a range of malignancies and can treat hypercalcaemia of carcinomatosis. Unfortunately one of their side-effects is necrosis of jaw bone, usually (although not always) associated with extractions or dento-alveolar surgery (Figure 8.2). Procedures dependent on bone remodelling (orthodontics) or pathology that causes it (infection, fractures) are also affected.

If asked to render 'dentally fit' someone who is to start bisphosphonates it is probably best to adopt a similar approach to those having head and neck radiotherapy—try to ensure they never need to have a tooth removed in the future. Obviously a balance has to be struck between inappropriately rendering everyone edentulous and the optimistic watch and wait approach that would be usual.

If you have to remove a tooth in a patient on bisphosphonates there will be many instances where patients have been started on these drugs and need teeth removed. If this can be avoided by endodontics, coronectomy etc. then do it. If not, warn the patient of risks (range from <1% for low risk drug in osteoporosis patient to 30% in a myeloma survivor at 10 years). Use prophylactic chlorhexidine and broad spectrum antibiotic, atraumatic extraction and alveolar septoplasty to ensure all bone lies well below gingival margin. This is on the basis that vascularized mucosal coverage will prevent superinfection of bone that will not remodel.

Treatment of established BRON There are no agreed effective treatments to date. Tactics that work for osteoradionecrosis do not seem to help. Limited sequestrectomy coupled with some form of coverage of the exposed bone seems to help and a variety of supplemental drug treatments are being used but there is no established evidence base for this. Refer to your local OMF department.

Fig. 8.2 Clinical example of bisphosphonate related osteonecrosis of the jaws (BRON).

Dento-alveolar surgery: removal of roots

Does the root need to be removed? If large, being extracted for pulpal or apical pathology, is symptomatic, is an impediment to denture construction, or is in a patient in whom risk of minor local infection is not tolerable (e.g. immunocompromised or at risk from IE) then the answer is yes.

Non-surgical methods The use of root forceps or elevators may allow simple removal of roots close to the alveolar margin. When using root forceps ensure the root can be seen to be engaged by the blades. Elevators can be used to direct a root along its path of withdrawal providing (a) one exists, and (b) an elevator can be introduced between bone and root. Do not waste time persisting with non-surgical methods if your initial attempt is unsuccessful.

Surgical methods Plan your operation. Do you know why the root cannot be delivered, exactly where it is, and about any adjacent structures? If not, get an X-ray.
- The flap: if edentulous incise along the crest of the ridge, if dentate in the gingival margin. Flaps may be envelope, two-sided (Figure 8.3), or three-sided. Relieving incisions make reflection of the flap easier but must be avoided in the region of the mental nerve ($\overline{45}$) and are better avoided around the buccal branch of the facial artery (mesial root $\overline{7}$). Include an interdental papilla at either side of the flap and start vertical cuts 2/3 of the way distal to the included papilla. Big flaps heal as well as small ones; the important consideration is access.
- Identify obstructions to the path of withdrawal of the root; these are either removed or the root is sectioned to create another path of withdrawal, depending on which approach is the least traumatic.
- Remove the minimum amount of buccal bone compatible with exposing the maximum diameter of the root and a point of application for an elevator (No. 8 round TC surgical bur).
- Elevate by placing an elevator between bone and tooth (remember to apply to the convex surface of curved roots) and direct the root along its natural path of withdrawal.
- Finally, debride and close the wound.

Special cases
- Small apical fragments: use an apicectomy approach.
- Multirooted teeth: always divide the roots, as this makes life much easier.
- Cannot find the root: re-X-ray and look in the soft tissues. The root may have been displaced into another cavity or even be in the aspirator; look carefully but remember discretion is the better part of valour. Tell the patient.
- Patient refuses operation: it's their body; record your advice and their decision.

Under GA Mallet and chisel can replace bur and the 'broken instrument' technique can be used. This involves using a straight instrument or elevator guided through the bone using the mallet, and either then being used as an elevator or being placed in contact with the tooth or fragment, which is delivered by a sharp blow. Use with care.

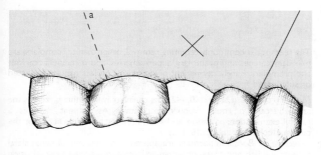

Fig. 8.3 Outline of two-sided flap in heavy shade.
X Retained root or similar.
a Line of additional incision to convert to three-sided flap.

Dento-alveolar surgery: removal of unerupted teeth

The teeth most commonly requiring removal, other than third molars, are maxillary canines and premolars, supernumaries, and mandibular canines and premolars. Rarely, permanent or deciduous molars may be impacted or submerged.

Maxillary canines (📖 pp. 140, 142) The canine may lie within or across the arch, buccally or, most frequently, palatally. Assessment requires a careful examination, palpation, and X-rays (either two films at 90° or the parallax technique, 📖 pp. 16, 142).

Techniques Buccal impactions are approached via a buccal flap, palatal via a palatal flap, and cross- or within-arch impactions need a combination of the two. Buccal flaps are as previously described (📖 p. 354). Palatal flaps involve the reflection of the full thickness of the mucoperiosteum of the anterior hard palate, the incision running in the gingival crevice from 6| to |6 for bilateral canines or to the contralateral canine region for single impactions. The neurovascular bundle emerging from the incisive foramen is often sacrificed, with no noticeable morbidity (if it bleeds use bone wax). **Never** incise the palate at 90° to the gingival crevice and **always** use an envelope flap, otherwise you will section the palatine artery. Remove bone over the bulge of the crown of the tooth until the maximum bulbosity of the crown and the incisal tip are exposed. If the root curvature and path of withdrawal are favourable, the entire tooth can be elevated out. If not, section at the cervical margin with a tapered fissure bur and winkle the pieces out separately. Debride the socket and close with vertical mattress sutures to minimize haematoma formation.

Mandibular canines Most lie buccally, and can be elevated or removed with root forceps. Unerupted, deeply impacted buccal or lingual canines rarely need to be removed. If necessary a degloving incision provides good access.

Maxillary premolars Most lie palatally. If partially erupted and conically rooted, they are simply elevated. Otherwise, a similar approach to that used for palatal canines is used. Premolars within the arch are approached buccally, sectioned, and removed piecemeal.

Mandibular premolars are often angled lingually. The 'broken instrument' technique can be invaluable. Otherwise, an extended buccal flap is raised to visualize and protect the mental nerve, buccal bone is removed, and the tooth sectioned at its cervical margin. The crown is then displaced downwards into the space created and the root elevated upwards.

Submerged deciduous molars If must be removed, they are approached buccally and sectioned vertically, then elevated along the individual roots path of withdrawal.

Supernumeraries (📖 p. 64) These are removed using the approach used for the tooth they impede or replace. This can be a surprisingly difficult operation, usually because of difficulty in finding and identifying the supernumary.

Dento-alveolar surgery: removal of third molars

Not all wisdom teeth need to be removed.[1] Those which have space to erupt into functional occlusion should be left to do so, and those which are deeply impacted and asymptomatic are best left alone. Decisions about surgery vary widely.[2]

Aetiology As the last tooth to erupt, the third molar is most liable to be prevented from doing so in a crowded mouth. *Causes:* soft Western diet doesn't create space by contact point abrasion, inherited tooth–jaw size incompatibility, and possibly an evolutionary tendency towards decreased jaw size.

Symptoms Pain, swelling, pericoronitis (🕮 p. 370), and sometimes a foul taste. Mostly due to localized infection, less commonly due to caries or resorption of second molar or cyst associated with third molar. Third molars covered by bone are very unlikely to become infected, whereas those where the crown has breached mucosa will almost inevitably do so. Infections in older, less vascular bone are more difficult to treat.

Indications for removal Recurrent pericoronitis, unrestorable caries in 7 or 8, external or internal resorption, cystic change, periodontal disease distally in 7. The prevention of LLS crowding on its own is **not** an indication, nor is vague TMJ pain.

Timing Symptoms are most common in the late teens and twenties; bone is soft, spongy and elastic in this age group, so this is the usual and most favourable time to operate. Prophylactic removal of symptomless third molars is currently hard to justify.[3]

Choice of anaesthetic Bilateral impacted third molars are more kindly treated under GA, as are those where surgery may be technically more difficult, e.g. disto-angular 8s. LA &/or sedation is appropriate for most unilateral impactions not presenting particular difficulty. Consider medical history.

Assessment Look first: unerupted or partially erupted? Take pre-op X-ray (DPT is ideal; see Figure 8.4).

Assess angulation (vertical, mesio-angular, disto-angular, horizontal, or transverse); depth of impaction from the alveolar crest to the maximum diameter of the crown; degree of impaction (and against what); root shape; bone density; the relationship to the ID canal; and the presence of any other pathology or complicating factors.

Plan the path of withdrawal (Figure 8.5). What impedes it? How much bone needs to be removed to provide a point of application for an elevator? How much to clear the path of withdrawal? Can this be done less traumatically by sectioning the tooth? In what direction?

Warn the patient about pain, trismus, swelling, and the possibility of damage to the ID and lingual nerves.

1 NICE 2000 🖲 www.nice.org.uk
2 M. Brickley 1993 *BDJ* **175** 102.
3 University of York 1998 *Effectiveness Matters* **3**(2).

Fig. 8.4 A DPT example of simple, vertically impacted, conically rooted third molars suitable for removal in the ambulatory setting.

Fig. 8.5 A schematic showing planning for third molar removal.

Bold arrow	natural path of withdrawal, this causes impaction against 2nd molar.
Dashed lines	lines of tooth sectioning.
Top curved arrow	rotational movement to disimpact.
Lower curved arrow	compensatory rotational movement which puts nerve at risk if tooth is not sectioned vertically.

Dento-alveolar surgery: coronectomy

This is used as an alternative to conventional surgical removal.[1] It involves removal of the crown of a lower 8, with deliberate retention of the roots. This may be indicated if the roots of the lower 8 are radiographically assessed as being closely involved with the ID canal. Radiographic signs of increased risk of nerve damage include:

- Proximity to nerve canal
- Narrowing or diversion of canal
- Darkening of root/interrupting white lines of canal
- Interruption of lamina dura
- Juxta-apical area

Technique (Figure 8.6):

Coronectomy involves transection of the tooth 3–4mm below the ADJ. The pulp is left untreated. The root is further reduced with a rose head bur to 3–4mm below the level of the alveolar crest. This may not be possible if there are defects in the lingual plate, due to risk of damage to the lingual nerve. Irrigate the socket with saline and close with a single suture.

Exclusion criteria:

- Predisposition to local infection/ medically compromised
- Mobile teeth
- Non-vital lower third molar
- Horizontal or distoangular impaction where sectioning crown puts nerve at risk
- If root becomes mobile during sectioning, it must be removed

Coronectomy compares favourably to surgical removal of lower wisdom teeth in terms of altered sensation, reported rates for conventional surgical removal are 8% temporary, and 3.6% permanent (personal rates vary). There is a similar incidence of dry socket (10–12%). Long-term data on late infection and cyst development are not yet available. If the coronectomy fails and the root is mobilized, there appears to be a reduced risk of nerve damage, although this probably reflects the fact that the nerve was not involved in the root in the first place. Post-coronectomy migration of the root may occur necessitating a second procedure. The root is likely to erupt away from the nerve thereby reducing the risk of damage. Failure of coronectomy may occur, particularly in women with conical roots that narrow into the ID canal.

1 T. Renton 2005 *BJOMS* **43** 7.

Fig. 8.6 A step by step illustration of coronectomy.
A   vertical impaction with high likelihood of nerve involvement.
B   gingival incision.
C   crown is sectioned through amelo-dentinal junction.
D   remaining root is reduced 3–4 mm below alveolar crest.
E   the residual roots (now lying below the surrounding bone) are then covered
    with the mucosal flap.

Dento-alveolar surgery: third-molar technique

(Figure 8.7)

Technique

Mandible A buccal flap is incised along the external oblique ridge (lies well lateral to the arch) over the crest of the ridge if unerupted, or in the gingival margin if partially erupted. Extend to the distal aspect of the second molar and down into the buccal sulcus. Cut on to bone to create a full thickness flap. If a mesio-angular or horizontal impaction, extend the incision around $\overline{7}$ to the mesial border, but beware the buccal branch of the facial artery. Reflect and retract flap. There is now good evidence to suggest that manipulation from the lingual aspect results in unnecessary lingual nerve morbidity. Bone and tooth removal should be from a buccal approach. An attached mucosa disto-lingual flap for visibility which does not encroach on the lingual nerve is reasonable. Wide exposure and sub-periosteal protection of the lingual nerve should therefore be undertaken by those using the lingual split technique. Remove bone to provide a point of application for an elevator and clear obstruction to the path of withdrawal. This can be done with chisels or a bur. With a bur this is done by creating a disto-buccal gutter, exposing the maximum bulbosity of the tooth. If needed the bur can then be used to section the $\overline{8}$ to provide an unimpeded path of withdrawal.

With chisels, place mesial and distal stop cuts around the tooth and split off a collar of buccal and distal bone to expose the bulbosity of the crown. This can then be extended into a lingual split, taking off a piece of lingual plate and allowing the tooth to be elevated lingually. Whichever technique is used, it is important to remember that if it has been done properly a minimum of directed force via an elevator will deliver the tooth or fragment out along its path of withdrawal. If this cannot be done, look carefully for another obstruction. Once the tooth is removed debride the socket, remove the follicle, and close the wound with loose sutures to allow for swelling. Achieve haemostasis with pressure.

Maxilla A flap similar to that in the mandible can be used for inaccessible wisdom teeth but many can be approached using a 'slash' incision (from disto-palatally on the tuberosity to disto-buccally at the second molar and into the buccal sulcus). Reflect and retract the flap. Bone removal can usually be effected with a hand-held chisel. The much softer bone rarely causes any problem with elevation, but care has to be taken to prevent displacement into the pterygoid space. The 'slash' incision often needs no closure, whereas a conventional incision will need repositioning with sutures.

Post-operatively

Pain can be quite severe and responds best to NSAIDs. Peri-operative LA works well and leaves patients pain-free but numb for the duration. Trismus is due to pain and muscle spasm and can be ↓ by adequate analgesia (📕 p. 546). It has obvious but often forgotten connotations for meals post-op. Swelling can also be ↓ by high-dose peri-operative steroids. There is no evidence that ice-packs help, although they are often used. Haemorrhage can usually be controlled by biting on pressure packs. Rarely, it may be necessary to re-explore the wound. Antibiotic prophylaxis is probably beneficial.[1]

Fig. 8.7

a   Outline of incision for raising a third-molar buccal flap.
b   Modification to create an envelope flap.
A   Vertically impacted third molar.
B   Horizontally impacted third molar.
C   Mesio-angular impaction of a third molar.
D   Disto-angular impaction of a third molar.

1 J. Piecuch 1995 *Journal Oral and Maxillofacial Surgery* **53**.

Dento-alveolar surgery: apicectomy

There are three surgical aids to endodontics: apicectomy, root hemisection, and removal of extruded endodontic paste.

Apicectomy (Figures 8.8 and 8.9)

This is by far the commonest. It is a *second line* treatment after failure of, or as a supplement to, orthograde endodontics (which has an 86–96% success rate in expert hands).[1]

Indications

- Impossible to prepare and fill apicial ⅓ of tooth, e.g. pulpal calcification, curved apex, open apex.
- Irretrievable broken instrument in canal.
- Post crown on tooth with apical pathology (only if post crown has sealed the coronal root and crown margin adequately).
- Root perforation.
- Fractured and infected apical ⅓.
- Persistent infection due to apical cyst or other lesion requiring biopsy, and repeat root canal therapy has been performed and is adequate or 'pull through' technique is planned. A coronal seal must be achievable.

Assessment IO X-ray, best possible root filling *in situ*, free from acute infection, crown sealed with good quality restoration.

Remember Non-surgical retreatment: 72% success; apicectomy and RRF: 60%, apicectomy no RRF: 51%.[1]

Technique This operation is best performed under LA. Ensure an area of two tooth widths either side of the tooth being treated is anaesthetized, and give palatal infiltration. In the mandible, give a block plus infiltration to aid haemostasis. If associated with infection, prophylactic antibiotics, e.g. amoxicillin 1g 1h pre-op and 6h post-op, or metronidazole 400mg 1h pre- and 6h post-op can help.

Flaps may be two- or three-sided, semilunar or sublabial; the latter two avoid post-op recession but give inferior access. Semilunar flaps are prone to breakdown. Reflect and retract well above the apex (there is often a bulge or perforation of the cortical plate to aid location of the apex). A bony window is created to visualize the apex, which is often found sitting in a mass of granulation tissue. Excise the apical 1–2mm and curette out the cystic and granulation tissue. Pack the cavity with bone wax or adrenaline-soaked ribbon gauze, identify the canal and prepare it with a 1/2-round bur or ultrasonics (depending on availability). Seal with 'super EBA', 'IRM' or 'MTA' and debride. Close, using interrupted or vertical mattress sutures.

Operating microscopes have become popular with those specializing in surgical endodontics (who would claim this to be 'gold standard'). It can minimize loss of tooth and allow visualization of accessory canals and precise preparation (with the right instruments) and seal of the apical canal. Cost and availability in relation to overall need for this procedure remains a significant issue in many countries.

---

1 N. Chandler 2002 *J. R. Coll. Surg. Edin.* **47** 600.

Special points in apicectomy

Warn patients about post-op swelling. Lower incisors present an access problem eased but not erased by a degloving incision and experience. Think twice about the mental nerve in lower premolar apicectomies. Think hard about alternatives to apicectomy of 6. Don't think at all about 7, 8. Remember the buccal and palatal roots in <u>4</u>; section the buccal root low to see the palatal. Apicectomy of <u>6</u> is fine provided the palatal root can be treated by an orthograde approach, is hemisected, or you are happy to deal with breaching the antrum.

Fig. 8.8
A An approach to apicectomy.
  a Outline of incision for three-sided flap, good access, best flap for the novice.
  b Outline of semilunar flap incision.
B An approach to apicectomy, a window is created in the buccal cortex to expose the apex, which is resected, leaving a smooth raw bony cavity.

Fig. 8.9 Clinical view of the apical preparation.

Dento-alveolar surgery: other aids to endodontics

Root perforations are approached as for apicectomy; however, multi-rooted tooth perforations, unroot-fillable roots, or untreatable periodontal pockets may be dealt with by

Root hemisection This simply involves raising a flap around the tooth, identifying and horizontally sectioning the root, and atraumatically elevating it out. The wound is closed and a cleanable undersurface sealed with Super EBA, IRM, or MTA left.

Removal of extruded paste Usually, all that is required is an apicectomy approach. However, careless use of 'paste only' techniques can result in paste in the floor of the nose, the antrum, or the ID canal. The nasal floor can be approached sublabially or intranasally, the antrum by standard methods (🕮 p. 384), and the ID canal by sagittally splitting the buccal cortex of the mandible.

Prognosis Single-rooted tooth apicectomies should succeed 58–96% of the time. The range is due to an ill-defined definition of 'success' and operator technique. Multirooted teeth, revision apicectomy, and perforation repair have a much lower success rate.

Dento-alveolar surgery: helping the orthodontist

Many minor oral surgical procedures, e.g. extraction of 4s or removal of 8s, are carried out at the instigation of an orthodontist. This page concerns itself with the specific procedures of frenectomy, pericision, tooth exposure, and tooth repositioning (see also Figures 8.10 and 8.11).

Frenectomy This is of value in closing a median diastema only if gentle traction on the upper lip and fraenum produces blanching in a palatal insertion around the incisive papilla. It follows that the excision of the fraenum must include those fibrous insertions, which leaves a raw area of alveolus after excision—this can be dressed with Surgicel, BIPP, or a periodontal pack. It is a different operation from preprosthetic fraenectomy and is performed for a different reason.

Pericision is simply incising supra-alveolar periodontal fibres to prevent relapse when derotating teeth.

Tooth exposure Orthodontic traction is the treatment of choice for malpositioned, unerupted canines and incisors if the apices are in good position for eruption. The essential aspect of the operation is to remove any sacrificable impediments to tooth movement. Bonding an eyelet and gold chain or other bracket technique has a lower incidence of reoperation; this is fiddly and requires use of composite in a hard to dry field.

Technique Palatal teeth are exposed by a palatal flap. Remove bone carefully with chisels; expose the greatest diameter of the crown and the tip. (Moving the tooth is counter-productive, therefore don't do it.) Excise palatal mucoperiosteum generously, it grows back; bond a bracket if you're going to. The wound may be packed firmly with, e.g. Whitehead's varnish and ribbon gauze and secure, or use an acrylic dressing plate with periodontal paste dressing, or cauterize and leave open. Close the remainder of the flap with vertical mattress sutures. Buccally located teeth are approached by a buccal flap, in order to preserve attached gingiva, and bonding should be done at operation. The flap can be repositioned coronally with the elastics or chain tunnelling subgingivally. Teeth within the arch are approached buccally removing crestal bone as needed.

Tooth repositioning (transplantation) Although there are claims of success rates as high as 93%, few people match this and most would transplant only when exposure and orthodontic movement were rejected. The most commonly transplanted tooth is the maxillary canine. It is essential to measure the available space and compare this with the erupted contralateral tooth or a good X-ray estimation, as it is not acceptable to grind down healthy teeth at operation to accommodate the retrieved tooth. If the tooth appears to be too big for the available space then orthodontic Rx is required to create space. As this is often the reason the patient rejected exposure, an impasse is sometimes reached.

Technique The tooth is exposed by buccal or palatal flap, and once it is certain that it can be removed atraumatically, the deciduous tooth, if present, is extracted and a new socket surgically prepared with a bur. The tooth is reimplanted without force, the flaps sutured, and a close-fitting but **not** cemented splint placed. Functional splinting is continued for 7–10 days and the tooth root-filled as soon as possible after surgery. Regular follow-up is essential to allow early detection of root resorption which is common.

Fig. 8.10 A Outline (heavy red line) of the incision for a palatal flap raised to expose a buried right maxillary canine.
P Position of the palatine arteries. Do not attempt a palatal 'relieving' incision; exposure is achieved by the length of the envelope flap.

Fig. 8.11 An apically repositioned flap allows access to the buccal surface without loss of attached gingivae.

Dento-facial infections

▶ Infection associated with teeth is rarely, if ever, treated *definitively* by antibiotics and analgesics.

Ask about the airway. Anyone having difficulty swallowing their own saliva should be admitted immediately as the airway is at risk. People can die from these infections.

The vast majority of infections in this area requiring surgical treatment are bacterial, usually arising from necrotic pulps, periodontal pockets, or pericoronitis. Can be life-threatening if allowed to progress, e.g. to the fascial spaces of the neck, mediastinum or the cavernous sinus, or as a focus for infective endocarditis (□ p. 493). There has been a substantial increase in the number of hospital admissions for severe cervicofacial infection of dental origin in the UK over the last decade.[1] This increase is greater in lower socio-economic groups.[2]

Microbiology Culture of dento-facial infections usually produces several commensal organisms, of which anaerobes are the most important. The predominant species *Bacteroides* (anaerobe) and streptococci (aerobe and anaerobe) are usually sensitive to the penicillins. Resistance is reported rarely. *Bacteroides* is nearly always sensitive to metronidazole. Remember the aerobic pathogens in established infection (don't just rely on metronidazole), and *Haemophilus* and *S. aureus* near the antrum (□ p. 384), *Strep. Milleri* is a particularly virulent pathogen present in aggressive potentially life-threatening infections.

Diagnosis Usually simple and clinical based on pain, swelling, temperature, and discharge.

Apical abscess Teeth with an apical abscess are TTP and non-vital. They may be discoloured or crowned and have a history of trauma or RCT. Pain and TTP are often diminished when the intrabony pus tracks through the soft tissues and discharges, usually in the buccal sulcus (exceptions are 2, and palatal roots of maxillary molars which discharge palatally, and 1̄2̄ which often discharge on the chin). May be associated periostitis with severe thickening.

Rx Drainage of pus either via the root canal, by incision of any fluctuant abscess, or by extraction under LA or GA. Palatal or buccal abscesses can be drained quite simply under LA by infiltrating a small amount of LA *between* the abscess cavity and the overlying mucosa, then incising the abscess. Explore using blunt closed forceps and keep patent either by excising an elipse of tissue or inserting and suturing a small rubber drain; this is particularly important in the palate. Cover the procedure with 'best guess' antibiotics such as amoxicillin 500mg tds PO for 5–7 days, or metronidazole 400mg tds PO for 5–7 days, or both. For severe infections, in-patient management with extraoral drainage may be needed.

---

1 S. Thomas 2008 *BMJ* **336** 1219.
2 D. Moles 2008 *BMJ* **336** 1323.

Periodontal abscesses arise in a pre-existing periodontal pocket (📖 p. 192). Initial treatment involves incision and drainage, followed by elimination of the pocket, unless extraction is considered the only option.

Pericoronitis is inflammation and infection of a gum flap (operculum) overlying a partially erupted tooth, usually an 8̄ often traumatized by an over-erupted 8. Rx: involves removal of the opposing 8̲, irrigation under the operculum with saline or chlorhexidine, and antibiotics (see above) if necessary. Nearly all third molars associated with pericoronitis need removal.

Dry socket is osteitis of a socket following tooth removal. Commonest in the mandible after removal of molars, especially 8̄ Predisposing factors are smoking, surgical trauma, LA, history, bone disease, oral contraceptives, or immunodeficiency.

Diagnosis Pain onset after (usually 2–4 days) extraction, similar in nature but worse than the preceding toothache. The socket looks inflamed and exposed bone is usually visible. Rx is to gently clean the socket by irrigation and dress the exposed bone with Alvogyl, BIPP, or ZOE packs (provide remarkable analgesia but are a horror to remove). Topical metronidazole is an alternative.[1] Chlorhexidine &/or hot salt mouthwashes may help. NSAIDs are the systemic analgesic of choice (📖 pp. 560, 562). Prophylactic anaerobicidals such as metronidazole reduce the incidence of this condition.[2]

Actinomycosis (📖 p. 174) Persistent low-grade infection, multiple sinuses. Rx: drainage and up to 6 weeks amoxicillin 500mg tds. Doxycycline 100mg od is an alternative.

Staphylococcal lymphadenitis Especially seen in children; small occult skin or mucosal breach allows ingress. May mimic a 'slapped face' due to exotoxin. Drain and give flucloxacillin 125–500mg qds (depending on age, 📖 p. 558).

Atypical mycobacteria Lymphadenitis with no obvious cause. Cold nodes, non-febrile patient. Drain or excise. Culture for up to 12 weeks. Do **not** start antituberculous therapy as many atypical mycobacteria are resistant and side-effects are common and significant. Clarithromycin most useful 'conventional' antibiotic. Excision of nodes is definitive Rx.

Ludwig's angin is a combination of abscess and cellulitis affecting both submandibular and sublingual spaces bilaterally. The floor of mouth is raised and the tongue pushed up and back. The floor of mouth, tongue and soft tissues of the neck are board hard. The patient is systemically unwell and often cannot swallow his own saliva. The airway is seriously at risk and this is an urgent case for admission.

Necrotizing fasciitis rare but life-threatening infection often with a highly virulent streptococci. Treatment involves wide local excision of necrotic tissue combined with resuscitation and IV antibiotics.

An abscess is a collection of pus (white cells, inflammatory exudates, tissue fluid and bacteria), it is relatively isolated from the circulation (and hence antibiotics). Treatment is drainage which continues until all pus is gone.

1 L. Mitchell 1984 *BDJ* **156** 132.
2 J. Rood 1979 *Br J Oral Surg* **17** 62.

Cellulitis is intra and intercellular oedema generated by inflammatory exudates. The overlying surface is red and hot and it allows the rapid migration of bacteria to surrounding areas (Figure 8.12). It has a good blood supply and high dose antibiotics are the treatment of choice.

Head and neck infections are usually a combination of both.

Fig. 8.12 A clinical example of spreading facial cellulitis—the blue markings allow the assessment of the impact of treatment.

Biopsy

A biopsy is a sample of tissue taken from a patient for histopathological examination.

Types of biopsy Biopsies may be incisional or excisional. Examples of incisional biopsies are fine-needle aspirate (really cytology), punch biopsy, trephines, and 'true-cut' needle biopsy. The commonest technique by far, however, is to excise an ellipse of tissue that includes a portion of the lesion and surrounding normal tissue. Excisional biopsy provides after the fact information on the excised sample (reserve for lesions <0.5mm).

What should be biopsied? Nearly everything that is worth excising is worth histological review, and so all excised specimens should be examined histopathologically. Any soft tissue lesion not amenable to accurate clinical Δ (by a reasonably trained eye) should be biopsied. All red lesions of oral mucosa and most white patches should be biopsied. If you think 'should I biopsy this?' then do it; you will always get some unpleasant surprises.

Special considerations Frozen sections are biopsy specimens taken during major surgery, either when the extent of the procedure will depend on the histological Δ of the lesion or to verify clearance of excision. It is essential to contact the pathology lab before the patient goes to theatre to warn them. Advance warning is also necessary for certain special tests, e.g. immunohistochemistry.

How it is done Tell the patient you need a piece of tissue to help make the Δ. LA or GA. For simple incisional biopsy, stabilize the tissue to be sampled. Transfixing with a 3/0 BSS helps avoid crush artefact, and orientates the specimen. Cut an ellipse of tissue, including lesion and normal surrounding tissue, lift up and dissect out, then close primarily with sutures.

Biopsy and oral cancer Incisional biopsy carries a (theoretical) risk of shedding malignant cells into the circulation. The alternative is to subject a patient to mutilating surgery before definitive Δ. If you suspect an oral malignancy, refer before biopsy because most consultants have a preferred approach. This also allows integrated Δ and counselling.

Specimens are best laid out on paper if small or pinned out on a cork board if large. This allows orientation and decreases shrinkage artefact, which can be considerable. Usual preservative is 10% formalin; ask if you are not sure, as some specimens are needed fresh. Consider a specimen for culture as well (e.g. lymph node biopsy). Make a diagram of the specimen on the pathology form to accompany the clinical details. A photograph of the operative site can help.

▶ Tell the pathologist what you are thinking!

Cryosurgery

Cryosurgery is the therapeutic use of extreme cold.

Equipment The coolants (usually nitrous oxide or liquid nitrogen) act via a cryoprobe, a tubing system in which the coolant is not in direct contact with the tissues. The probe tip is applied to the lesion with an intervening layer of lubricant jelly; this gives rise to an 'iceball', which is essential for success. Liquid nitrogen can also be directly sprayed onto lesions and, rarely, bone can be immersed into liquid nitrogen prior to reuse as a framework for grafting.

Mechanism Cell death and subsequent tissue necrosis by cellular disruption, dehydration, enzyme inhibition, and protein denaturation follow application of extreme cold. Indirect effects include vascular stasis and an immune response.[1] There is a curious lack of infection and scarring following cryosurgery.

Indications Some vascular malformations and haemangioma (not the same thing) respond very well. Areas of leukoplakia unsuitable for excision, and provided they have not already undergone malignant change, may respond. Occasionally, malignant change following cryosurgery of leukoplakia is reported, so some controversy surrounds the technique. Extensive hyperplastic lesions, e.g. palatal hyperplasia under F/-, may respond. Viral warts respond in most instances and some advocate its use for mucoceles. Superficial basal cell carcinoma is frequently treated with cryosurgery, usually liquid nitrogen spray, although its use in more aggressive malignancy is controversial, as is its use following enucleation of keratocysts. Intractable facial pain is one of the more accepted uses, the freezing of peripheral nerves being followed by a period of analgesia which extends beyond the original post-op numbness.

Technique
1) Warn the patient about the procedure, post-op oedema (which can be severe), and a slough which forms over frozen sites. There is sometimes depigmentation of skin lesions.
2) LA for larger lesions or if biopsy needed. (LA may ↑ effectiveness of iceball.)
3) Select a probe tip suitable for the lesion; overlap ice zones if the lesion is large.
4) Use KY jelly to improve contact between probe and tissues.
5) Usual freeze–thaw cycles are 1 min, repeated at least twice.
6) Do not remove probe until defrosting has occurred.
7) Careful follow-up and check the histology of the lesion, except when using cryoanalgesia.

Simple analgesics and chlorhexidine mouthwash post-op often help.

The treatment of frank malignancy by cryosurgery remains controversial, but freeze–thaw cycles used must be in excess of the usual (up to 3min) and tissue temperatures monitored.

1 V. Popescu 1980 *J Max-fac Surg* **8** 8.

Non-tumour soft-tissue lumps in the mouth

Abscess (📖 p. 370). Generalized gingival swelling and gingivitis (📖 p. 187).

Brown 'tumour' Not a tumour but a giant cell lesion sometimes found in soft tissue but more commonly within bone (📖 p. 378). It occurs 2° to hyperparathyroidism, although this is usually suggested after enucleation on finding giant cells in a fibrous stroma histologically. Check bone biochemistry (Ca^{2+}, PO^{4+}↓, alkaline phosphatase ↑, PTH ↑). If hyperparathyroidism is confirmed and treated, these lesions regress.

Dermoid cyst Developmental cyst commonest at the lateral canthus of the eye, but next most often found in the midline of the neck above mylohyoid, where it causes elevation of the tongue. Rx: complete but conservative excision.

Congenital epulis By definition present at birth; usually presents as a pedunculated nodule. Histology reveals large granular cells. Rx: complete but conservative excision.

Peripheral giant cell granuloma (giant cell epulis) Deep red gingival swelling, probably caused by chronic irritation. Histology reveals a vascular lesion with multinuclear giant cells. Rx: excision with stripping of periosteum and curettage of underlying bone.

Pregnancy epulis An ↑ inflammatory response to plaque during pregnancy causes a lesion indistinguishable from a pyogenic granuloma. Onset usually in third month. Rx: none (other than OHI) if possible, as it regresses after delivery. If very troublesome, simple excision; but it may recur.

Pyogenic granuloma Red fleshy swelling, often nodular, occurring as a response to recurrent trauma and non-specific infection. Histology shows proliferation of vascular connective tissue, therefore bleeds easily. Rx: excision, debride area, good OH.

Fibroepithelial polyp An over-vigorous response to low grade recurrent trauma. May be cessile or pedunculated and range from small lumps to lesions covering the entire palate. Excise with base. Histology shows dense collagenous fibrous tissue lined by keratinized stratified squamous epithelium.

Irritation (denture) hyperplasia A very common hyperplastic response to repeated trauma, e.g. following denture-induced ulceration. Classically, seen as rolls of tissue in the sulcus related to a denture flange. Histology is similar to fibroepithelial polyp. Rx: complete excision with temporary removal of dentures allows healing. Consider simple preprosthetic measures and replace F/F.

Mucoceles Usually mucous extravasation cysts, where saliva leaks from a traumatized duct and pools, creating a compressed connective tissue capsule. Rarely, they are mucous retention cysts. Mostly affect lower lip—similar swellings in the upper lip are often minor salivary gland tumours (📖 p. 477). Rx: excision with associated damaged glands and duct.

Ranula Mucoceles of the floor of the mouth, arising from the sublingual gland. Tend to recur if marsupialized. A plunging ranula crosses deep to mylohyoid and appears as a neck and floor of mouth swelling. Rx: excision of cyst and associated sublingual gland, submandibular gland may have to be excised if the duct is damaged.

Granulomata Lumps characterized by the histological finding of granulomata may be caused by Crohn's disease (📖 p. 432) or its localized variant orofacial granulomatosis, sarcoidosis (📖 p. 419), or implanted foreign bodies such as amalgam.

Haemangioma Developmental lesion of blood vessels. Present at birth, they can grow with the child, remain static, or regress. Blanch on pressure. Do **not** biopsy. 80% spontaneously regress; Rx for those that don't: laser or cryotherapy.

Lymphangioma Rarer developmental lesion, this time of lymphatics. Can be microcystic or macrocystic. May present as an enlarged tongue, cheek or lip (usually microcystic) or neck swellings (usually macrocystic). Rx microcystic difficult as no clear plane of excision although some can be beneficially excised. Macrocystic lymphangiomas do have definable planes in most cases and can be excised with little damage to surrounding structures. Sclerosant picinabil can be used in the larger cyst cavities.

Vascular malformations Developmental lesions of blood vessels which *do not* regress but grow with patient. Characterized by rate of blood flow in lesion. Rx: interventional radiology and surgery.

Warts/squamous papillomata Main aetiological factor is HPV. True warts are rare in the mouth and usually transmitted from skin warts. Found in those with STD or AIDS, but most have no such link.

Papillomas are common in the mouth; appear as multiply papillated pink or white asymptomatic lumps. Rx: excision biopsy (if on a stalk—ligate or diathermy base as they contain a prominent vessel).

Non-tumour hard-tissue lumps

Cysts (📖 p. 380); benign tumours (📖 p. 382); malignant tumours (📖 p. 416).

Tori are bony exostoses found in both *jaws*. *Torus palatinus* is found in the centre of the hard palate; *torus mandibularis* on the lingual premolar/molar region of the mandible. Rx: reassurance that these developmental anomalies cause no harm (they are *not* part of the Gardener syndrome, p. 728). Rarely, excision for denture construction is indicated.

Giant cell granuloma (📖 p. 376) This can present as an intrabony swelling or symptomless radiolucency. Carefully enucleate.

Brown 'tumour' (📖 p. 376) Again, imitates the giant cell granuloma; difference is in bone biochemistry.

Paget's disease of bone Relatively common over the age of 55yrs and affects the skull, pelvis, and long bones, as well as the jaws. Although aetiology is uncertain both the measles and respiratory syncytinal virus have been implicated. The maxilla is more frequently affected than the mandible. Hypercementosis of roots makes extractions difficult in this group. There is a replacement of normal bone remodelling by a chaotic alternation of resorption and deposition, with resorption dominating in the early stages. Bone pain and cranial neuropathies can occur. X-rays show a 'cotton wool' appearance. Biochemistry shows an ↑ alkaline phosphatase and urinary hydroxyproline. Avoid GA; use prophylactic antibiotics and plan extractions surgically. Bisphosphonates (📖 p. 581) and calcitonin are used in treatment.

Fibrous dysplasia Areas of bone are replaced by fibrous tissue. Onset in childhood; ossifies and stabilizes with age. Jaw involvement usually presents as a painless hard swelling. Characteristic X-ray appearance is of 'ground glass' bone. Histology shows fibrous replacement of bone with osseous trabeculae which look like irregular 'Chinese characters' Rx: skeletal resculpting after stabilization of growth &/or orthognathic surgery/orthodontics.

Cherubism Hereditary, and presents at 2–4yrs. It is a bilateral variant of fibrous dysplasia. In addition to the histological pattern for fibrous dysplasia there are also multinucleated giant cells. Natural history is not well understood, may burn out or regress. Skeletal resculpting after cessation may be necessary.

Cysts of the jaws

Cysts are abnormal epithelium-lined cavities which often contain fluid but only contain pus if they become infected. Jaw cysts predominantly arise from odontogenic epithelium and grow by a means not fully understood but involving epithelial proliferation, bone resorption by prostaglandins, and variations in intracystic osmotic pressure.

Diagnosis

Many are detected as asymptomatic radiolucencies on X-ray; others present as painless swellings, almost always of the buccal cortex. Infected cysts present with pain, swelling, and discharge. Vitality test associated teeth. Take a DPT and a periapical film when possible to screen for size and coexisting pathology. Transillumination rarely helps, but aspiration is sometimes useful and can help distinguish some lesions. Rarely, cysts may present with a pathological #, especially of the mandible.

Treatment

- Enucleation with 1° closure is commonest and generally the Rx of choice. It consists of removing the cyst lining from the bony walls of the cavity and repositioning the access flap. Any relevant dental pathology is treated at the same time, e.g. by apicectomy.
- Enucleation with packing and delayed closure is used when badly infected cysts, particularly very large ones, are unsuitable for 1° closure. Pack with Whitehead's varnish or BIPP.
- Enucleation with 1° bone grafting. Rarely useful.
- Marsupialization. This is the opening of the cyst to allow continuity with the oral mucosa; healing is slower than with enucleation and a cavity persists for some time. It is useful to allow tooth eruption through the cyst or where enucleation is C/I.

▶ Always submit cyst lining for histopathology.

Types of cysts

Many classifications exist, few are helpful.

Inflammatory dental cysts are very common, and may also be called radicular cysts. Described as apical or lateral depending on position in relation to tooth root, or residual if left behind after tooth extraction. Necrotic pulp is the stimulus, and the epithelium comes from cell rests of Malassez. Rx: enucleation plus endodontics or extraction.

Eruption cysts, 🕮 p. 62.

Dentigerous cysts form around the crown of an unerupted permanent tooth and arise from reduced enamel epithelium. May delay eruption. Rx: marsupialization or enucleation, depending on position and desired fate of the tooth.

Keratocysts are lined by parakeratinized epithelium derived from the remnants of the dental lamina and are thought to replace a missing tooth. They have a fluid filling with a protein content <4g/dl. Aspiration of samples for biochemistry and cytology for parakeratinized squames can be helpful. It is important to identify these cysts, as outpouching walls and 'daughter' or 'satellite' cysts make them more liable to recur. Their multiloculated appearance on X-ray may confuse them with an ameloblastoma (p. 382). Rx: careful enucleation, &/or cryotherapy &/or Carnoy's solution, or aggressive curettage of the cavity. Rarely, excision is needed if recurrent.

Calcifying epithelial odontogenic cysts are rare and distinguished by areas of calcification and 'ghost cells' on histology. Rx: enucleate.

Solitary bone cysts are usually an incidental finding on X-ray and devoid of a lining, but may contain straw-coloured fluid. They probably arise following breakdown of an intraosseous haematoma, and are distinguished by a scalloped upper border on X-ray where the cyst pushes into cancellous bone between teeth but spares the lamina dura. Opening the cyst, gentle curettage, and closure heals these 'cysts'; associated teeth need no Rx.

Aneurysmal bone cysts are expansile lesions full of vascular spongy bone. Present as a symptomless swelling, unless traumatized, when bleeding causes pain and rapid expansion. Small ones can be carefully enucleated, but larger aneurysmal bone cysts need excision and possible reconstruction since they will recur if incompletely excised.

Fissural cysts are not associated with dental epithelium but arise from embryonic junctional epithelium. They are rare and include incisive canal cysts, incisive papilla cysts, and nasolabial cysts. Rx: enucleation.

Benign tumours of the mouth

Non-odontogenic tumours

Epithelial

Squamous cell papilloma (📖 p. 377) Resembles a white or pink cauliflower and is caused by papilloma virus. Usually presents on the palate. Does not undergo malignant change. Excise.

Connective tissue

Fibroma Very rare. Benign fibrous tumour, usually pink and pedunculated. Excise with a narrow margin.

Lipoma Soft, smooth, slow growing yellowish lump composed of fat cells. Enucleate or excise with narrow margin.

Osteoma Smooth, hard, benign neoplasm of bone. Usually unilateral and covered by normal oral mucosa. Not situated in the classical position of tori (📖 p. 378). Gardener syndrome (📖 p. 728).

Neurofibroma Rare tumour of the fibroblasts of a peripheral nerve. Usually affects the tongue; may be part of von Recklinghausen disease (📖 p. 732). Can undergo sarcomatous change. Excise with a small margin.

Neurolemmoma (schwannoma) Tumour composed of Schwann cells (cells of the axonal sheath). Rx: excision; nerve fibres can sometimes be preserved due to eccentric tumour growth.

Granular cell myoblastoma Rare tumour of histiocyte origin, usually arising as a nodule on the tongue. Excise with a margin.

Ossifying fibroma May be neoplasm or developmental anomaly. It is a well-demarcated fibro-osseous lesion of the jaws. Presents as a painless slow-growing swelling, expanding both buccal and lingual cortices. X-ray shows a radiolucent area, circumscribed by a radio-opaque margin. Histology is similar to fibrous dysplasia. Enucleation or conservative excision is curative. A faster-growing but equally benign version occurs in children.

Odontogenic tumours

Many of these are fascinating (to some) rarities. Only the more important are discussed.

Ameloblastoma One of the commoner odontogenic tumours. Common-est in men and Africans, and in the posterior mandible. There are three basic types: unicystic, polycystic, and peripheral. The unicystic type is the least aggressive; the polycystic and peripheral types show a tendency to invade surrounding tissue, whereas the unicystic expands it. Metastases are very rare. Histologically, two types are seen: plexiform and follicular. Rx: unicystic can be enucleated provided a rim of enclosing bone is removed as well; the other types require excision with a margin.

Adenoameloblastoma Tends to occur in the anterior maxilla in females. Rx: conservative excision, as recurrence is not a problem.

Calcifying epithelial odontogenic tumour (Pindborg tumour) Characteristically, a radiolucency on X-ray with scattered radiopacities. Needs excision with a margin.

Myxoma Occurs in both hard and soft tissues. Those arising in the jaws are tumours of odontogenic mesenchyme. This is a tumour of young adults arising within bone and can invade the surrounding tissue extensively. Characteristically, has a 'soap bubble' appearance on X-ray. Histology reveals spindle cells in a mucoid stroma. These tumours need excision with a margin of surrounding normal bone.

Ameloblastic fibroma Rare; affects young adults and appears as a unilocular radiolucency on X-ray, causing painless expansion of the jaws. Enucleation is usually curative.

Odontomes Not true neoplasms, but malformations of dental hard tissues. Classically, they are classified as *compound* when they are multiple small 'teeth' in a fibrous sac, and *complex* when they are a congealed irregular mass of dental hard tissue. These are best regarded and treated as unerupted, malpositioned, or impacted teeth, and removed using standard dento-alveolar techniques when required (📖 p. 356).

Disturbances in tooth formation can lead to isolated abnormalities of enamel, dentine, and cementum. Cementomas are worthy of mention because they create extreme difficulty in tooth removal. Dens in dente, 📖 p. 70.

The maxillary antrum

These are the largest of the four paired paranasal air sinuses, lying in each half of the maxilla between the alveolus inferiorly, nasal cavity medially, and orbits superiorly.

Antral pathology often mimics symptoms attributable to maxillary teeth. Δ is by exclusion of dental pathology, nasal discharge or stuffiness, tenderness over the cheeks, and pain worse on moving the head. Occipito-mental X-rays (15° and 30°) may reveal antral opacity, fluid level, or # (📖 p. 462). To define fluid level, repeat film with head tilted. Other X-rays: DPT for cysts and roots and CT scans for tumours, pansinusitis, and blow out #.

Extractions and the antrum The proximity of maxillary cheek teeth to the antral floor makes it easy for roots and even teeth to be displaced into the antrum. It also predisposes to # of the alveolar process during 6,7,8 extraction. Displaced roots can be retrieved either by an extended transalveolar approach similar to that for removing roots (useful when the roots are lying under the antral lining) or via a *Caldwell–Luc* approach.

Maxillary sinusitis

Acute sinusitis usually follows a viral URTI which has ↓ cilia activity, and is due to bacterial superinfection (usually mixed; anaerobes, haemophilus, staphylococci, and streptococci). Less common, due to foreign body, e.g. roots, water. Poor drainage via the osteum exacerbates the situation. Δ as above and confirmed by proof puncture if necessary. Rx: erythromycin 500mg PO qds or doxycycline 100mg PO od. Decongestants, e.g. oxymetazoline or xylometazoline spray.

Chronic sinusitis may then develop, particularly if a foreign body or poor drainage is present. Mucosal lining hypertrophies and may form polyps. A post-nasal discharge (drip) is often present. Rx: aimed at reventilation of the sinus. Foreign bodies, if present, should be removed via an incision in the canine fossa (above the premolars) and creation of a bony window into the antrum (Caldwell–Luc). Ventilation is provided either by intra-nasal antrostomy or (ideally) by endoscopic enlargement of the osteum &/or drainage of anterior ethmoids, depending on cause (functional endoscopic sinus surgery—FESS, 📖 p. 393).

Oro-antral fistula

Is the creation of a pathological epithelium-lined tract between the mouth and maxillary sinus. This most often occurs following the extraction of isolated molar teeth when the fistula tends to persist. Post-extraction reflux of fluids into the nose or minor nosebleeds are a diagnostic pointer. Confirm by getting patient to attempt to blow out against a closed nose; air bubbles through the fistula. Occasionally antral mucosa prolapses through the socket. Rx: many small fistulae are asymptomatic and close spontaneously. Closure if Δ is made at time of extraction: close the socket by suture or buccal advancement flap (Figure 8.13), give antibiotics and decongestants as above, and advise not to blow nose. Closure if Δ is made

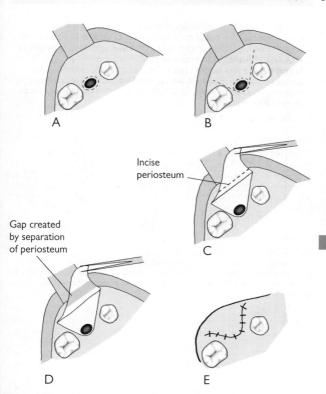

Fig. 8.13 The buccal advancement flap (after Rehrmann).
Steps:

A Excise the fistulous tract; easiest with a No.11 blade.

B Outline (dashed) of incision for a full thickness mucoperiosteal buccal flap.

C Reflect full thickness mucoperiosteal flap and incise the periosteal layer ONLY.
This makes it possible to mobilize the flap.

D 'Stretch' the flap to assess the degree of elasticity once the restraining effect of
    the periosteum is lost.

E The flap is advanced across the fistula and sutured to palatal mucosa *over* bone.

>2 days after extraction: place on antibiotics, etc., for 2 weeks and review
after 6. Many will have closed. If not, repair by:

- *Buccal advancement flap* Excise fistula to prepare a line of closure
  over bone and raise a broad-based buccal flap. Incise periosteum to
  allow mucosa to stretch over the socket and close, **over bone**, with
  vertical mattress sutures. Use antibiotics, etc., remove sutures at 10 days.
  Disadvantages: thin tissue may break down; reduces sulcus depth.

- *Palatal rotation flap* Excise fistula as above. Dissect a palatal mucoperiosteal flap based on palatine artery, rotate over socket, and suture in similar fashion (Figure 8.14). *Disadvantages*: bare bone left to granulate; difficult flap to rotate without distortion.
- *Buccal fat pad flap* If after raising the buccal advancement flap the periosteal incision is opened with artery forceps, the buccal fat pad is exposed. This can be easily mobilized as a pedicled flap to suture into and obtund the defect.

Sinus lift operation (📖 p. 470)

Fig. 8.14 The palatal rotation flap (after Ashley).
A Excise fistula; outline palatal flap based on greater palatine artery.
B Mobilize and rotate palatal flap, suturing its leading edge to buccal mucosa over bone. Leave donor site to granulate under surgical dressing or pack.

Minor preprosthetic surgery

When teeth are extracted alveolar bone resorbs, therefore should aim to preserve alveolar bone whenever possible, either by not extracting teeth (overdentures, 📖 p. 328) or by using a minimally traumatic technique.

At time of extraction of remaining teeth Extract carefully, compress the sockets, remove only small unattached pieces of bone, cover any exposed areas of bone with gingival flaps, and surgically remove roots *only* when necessary (infected, loose, >1/3 root length). Consider interseptal alveolotomy if ridge is prominent and heavily undercut (e.g. Class II). This consists of creating a labial osteomucosal flap by dividing the septae and extending bone cut at the <u>3</u> region through the buccal plate and collapsing-in the bone flap. Prominent frena should simply be excised. Attempts at decreasing the rate of ridge resorption have been made by leaving roots under mucosal flaps and by implanting hydroxyapatite or biocoral cones into extraction sockets.

Problems in denture wearers

▶ Only use surgery when denture faults and psychogenic disorders have been excluded. Screen jaws with DPT.

Retained roots and bone sequestrae are removed using standard transalveolar technique, except in the maxilla where buried canines may be removed using an osteoplastic flap (where bone is raised on a mucoperiosteal hinge).

Small bony irregularities can be smoothed with a bur but consider ridge augmentation if extensive.

Fibrous (flabby) ridges ↓ by raising a flap of attached gingiva to repair the defect, excise remaining soft tissue ridge, and repair with flap raised first. Fibrous tuberosities can be dealt with similarly.

Fibrous bands and irritation hyperplasia (Figure 8.15) should be excised. Results are improved if palatal mucosal grafts are used to repair the defects and minimize scarring.

Tori can be reduced with a bur under a local flap. Or resected with a combination of bur and chisel.

Muscle attachments to the mylohyoid ridge or genial tubercles can be displaced by resecting the bone from the mandible with a chisel and dissecting away the muscles. Genioglossus and geniohyoid should be reattached to the labial sulcus.

Ridge augmentation (📖 p. 470) The use of subperiosteally injected porous hydroxyapatite as an out-patient procedure under LA is useful in a very limited number of cases, mainly due to ridge type. In this technique, a subperiosteal tunnel is raised along the crest of the ridge and filled swith hydroxyapatite/saline sludge. It is very dependent on the shape of the ridge, and works best with concave ridges as opposed to the more often seen feather-edge ridge. *Problems*: migration of particles after periosteal elevation.

Sulcus deepening (📖 p. 470) When adequate vertical and horizontal basal bone exists but there is a shortage of ridge &/or attached gingiva, these procedures can help. Depends on: (a) dissecting away non-attached mucosa to leave a raw 'new' sulcus; (b) lining this new sulcus with skin or mucosa; (c) *securing the new depth with a 'stent'*—a denture or baseplate lined with tissue conditioner or impression compound, which is held in place by nylon sutures for 10–14 days, then replaced immediately by a new denture with a soft lining extended to the new sulcus and worn continually for the first 3 months.

Fig. 8.15 A clinical example of irritation hyperplasia caused by an ill-fitting lower denture.

Implantology

Single or multiple dental implants have become a well accepted method of restoration of missing teeth. They have the advantage of replacing teeth often using available bone without preparing healthy remaining teeth. Single tooth implants are an attractive alternative to anterior bridgework for this reason.

History Numerous procedures for oral implants have been described; all had advocates but most failed. Genuine advances in the discipline have come about, thanks to a major contribution by Bränemark: 'osseointegration'. All current implants are based on this now well-accepted concept.

Osseointegration is the direct abutment of bone to implant surface such that osteoblasts can be seen on electron micrographs to be growing on the implant surface. In addition, a tight fibrous/epithelial attachment above the crestal bone between gingiva and implant is essential. Finally, the implant must be designed to resist displacement and evenly dissipate occlusal loads.

Types of implant Large range. Materials are usually titanium alloys with different surface treatments to increase surface area and improve initial integration. Bioceramic is less common. They may be inserted transmucosally or in two stages (see below). Attached mucoperiosteum is 'best' perimplant tissue.

Indications Edentulous mouths unable to retain dentures, partially dentate for bridge abutments, single anterior tooth replacement, and maxillofacial prostheses post cancer surgery or trauma. If implants survive first 2yrs there is a 98% success rate with dramatic improvement in all functional parameters.[1] Success mandible > maxilla (bone quality). Irradiated bone should receive hyperbaric O_2 preoperatively.

Techniques Joint planning between surgeon and restorative dentist is essential for success.[2] If a single dentist is trained in both components of treatment the approach is simplified ('implantologist'). A balanced occlusion should be creatable, and a high standard of OH is mandatory. The surgical procedure is highly equipment-dependent, and the surgeon needs to be trained in the particular technique used. Most commonly, this involves:

- Fixture installation. A gingival–mucosal flap is raised, and a receiving channel is prepared in bone, using drills matched to the implant size and type. The fixture, depending on the type of implant is either pressed or screwed into place. In two-stage procedures the implant is covered by the flap at the end of the procedure. When placing multiple implants a direction indicator is helpful for achieving parallelism. Bone overheating must be avoided by constant irrigation. In two-stage procedures, healing periods as short as 1.5 months (mandible) and 2 months (maxilla) are now recommended. In one-stage procedures the implant heals partially exposed to the mouth for the same time period.

1 R. Adell 1983 *J Prosthetic Dent* **49** 251.

2 BAOMS/BSSPD 1995 Guidelines on Standards for the Treatment of Patients Using Endosseous Dental Implants, BDJ.

- In two-stage procedures, abutment connection is then carried out by punch excision of mucosa overlying the implants, removal of cover screws and insertion of the abutment. Prosthetic procedures start at abutment connection.

Implant salvage/bone augmentation The principles of GTR (📖 p. 208) can be used to allow bone formation around osseointegrated implants either to height or bulk, or to cover an exposed side of the implant.

Computer-aided design and computer-aided manufacturing (CAD/CAM) systems are used for implant placement and restoration on the same day.

Craniofacial implants (📖 p. 485)

Transmandibular implants (📖 p. 470)

Lasers

Definition Light amplification by the stimulated emission of radiation. Light consists of packets of photons transmitted in electromagnetic waves (visible light 400–700nm). Laser energy is produced by light stimulation of active media to generate collimated light energy at a specific frequency. The active media determines the characteristics of the laser.

Clinical lasers

These consist of two main groups, *hard* and *soft* lasers.

Hard lasers work principally by thermal effect, although certain benefits such as decreased scarring and pain are thought to be due to the photo-chemical effects of the laser beam.

Carbon dioxide laser A hard laser in common use in the hospital service. Main role is as a cutting beam which seals small vessels as it cuts. Also used to evaporate benign white patches of oral mucosa. Used as continuous wave or pulsed beam at 10–20 watts of energy.

KTP laser Similar to carbon dioxide laser, giving initially painless wounds. Becomes painful after 48–72h, however.

Argon laser Produces a light beam which is selectively absorbed by haemoglobin and melanin, therefore particularly useful for pigmented and vascular lesions.

Neodymium–Yttrium aluminium garnet (Nd–Yag) laser Originally marketed as a hard laser with a relatively low power output; now available as a soft dental laser.

Tuneable dye laser Expensive variable frequency laser.

Soft lasers Thought to work by stabilizing cell membranes by a non-thermal photochemical process, increasing cellular metabolism by a minor thermal change, and possibly by inducing endorphin release.

Helium–Neon The red aiming beam on hard lasers, classroom pointers, and the 'Terminator's' weaponry. Part of the soft laser group, it has no cutting effect but seems to act photochemically on cells. A similar non-thermal red light laser at highly specific frequency is used to active photosensitive chemicals as part of photodynamic therapy (PDT).

Neodymium–Yag A system using this active media is now marketed for use in dentistry and is purported to ↑ cell turnover, ↑ inflammatory response; inhibit oedema, ↑ rate of cell regeneration, e.g. peripheral neurones, and ↑ wound scarring. All this without any recognized side-effects. Many of these claims have yet to be widely validated.

Summary

Lasers are available for a range of uses in dentistry; they are expensive and require special safety precautions. Some benefits can be achieved in other ways and some have yet to be proven. They are a tool, not a magic wand.

Minimally invasive surgery

While some specialties such as orthopaedics and gynaecology have been using endoscopic technology for many years, a recent surge in fibre-optic technology coupled with the 'discovery' of the laparoscope by general surgeons made minimally invasive (minimal access) surgery one of the hot topics of the late 1990s.

One of the spin-offs of the sudden uncontrolled ↑ in the number of laparoscopic operations was bad publicity about some of the adverse outcomes following this type of surgery, and questions about surgeons' training. One very positive result of this has been the development of surgical skills laboratories, structured courses, and a real interest in training and education.

In the field of oral and maxillofacial surgery minimally invasive surgery has yet to make a significant impact. Current examples include:

Temporomandibular joint arthroscopy Uses specialized small rigid endoscopes with a fibre-optic light source which can be placed in the TMJ space (usually upper joint space) through a tiny incision in the preauricular skin. The joint is distended by a throughflow of sterile irrigant which exits via a needle placed about 1cm anterior to the arthroscope. Reasonable visualization is possible but significant surgery is fairly limited.

Functional endoscopic sinus surgery (FESS) Rigid endoscopes with angled viewing ports allow visualization and a certain amount of surgery of the paranasal sinuses. Biopsy and sampling of a wide range of paranasal tissues is possible and specific surgical expansion of the osteum may prove to be the ideal treatment for resistant chronic sinusitis. This technique has been rapidly developed by many ENT enthusiasts; however its evidence base is still being established.

Endoscopically assisted internal fixation Internal fixation of facial # is now widely accepted and standard practice; however, some areas, particularly of the mandible, are very difficult to access safely. Condylar neck # and some angle # may be more easily treated using a modified trocar system and an endoscope with light source.

Endoscopically assisted face and brow lifting Aesthetic facial surgery by its very nature requires distant and minimalist scars. Endoscopic brow lifting from the anterior scalp is reasonably straightforward and has become standard. Endoscopic facelifting makes a tedious operation more so.

NB While flexible fibre-optic scopes play quite an extensive role in examination of the upper aerodigestive tract, the extent to which significant head and neck surgery can be performed is currently limited.

Oral medicine

Contents

Principal sources Much of the skill of oral medicine lies in the clinical recognition of lesions, therefore a colour atlas of oral mucosal disease is invaluable, e.g. M. Lewis & R. Jordan 2004 *A Colour Handbook of Oral Medicine,* Blackwell Publishing. Other useful sources of information are A. Field & L. Longman 2003 *Tyldesley's Oral Medicine (Ed 5),* OUP. C. Scully 2008 *Oral & Maxillofacial Medicine—The Basis of Diagnosis and Treatment (Ed2),* Churchill Livingstone.   Related subjects are **Oral Pathology**: J. Soames and J. Southam 2004 *Oral Pathology,* 4 edn OUP; R. Cawson and E. Odell 2008 *Cawsons essentials of oral pathology & oral medicine (Ed 8—the most recent version of my 'best buy' book when I was in dental school),* Churchill Livingstone. **Temporomandibular joint**: R. Gray 1995 *Temporomandibular Disorders: A Clinical Approach, BDJ.* Although the authors of the latter have a slightly different approach, this is a thoughtful, informative, and useful book.

Bacterial infections of the mouth

Caries (📖 p. 24); periodontal disease (📖 Chapter 5); dento-facial infections (📖 p. 370). This page refers primarily to mucosal infections.

Scarlet fever May be due to a delayed type hypersensitivity to streptococcal erythrogenic toxin. Usually causes an URTI. The sore throat is accompanied by a skin rash, general malaise, and fever. The oral mucosa is reddened and the tongue undergoes pathognomonic changes; the dorsum develops a white coating through which white oedematous fungiform papillae project—the 'strawberry tongue' of scarlet fever. Later the white coating is shed and the dorsum becomes smooth and red with enlarged fungiform papillae—'raspberry tongue'. Rx is directed towards the systemic condition with high-dose penicillin. The oral manifestations resolve within 14 days.

Tuberculosis A re-emerging infectious disease caused by *Mycobacterium tuberculosis*. It is commonly seen in immunocompromised patients, including elderly persons. TB is rare in Western countries, however, it is being reported more frequently in recent years. This has been attributed to increased migration and spread of HIV. Although 1/3 of global population is affected by TB, oral involvement with it is rare. When it does occur it is usually due to open pulmonary infection or coexisting HIV. The oral lesion presents as a deep painful ulcer with raised borders, gradually increasing in size. Any part of the oral mucosa may be involved, although the posterior aspect of the dorsum of the tongue is the commonest site. PCR may facilitate definitive Δ, especially in cases with unusual presentation. Histopathology shows necrotizing granuloma with Langhan's giant cells and epithelioid cells and a Ziehl–Nielsen stain reveals mycobacteria. Previous infection can sometimes be seen on facial views as radio-opacities due to calcifications within lymph nodes. Refer to a chest physician for management as combination chemotherapy is required.

Syphilis All phases (1°, 2° and 3°) affect the mouth.

1° lesion A chancre (a firm, painless ulcerated nodule) develops at the site of inoculation, usually the lips or tongue. This lesion is highly infectious and *Treponema pallidum* can easily be isolated. There is usually marked cervical lymphadenopathy which resolves spontaneously in 1–2 months.

2° lesion Develops 2–4 months after the 1° with a cutaneous rash, condylomata and ulceration of the oral mucosa. This oral involvement occurs regardless of the site of 1° infection, with superficial grey, sloughy ulcers known as mucous patches or snail-track ulcers. These are also highly contagious and *T. pallidum* can be easily isolated. Syphilis serology is positive at this stage. The ulcers generally clear up within a few weeks, although there may be recurrences.

3° lesion Develops several years later in 30% of patients and is marked by gumma formation. This is a necrotic granulomatous reaction usually affecting the palate or tongue, which enlarges and ulcerates and may lead to perforation of the palate. In the past, syphilis of the tongue was associated with malignant change, often presenting as a leukoplakia. It is not entirely clear whether it was the condition or its Rx which caused this. Lesions are non-infectious.

Congenital syphilis Due to *Treponema pallidum* crossing the placental barrier leading to classical appearance of saddle nose, frontal bossing, Hutchinson incisors (peg-shaped with notch), and mulberry (Moon) molars.

Gonorrhoea 15 times more common than syphilis. This is a result of oro-genital contact with an infected partner and presents as a non-specific stomatitis or pharyngitis with frequent persisting superficial ulcers and purulent gingivitis caused by *Neisseria gonorrhoeae*. Swabs may reveal Gram −ve intracellular diplococci. Rx is with high-dose penicillin; STD should be referred to a genitourinary medicine specialist.

Viral infections of the mouth

Herpes simplex (human herpesvirus type 1 and 2) Most common viral infection affecting the mouth. Although oral infection with herpes simplex types 1 and 2 has been described, type 1 remains the dominant pathogen. Antibodies indicating past infection are virtually ubiquitous in adults. There are two oral manifestations.

Primary oral infection. Varies widely in severity (↑ with age). In infancy is often mistakenly attributed to 'teething'. Presents with a single episode of widespread stomatitis and unstable mucosa with vesicles which break down to form shallow painful ulcers , enlarged, tender cervical lymph nodes, halitosis, coated tongue, fever, and a general malaise for 10–14 days. Although generally self-limiting, rare complications include herpetic encephalitis and menengitis. Δ: based on the clinical features and history, although the virus can be grown in cell culture. Microscopically ballooning degeneration of epithelial cells with intranuclear viral inclusions 'Lipshutz bodies' are seen. A fourfold ↑ in convalescent phase antibodies is also diagnostic, *but* give the Δ only retrospectively. Rx: topical and systemic analgesia (benzydamine, paracetamol), a soft or liquid diet with extra fluid intake, and prevention of 2° infection (chlorhexidine mouthwash) is usually adequate in healthy patients. Severely ill or immunocompromised patients should receive systemic aciclovir.

Recurrent infections seen in up to 30% of patients affecting mucocutaneous junction of the lips (herpes labialis, cold sore) is a reactivation of the 1° infection which is believed to lie dormant in the trigeminal ganglion. Precipitating factors include trauma, e.g. during removal of 8 and immunosuppression and, less commonly, exposure to sunlight, stress, or other illness. Usually recurs on the skin of lip or nose supplied by one branch of trigeminal nerve, classically at the mucocutaneous junction, or rarely as an IO blister. Prodromal phase over 24h where there is a prickling sensation on the lips followed by vesiculation and pain. Lesions may respond to 1% penciclovir or aciclovir 5% cream if used in the prodromal stage at least 5 times a day. Should consider systemic aciclovir (🕮 p. 573) in the immunosuppressed.

Varicella zoster (human herpes virus 3) is neurogenic DNA virus which causes chickenpox as a 1° infection and shingles as a reactivation.

Chickenpox Classically an itchy, vesicular, cutaneous, centripetal rash which may rarely affect the oral mucosa. Patients are infectious from 1 to 2 days before the rash, until rash scabs.

Shingles is confined to the distribution of a nerve, the virus staying either in the dorsal root ganglion of a peripheral nerve or the trigeminal ganglion. Always presents as a unilateral lesion never crossing the midline. Facial or oral lesions may arise in the area supplied by the branches of the trigeminal nerve. Δ: pre-eruption pain, followed by development of painful vesicles on skin or oral mucosa, which rupture to give ulcers or crusting skin wounds, in the distribution outlined above. These usually clear in 2–4 weeks, with scarring and pigmentations and is often followed by severe postherpetic neuralgia which may continue for years. Rx: symptomatic relief for chickenpox. There is some evidence to suggest that aggressive early Rx of shingles with aciclovir ↓ the incidence and severity of post-herpetic neuralgia in immunocompromised patients. Urgent referral to an ophthalmologist if the eye is involved.

Coxsackievirus is an RNA virus causing 2° oral mucosal conditions.

Herpangina Caused by Coxsackie A virus (A1 + A6, A8, A10, A12, A16, or A22) is confined to children and presents with widespread small ulcers on the oral mucosa with fever and general upset. Clinically it resembles herpetic stomatitis, but with no *gingivitis* and mainly affecting posterior mouth and soft palate with only moderate cervical lymphadenitis. May be preceded by sore throat and conjunctivitis. Can also be mistaken as 'teething'. Self-limiting in 10–14 days. Fairly rare.

Hand, foot, and mouth disease Caused by Coxsackie virus (usually A16, but less commonly types 5 and 10) and is also confined to children. A papular, vesicular rash appears on the hands and feet in conjunction with nasal congestion and oral mucosal vesicles. These break down, leaving painful superficial ulcers, particularly on the palate. The gingivae are rarely involved. It is self-limiting in 10–14 days. Rx as herpetic stomatitis. Quite common.

Human papilloma virus has been associated with squamous cell papilloma (📖 p. 376), condyloma acuminatum (multiple white/pink nodules), focal epithelial hyperplasia (multiple painless papules), and verruca vulgaris (white exophytic lumps). HPV may be associated with oropharyngeal cancer although this remains inconclusive. This group of viruses are linked with cervical cancer. Rx: local surgery and possibly interferon for benign growths. Conventional treatment for cancer 📖 p. 480.

Measles The prodromal phase of measles may be marked by small white spots with an erythematous margin on the buccal mucosa, known as Koplik spots. A few days later the maculo-papular rash of measles appears, usually behind the ears, then spreading to the face and trunk. Complications include pneumonia and encephalitis which may lead to neurological deficits in 40% and has a 15% mortality.

Glandular fever (infectious mononucleosis) is seen mostly in children and young adults and spread by infected saliva. It varies widely in severity and presents with sore throat, generalized lymphadenopathy, fever, headaches, general malaise, and often a maculo-papular rash. There may be hepatosplenomegaly. Oral manifestations may mimic 1° herpetic gingivostomatitis, with widespread oral ulceration, and in addition petechial haemorrhages, especially at the junction of hard and soft palate (pathognomonic), and bruising may be present. The cause is usually Epstein–Barr virus (EBV) and, less commonly, cytomegalovirus (CMV). Toxoplasmosis can give a similar picture. Δ: initially monospot test, Paul–Bunnell test to exclude EBV, and acute and convalescent titres for CMV and toxoplasmosis. Be aware that early HIV infection can mimic this condition. Rx: symptomatic as for 1° herpes, except toxoplasmosis, which may respond to sulfa drugs; seek expert advice. **NB** Ampicillin should not be given to patients with a sore throat who may have glandular fever as it inevitably produces an unwanted response, ranging from a rash to anaphylaxis.

Opportunistic infection on the tongue mucosa by EBV is thought to be the pathological mechanism behind 'hairy leukoplakia'.

Reiter's disease (reactive arthritis) Causative agent unknown but appears to be 2 to 3 weeks post-infective response. Consists of urethritis, arthritis, conjunctivitis &/or oral ulcers or erosions. Predominantly affects young males and is associated with HLA B27 in 80% of patients—leukocytosis and ↑ ESR are common.

Oral candidosis (candidiasis)

Although over 100 *Candida* species can be isolated only a handful are clinically important. *C. albicans* and *C. dubliniensis* are by far the most important. It is found in the mouths of more than 40% of the symptom-free population. Overt infection occurs when there are local or systemic predisposing factors, therefore the prime tenet of management is to look for and treat these factors. Candidosis is conveniently divided into:

Acute candidosis

Pseudomembraneous candidosis (thrush) Commonest in infancy, old age, and the immunosuppressed or debilitated (e.g. radiotherapy, cytotoxics, steroids, diabetes, cancer, HIV, and haematological malignancy), or those on broad spectrum antibiotics (disease of the diseased). Δ: appears as creamy lightly adherent plaques on an erythematous oral mucosa, usually on the cheek, palate, or oropharynx. Occasionally symptomless, but more commonly cause discomfort on eating. These plaques can be gently stripped off, leaving a raw under-surface and, with Gram staining, show candidal hyphae. In infancy, widespread oral candidosis can be associated with a livid facial rash and an associated nappy rash. Colonization of a breast-feeding mother's nipples can lead to mutual recolonization. Rx: in addition to treatment of predisposing factors, nystatin SF suspension 100 000 units rinsed then swallowed qds 10 days, or nystatin pastille 1qds, are cheap and usually effective preparations. Chlorhexidine mouthwash is an effective adjunct to Rx. Amphotericin and miconazole are more expensive (and mutually antagonistic) alternatives. Fluconazole 50mg od or itraconazole 100mg od (caution in patients at risk of heart failure) are the systemic drug of choice. *C. glabrata*, *C. tropicalis*, and *C. knusel* are fluconazole resistant, therefore, candida subtyping should be performed for resistant cases. Most antifungals especially azole group interact with number of drugs including warfarin.

Acute erythematous candidosis (formerly called denture sore mouth) is an opportunistic infection following the use of broad-spectrum antibiotics, sometimes inhaled steroids, and in patients with HIV as well as those with xerostomia. It is red and painful and exacerbated by hot or spicy foods. The oral mucosa has a red, shiny, atrophic appearance and there may be coexisting areas of thrush. Rx: eliminate cause (if due to inhaled steroids rinse mouth with water after inhaling and/or use a spacer device), otherwise as above.

Chronic candidosis

Chronic atrophic candidosis (denture stomatitis) (📖 p. 324) Reported prevalence of denture stomatitis: 10–75%.

Angular cheilitis is a combined staphylococcal, β-hemolytic streptococci and candidal infection, involving the tissues at the angle of the mouth (Figure 9.1). Aetiology is multifactorial with local and systemic precipitating factor, e.g. trauma, inadequate vertical dimension of denture, iron deficiency and B$_{12}$ deficiency anaemia. Therefore, haematological deficiency should be investigated with a FBC, red cell folate, B$_{12}$, and glucose. Often associated with chronic atrophic candidosis. Clinically, see red, cracked, macerated skin at angles of the mouth, often with a gold crust. Infecting organisms can be identified on culture of swabs of the area, although it is usual to make a clinical Δ. Rx: miconazole cream, which is active against all three infecting organisms. Rx needs to be prolonged, up to 10 days after resolution of clinical lesion, and carried out in conjunction with elimination of any underlying factors. Mupirocin cream applied to the anterior nares helps eradicate sources of S. aureus.

Median rhomboid glossitis is no longer considered to be an anatomical abnormality but a form of chronic atrophic candidosis affecting the dorsum of the tongue. Seen in patients using inhaled steroids and smokers. Some patients have lesions in the centre of the dorsum of tongue and palate (kissing lesions). Rx only if symptomatic as discomfort can be improved with topical antifungals, but the appearance cannot. Exclude haematinic deficiency and diabetes.

Chronic hyperplastic candidosis (candidal leukoplakia) More commonly seen in middle aged men who are heavy smokers. Typically presents as white patch on the oral commissural buccal mucosa bilaterally or dorsum of tongue. Although there is an ↑ risk of malignant change (see 📖 p. 416), the initial approach *after ensuring the diagnosis microbiologically and histopathologically* is to eradicate the candidal infection. Candidal hyphae can be seen in the superficial layers of the epidermis, one reason why eradication is so difficult. Rx: systemic antifungals such as fluconazole and itraconazole, while expensive, are indicated in an attempt to remove the infecting organism. Often associated with iron, folate, and B_{12} deficiency, and smoking, which should be corrected. Most lesions will resolve after such Rx; if not, reassess degree of dysplasia. Patients should be encouraged to stop smoking to avoid recurrence.

Chronic mucocutaneous candidosis A rare syndrome complex with several subgroups, including: **candidal endocrinopathy**, where skin and mouth lesions occur in conjunction with endocrine abnormalities, **granulomatous skin candidosis**, a **late-onset predominantly male-affecting group**, and an **AIDS-associated group**. Rx: difficult, fluconazole 100mg od for 3 weeks or itraconazole 200mg od for 3 weeks (📖 p. 573). Voriconazole has recently been introduced as a treatment.

Histoplasmosis This and other rare fungal infections have occasional oral manifestations.

Fig. 9.1 Clinical example of severe angular cheilitis associated with chronic oral candidosis.

Recurrent aphthous stomatitis (ulcers)

This is the term given to a fairly well-defined group of conditions characterized by recurrent oral ulceration. There are three subgroups:

Minor aphthous ulcers A very common condition (~25% of population) affecting ~80% of RAS patients. Start at childhood or adolescence. Usually appears as a group of 1–6 ulcers at a time, of variable size (usually 2–5mm diameter) (Figure 9.2). Mainly occur on non-keratinized mucosa and heal within 1–2 weeks without scarring. Usually recur at an interval of 1–4 months. Prodromal discomfort may precede painful ulcers. Exacerbated by stress, local trauma, menstruation (fall in progesterone level), sodium lauryl sulfate (in some toothpastes), drugs (NSAID, alendronate and nicorandil), smoking, allergy to some foods and may be an oral 'marker' of iron, B$_{12}$, or folate deficiencies. In some cases are a manifestation of Crohn's disease, ulcerative colitis, or gluten enteropathy. Aetiology, although not fully understood, is almost certainly autoimmune in patients with genetic predisposition (HLA A1, A11, B12 and DR2). There is a familial history in 45% of cases. Rx: prevent superinfection with chlorhexidine mouthwash and relieve pain (simple analgesics, benzydamine mouthrinse). Topical tetracycline and steroid preparations are sometimes useful (📖 p. 576). It is important to look for and treat any underlying deficiency or coexisting pathology (FBC, Haematinics, B12 and red cell folate, serum antiendomysium and transglutaminase assay).

Major aphthous ulcers Seen in 10% of RAS patients. A more severe and more frequent variant with fewer, but larger ulcers >10mm which may last 5–10 weeks and most commonly affect keratinized mucosa. Associated with tissue destruction and scarring, and any site in the mouth and oropharynx may be affected. There is an even higher association between major aphthae and gastrointestinal and haematological disorders. They are also seen in AIDS. Seldom a cyclical pattern. Rx: as for minor aphthae, plus topical or systemic steroids (📖 p. 576).

Herpetiform ulcers Least common. A descriptive term, as these ulcers have nothing whatsoever to do with infection with the herpesvirus. Commoner in older females. Manifest as a crop of small but painful ulcers which usually last 1–2 weeks, the commonest site being the floor of mouth, lateral margins, and tip of tongue. They heal without scarring and may occur on both keratinized and non-keratinized surfaces. Rarely, merge to form a large ulcer which heals with scarring. Rx: as for minor aphthous ulceration.

Behçet disease A severe refractory systemic vasculitis of unknown aetiology, characteristically affecting venules. All organs of the body can be concurrently or consecutively affected. It has a world wide distribution but is most prevalent in the Far East, along the *Silk Route*, and in the Middle East. In the UK a prevalence of 0.064 in 10 000 has been reported from Yorkshire. It is a disease of young adults, and rare before age of 10yrs and after 50yrs. More common and more severe in young males. It is associated with HLA subtype Δ clinical due to absence of laboratory tests and based on presence of recurrent oral ulcers and two of the following: recurrent genital ulceration, eye lesions (uveitis), or skin lesions (erythema nodosum, folliculitis). Good evidence that prophylactic Rx with azathioprine can prevent blindness. Steroids are mainstay. Rx: ophthalmic referral if eye involved. Monoclonal anti-TNF (etanercept and infliximab) are helpful in severe mouth ulcers. Thalidomide is also effective but neuropathy is a major side-effect.

Oral ulcers See 📖 p. 444.

Fig. 9.2 Classically aphthous ulceration affects the non-keratinized mucosa although it is not an exclusive finding.

Vesiculo-bullous lesions—intraepithelial

Vesicle is a small blister a few millimetres in diameter.

Bulla is a larger blister.

Intraepithelial bullae are caused by loss of attachment between individual cells (acantholysis).

Subepithelial bullae separate the epithelium from the underlying corium.

Ulcer is a breach in the mucous membrane.
Immunopathology: immunofluorescence is a prime diagnostic test. Direct immunofluorescence is performed on fresh biopsy specimen. Indirect is performed on a serum sample.

Erosions are shallower than ulcers.
   Because the vesiculo-bullous lesions constitute a defined group with examples from several different pathological processes, they are a favourite examinations topic. One method of classifying this group is into intraepithelial and subepithelial, according to where the blisters form.

Pemphigus is a chronic skin disease which is lethal if not Rx. Oral mucosa is affected in 95% of patients with pemphigus vulgaris and may be the initial presentation of pemphigus in 50%. Autoimmune in aetiology, there are circulating autoantibodies to epithelial intercellular substance. Acantholysis and intercellular IgG &/or C3 are typical (autoantibodies against desmoglein 1 and 3 adhesion molecules of squamous epithelium) and cause separation of epithelium above the basal cell layer, and oedema into this potential space produces a superficial, easily burst, fluid-filled bulla. Rupture leaves a large superficial, easily infected ulcer. The first identifiable lesions are quite often found in the mouth, especially on the palate, although these are usually seen as ulcers because the bullae break down rapidly. It is mainly a disease of middle age (F > M), with ↑ incidence in Jews and Arabs. Rarely, it may be drug-induced. Δ: stroking the mucosa produces a bulla (Nikolsky's sign), but this is inducing pathology for the sake of Δ. Other methods are by direct or indirect immunofluorescent techniques (biopsy samples need to be fresh). Rx: systemic steroids &/or azathioprine, dapsone, mycophenolate mofetil, or gold; also cyclophosphamide, especially in refractory and severe cases. Newer therapies include biologic agents (rituximab) and calcineurin inhibitors appear promising.

Benign familial chronic pemphigus (Hailey-Hailey disease) differs from the above by having a strong family history, with onset of the disease in young adults.

Viral infections, 📖 p. 398.

Epidermolysis bullosa (simplex is most common form) Other variants are subepithelial. Due to genetic defect in basement membrane proteins. Skin blisters due to mild trauma, leading to scarring and disfigurement. Caries and periodontal disease are common due to inability to maintain good OH. Simplex type is due to mutations in *K5* or *K14* gene, leading to disruption of basal cells and formation of bullae. No cure and treatment is symptomatic and preventive.

Vesiculo-bullous lesions—subepithelial

Angina bullosa haemorrhagica A fancy name for an acute, localized oral blood blister of unknown aetiology, although trauma may cause break in epithelium–connective tissue junction leading to bleeding from superficial capillaries and formation of bulla. Most common in elderly and rare below 10 years of age. Steroid inhalers may predispose. Soft palate, cheeks and tongue most common sites. Δ: exclude other bullous conditions. Rx: puncture &/or reassure (must differentiate from pemphigus/pemphigoid).

Mucous membrane pemphigoid Commonest in females >60yrs. Presents as mucous membrane bullae which rupture and heal with scar formation. Rare to see skin bullae. Conjunctiva may be affected and if scarring occurs can lead to loss of vision, therefore regard oral signs as a warning to prevent ocular damage. The natural history is of a long-lasting disease which persists with periods of activity and inactivity alternating and may be quiescent for several years. More common than pemphigus and pemphigoid. Δ: again direct (biopsy vesicle or perilesional tissue rather than erosion) and indirect immunofluorescence is used, the antibodies (mainly IgG and C3) being found at the level of the basement membrane or hemidesmosomes. The bullae are blood-filled and tense and may be found in conjunction with desquamative gingivitis. Rx: topical steroids, systemic steroids with or without azathioprine, or dapsone. Refer to ophthalmology.

Pemphigoid affects >60-yr age group. Subepithelial bullae form which are firm and less likely to break down than those in pemphigus due to autoantibodies to epithelial basement membrane. The oral mucosa is only affected in ~20% of patients. May be an external 'marker' of internal malignancy or a drug-related immune response.

Dermatitis herpetiformis is a rare chronic condition of unknown aetiology, but often associated with gluten sensitivity with autoantibodies against reticullin, gliadin, endomysium, and transglutaminase. Oral lesions seen in 70% of patients with skin lesion. Commoner in middle-aged men; it affects both skin and mucous membranes; bullae in the mouth break down to leave large erosions. Rx: dapsone may be used both diagnostically and therapeutically. Gluten-free diet helps. Sulfapyridine is an alternative to dapsone.

Lichen planus affects both skin and mucous membranes. Bullous lichen planus is a rare variant in which subepithelial bullae form and break down, leaving large erosions. See also 📖 p. 430.

Epidermolysis bullosa This is a rare skin disease which exists in numerous different forms. The dystrophic autosomal recessive form is most likely to present with oral manifestations and appears shortly after birth. Associated with bullae formation after minor trauma to skin or mucosa; these break down leaving painful erosions. Dentine may be affected leading to hypoplasia and high susceptibility to caries. Healing is with scarring, resulting in difficulty in eating, speaking, and swallowing as scar tissue limits movement.

Skin involvement can lead to destruction of extremities and may be overtaken by carcinomatous change. Prognosis varies widely depending on type. Phenytoin and steroids may help some varieties.

Erythema multiforme This is a group of signs and symptoms of multifactorial aetiology; minor form (only mouth with target lesions on skin) or major (2 or more mucous membranes with more variable skin involvement) the most severe form is known as Stevens–Johnson syndrome (📖 p. 731). Affects skin and mucous membranes with an acute onset, usually in young adult males, and is probably due to deposition of immune complexes. It is associated with exposure to certain drugs (sulfas, barbiturates and cephalosporins) or infecting organisms (herpes simplex, mycoplasma) in a susceptible individual (hormonal changes). Δ: from clinical features which include 'target lesions', concentric rings of erythema on the palms, legs, face, or neck. Oral lesions seen in 70% in which the oral mucosa is covered in bullae which break down, the lips and gingivae becoming crusted with painful erosions. There is usually a fever. It is a self-limiting condition in 3–4 weeks but can recur once or twice a year.

Management Hospitalization may be required in severe forms. Biopsy; virological studies to exclude herpes; identify and avoid precipitating factors; aciclovir may be needed if it is related to herpes. Improve OH with 0.2% chlorhexidine mouthwash. Severe form: Rx with steroids and azathioprine. Minor form: Rx with topical steroids.

Linear IgA disease is rare, identified pathologically. May be variant of dermatitis herpetiformis.

White patches

Numerous conditions manifest as white patches of the oral mucosa; some of these are transient, such as thrush (📖 p. 400) or chemical burns (e.g. aspirin). May be localized (due to trauma or neoplasia) or wide spread (hereditary or systemic).

White spongy naevus This is a rare condition affecting keratin. A benign, familial disorder inherited as autosomal dominant. It appears as asymptomatic diffuse soft, uneven thickening of the superficial layer of the epithelium, which characteristically has no definite boundary and may affect any part of the mouth. Histology shows hyperplastic epithelium with gross intraepithelial oedema. Rx: neither exists nor is required.

Frictional keratosis This is a white patch due to hyperplastic hyperkeratotic epithelium induced by local trauma, e.g. sharp tooth and cheek biting. It is managed by removal of the source of the friction, which will generally allow complete resolution of the lesion. If this doesn't happen, biopsy is indicated. Can be seen as self-mutilation in psychiatric disorders or learning disability.

Smokers' keratosis Characteristically a white patch affecting buccal mucosa, tongue, or palate. Appears as discrete white patch. Due to a combination of low-grade burn and the chemical irritants of smoke, and seen particularly in pipe smokers. There is little evidence that these patches are premalignant and they resolve on stopping smoking.

Stomatitis nicotina Affects palate; numerous red papules on a white/grey base. The papules have a dark 'head' which is the opening of a distended minor salivary gland.

'Syphilitic leukoplakia' A white patch on the dorsum of the tongue is one of the classical appearances of tertiary syphilis (📖 p. 396). Active disease must be treated; however, this will not resolve the area of leukoplakia, which has a propensity to undergo malignant change. Δ is usually suggested by histology, serology, or dark ground microscopy of smears.

Chronic hyperplastic candidosis/candidal leukoplakia, 📖 p. 401.

Lichen planus, 📖 p. 430 (Figure 9.3).

Lupus erythematosis, 📖 p. 430.

Leukoplakia, 📖 p. 414.

Hairy leukoplakia, 📖 p. 440.

Panoral leukoplakia is where the entire oral mucosa appears to be undergoing hyperplastic field change. Risk of malignant change.

Oral carcinoma Occasionally, oral cancer may appear as a white patch, as distinct from a leukoplakia becoming malignant.

Skin grafts may appear as a white patch in the mouth—and are a trap for the unwary in exams.

Renal failure can produce soft, oval white patches which resolve on Rx of renal failure.

Darier's disease A rare skin condition whose oral lesions (present in ~50%) are coalescing white papules on gingivae and palate.

Pachyonychia congenita A rare genetic condition affecting nails, skin, and sweat glands. Oval, benign white patches on tongue are common.

Proliferative verrucous leukoplakia hard to define white patch which appears to have a high incidence of long-term malignant transformation. F>M

Fig. 9.3 The typical appearance of reticular pattern oral lichen planus, a condition with no premalignant potential (this is found in the erosive variant, see 📖 p. 415).

Pigmented lesions of the mouth

In many respects the pulling together of pigmented lesions of the oral mucosa is artificial, as they are not related by pathology or Rx. Pigmented lesions are, however, a popular exam question and with this in mind we offer the following well-recognized conditions.

Δ is aided by whether the pigmentation is localized, or generalized throughout the mouth.

Localized

Foreign body amalgam tattoo is the commonest, a localized dense blue/black area of mucosal pigmentation. May result from implantation at time of restoration or from broken filling. Radio-opaque. May be palpable but often not. Amalgam tends to become granular and fragmented and if removal is planned, cut out as full thickness wedge. If asymptomatic, diagnose and reassure. 'Road rash' from grit after road traffic accident or graphite from pencils can cause similar.

Local response to chronic trauma usually presents as an area of keratosis but sometimes can appear pigmented.

Ephelis a freckle of the oral mucosa. Harmless.

Pigmented naevi Rare and benign. Analogous to a mole. Mostly harmless. Most commonly seen on vermilion border of lips and palate. If <1cm, they do not change in size or colour.

Peutz–Jegher syndrome (🔲 p. 730) Multiple small perioral naevi.

Kaposi's sarcoma (🔲 p. 440) A radiosensitive tumour associated with AIDS.

Malignant melanoma Potentially lethal, relatively rare IO malignancy. Very dark, irregular outline, enlarges rapidly; poor prognosis. Rare variant is non-pigmented.

Generalized

Racial pigmentation of the oral mucosa varies with skin type and is obviously not pathological.

Foodstuffs A variety can cause superficial mucosal discoloration. Tobacco is the major offender, and paan in some Asian cultures.

Drugs Antimalarials, phenothiazines, cisplatin, zidovudine, busulfan, and oral contraceptives can all cause mucosal pigmentation. Commonest offender is chlorhexidine mouthwash, especially if 'blended' with tea and tobacco.

Heavy metal salts Now rare; classically deposited along the gingival margin in lead or mercury poisoning.

Endocrine associated Addison's disease, ACTH-secreting tumours, adenomatous pituitary dysfunction (Nelson syndrome), ACTH Rx.

Diagnose: BP, electrolytes, cortisol levels, and response to ACTH stimulation (synacthen test).

Haemochromatosis Haemosiderin deposits cause hyperpigmentation. Rare.

Black hairy tongue Caused by overgrowth of pigment-producing microorganisms combined with benign overgrowth of the filiform papillae of the dorsum of the tongue and a lack of normal desquamation. Rx: reassurance, improve OH, tongue scrape or tongue shave depending on patient need/severity.

Premalignant lesions

There exists a group of conditions which have an ↑ risk of malignant transformation of the oropharyngeal mucosa. Although a great deal of attention has been paid to these premalignant conditions, it should be remembered that only a small number of oral cancers are preceded by them, and also that the designation 'premalignant' does not necessarily imply certain malignant transformation. Indeed, the majority of patients with so-called premalignant lesions will not go on to develop oral cancer. The ↑ risk of progression to carcinoma necessitates accurate Δ, Rx if indicated, and long-term follow-up in an attempt to pre-empt life-threatening disease.

Leukoplakia 'White patch or plaque which cannot be characterized clinically or pathologically as any other disease and is not associated with any physical or chemical agent except the use of tobacco' (WHO).

The histopathology of these lesions varies widely from the essentially benign to carcinoma-in-situ. They are usually characterized by a thick surface layer of keratin with thickening of the prickle cell layer of the epithelium, acanthosis, and infiltration of the corium by plasma cells; however, the most important variable is cellular atypia amongst the epithelial cells. Pointers to look for are: nuclear hyperchromatism, an ↑ nuclear/cytoplasmic ratio, cellular and nuclear pleomorphism, ↑ &/or atypical mitoses, individual cell keratinization, and focal disturbance in cell arrangement and adhesion. The degree of cellular atypia is one of the most important factors to be considered in the management of a leukoplakia. However, histology of epithelial dysplasia is not reliable, and in one study pathologists in 20% of cases could not confirm or refute their own earlier Δ of dysplasia. Furthermore there is no guarantee that the biopsy specimen is representative of the whole lesion. The second major consideration is the site, e.g. floor of mouth and ventral surface of tongue are more likely to undergo malignant change than most. Thirdly, relation to cause, e.g. buccal leukoplakia, the preferred site for a paan quid is at high risk of malignant change if the habit is not discontinued.

On average 5% of leukoplakias progress to carcinomas; however, in certain sites, e.g. floor of mouth, >25% may progress and certain variants, e.g. 'candidal leukoplakia', have a claimed 10–40% incidence of malignant change. Δ and Rx: specialist referral is indicated—biopsy (possibly guided by toluidine blue to select most appropriate area) and Rx as appropriate. Malignant transformation is more common among non-smokers (idiopathic leukoplakia): 2.4% are malignant in 10yrs, 5% are malignant in 20yrs, a 50–100 times greater risk than normal mouth.

Erythroleukoplakia (speckled leukoplakia) This is basically leukoplakia with areas of erythroplakia. Exhibits an ↑ risk of malignant transformation.

Erythroplakia is generally a well-demarcated, red velvety patch of the oral mucosa which histologically shows marked cellular atypia, no surface keratinization, and a degree of atrophy of the surface layer. Most of these lesions are carcinoma-in-situ or frank carcinoma and are found at high risk sites (at least 85%).

Erosive lichen planus is a comparatively rare variant of lichen planus, which some authorities believe to be premalignant (<1%). The common forms of lichen planus have no premalignant potential.

Submucous fibrosis is a condition found particularly in those of South Asian extraction, and is thought to be a tanning of the oral mucous membrane induced by betel-quid chewing *without* the addition of tobacco (some cultures use a quid of betel leaf, areca nut, and slake lime; others add tobacco to this; the first seems to produce submucous fibrosis, the second carcinoma). The mucosa is pale, with constraining fibrous bands, and fibrosis of the submucosa occurs, making the lips and cheeks immobile and resulting in trismus. Histology shows hyalinization and acellular dense fibrous tissue with narrowed blood vessels and a lymphocytic infiltrate. There is epithelial atrophy and cellular atypia. Pathogenesis unclear; ↑ levels of copper due to areca nut chewing leading to cross-linking of collagen by upregulation of lysyl oxidase and thus ↑ fibrosis and DNA damage.

Malignant transformation is seen in 10% in 10–15yrs. Rx: stop habit, intralesional steroids/exercise, surgery with flap reconstruction.

Dyskeratosis congenita A rare autosomal dominant condition of pigmented skin, nail dystrophy, and leukoplakia evident in childhood. White plaques have premalignant potential (📖 p. 430).

Patterson–Brown–Kelly syndrome (Plummer–Vinson syndrome), 📖 p. 730.

Management of premalignant lesions Record site, preferably photographically. Consider site, histology, age, and health of the patient, in conjunction with aetiological factors, before deciding on long-term observation or active intervention. Completely stop patient from smoking and 60% will disappear.[1] Observation may consist of clinical examination with repeated cytology (although cytology has generally been disappointing), or biopsy if change is seen. Guided biopsy with toluidine blue may ↑ diagnostic accuracy. Rx options: laser excision, cryotherapy, surgical excision, topical bleomycin, photodynamic therapy after removal of any identifiable aetiological factors. Follow-up at 3-monthly intervals.

▶ It is impossible to predict the behaviour of a patch of leukoplakia with precision.

1 J Pindborg 1980 *Oral Cancer and Precancer.* Wright, Bristol.

Oral cancer

Cancer of the mouth (Figure 9.4) accounts for ~2% of all malignant tumours in northern Europe and the USA, but ~30–40% in the Indian subcontinent. >90% of these are SCCs. Globally it is the 6th commonest cause of cancer-related death. >2000 new cases of oral cancer are registered per year in the UK and each year half that number dies from or with the disease. Oral cancer is preventable in 75% of cases. Overall mortality rate is just over 50% despite treatment. Recent survival data suggests that the UK has the best survival figures for diagnosed oral cancer at all stages.

Site The floor of the mouth is the commonest single site, and when combined with lingual sulcus and ventral surface of tongue, creates a horseshoe area (coffin area), accounting for over 75% of carcinomas seen in European or American practice. M>F, although this difference is less than it has been in the past, partly due to changes in smoking habits. There appears to be an increasing incidence in younger patients and those who do not use tobacco. Currently 95% of patients are >40yrs.

Aetiology Main aetiological factor in cancer of the lip is exposure to sunlight, as with skin cancer. It is estimated that the risk of developing lip cancer doubles every 250 miles nearer the equator. Excessive alcohol and tobacco use are the important factors in the aetiology of cancer of the mouth showing a 'synergistic effect'. Perhaps the most clear-cut aetiological factor is the chewing of tobacco and paan. Late-stage syphilis is now an exceedingly rare risk factor. One paper has linked the disease with the number of oral sex partners although the link with HPV remains unconfirmed. Immunosuppression, e.g. renal transplant, HIV patients have ↑ risk of this and other tumours.

Clinical appearance Most often seen as a painless ulcer, although may present as a swelling, an area of leukoplakia, erythroleukoplakia or erythroplakia, as malignant change of long-standing benign tumours or rarely in cyst linings or a non-healing extraction socket. Malignancy should be suspected if any of the above lesions persists for more than 3 weeks. Pain is usually a *late* feature when the lesion becomes superinfected or during eating of spicy foods. Referred otalgia is a common manifestation of pain from oral and particularly tongue or oropharyngeal cancer. The ulcer is described as firm with raised edges, with an indurated, inflamed, granular base and is fixed to surrounding tissues.

Staging The **TNM** classification is most commonly used;

T	primary tumour	N	cervical nodes
T1	<2cm diameter	N0	no nodes
T2	2–4cm diameter	N1	single node <3cm
T3	>4cm diameter	N2	single 3–6cm node (N2a), multiple nodes (N2b) or contralateral node(s) (N2c)
T4	massive, invading other structures		
		N3	node >6cm
		M	distant metastases
		M0	absent
		M1	present

Survival Dependent on site, stage (prognosis for stage I is >85% and for stage IV is 10%), and comorbidity. The presence or absence of extracapsular spread of tumour in metastatic cervical nodes is the most important single prognostic factor. Nodal involvement decreases cure rates by 50%.

Histopathology Mostly SCC. Characteristically shows invasion of deep tissues with cellular pleomorphism and ↑ nuclear staining. The presence of a lymphocytic response may have prognostic value, as does the manner of invasion (pushing or spreading). Can spread via local infiltration or lymphatic system (cervical nodes), and late spread via blood stream. However, histologically similar tumours can show quite different biological behaviour and this is a focus of current research.

Verrucous carcinoma A distinctive exophytic, wart-like lesion which grows slowly, spreading laterally rather than deeply is locally invasive, and is regarded as a lower-grade SCC, characterized by folded hyperplastic epithelium and a lower degree of cellular atypia. Surgical excision &/or radiotherapy is the Rx. Historically inadequate radiotherapy has been reported to induce more aggressive behaviour.

Other tumours Malignant connective tissue tumours (sarcomas) are rare in the mouth, but fibrosarcoma and rhabdomyosarcoma are seen in children. Osteosarcoma of the jaws has a slightly better prognosis than when found in long bones.

Salivary gland tumours, 📖 p.477. Malignant melanoma, 📖 p.479.

Management of oral malignancy, 📖 p.480.

Fig. 9.4 A typical location for an oral cancer which presents as a slow growing, painless non-healing ulcer or granular lesion, refer immediately for investigation and management through your local urgent cancer referral service.

Abnormalities of the lips and tongue

Although many diseases of the oral mucosa will involve the lips and tongue, there are a number of conditions specific to these structures, due in part to their highly specialized nature. The tongue is a peculiar muscular organ covered with specialized sensory epithelium and the lips form the interface between skin and mucosa.

The tongue

Ankyloglossia (tongue tie) The commonest of the developmental variations of the tongue and may be associated with microglossia. Rx: frenectomy.

Macroglossia Congenital; Down syndrome, Hurler syndrome, Beckwith–Weidemann syndrome. Benign tumours (e.g. lymphangioma), or acquired; acromegaly, amyloidosis, 🕮 p. 491. Surgical reduction of the tongue is bloody, but sometimes worthwhile.

Fissured tongue Deep fissuring of the tongue is not pathological in itself (affects 3% of tongues) but may harbour pathogenic microorganisms. Commoner in Down syndrome patients than average population. Different fissure patterns are identified by various delightful names such as scrotal tongue. The Melkerson–Rosenthal syndrome is a deeply fissured tongue in association with recurrent facial nerve palsy and swelling. Sjogrens syndrome can have a tongue with a lobulated appearance. Rx: reassurance for most, referral for Melkerson–Rosenthal.

Hairy tongue A peculiar condition of unknown aetiology probably due to elongation of the filiform papillae, which may or may not be accompanied by abnormal pigmentation. More common in smokers and people with poor oral hygiene and hyposalivation. Sometimes responds to podophylin paint, a thorough scrape, eating pineapple chunks, sucking a peach stone or surgical shave.

Median rhomboid glossitis, 🕮 p. 401.

Geographic tongue (benign migratory glossitis, erythema migrans) This is a peculiar inflammatory condition of unknown aetiology. Seen in 1–2% of adults. Involves the rapid appearance and disappearance of atrophic areas with a white demarcated border on the dorsum and lateral surface of the tongue, giving it the appearance of moving around the tongue surface. It is due to temporary loss of the filiform papillae. Pain is usually secondary to other stimuli e.g. acid foods (e.g. tomatoes or fruits) or cheese. Several clinical variants exist. Familial pattern is common. 4% have psoriasis. Rx: reassurance about benign self-limiting nature.

Depapillation of the tongue also appears in a number of haematological and deficiency states and in severe cases may also appear lobulated.

Sore tongue (glossodynia) May occur in the presence or absence of clinical changes; however, it should be remembered that even the presence of glossitis may not explain the symptoms of sore or burning tongue. Main causes of glossitis are iron deficiency anaemia, pernicious anaemia, candidosis, vitamin B group deficiencies, and lichen planus. Sore, but clinically normal tongue is a common problem and often psychogenic in origin; however, the first line of Rx is to exclude any possible organic cause, e.g. haematological deficiency states and unwanted reactions to self-administered or professionally administered medicines or mouthwashes.

The lips

Granulomatous cheilitis (orofacial granulomatosis) This is characterized by swelling of the lips and is histologically similar to Crohn's disease (non-caseating granuloma being found on biopsy but no systemic features). It may be the initial manifestation of Crohn's disease or completely isolated. Intralesional steroids, e.g. triamincinolone, 40mg into affected lip, anti-TNF therapies or clofazimine 100–200mg daily for 3–6 months may help.

Persistent median fissure This may be found as a developmental abnormality but is usually secondarily infected, which is extremely difficult to eradicate. May be associated with granulomatous cheilitis. Rx excision ± intralesional steroid.

Sarcoidosis A chronic granulomatous condition which can affect any body system. Lip swelling, and gingival and palatal nodules occur. Heerfordt syndrome 📖 p.728. Biopsy reveals non-caseating granuloma with inclusion bodies in 20 to 50%). CXR: hilar lymphadenopathy. Serum adenosine deaminase, angiotensin converting enzyme level is ↑. Ask an ophthalmologist to exclude uveal tract involvement. Mortality rate for disseminated systemic disease is 10–20%. Rx: steroids, intralesional or systemic.

Actinic cheilitis Sun damage to the lower lip causes excessive keratin production and ↑ mitotic activity in the basal layer. Premalignant. Advise sun blocks.

Exfoliative cheilitis Similar to above but of unknown aetiology.

Dry sore lips Except when accompanied by frank cheilitis, this is usually entirely innocent and can be treated symptomatically. Common causes are lip licking, exposure to wind or sunlight. It is also a manifestation of viral illness. Rx: lip salves.

Peutz–Jegher syndrome, 📖 p. 730.

Herpes labialis, 📖 p. 398.

Mucocele, 📖 p. 376.

Allergic angio-oedema Severe type I allergic response affecting lips, neck, and floor of mouth. Usually an identifiable cause. Rx: mild—antihistamine PO; severe—as anaphylaxis, 📖 p. 528.

Hereditary angio-oedema Defect of C_1-esterase inhibitor. Lip, neck, floor of mouth swelling, and swelling of feet and buttocks. Precipitated by trauma. Diagnosis from family history, bloods: low C4, normal C3 and absence of C1 esterase inhibitor activity. Rx: acute attacks—fresh frozen plasma (contains C_1-esterase inhibitor) or partially purified (seek advice in your locality). Prophylaxis; long term, tranexamic acid, short term, (procedures) danazol.

Kawasaki disease This systemic vasculitis affecting children <5yrs causes death in the UK in <4% (USA and Japan ~0.1%).[1] It can be treated if Δ. The criteria include red, dry cracked lips, strawberry tongue, and erythematous oropharyngeal mucosa, bilateral conjunctivitis, cervical lymphadenopathy, generalized rash, desquamation of hands and feet and fever. If suspected refer to a paediatrician.

1 N. Curtis 1997 *BMJ* **315** 322.

Salivary gland disease—1

The salivary glands consist of the major glands, the paired sublingual, submandibular, and parotid glands, and the minor salivary glands present throughout the oral mucosa, but particularly dense in the posterior palate and lips.

Xerostomia Dry mouth can be both a sign and a symptom. Note that some patients complain of a dry mouth when, in fact, they have an abundance of saliva. True xerostomia predisposes the mouth, pharynx, and salivary glands to infection (candidosis, ascending sialadenitis) and caries. Common causes include irradiation of the head and neck, drugs (e.g. tricyclic antidepressants, atropine, antihistamines), anxiety states, and salivary gland diseases (Sjögren syndrome, sarcoidosis). Rx is aimed at the underlying cause. Symptomatic relief with frequent sips of water or ice chips, carboxymethylcellulose saliva, e.g. Glandosane® spray or Saliva-Orthana®, helps. Optimal OH is essential. SF (containing sorbital) chewing gum may help. Pilocarpine systemically ↑ salivary flow at expense of unwanted effects.

Sialorrhoea/ptyalism Rare, although apparent sialorrhoea can occur with drooling due to inflammatory conditions of the mouth, or neurological disorders which inhibit swallowing. Rare causes include mercury poisoning and rabies. Problems with swallowing may be overcome by surgical repositioning of the major salivary ducts. Propantheline 15mg tds will reduce salivary flow.

Sialadenitis Inflammation of, usually, the major salivary glands. **Acute bacterial sialadenitis** presents as a painful swelling, usually with a purulent discharge from the duct of the gland involved. It may also develop as an exacerbation of **chronic bacterial sialadenitis**, which often exists as a complication of duct obstruction. Both conditions are almost always unilateral and common infecting organisms are oral streptococci, oral anaerobes, and *Staph. aureus*. Rx: exclusion or removal of an obstructing calculus. Plain radiographs with reduced exposure may reveal calculus, but 50% are radiolucent. (📖 p. 478). Culture of pus from the duct and aggressive antibiotic therapy (Co-amoxiclav and metronidazole) for unclearable ducts. Stimulation of salivary flow by chewing or massage helps chronic recurring sialadenitis. Rarely, loculated pus collection within the gland necessitates incision and drainage; USS can localize collection. Once the acute symptoms have resolved, sialography is indicated to define duct structure and may prove therapeutic. Other treatments include irrigating the gland with antibiotics &/or steroids. Recurrent chronic sialadenitis is an indication for removal of the gland (📖 p. 478). **Viral sialadenitis**, commonly mumps (serum amylase and lipases), an acute, infectious viral disease which primarily affects the parotid (10% submandibular gland). It is transmitted by direct contact with droplets of saliva and usually affects children and young adults with sudden onset of fever, pain, and parotid swelling. Classically, one gland is affected first, although bilateral swelling is the norm. In adults, the disease is more severe, with multisystem problems such as orchitis. Protection is now conferred by the measles, mumps, rubella vaccine. Rx: supportive, isolate patent for 7–10 days.

Rarely, sialadenitis can occur as a manifestation of allergy to various drugs, foodstuffs, or metals.

Sialolithiasis, 📖 p. 478.

Recurrent parotitis of childhood Unknown aetiology; congenital malformation of portions of ducts and infections ascending from mouth following dehydration. Ages 5–9yrs; recurrent unilateral parotitis with malaise. Eased by antibiotics. Resolves by puberty. EBV implicated in aetiology, possibly by structural damage to ducts. Rx: antibiotics, duct irrigation, sialogram (if tolerated).

Salivary duct and salivary gland fistulae Communications between the duct or gland and the oral mucosa or skin may occur post-traumatically or post-operatively. Although most stop spontaneously after 10 days, duct repair or gland excision may be needed. Propantheline 15mg tds before food can ↓ salivary flow and dry up small fistulae.

Mucocele, ranula, 📖 p. 376.

Salivary gland disease—2

Sialosis A non-inflammatory, non-neoplastic swelling of the major salivary glands, usually the parotids and usually bilateral. Of unknown aetiology, although linked with endocrine abnormalities, nutritional deficiencies, and alcohol abuse. Sialography is essentially normal. Histology is of serous acinar cell hypertrophy. Rx: aimed at any aetiological factors. Δ: exclusion of underlying organic disease by history, haematology, and biochemistry.

Sjögren syndrome (secondary Sjögren syndrome) 90% female. The triad of xerostomia, keratoconjunctivitis sicca, and a connective tissue disorder, usually rheumatoid arthritis. When the connective tissue component is absent the condition is called **primary Sjögren syndrome (sicca syndrome)**. The aetiology is probably autoimmune and there is a 5% risk of malignant lymphomatous transformation of the affected gland. Δ: antinuclear antibodies (70% +ve), SSA (70% +ve), SSB (40% +ve). Rheumatoid factor (70% +ve), ESR (↑), immunoglobulins (↑), labial gland biopsy shows lymphocytic infiltrate. Parotid gland flow, sialography, schrimer test, and slit lamp exam are all advocated, but once a Δ is established all that can be done for the patient is symptomatic Rx and an awareness of complications. Synthetic saliva (🕮 p. 576), synthetic tears, meticulous OH, Rx of candida, and patient awareness of the risk of lymphomatous change. See also 🕮 p. 731 and British Sjögren Syndrome Society (℘ www.bssa.uk.net)

Salivary gland tumours. 80% are benign; 80% occur in the parotid and 80% of these are in the superficial lobe. The majority are **pleomorphic adenomas** (PSA) have a mixed cellular appearance on histopathology. Although benign, the cells lie within the capsule of the tumour and satellite cells may lie outwith the capsule, creating a tremendous propensity for recurrence if simply enucleated. Tumour in the parotid should therefore be removed by parotidectomy, taking a safe margin of normal tissue (🕮 p. 478). **Lymphangiomas and haemangiomas** are the commonest tumours found in salivary glands in children. **Adenolymphoma** is found almost exclusively in the parotid, and **adenoid cystic carcinoma** is more commonly found in the minor than the major salivary glands. Tumours of the submandibular, sublingual, and minor salivary glands are more likely to be malignant than those found in the parotid. Pointers to malignant change in salivary gland tumours are: fixation to surrounding tissues, nerve involvement (particularly the facial nerve in parotid tumours), pain, rapid growth, and lymphadenopathy. For management, see 🕮 p. 478.

Other salivary tumours include mucoepidermoid carcinoma and acinic cell carcinoma, both of which can behave indolently or aggressively. Monomorphic adenomas are benign, with many histological varieties.

Miscellaneous Lymphoepithelial lesion (Miculicz disease) is essentially an aggressive form of the Sjögren syndrome without the eye or connective tissue component. **NB** Miculicz syndrome is salivary enlargement of known cause.

Frey syndrome, 🕮 p. 728.

Drug-induced lesions of the mouth

One way of thinking of these reactions is to divide them into local and systemic effects.

Local reactions

Chemical burns, e.g. from an aspirin tablet being held against the oral mucosa beside a painful tooth, are still seen and make one despair of the public at times. The burns are superficial necrosis of the epithelium and can appear as a transient white patch. Rx: re-education and removal of the irritant. The mucosa will spontaneously heal. Iatrogenic causes include trichloracetic acid and phenol. Also caused by accidental ingestion of corrosives (e.g. paraquat).

Interference with commensal flora Prolonged or repeated use of antibiotics, particularly topical antibiotics can lead to the overgrowth of resistant organisms, especially candida. Corticosteroids can cause a similar problem by immunosuppression.

Oral dyaesthesia A sore but normal-appearing tongue can be caused by certain drugs (e.g. captopril).

Systemic effects

Depressed marrow function There are a wide range of drugs which will depress any or all of the cell lines of the haemopoietic systems and these in turn can affect the oral mucosa, e.g. phenytoin. Long-term use can result in folate deficiency and macrocytic anaemia which can produce severe aphthous stomatitis. Chloramphenicol and certain analgesics can induce agranulocytosis, leading to severe oral ulceration. Chloramphenicol can also induce aplastic anaemia, which affects haemostasis, although spontaneous oral purpura and haemorrhage are a rare presentation.

Immunosuppression Steroids and other immunosuppressants (azathioprine) predispose to viral and fungal infection.

Lichenoid eruption Classically associated with the use of gold in the Rx of rheumatoid arthritis (📖 p. 506). NSAIDs, oral hypoglycaemics, and beta blockers are commoner offenders.

Erythema multiforme (Stevens–Johnson syndrome), 📖 p. 731.

Fixed drug eruptions Recurrent, sharply circumscribed lesions at the same site occurring on exposure to a specific drug. Extremely rare in the oral mucosa.

Exfoliative stomatitis Simply an oral manifestation of the very dangerous drug reaction known as exfoliative dermatitis, in which the skin and other membranes are shed. Again, gold has been implicated.

Gingival hyperplasia Common in patients on phenytoin, ciclosporin A, nifedipine, and certain other calcium channel-blockers; less commonly the OCP can have this effect. It is characterized by progressive fibrous hyperplasia and, while improved by OHI, will occur even in the presence of meticulous OH. Rx: Ask if drug can be safely changed and improve oral hygiene (if possible). Gingival surgery may be needed.

Oral pigmentation Black lines in the gingival sulcus are described as being a sign of heavy metal poisoning. Chlorhexidine causes a black or brown discoloration of the dorsum of the tongue, and some antibiotics can also do this. Tetracycline discoloration of teeth is well known.

Xerostomia, 📖 p. 420.

Allergic reactions Penicillin is a common offender.

There are a host of conditions affecting the oral mucosa which may be ascribed to the use of drugs. Recognition by history and patch testing of these is, of course, important, providing the drug can be withdrawn, but one has to pay attention to the reason the drug was given in the first place, and it may be that minor oral symptoms have to be tolerated when the drug is essential for the overall well-being of the patient.

Facial pain

Pain is an unpleasant sensory and emotional experience caused by actual or potential tissue damage, or described in terms of such damage. It is a complex and multifaceted symptom and several other sections of this book are relevant. The commonest source of pain in the region of the jaws and face is the tooth pulp. Pain not directly related to the teeth and jaws is dealt with here.

Trigeminal neuralgia Most common neurological cause of facial pain, it is an excruciating condition affecting mainly the >50s, F>M. It presents as a shooting 'electric shock' type of pain of rapid onset and short duration (few seconds to less than 2min), affecting one side of the face in the distribution of the trigeminal nerve. Often stimulated by touching a trigger point in the distribution of the trigeminal nerve. Patients may refuse to shave or wash the area which stimulates the pain although, strangely, they are rarely woken by it. In the early stages of the disease there may be a period of prodromal pain not conforming to the classical description and it may be difficult to arrive at a Δ; patients often have multiple extractions in an attempt to relieve the symptoms. It is thought to be a sensory form of epilepsy, although some cases are due to vascular pressure intracranially. Δ is by the history, and carbamezipine is useful both therapeutically and diagnostically, with an 80% response rate. Injection of LA can break pain cycles and be useful diagnostically. Cryotherapy can induce protracted analgesia, but sectioning the nerve rarely helps. For intractable cases, radiofrequency ganglionolysis or decompression of trigeminal nerve intracranially may be required.

Glossopharyngeal neuralgia A similar condition to trigeminal neuralgia but much less common. Affects the glossopharyngeal nerve, causing a sharp shooting pain on swallowing. There may be referred otalgia. Again, carbamezipine is the drug of choice.

▶ Patients under the age of 50yrs presenting with symptoms of cranial nerve neuralgia require full neurological examination and investigation, as these may be the presenting symptoms of an intracranial neoplasm, skull base metastases, HIV, syphilis, or multiple sclerosis.

Temporal arteritis (cranial arteritis) A condition affecting older age groups. The pain is localized to the temporal and frontal regions and usually described as a severe ache, although it can be paroxysmal. The affected area is tender to touch. Jaw claudication is seen in 20%. Major risk is involvement of retinal arteries, with sudden deterioration and loss of vision; underlying pathology is inflammatory arteritis. Tongue necrosis following lingual artery involvement has been described. Biopsy shows the arterial elastic tissue to be fragmented with giant cells. Δ: pulseless temporal arteries, classical distribution of pain, and massively raised ESR. Rx: aim is to relieve pain and prevent blindness and involves systemic prednisolone, guided by symptoms and ESR.

Migraine, 📖 p. 509.

Periodic migrainous neuralgia (cluster headache) Similar aetiology to migraine but with different clinical presentation: periodic attacks of severe, unilateral pain, boring or burning in character, lasting 30–60min, located around the eye, associated with watering of eye on affected side; congestion of conjuctiva and nasal discharge common. Attacks often occur at a particular time of night (early morning 'alarm clock wakening'), and tend to be closely concentrated over a period of time, followed by a longer period of remission. Most sufferers describe alcohol intolerance. Rx: O_2 inhalation, NSAID drugs, ergotamine or sumatriptan, intranasal lidocaine. Pizotifen is used prophylactically.

Pain associated with herpes zoster, ▢ p. 398.

Glaucoma Gives rise to severe unilateral pain centred above the eye, with a tense, stony hard globe. Due to raised intraocular pressure. Acute and chronic forms are recognized. The acute form presents with pain and responds to acetazolamide. Will need ophthalmological referral.

Myocardial infarction and angina May on occasion radiate to the jaws.

Multiple sclerosis May mimic trigeminal neuralgia or cause altered facial sensation. Differs from V neuralgia in that different neurological signs and symptoms in time and place are evident from the history. Eye pain (retrobulbar neuritis) is associated. Δ: depends upon finding multiple focal neurological lesions, disseminated in time and place. MRI reveals typical appearance of brain.

Atypical facial pain This constitutes a large proportion of patients presenting with facial pain (1–2%). Mostly middle aged women (70%). Classically, their symptoms are unrelated to anatomical distribution of nerves or any known pathological process, and these patients have often been through a number of specialist disciplines in an attempt to establish a Δ and gain relief. This Δ tends to be used as a catch-all for a large group of patients, with the connecting underlying supposition that the pain is of psychogenic origin. There may be a florid psychiatric history or undiagnosed depression (50% are depressed or hypochondriacal); alternatively, the patient may simply be overreacting to an essentially minor discomfort or recently noticed anatomical variant as part of a general inability to cope with life. Pointers to a psychogenic aetiology include imprecise localization, often bilateral pain or 'all over the place'. Bizarre or grossly exaggerated descriptions of pain. Pain is described as being continuous for long periods with no change, and none of the usual relieving or exacerbating factors apply. Sleeping and eating are not obviously disturbed, despite continuous unbearable pain. Most analgesics are said to be unhelpful, although many will not have tried adequate analgesia. No objective signs are demonstrable and all investigations are essentially normal. After exclusion of any possible organic cause the introduction of an antidepressant, e.g. dosulepin, may (or may not) produce dramatic improvement in the pain.

Oral dysaesthesia or burning mouth syndrome is an unpleasant abnormal sensation affecting the oral mucosa in the absence of clinically evident disease. Five times more common in women aged 40–50yrs than other groups. Related to atypical facial pain. Δ: by exclusion of haematological, metabolic, nutritional, microbiological, allergic, and prosthetic causes. With experience the patient type often becomes obvious. Rx: 50% achieve remission in 6-7 years. Dosulepin if sleep disturbance is prominent; paroxetine or fluoxetine if daytime stimulus is needed.

Bell's palsy Caused by inflammation of VII in the stylomastoid canal. Although the main symptom is facial paralysis, pain in or around the ear, often radiating to the jaw, precedes or develops at the same time in ~50% of cases. Rx: steroids improve chance for full recovery if Rx early (within 3 days of onset). If no Rx, 20% of patients will not completely recover. Protect cornea with eye pad. Combining aciclovir with steroid or aciclovir alone does not appear to improve recovery over steroid alone.[1]

Ramsey Hunt syndrome, 🕮 p. 730 Pain is associated with herpes zoster virus in the facial nerve. Systemic aciclovir and steroids improve recovery.

1 D. Gilden 2007 *N Eng J Med* **357** 1598.

Oral manifestations of skin disease

Lichen planus A chronic inflammatory disease of adults involving skin and mucous membranes. It effects up to 2% of the general population. 50% of patients with skin lesions have oral lesions, whereas 25% have oral lesions alone. The oral lesions persist longer than the skin lesions. It affects females more commonly than males at the ratio of 3:2. It is an autoimmune condition mediated by a T lymphocyte attack on stratified squamous epithelia which leads to hyperkeratosis with erythema or striations. 'Lichenoid eruptions' are an unwanted reaction to some drugs. Usually the oral lesions are bilateral and posterior in the buccal mucosa; it is not seen on the palate but can, however, affect the tongue, lips, gingivae, and floor of mouth. The most common oral lesion is a lacey reticular pattern of hyperkertotic epithelia seen bilaterally on the buccal mucosa. Other variants include coalesced plaque-like lesions. Six types are recognized: the reticular pattern just described, papular pattern, plaque-like pattern, erosive pattern, atrophic pattern, and bullous pattern. The skin lesions affect the flexor surfaces of the arms, and wrists and legs, and are particularly common on the shin as purple papules with fine white lines (Whickham's straie) overlying them. Histology shows hyperparakeratosis, with elongated rete ridges with a saw-tooth appearance, a prominent granular cell layer, acanthosis, and basal cell liquefaction. There is usually a dense band of lymphocytes directly beneath the epithelium. Lichen planus can last for months or years. It can always be distinguished histologically and usually clinically from leukoplakia. Lichen planus is essentially benign. Some controversy exists about the risk of malignant transformation; this risk has only really been identified in the *erosive* forms of lichen planus, and Rx of the erosive form is based around transforming it to the completely benign reticular pattern. Rx: distinction from leukoplakia, sytemic lupus erythematosus, or malignancy is needed; if there are lichenoid eruptions the implicated drugs should be identified and avoided if possible. If the condition is symptomatic superinfection should be treated or prevented with chlorhexidine mouthwash. If severe atrophic or erosive components are present topical steroids may be used, such as triamincinolone in carboxymethylcellulose paste, betamethasone pellets 1mg in 10ml of water used as a mouthrinse and expectorated in an increasing dose until symptoms are resolved, systemic steroids, or topical tacrolimus. These should all be used in a specialist environment. Symptomatic reticular lichen planus can usually be safely managed with a low-dose topical steroid.

Dyskeratosis congenita A rare autosomal dominant condition, characterized by oral leukoplakia, dystrophic changes of the nails, and hyperpigmentation of the skin; the oral lesion is prone to malignant change (🕮 p. 414).

Vesiculo-bullous lesions, 🕮 p. 406.

Oral manifestations of connective tissue disease

Ehlers–Danlos syndrome rare inherited connective tissue disease characterized by hyperextensible skin, hypermobile joints, and fragile vessels due to mutations in collagen. This results in very easy bruising and bleeding of skin as well as hypermobility. Oral features include severe early onset periodontal disease, small teeth with short roots, pulp stones, and occasional hypermobility of the TMJ. Bleeding during surgery, weak scars, sutures 'pulling through', and difficulty with root canal Rx are the main practical points. Some types of Ehlers–Danlos syndrome can lead to an ↑ susceptibility to infective endocarditis and significant heart damage due to mitral valve prolapse, and some types are prone to cerebrovascular accident due to weakness of intracranial blood vessels. Rx: aimed at the symptoms.

Rheumatoid arthritis (📖 p. 506) Main associations are Sjögren syndrome (15%) and rheumatoid of the TMJ (10% cases), which may cause pain, swelling, and limitation of movement. Rarely, pannus formation within the joint may occur. Rx: as for systemic rheumatoid arthritis, which may include methotrexate or tumour necrosis factor alpha.

Systemic lupus erythematosus (SLE) A systemic multisystem disease of uncertain aetiology, although viruses, hormonal changes, and drug therapy have all been implicated. The association with the presence of antinuclear factor is more common in females. Gives rise to skin lesions, classical malar 'butterfly' rash, and oral mucosal lesions in 30%, which include ulceration and purpurae. Antinuclear antibodies are present. F>M. Arthritis and anaemia frequent.

Chronic discoid lupus erythematosus The lesions of this condition are limited to skin and mucosa. May present as disc-like white plaques in the mouth and can progress to SLE, although more likely to remain as a chronic and recurring disorder. Lip lesions in women may be premalignant. Rx: SLE—systemic steroids; DLE—topical steroids. Butterfly rash may be present. DLE can be distinguished from SLE by the presence of specific double-stranded DNA antinuclear antibody in serum. Rx: DLE recalcitrant lesions may respond to dapsone or thalidomide.

Systemic sclerosis A chronic disease characterized by diffuse sclerosis of connective tissues. F>M (30–50 years). It has an insidious onset and is often associated with Raynaud's phenomenon (painful reversible digital ischaemia on exposure to cold). Classically, the face has a waxy mask-like appearance (Mona Lisa face). Eating becomes difficult due to immobility of underlying tissues, and dysphagia occurs due to oesophageal involvement. Autoantibodies are present. Circulating levels of E-selectin and thrombomodulin are useful markers in monitoring disease activity. Rx: combination of cyclophosphamide and steroids may help in early disease; penicillamine has always been used but has numerous unwanted effects. 5-year survival is 70%.

Polyarteritis nodosa Characterized by inflammation and necrosis of small and medium-sized arteries; necrosis at any site may occur and is seen as ulceration in the mouth. Up to 60% of patients die in the first year; Rx with systemic steroids ↑ the 5-year survival to 40%.

Dermatomyositis Inflammatory condition of skin and muscles; 15% are associated with internal malignancy. May occasionally present with mouth ulcers and soreness of tongue, palate or gingiva.

Reiter syndrome, 📖 p. 730.

Oral manifestations of gastrointestinal disease

Patterson–Brown–Kelly syndrome, 📖 p. 730

Coeliac disease (gluten-sensitive enteropathy) This common form of intestinal malabsorption may present with oral ulceration as the only symptom in adults. Although children also present with ulceration, they are more likely to show weight loss, weakness, fatty diarrhoea and failure to thrive. Other findings are glossitis, stomatitis, and angular cheilitis. Up to 5% may have RAS without anaemia. Rx: haematological and gastrointestinal investigations are required, blood picture, and haematenic assay. ↑ malabsorption. Antibodies to gluten, reticulin, endomysium (antiendomysial Ab is marker for coeliac disease); small bowel biopsy required for definitive Δ. B₁₂, folate, iron ↓ should be corrected. Rx: gluten-free diet.

Ulcerative colitis Rarely, pyostomatitis vegetans, a papilliferous, necrotic mucosal lesion can occur; more commonly ulcers indistinguishable from aphthae are seen. Gastrointestinal symptoms predominate. Arthritis, uveitis, and erythema nodosum also occur. Topical steroids and systemic sulfasalazine are used in Rx; low doses of azathioprine are effective in maintaining remission. Most of these patients are managed by gastrointestinal specialists.

Crohn's disease Chronic inflammatory disease affecting any part of the gut from mouth to anus. Primarily affects the terminal ⅓ of the ileum, although ~1% of cases will present with oral ulceration predating any other symptoms. These tend to affect the gingiva, buccal mucosa, and lips with purplish-red non-haemorrhagic swellings, linear long-standing ulcers, and granulations (Figure 9.5). Granulomatous cheilitis is probably a variant. Painful oral lesions seem to respond well to simple excision but Rx is aimed at the systemic disease.

Orofacial granulomatosis Clinically and histologically identical to oral manifestations of Crohn's disease. Δ of exclusion (Crohn's, sarcoid). Probable aetiology is as a hypersensitivity response to certain foods, additives such as benzoates, cinnaminides in toothpaste, etc. Δ is biopsy to demonstrate granulomata histically and exclusion of systemic disease 📖 p. 496. Rx: specific to the local problem; intralesional steroid. Most beneficial Rx is to identify and avoid the irritant factors. Patients who have generalized Crohn's or very severe orofacial granulomatosis may benefit from systemic Rx with sulfasalazine or infliximab.

Gardener syndrome, 📖 p. 728.

Peutz–Jegher syndrome, 📖 p. 730.

Cirrhosis Glossitis occurs in ~50% of patients. Sialosis is another association.

Fig. 9.5 An extreme case of lip swelling secondary to severe orofacial granulomatosis associated with Crohn's disease.

Oral manifestations of haematological disease

Anaemia The nutritional deficiencies associated with anaemia, iron, B_{12}, and folate, are all associated with **recurrent oral ulceration** (📖 p. 404) and specific deficiencies may be present, even in the absence of a frank anaemia. **Atrophic glossitis** was formerly the commonest oral symptom of anaemia but is less often seen now. Red lines or patches on a sore, but normal-looking tongue, may indicate B_{12} deficiency. **Candidosis** (📖 p. 400) may be precipitated or exacerbated by anaemia, particularly iron deficiency, and **angular cheilitis** is a well-recognized association. The sore, clinically normal tongue (**burning tongue**) is sometimes a manifestation or even precursor of anaemia.

Patterson–Brown–Kelly syndrome, 📖 p. 730.

Leukaemia This and other haematological malignancies are associated with a ↓ in resistance to infection. The mouth may be involved, either secondarily to this tendency to infection or as a direct consequence of infiltration of the oral tissues. The oral lesions of leukaemia are painful and can lead to difficulty in swallowing. Prevention of superinfection with chlorhexidine mouthwashes and aggressive appropriate Rx of infections which arise are of real help. There is an ↑ tendency to bleed manifested as fine petechial haemorrhages or bruising around the mouth, and the gingiva may bleed heavily in the presence of only negligible trauma. Management of the bleeding is aimed at the underlying disorder; local techniques include improving OH, avoiding extractions, and using local haemostatic methods (📖 p. 348). Spontaneous gingival bleeding may be controlled by using impressions as a made-to-measure pressure dressing.

Cyclical neutropenia This condition may manifest as oral ulceration, acute exacerbations of periodontal disease, or NUG. As name suggests, recurs in 3–4 week cycles.

Myeloma Macroglossia is an occasional finding. Multiple osteolytic punched out lesions in skull and jaws are a classic appearance. Also, pain, paraesthesia and pathological fracture. Bisphosphonates form part of these patients' treatment and 10-year survivors have a 30% risk of BRON (📖 pp. 352, 581).

Purpura is due to platelet deficiency. Commonest as idiopathic thrombocytopenic purpura (ITP) in children. Palatal petechiae or bruising may be seen. Palatal petechiae are also seen in glandular fever, rubella, HIV, and recurrent vomiting.

Angina bullosa haemorrhagica Oral blood blisters; irritating but of no known significance (📖 p. 408).

Oral manifestations of endocrine disease

Acromegaly Oral signs of acromegaly include enlargement of the tongue and lips, spacing of the teeth, and an ↑ in jaw size, particularly the mandible resulting in a Class III malocclusion. Jaw pain is sometimes described, which can respond to Rx of the growth-hormone-secreting pituitary tumour responsible for the disease. Rx: trans-sphenoidal hypophysectomy.

Addison's disease (see 🕮 p. 540) (adrenocortical hypofunction) Classically, causes melanotic hyperpigmentation of the oral mucosa, commonly of the cheek. May also be part of the endocrine–candidosis syndrome.

Cushing syndrome A 'moon face' and oral candidosis are the common head and neck manifestations. Facial acne is also seen. Note a need for steroid prophylaxis.

Hypothyroidism Congenital hypothyroidism is associated with enlargement of the tongue, with puffy enlarged lips and delayed tooth eruption. In adult hypothyroidism, puffiness of the face and lips also occurs, but there are no particular oral changes. Rx of hypothyroidism with carbimazole is a rare cause of oral ulceration.

Hyperthyroidism Not associated with any particular oral changes. Occular proptosis characteristic of Graves' disease.

Hypoparathyroidism May be a component in the endocrine–candidosis syndrome; facial twitching and paraesthesia due to hypocalcemia can be seen. Occasionally delayed eruption and enamel hyperplasia can be seen.

Hyperparathyroidism Rare. Caused by hyperplasia or adenoma of the parathyroids. ↑ parathormone causes ↑ plasma Ca^{2+} liberated from bone. Irreversible renal damage in absence of treatment so worth detecting (diagnosis confirmed by ↑Ca, ↓ph, ↑PTH, ↑alk. Phos.) Appears in the jaws as loss of lamina dura; a 'ground glass' appearance of bone and cystic lesions (often looking multilocular), which contain dark-coloured tissue; 'brown tumour' histologically indistinguishable from a giant cell granuloma (🕮 p. 378).

Diabetes No specific oral changes, although manifestations of ↓ resistance to infection can be seen if poorly controlled (e.g. severe periodontal disease). Xerostomia and thrush are prominent features of ketoacidosis. Sialosis is sometimes seen as a late feature of diabetes. Burning mouth may be a presenting feature, and oral or facial dysaesthesiae may reflect the peripheral neuropathies seen in diabetics. There is a tendency to slower healing following surgery. Lichenoid reactions due to oral hypoglycemic drugs may be seen.

Sex hormones There is a well-recognized ↑ in the severity and frequency of gingivitis at puberty and in pregnancy. Some females have recurrent aphthae clearly associated with their menstrual cycle, and several symptoms, usually burning tongue or mouth or general soreness of the tongue or mouth, have been described during the menopause. It should be remembered, however, that there are profound psychological changes at this time of life in many women, and these symptoms may be a manifestation of atypical facial pain rather than a directly hormonally-mediated effect. Hormone replacement does not seem to help.

Oral manifestations of neurological disease

Examination of the cranial nerves: 📖 p. 508; general concepts of neurological disease: 📖 p. 510. Of the cranial nerves, the trigeminal and facial nerves contribute most to disorders affecting the mouth, face, and jaws.

Trigeminal nerve Ophthalmic lesions result in abnormal sensation in skin of the forehead, central nose, upper eyelid, and conjunctivae. *Maxillary* lesions affect skin of cheek, upper lip and side of nose, nasal mucosa, upper teeth and gingiva, palatal and labial mucosa. The palatal reflex may be lost. *Mandibular* lesions affect skin of lower face, lower teeth, gingivae, tongue, and floor of mouth. Lesions of the motor root manifest in the muscles of mastication. Taste sensation is *not* lost in such lesions, although other sensations from the tongue are. Testing is performed by having the patient close his eyes and report on sensations experienced, in comparison to each other, while the areas of superficial distribution of the nerve are stimulated by light touch (cotton wool) and pin-prick (probe or blunt needle). The motor branch is tested by moving the jaws against resistance. A blink should be elicited by stimulating the cornea with a wisp of cotton wool (corneal reflex).

Facial nerve is motor to the muscles of facial expression and stapedius, secretomotor to the submandibular and sublingual salivary glands, and relays taste from anterior ⅔ of tongue via the chorda tympani. Tested by having the patient raise eyebrows, screw eyes shut, whistle, smile, and show their teeth. Upper and lower motor neurone lesions can be distinguished because the forehead has a degree of bilateral innervation and is relatively spared in upper motor neurone lesions. Taste is tested using sour, salt, sweet, and bitter solutions. If taste is intact, flow from the submandibular duct can be assessed by gustatory stimulation. Test hearing to assess stapedius.

Neurological causes of facial and oral pain, 📖 p. 426.

Neurological conditions causing altered sensation Intracranial: e.g. CVA, multiple sclerosis, polyarteritis, cerebral tumours, infection, trauma, sarcoidosis; *extracranial:* nasopharyngeal or antral carcinoma, trauma, osteomyelitis, Paget's disease, viral or bacterial infection, leukaemic infiltrate. Psychogenic causes include hyperventilation syndrome and hysteria.

Neurological causes of facial paralysis Upper motor neurone or lower motor neurone; of the former, strokes are the commonest. Combination lesions can be caused by amyotrophic lateral sclerosis of the cord. Lower motor neurone paralysis can be caused by Bell's palsy (📖 p. 427), trauma, infiltration by malignant tumours, Ramsay Hunt syndrome, Guillain–Barré syndrome (post-viral polyneuritis, may even appear to be bilateral). Apparent paralysis may occur in myaesthenia gravis where abnormally ↑ fatigue of striated muscle causes ptosis and diplopia. Therapeutic paralysis may be induced for facial spasm, using botulinum toxin injected locally (as used for facial aesthetics!). Horner syndrome results in ptosis.

Neurological causes of abnormal muscle movement Tetanus is an obvious cause. Muscular dystrophy may present with ptosis and facial paralysis. Hemifacial spasm and other tics may be caused by a tumour at the cerebello-pontine angle. Orofacial dyskinesia can be a manifestation of Parkinson's disease or an unwanted effect of major tranquillizers. Phenothiazines and metoclopramide are notorious for causing dystonic reactions in young women and children. Bizarre attacks of trismus due to masseteric spasm have been ascribed to metoclopramide.

Oral manifestations of HIV infection and AIDS

AIDS is the terminal stage of infection with the human immunodeficiency virus (HIV), which is recognized as undergoing a number of mutations. It is discussed in general terms on 📖 p. 578. The underlying severe immunodeficiency leads to a number of oral manifestations (75% have orofacial disease) which, although not pathognomonic, should raise the possibility of HIV infection. They have been classified.[1]

Group I **Strongly associated with HIV**

Candidosis Seen in 70% of HIV patients as early manifestation (📖 p. 400). Erythematous (early), hyperplastic, pseudomembraneous (late), and angular cheilitis in young people (most common oral feature of HIV). 50% of patients with HIV-associated thrush develop AIDS in 5 years.

Hairy leukoplakia Bilateral, white, non-removable corrugated lesions of the tongue, unaffected by antifungals but usually resolve with aciclovir or valaciclovir, and associated with EBV. It is a predictor of bad prognosis and possible development of lymphoma.

HIV gingivitis Unusually severe gingivitis for the general state of the mouth. Often characterized by linear gingival erythema, intense red band along gingival margin.

Acute ulcerative gingivitis (📖 p. 191) Occurs in young, otherwise healthy mouths.

HIV periodontitis Severe localized destruction out of place with OH.

Kaposi's sarcoma (KS) Commonest malignancy among HIV patients. Rx: radiotherapy is effective. One or more erythematous/purplish macules or swelling, frequently on the palate. 50% occur intra- or perorally. It is pathognomonic if seen in young male who is not receiving immunosuppression.

Non-Hodgkin's lymphoma Similar to the above. Burkitt's lymphoma is 1000 times more common than in HIV-negative persons in the west.

Group II **Less strongly associated with HIV**
Atypical oropharyngeal ulceration
Idiopathic thrombocytopenic purpura
HIV associated salivary gland disease HIV children > adults. Similar to Sjögren syndrome.
Wide range of common viral infections

Group III **Possible association with HIV**
Wide range of rare bacterial and fungal infections
Cat scratch disease
Neurological abnormalities
Osteomyelitis/sinusitis/submandibular cellulitis
Squamous carcinoma

1 S. Challacombe 1991 *BDJ* **73** 305.

Clearly, the conditions in *Group III* are likely to be seen in patients who are HIV −ve at least as often as in patients who are HIV +ve.

Persistent generalized lymphadenopathy Otherwise inexplicable lymphadenopathy >1cm persisting for 3 months, at two or more extrainguinal sites. Cervical nodes particularly commonly affected. May be prodromal or a manifestation of AIDS.

Rx for AIDS AIDS is currently incurable, but then again so is life. Antiretroviral drugs prolong and improve quality of life in those with active AIDS. Rx with antiretroviral agents (HAART – Highly Active Anti Retroviral Therapy) has revolutionized the medium-term prognosis, these are changing regularly and the combinations used are complex. Facial manifestations of their use include a severe lipodystrophy. Early detection and Rx of opportunistic infections and neoplasms also has a major impact on quality of life.

Dental Rx for patients with AIDS This group present two risks with regard to dental Rx.

- To personnel carrying out the Rx. Affected patients carry an infectious disease with no known cure, which is transmitted by blood and blood products. As it is impossible to adequately identify all such patients, routine cross-infection control is now a necessity.
- As these patients are immunocompromised, any Rx with a known risk of infective complications, e.g. extractions, should be covered with antiseptic and antimicrobial prophylaxis, and any surgery should be as atraumatic as possible. There may also be a slight tendency to bleeding in these patients, and local haemostatic measures (◻ p. 348) may be needed.

Prophylaxis after contaminated needlestick injury, e.g. hollow point needlestick from AIDS patient. Should be given within 24 hours. Combination therapy offers best chance of preventing HIV seroconversion.[1]

---

1 CMO expert advisory group on AIDS (🖑 www.dh.gov.uk).

Cervico-facial lymphadenopathy

You cannot palpate a normal lymph node, therefore a palpable one must be abnormal (Figure 9.6). The most important distinction to make is whether this is part of the node's physiological response to infection or whether it is undergoing some pathological change. The finding of an enlarged node or nodes in children is relatively common and can be reasonably managed by watchful waiting. Undiagnosed cervical lymphadenopathy in adults mandates biopsy-establishing definitive Δ.

Investigations Routine EO and IO examination (📖 p. 9) to exclude the common causes: apical and periodontal abscesses, pericoronitis, tonsillitis, otitis, etc. The fundamentals are history and palpation.

History Ask about pain or swelling in the mouth, throat, ears, face, or scalp. Was there any constitutional upset when the lump appeared? Has it been getting bigger progressively or has it fluctuated? Is it painful, and how long has it been present?

Palpation Fully expose the neck and palpate from behind, with the patient's head bent slightly forward to relax the neck. Examine systematically, feeling the submental, facial, submandibular, parotid, auricular, occipital, the deep cervical chain, supraclavicular, and posterior triangle nodes. Differentiating between the submandibular salivary gland and node can be a problem, made simpler by palpating bimanually; the salivary gland can be felt moving between the external and internal fingers. Supraclavicular nodes are more liable to be due to occult tumour in the lung or upper gastrointestinal tract, whereas posterior triangle nodes are more liable to be haematological or scalp skin in origin.

If a node is palpable, note its texture, size, and site, and whether it is tender to touch or fixed to surrounding tissues.

Acutely infected nodes tend to be large, tender, soft, and freely mobile.

Chronically infected nodes are soft to firm and less liable to be tender.

Metastatic carcinoma in nodes tends to be hard and fixed.

Lymphomatous nodes are described as rubbery and have a peculiar firm texture.

Supplementary investigations Examine axillary and inguinal nodes, liver, and spleen. Carry out a FBC to look for leukocytosis and a monospot test for glandular fever. Once infection is excluded it is essential to exclude, as far as possible, an occult primary malignancy of the head and neck; the best way to do this is by direct examination, flexible nasendoscopy, and CXR. If access for examination is limited, EUA.

Ultrasound-guided fine-needle aspiration cytology in specialist units is probably the gold standard minimalist investigation. MRI and CT scanning will confirm the presence, shape, size of, and presence of necrosis within nodes and may reveal occult tumour. MRI/CT cannot, however, confirm the pathological process within the node.

If the Δ has still not been established it is reasonable to proceed to excision biopsy of the node, which should be cultured for mycobacteria as well as examined histologically. Find out how your pathology department likes the nodes sent; some want them fresh.

Common causes Dental abscesses, pericoronitis, tonsillitis, glandular fever, lymphoma, metastatic deposits, and leukaemia.

Rare causes Brucellosis, atypical mycobacteria (although commoner in children), TB, AIDS, toxoplasmosis, actinomycosis, sarcoidosis, cat scratch fever, syphilis, drugs (e.g. phenytoin) mucocutaneous lymph node syndrome (Kawasaki disease) and Crohn's disease. Other neck lumps: 📖 p. 482.

Fig. 9.6 A prominent palpable cervical lymph node arising at the junction of levels I and II in the neck; all such masses should be rapidly and fully investigated prior to any form of open biopsy. Biopsy is often requested by haematologists to diagnose lymphoma but carries the risk of decreasing the patient's prognosis if the diagnosis is squamous or salivary cancer of the head and neck.

An approach to oral ulcers

Oral ulceration is probably the commonest oral mucosal disease seen; it may also be the most serious. It is important, therefore, to have an approach to the management of oral ulcers firmly established in your mind.

Duration How long has the ulcer been present?

▶ If >3 weeks, referral for appropriate specialist investigation, including biopsy, is mandatory.

If of recent onset, ask whether it was preceded by blistering. Are the ulcers multiple? Is any other part of the body affected and have similar ulcers been experienced before? Then look at the site &/or distribution of the ulcer(s).

Blistering preceding the ulcer suggests a vesiculo-bullous condition (📖 p. 406) such as herpetic gingivostomatitis. Blistering with lesions elsewhere in the body suggests erythema multiforme, or hand, foot, and mouth disease.

Distribution If limited to the gingivae, suggests NUG (📖 p. 191). Unilateral distribution suggests herpes (📖 p. 398). Under a denture or other appliance suggest traumatic ulceration.

Recurrence of the ulcers after apparent complete resolution is characteristic of RAS (📖 p. 404).

Pain Its presence or absence is not particularly useful diagnostically, although the character of the pain may be of value. Pain is often a late feature of oral carcinoma and the fact that an ulcer may be painless *never* excludes it from being a potential cancer.

For most ulcers of recent onset, and a few present for an indeterminate period, a trial of therapy is often a useful adjunct to Δ. This is especially useful in RAS, viral conditions (where Rx is essentially symptomatic), and lesions probably caused by local trauma (Rx being removal of the source of trauma and review after 1 week).

Ulcers which need early diagnosis include:

Herpes zoster As early aggressive Rx with aciclovir may reduce post-herpetic neuralgia.

Erythema multiforme In order to avoid re-exposure to the antigen.

Erosive lichen planus As this may benefit from systemic steroids or other specialist Rx and will require specialist long-term follow-up.

Traumatic Ulcerative Granuloma with Stromal Eosinophilia (TUGSE) because it can be clinically indistinguishable from SCC but spontaneously resolves in most cases (after up to 6 weeks).

Oral squamous cell carcinoma For obvious reasons.

Temporomandibular pain—dysfunction/ facial arthromyalgia

The allocation of this section to a speciality chapter created problems in just the same way as the referral of the 'TMJ' patient to a specialist is fraught with confusion. We have selected this site because we feel it is important to look at these patients from a physician's approach rather than a dental or surgical one.

What is it? The problem being addressed is pain in the preauricular area and muscles of mastication with trismus, with or without evidence of internal derangement of the meniscus. Conditions which can otherwise be classified as facial pain syndromes or other forms of joint disease are excluded and can be found in the relevant pages (📖 pp. 426, 468).

Prevalence Affects ~40% of the population at some time in their lives. F>M. 20–30 years of age.

Aetiology Idiopathic. Multiple theories put forward regarding occlusion, trauma, stress, habits, joint hypermobility. To date, the concept of stress-induced parafunctional habits (bruxism, clenching) causing pain and spasm in the masticatory apparatus coupled with a ↓ pain threshold has seemed the most reasonable. This is compatible with the observed high association with back pain, headaches, and migraine. It does not explain the cause in those patients who can identify no different levels of stress in their lives nor does it help explain the high incidence of internal derangement of the meniscus. The discovery of a biochemical marker (tyramine sulfate in the urine) in non-depressed TMJ patients has suggested that these patients are somehow biochemically sensitive to both mediators of damage in the joint, such as neuropeptides, and centrally (via serotonin) resulting in a lowered ability to cope with the local discomfort. The neuropeptide release can explain both joint pain and internal derangement (see Figure 9.7).[1]

Clinical features Pain, clicking, locking, crepitus, and trismus are the classical signs and symptoms. Some patients may be clinically depressed but most are not. Pain is elicited by palpation over the muscles of mastication &/or the preauricular region. Clicking commonly occurs at 2–3mm of tooth separation on opening and sometimes closing. This is due to the meniscus being displaced anteriorly on translation of the head of the condyle and then returning to its usual position (the click). A lock is when it does not return.

Management Success has been claimed for a wide range of treatments, reflecting confusion over Δ and the multifactorial and self-limiting nature of the condition. Simple conservative Rx within the range of every dentist is successful in up to 80% of cases (see Figure 9.8).

---

1 M. Harris 1993 *BDJ* **174** 129.

Fig. 9.7

Fig. 9.8 Practice-based protocol for 'TMJ' patient.

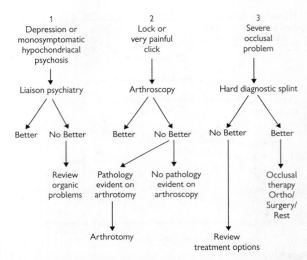

Fig. 9.9 Specialist-based protocol (Once Rx 1,2,3 have been clearly exhausted and tricyclics instituted, residual problem is usually one of three).

1) *Reassurance and explanation* Advice as to the nature of the problem and its benign and frequently self-limiting course is all that many patients require. Do not create a problem where there is none! This is also the time to take a gentle but thorough social and family history to identify clinically depressed patients or those with significant stress. An information leaflet is helpful.

2) *Simple analgesia, rest, gentle heat, and remedial exercises* Whether these are given by dentist, physiotherapist (in the form of short-wave diathermy and ultrasound) or ancillary staff is unimportant, as the crucial part is that carried out by the patient at home by taking the analgesics and performing the exercises as instructed.

3) *Splint therapy* Upper/lower, hard/soft have all been used with varying success. The initial aim of a splint is to: (a) show something is being done (placebo); (b) ↓ bruxism and joint load; and (c) ↑ the gap between condyle and fossa, whereby the disc may be freed. A simple, full-coverage upper or lower splint should be worn as often as possible, nights and evenings especially, and reassessed after 4–6 weeks.

These three simple measures should relieve symptoms in ~80% of patients and identify those needing referral to a specialist (Figure 9.9). **Do not** persist with ineffective Rx if symptoms have not improved within 3 months.

4) *Drug therapy* There is a natural reluctance among many patients to take drugs, particularly those associated with psychiatry. There is also a misconceived reluctance among clinicians to use the tricyclics and related compounds. They are non-addictive and the commoner side-effects of weight gain, constipation, and dry mouth can be overcome. Benzodiazepines are not recommended but nortriptyline, dosulepin, and related compounds have been demonstrated to have analgesic and muscle relaxant effects independent of their antidepressant effect, and probably work via the central biochemical sensitivity identified by the presence of urinary conjugated tyramine sulfate.

5) *Occlusal adjustment* There are a group of patients where a significant occlusal problem exists. In these cases a hard diagnostic occlusal splint can be constructed for the mandible (Tanner) or for the maxilla (Michigan), and should be made to give multiple even contacts in centric relation and anterior guidance. The patient attempts to wear this full-time for up to 3 months. If pain is abolished while wearing the appliance, returns when it is removed, and is abolished on reinstitution, then occlusal adjustment by orthodontic, surgical, or restorative means is a reasonable option.

6) *Surgery for internal derangement* If pain can be abolished by other methods and the patient continues to be bothered by a painful click, particularly with recurrent locking, Rx aimed specifically at the meniscus is justified. The first line which may be useful diagnostically and improve pain due to capsulitis is arthroscopy. This is examination and irrigation of the upper joint space by a rigid endoscope, through which lysis and lavage of adhesions and synovial inflammatory mediators can be performed. Menisci damaged beyond the scope of arthroscopy can be repositioned at open arthrotomy. Consensus dictates that the minimum of interference to the articulatory surfaces and the avascular meniscus is carried out. Rarely, completely ruined joints will benefit from total joint replacement.

Chapter 10

Maxillofacial surgery

Contents

Relevant sections; *Oral cancer* 📖 *p. 416, neck lumps* 📖 *p. 442, TMJ* 📖 *p. 446, Salivary glands* 📖 *p. 420, Clefts* 📖 *p. 170, orthognathic surgery* 📖 *p. 168 Preprosthetic surgery* 📖 *p. 330 &* 📖 *p. 388.*

Principal sources and further reading D. Mitchell 2006 *An Introduction to Oral and Maxillofacial Surgery*, OUP. J. Watkinson 2000 *Head & Neck Surgery*, Butterworth-Heinemann. ACS 2004 *ATLS Core Course Manual*. M. Yaremchuk 1992 *Rigid Fixation of the Craniomaxillofacial Skeleton*, Butterworth-Heinemann. J. Shah 2003 *Oral Cancer*, Dunitz. R. Cawson 1997 *Pathology and Surgery of the Salivary Glands*, Isis Medical Media. K Wolfe, F Holzle. 2005 *Raising of Microvascular Faps*, Springer. B. Jones 2008 *Facial Rejuvenation Surgery*, Mosby. L. Peterson 2004 *Contemporary Oral and Maxillofacial Surgery*, Mosby. Personal experience.

In general, maxillofacial surgery is a postgraduate subject which has evolved from oral surgery, with foundations in medicine, dentistry, and surgery. It is included here as an introduction to students, an *aide-mémoire* for junior hospital staff, and a guide for those who will be referring patients.

Advanced trauma life support (ATLS)

ATLS is a system providing one safe way of resuscitating a trauma victim. It was first conceived in Nebraska, subsequently developed by the ACS, and has now reached international acceptance. It is not the only approach but it is one which works. It is highly recommended.

Trauma deaths have a trimodal distribution. The first peak is within seconds to minutes of injury. The second is within the first hour, the 'golden hour', and is the area of main concern. The third is days to weeks later but may reflect management within the golden hour.

The core concept behind ATLS is the **primary survey** with **simultaneous resuscitation**, followed by a **secondary survey** leading to definitive care.

Primary survey

This uses the mnemonic **ABCDE** on the basis of identifying and treating the most lethal injury first.

1) *Airway with cervical spine control* Establish a patent airway and protect the cervical spine from further injury. Chin lift, jaw thrust, oral airway, nasopharyngeal airway, intubation, surgical airway as needed, coupled with manual inline immobilization of cervical spine or rigid cervical collar, sandbags, and tape.

2) *Breathing and ventilation* Inspect, palpate, and auscultate the chest. Count respiratory rate. Give 100% O_2. Chest decompression by needle puncture in 2nd intercostal space mid-clavicular line if indicated for tension pneumothorax. Chest drain 5th intercostal space anterior axillary line if needed.

3) *Circulation with haemorrhage control* Assess level of consciousness, skin colour, pulse and BP, manual pressure control of extreme haemorrhage. Establish two large venous cannulae, take blood for X-match and baseline studies. Give 2l of prewarmed Hartmann's solution. Establish ECG, seek help for operative control of bleeding if needed. Establish urinary catheter unless urethral transection is suspected, and oro- or nasogastric tube.

4) *Disability* (neuro-evaluation) Glasgow coma score. Pupillary response to light, visual acuity. Prevent hypotension and hypoxia.

5) *Exposure* Remove all clothing to allow full assessment of injuries. Ensure monitoring: respiratory rate, BP, pulse, arterial blood gases, pulse oximetry, and ECG. Prevent hypothermia.

If all these can be established and monitored parameters are normalized, the patient's chances of living are optimized.

X-rays At this stage obtain a chest and pelvis film in the resuscitation room. Cervical spine film may help but cervical spine should remain immobilized until fully assessed if mechanism of injury suggests spinal trauma.

Reassess the ABCs

If all is stable move to the **secondary survey**, which is a head-to-toe examination of the patient. It is at this stage *only* that specific non-immediately life-threatening conditions should be identified and dealt with in turn.

Maxillofacial injuries Other than those with a direct effect on the airway or cervical spine, or causing exsanguinating haemorrhage, should not be dealt with until the **ABCs** have been completed and this question should be asked of all referring doctors prior to accepting responsibility for a patient. Remember to exclude intracranial, visceral, and major orthopaedic injuries.

While ATLS is designed primarily for front-line physicians, modified courses for dental graduates are available, and strongly recommended to anyone who may undertake care of the trauma patient.

Primary management of maxillofacial trauma

The first consideration is whether the patient has suffered polytrauma, which may have multiple and life-threatening ramifications, or, as is more commonly the case, trauma confined to the face. In the former the prime concern is keeping the patient alive, and the maxillofacial injuries can await Rx (📖 p. 452). Remember that isolated facial injuries rarely cause sufficient bleeding to induce hypovolaemic shock. Ask yourself: Can they see?

Airway The brain can tolerate hypoxia for ~3min. Most conscious patients can maintain a patent airway if the oropharynx is cleared. Give all traumatized patients maximal O_2 initially. Oral airways are not tolerated unless patient is unconscious. Nasopharyngeal airways are only of value if they can be inserted safely and kept patent. If the patient is unconscious and the airway is obstructed they should be intubated. If this is not possible, an emergency airway can be maintained by cricothyroid puncture with a wide-bore cannula. Long-term security of the airway can be achieved by surgical cricothyroidotomy as an emergency, or tracheostomy as a planned operation. Conscious patients with severe isolated facial trauma maintain their airway by sitting leaning forward; let them.

Cervical spine injuries Until these are excluded, the patient should be immobilized; must balance with need to remove from spine boards ASAP (painful, prevent pressure sores). Use common sense to decide between immobilization and sitting leaning forward.

Bleeding As above. Gunshot wounds and lacerated major vessels are exceptions which can cause extensive bleeding. Specific techniques to control naso- and oropharyngeal bleeding are: bilateral rubber mouth props to immobilize the maxilla; bilateral balloon catheters passed into the post-nasal space, inflated then pulled forward; and bilateral anterior nasal packs.

Scalp wounds Can exsanguinate children; control with pressure and heavy full thickness sutures.

Head injuries The main cause of death and disability in patients with isolated maxillofacial trauma. Assessment: 📖 p. 456. Do no further harm.

CSF leaks Facial and skull # can create dural tears, leading to CSF rhinorrhoea (from the nose) or otorrhoea (from the ear). Although controversial, prophylactic antibiotics are used by many. A combination penicillin in high dose is often used, despite the fact that conventional antibiotics do not cross the healthy blood–brain barrier in adequate levels, the rationale being that the blood–brain barrier is damaged in these cases. It was the concern that low levels of antibiotic in the CSF would only suppress *signs* of meningitis whilst selecting resistant organisms that prompted influential recommendations against prophylaxis.[1]

Tetanus immunity If in doubt give tetanus toxoid.

---

[1] Working Party of the British Society for Antimicrobial Chemotherapy 1992 *Lancet* **344** 1547.

Analgesia May not be needed. Avoid opioids if possible as they interfere with neuro-observations. If needed, use diclofenac 75mg IM bd or codeine phosphate 60mg IM 6 hourly.

Patients to admit Any question of danger to the airway, skull #, history of unconsciousness, retrograde amnesia, bleeding, middle 1/3 #, mandibular # (except when very simple), malar # if +ve eye signs, children, and those with domestic or social problems. If in doubt *admit*. Place on, at least, initial hourly neurological observations (most will need 1/4 hourly obs initially). IV access and antibiotic. If not admitting, give the patient a head-injury card.

If teeth have been lost ensure they are not in the chest (CXR) or soft tissues.

X-rays 📖 pp. 458, 460, 464.

Assessing head injury

▶ All patients with recent facial trauma warranting hospital admission need at least initial assessment for head injury.

Change in the level of consciousness is the earliest and most valuable sign of head injury.

A combination of the following is generally used.

Glasgow coma scale (GCS)

Eyes open

- spontaneously   4
- to speech   3
- to pain   2
- do not open   1

Best verbal response

- orientated   5
- confused   4
- inappropriate   3
- incomprehensible   2
- none   1

Best motor response

- obeys commands   6
- localizes pain   5
- normal flexion   4
- abnormal flexion   3
- extension   2
- none   1

Pulse and BP ↓ pulse and ↑ BP is a late sign of ↑ intracranial pressure.

Pupils Measure size (1–8mm) and reaction to light in both pupils.

Respiration ↓ rate is a sign of raised intracranial pressure.

Limb movement

Indicate   normal
mild weakness
severe weakness
extension
no response

for arms and legs (record right and left separately if there is a difference).

CT scan The definitive investigation. However, patients must never be transferred before correcting hypoxia and hypovolaemia.

Using GCS

Severe head injury &/or deterioration = call for help.

One accepted method of categorizing head-injured patients by severity using GCS is:[1]

Severe	<8
Moderate	9–12
Minor	13–15

In addition:

A severe head injury is present if the following are seen:
- Unequal pupils (except traumatic mydriasis).
- Unequal limb movement (except orthopaedic injury).
- Open head injury (i.e. compound to brain).
- Deterioration in measured parameters.
- Depressed skull #

Subtle signs of deterioration include:
- Severe &/or worsening headache.
- Early unilateral pupillary dilatation.
- Early unilateral limb weakness.

A GCS of <6 in the absence of drugs has a dismal prognosis.
A change in GCS of 2 or more is significant. Beware changes in monitoring staff!

Optimizing outcome You are preventing 2° brain injury:
- Oxygenate.
- Moderate hyperventilation to control PCO_2.
- Control haemorrhage and optimize fluid balance.
- Contact neurosurgery and ask advice.
- Only use mannitol under expert advice.
- Do not use steroids at all.[1]

1 ACS 2004 *ATLS Core Course Manual.*

Mandibular fractures

These are the commonest # of the facial skeleton (Figure 10.1). Most are the result of fights and road traffic accidents (the former appear to be increasing whereas the latter are decreasing as a result of seat belts, etc.). Rarely, they may be comminuted with hard and soft tissue loss, e.g. gunshot wounds.

Classification The most useful is based on site of injury: dento-alveolar, condyle, coronoid, ramus, angle, body, symphyseal, or parasymphyseal. Further subclassification into unilateral, bilateral, multiple, or comminuted aids Rx planning. In common with all # they can be grouped into simple (closed linear #), compound (open to mouth or skin), pathological (# through an area weakened by other pathology), or comminuted; again, this influences Rx.

Muscle pull Pull on # segments renders the # favourable or unfavourable depending on whether or not the # line resists displacement. This is of less importance than recognizing the # and its associated injuries.

Common # Condylar neck # are commonest and range from easiest to most difficult. Often found with a # of the angle or canine region of the opposite side of the jaw. Rarely, bilateral condylar # is found with a symphyseal #—'guardsman's #' from falling on the point of the chin. Angle # usually occurs through wisdom-tooth socket, and body # commonly through canine socket.

Diagnosis History of trauma. Ask if the patient can bite their teeth or dentures together in the manner which is normal to them. Inability to do this and a lingual mucosal haematoma is pathognomonic of a mandibular #. Look at the face; there is usually bruising and swelling over the # site and sometimes lacerations. If the # is displaced, there may be gagging on the posterior teeth and the mouth hangs open. The saliva is usually blood-stained. The patient may complain of paraesthesia in the distribution of the IDN. Gentle palpation over the mandible will reveal step deformities, bony crepitus, and tenderness. All have trismus.

Examination of the mouth May reveal broken teeth or dentures which should be removed. Suction the mouth to clean away blood clots prior to examining both the buccal and lingual sulcus. Look for step deformities in the occlusion, and examine the teeth. Palpate for steps in the lingual and buccal sulcus. If Δ is uncertain it is sometimes worth trying to elicit abnormal mobility across the suspected # site, using gentle pressure. In cases where you are very unsure, place one hand over each angle of the mandible and exert gentle pressure; this will produce pain if there is a #, even if it is only a crack #. Never perform this if you have proved otherwise that there is a #.

X-rays DPT and PA mandible are the essentials. Right and left lateral obliques if DPT is unobtainable. Rotated PA (helpful for # between the symphysis and canine region), IO periapicals, occlusal, high DPT, or reverse Townes for condyles, and CT are all second-line investigations which may help.

Preliminary Rx (📖 p. 454) Most patients will be admitted to hospital, nursed sitting up and leaning forward as this is the most comfortable position. Barrel bandages are a waste of time. Keep nil by mouth and maintain hydration by IV crystalloid. Compound # need antibiotics. Assess need for analgesia; LA, temporary immobilization with circumdental wire (bridle wire), parenteral NSAIDs, or opioids may be needed.

Fig. 10.1 Malocclusion and abnormal mobility are pathognomonic of a fractured mandible.

Mid-face fractures

The mid-facial skeleton is a complex composite of fine fragile bones, which rarely # in isolation. It forms a detachable framework which protects the brain from trauma. Severe trauma can move the entire mid-face downwards and backwards along the base of the skull, lengthening the face and obstructing the airway (clot and swelling exacerbates this). Most *conscious* patients, however, can compensate for this. # of the cribriform plate of the ethmoids can lead to dural tears and CSF leak (🕮 p. 454).

Orbit The globe and optic nerve are well-protected by the bony buttress of the orbit. Most # lines pass around the optic foramen; however, swelling can cause proptosis. Late changes can include tethering and enopthalmos. *Retrobulbar haemorrhage* is an arterial bleed behind the globe following trauma. It presents as a painful, proptosed eye with decreasing visual acuity, and is a surgical emergency. The clot must be decompressed and evacuated. Medical management with mannitol 20% 2g/kg, acetazolamide 500mg and prednisolone at least 1mg/kg all IV may help while theatre is being arranged.

Bleeding Severe bleeding is rare, but severe mid-facial trauma may lacerate the 3rd part of the maxillary artery, resulting in profuse bleeding into the nasopharynx which requires anterior and posterior nasal packs and possibly direct (endoscopic) ligation.

Classification Mainly based on the experimental work of Rene Le Fort. Le Fort I # detaches the tooth-bearing portion of the jaw via a # line from the anterior margin of the anterior nasal aperture running laterally and back to the lower ⅓ of the pterygoid plate. Le Fort II detaches the true mid-face in a pyramidal shape (see Figure 10.2). Le Fort III detaches the entire facial skeleton from the cranial base, as Figure 10.2.

Diagnosis Le Fort I may occur singly or associated with other facial #. The tooth-bearing portion of the upper jaw is mobile, unless impacted superiorly. There is bruising in the buccal sulcus bilaterally, disturbed occlusion, and posterior 'gagging' of the bite. Grasp the upper jaw between the thumb and forefinger anteriorly, place thumb and forefinger of other hand over the supraorbital ridges, and attempt to mobilize the upper jaw to assess mobility. Spring the maxillary teeth to detect a palatal split. Percussion of the upper teeth may produce a 'cracked cup' sound. Le Fort II and III # produce similar clinical appearances; namely, gross oedema of soft tissues, bilateral black eyes (panda facies), subconjunctival haemorrhage, mobile mid-face, dish-face appearance, and extensive bruising of the soft palate. Look for a CSF leak and assess visual acuity. Le Fort II # may also show infra-orbital nerve paraesthesia and step deformity in the orbital rim. Peculiar to Le Fort III # are tenderness and separation of the frontozygomatic suture, deformity of zygomatic arches bilaterally, and mobility of entire facial skeleton.

X-rays Occipito-mental 10° and 30°, submento-vertex, lateral skull, postero-anterior skull **only** if C-spine is confirmed to be intact. Otherwise secure C-spine and await CT scan as the definitive imaging technique.

Preliminary Rx as 🕮 pp. 452, 454; **definitive Rx**, 🕮 p. 464.

Fig. 10.2 Each line represents a different fracture line although these lines are in reality more often produced surgically, trauma being less predictable.

Nasal and malar fractures

Malar (or zygoma) # A common and easily missed injury, usually the result of a blow with a blunt object (e.g. fist). The malar forms the cheekbone and resembles a four-pointed star on occipito-mental X-ray. The 'star' points to the maxilla (orbital margin and lateral wall of antrum), frontal bone, and temporal bone. # can involve the arch alone or the whole malar, which may or may not be displaced. The nature of the displacement is of value in planning the Rx.

Diagnosis From history, examination, and X-ray. Bruising around eye with subconjunctival haemorrhage (unilateral) (Figure 10.3). Diplopia, a step deformity of the orbital rim, sometimes paraesthesia of the infra-orbital nerve, limitation of lateral excursion of the mandible on mouth opening, and unilateral epistaxis. There is often tenderness on palpation of the zygomatic buttress IO and usually some flattening of the cheek prominence.

Orbital floor # Main signs are those of the malar # (or middle 1/3 # if that is the presenting injury). Late signs are enopthalmos and tethering of inferior rectus, causing diplopia in upwards gaze. Also known as orbital blowout #; fat and muscle herniates through the thin orbital floor (a similar injury can occur to the medial wall). Classically, seen on X-ray as 'hanging drop sign' (radiolucent fat hanging into antrum) (Figure 10.4). Confirm with coronal CT scan. Lateral wall &/or roof # are much less common.

Nasal # Simple nasal trauma is seen by a number of different specialities and considered rather trivial. This is unfair to the patients, as long-term results of nasal # leave a lot to be desired. Nasal # are frequently associated with deviation or crumpling of the septum, obvious nasal deformity, epistaxis, and a degree of nasal obstruction. Rx: often consists of simply manipulating the nasal bones with the thumb and splinting. This leaves the septum untreated and contributes to poor long-term results, many needing septorhinoplasty later.

Nasoethmoid # Consists of nasal bones, frontal process of maxilla, lacrimal bones, orbital plate of ethmoid, and displacement of the medial canthus of the eye. These # require accurate reduction, stabilization, and fixation of the medial canthus. Δ: bilateral black eyes, obvious nasal deformity (particularly depression of the nasal bridge), septal deviation, epistaxis, and obstruction. Look for CSF leak.

Septal haematoma A comparatively uncommon complication of nasal trauma which demands immediate evacuation as, if ignored, it can lead to septal necrosis.

Fig. 10.3 Presence of subconjunctival haemorrhage (seen here medially and laterally) is usually indicative of underlying fracture.

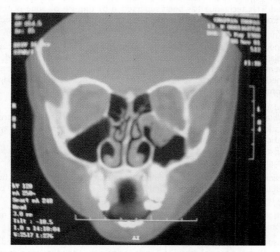

Fig. 10.4 A coronal CT scan demonstrating prolapse of the contents of the left orbit into the maxillary antrum—the 'hanging drop' of a blow out fracture.

Treatment of facial fractures

Essentially involves reduction, fixation, and immobilization of the # segments. In mandibular and maxillary #, this was traditionally achieved by IMF, i.e. immobilizing the jaws in occlusion. Nowadays, elastic traction is sometimes used to supplement internal fixation. Wisdom teeth, and grossly broken down or periodontally infected teeth in the # line should be removed. Otherwise, provision of antibiotics and adequate reduction and immobilizatiion with good follow-up (including endodontics as a 2° procedure) often allows preservation of teeth in the # line.

Open reduction and internal fixation (ORIF) of facial bone # has revolutionized Rx. # sites are exposed, usually via mucosal incisions, and reduced under direct vision; the teeth are placed in temporary IMF &/or a wire around the tooth on either side of the # (tension band or bridle wire) and small bone plates fixed by monocortical screws are placed to immobilize the reduction. IMF can then be released for recovery and elastics placed instead on the ward if needed. Very rarely interosseous wires replace plates, or IMF alone may be used. Resorbable plating systems are now on the market (polylactic & polyglycolic acid) but are yet to match titanium's reliability.

Edentulous mandible The absence of teeth in occlusion created problems when relying on IMF, and modified dentures called Gunning splints were used. This technique has been superseded by the use of bone plates in virtually all cases. Pencil-thin edentulous mandibles are best managed by thick (2.4mm) plates with bicortical screws inserted transcutaneously.

Condylar # Management depends on age and type of injury. <12yrs: analgesia, soft diet, and intermaxillary elastic guidance (if needed) produces optimal results. >12yrs: pain-free, pre-injury occlusion should be established (by elastic traction if need be), and the patient reassessed at 7 days. If spontaneous pain-free occlusion not possible at this stage: ORIF.[1]

Mid-face # Use one of the following methods:

Internal fixation Interosseous plating (by far commonest), wiring, transfixation with Kirschner wires. Plating to recreate the pyriform and zygomatic buttress system is currently most widespread.

External fixation E.g. Levant frame, box frame, which fix the mid-face to the cranium.

Malar # Are elevated by a temporal approach (Gillies) or bone hook percutaneously and supplemented by internal fixation with a range of plating techniques through small eyelid incisions.

Nasal bones Are manipulated and splinted. Some benefit from mini-submucous resection of the septum.

Nasoethmoidal # Are openly reduced and wired or microplated to reposition the medial canthi and restore anatomy often through a coronal flap incision.

---

1 Faculty of Dental Surgery 1997 *National Clinical Guidelines* (⅋ www.rcseng.ac.uk).

Fractures in children Considerably rarer. Plates and pins tend to be avoided because of risk to unerupted teeth. Patients <10yrs may require a form of Gunning splint which fits over the mixed dentition. # are usually firmly united within 3 weeks. Microplates can sometimes be used, or heavy resorbable sutures at the lower border of the mandible.

Post-op care Antibiotics and scrupulous OH are required. The main problems are presented by IMF, and the risk to the airway post-operatively. IMF requires a liquidized diet of at least 2500 calories (2000 for F) and 3l of fluid daily. Do not discharge until this can be maintained at home. ORIF requires a soft diet for up to 3 weeks.

Complications **Mandible** Infection, paraesthesia, damage to teeth, TMJ pain, malunion, delayed union, non-union, bony sequestration, plate and wire infection. **Maxilla** Post-op deformity, epiphora, diplopia, late enophthalmus, anosmia. Failure of union is very rare, although malunion is a problem with poor reduction or late referral. **Malar** Diplopia, retrobulbar haemorrhage, enophthalmos, paraesthesia. **Nasal** Deformity, nasal obstruction.

Composite tissue loss Gunshot wounds have led to more facial # presenting as composite defects of hard and soft tissue with tissue loss. These patients need to be stabilized, often with surgical debridement and external fixation prior to free-tissue transfer as part of definitive Rx.

Facial soft-tissue injuries

The face is highly visible and once cut no one can make the scar disappear. You can, however, give the patient the best possible scar by following certain principles. Definitive closure of soft tissue wounds should be done in tandem with fixation of bones or after exclusion of underlying bony injury.

Assessment ABCs, mechanism of injury, allergies, and PMH, need for tetanus and rabies prophylaxis. Wounds should be closed within 24h.

Examination Type of patient, type of wound (cut, burst, flap, tissue loss), special anatomy, eye, eyelid, lip, V/VII, parotid/lacrimal duct.

Investigation X-ray for FB.

Plan treatment Clean simple wounds in cooperative patient are best closed under LA. Otherwise admit for GA in theatre.

Clean wound Irrigate clean wounds with saline or aqeuous chlorhexidine. Bites or dirty wounds with ingrained FB need aggressive scrubbing with 50:50 water:betadine. Minimal or no excision of tissue for debridement. Explore all wounds for FB, #, nerve, duct, or vessel damage. Get haemostasis.

Wound closure In layers, mucosa, and muscle: resorbable 3/0–4/0; skin: monofilament 4/0–6/0. (Suturing: 📖 p. 350.) Avoid tension on skin edge.

Types of wound

Simple lacerations Close in layers with accurate anatomical apposition. Approximate, don't strangulate. Use minimum number of sutures to achieve intact wound with slight eversion. Remove facial sutures in 6 days.

Crush lacerations Skin has burst: minimal edge excision, deep closure, and light skin approximation. Tends to swell. Remove sutures at 3–4 days.

Slicing/shelving lacerations Convert to simple where possible by excision, as tends to 'trap door' otherwise. If excision would be excessive, tack down carefully.

Avulsion If flap, and seems viable: reposition and avoid haematoma. If complete: skin graft or local flap.

Penetrating injuries especially through platysma should be explored by senior surgeon in theatre, phone your next in line.

Anatomical sites

Eye Exclude globe injury.

Ear Drain haematoma if present to avoid 'cauliflower'.

Septum Drain haematoma to prevent perforation/collapse.

Eyelid, pinna, eyebrow, and vermilion Require precise matching. Test pre-anaesthetic for facial and trigeminal nerve function.

Special wounds

Abrasions Heal spontaneously but must be cleaned thoroughly; dress with chloramphenicol ointment.

Bites Easily get infected. Use co-amoxiclav,[1] clean very carefully, and close primarily. Small twist or finger drain helpful.

Burns Need specialist referral.

Tissue loss Nasal tip, pinna, and lip commonest. Skin graft or local flap repair is more likely to succeed than stitching severed part back on.

Gunshot wounds, 📖 p. 465.

---

1 Editors (2004) *Drugs & Therapeutics Bulletin* **42** 67.

Surgery and the temporomandibular joint

TMPDS 📖 p. 446.

Ankylosis May be true or false.

True ankylosis is restriction of movement caused by a pathological joint condition, usually due to trauma (intracapsular # in childhood) or infection. Extreme limitation of movement and X-rays will confirm degree of bony union. In fibrous union, exercises are of value. In bony union, interpositional arthroplasty or condylectomy with reconstruction is needed. Post-op exercise is crucial.

False ankylosis Restriction of movement imposed by extra-articular abnormalities is very rare. Rx depends upon cause. **Trismus** (limitation of movement due to spasm of muscles of mastication) may be confused with ankylosis but does not affect the joint. It is much more common and complicates many oral surgical procedures; may follow trauma or infection, or may be a manifestation of occult malignancy.

Trauma Condylar #, 📖 p. 458.

Intracapsular # Essentially a childhood injury (relatively shorter, thicker condylar neck) keep in function to prevent ankylosis. Condyle # are the subject of UK clinical guidelines (📖 p. 464).

Dislocation Occurs in normal joints due to exceptional circumstances, or in lax joints where dislocation is recurrent. May be unilateral or bilateral. Condyle can be palpated anterior to articular eminence, X-rays confirm position, mouth is gagged open. Rx: immediate reduction; the vast majority can be performed with LA around the dislocated joint &/or sedation. Place thumbs over molar teeth and exert downward and backward pressure (if LA is used, less force is needed and thumbs can be placed in buccal sulcus, avoiding the risk of being bitten). Advise jaw support when yawning, etc.; this is usually enough, and avoids IMF. In chronically recurring dislocations, patients can be taught to self-reduce. Exercises are of limited benefit but may avoid surgery. Sclerosant injections are unpleasant and no longer used. Operations are legion; capsular plication, pins to augment articular eminence, Dautrey downfracture of zygomatic arch, obliteration of upper joint space, eminectomy, high condylectomy. No one operation has gained pre-eminence.

Condylar hyperplasia Rare. Rx: high condylectomy if active (bone scan, but interpretation variable and condylar replacement, e.g. with costochondral cartilage, is unpredictable) or wait for it to 'burnout', then definitive orthognathic surgery.

Tumours Rare. Rx: ablation, reconstruction, and radiotherapy if malignant.

Arthritides Rheumatoid, psoriatic, and gouty arthritides all manifest in the TMJ but in <15% of patients with the systemic disease. The signs and symptoms are joint stiffness, pain, tenderness, and crepitus. Δ: knowledge of systemic disease and local signs. Rx: treat systemic condition. Symptomatic

Rx of joint with appliances, physiotherapy, exercises, NSAIDs and intra-articular steroids. Main long-term problem is limitation of function.

Osteoarthrosis A distinct entity of the TMJ, with a different clinical course from that seen in other joints. Appears to be a degenerative condition of articular cartilage. Δ: crepitus, limitation, and pain on movement, tenderness over condyle, often with X-ray evidence of condylar erosions. Most have symptoms for ~1yr which gradually ↓ over the next 2yrs. X-rays show condylar remodelling to a flat smooth surface. Patients then enter a long period of remission. Rx is therefore aimed at pain relief, using standard TMPDS measures (📖 p. 446). Those remaining unresponsive may benefit from intra-articular steroids (📖 p. 564), which probably accelerate natural remodelling. A small group will remain with pain 3–4 months after steroids, usually with X-ray abnormalities. They should be considered for high condylar shave or high condylectomy.

Surgery and TMPDS Approximately 20% of patients with TMPDS remain unresponsive to conservative Rx. They may benefit from arthrography or arthroscopy both as an investigation and a Rx (distension of the joint space-releasing adhesions). Surgery for pure TMPDS in patients unresponsive to the above may be of benefit (probably by cutting the nerve supply to the joint), although clicking can certainly be eliminated by meniscal plication &/or pterygoid myotomy, and irrevocably damaged menisci can be removed but require some form of interpositional reconstruction.

Joint replacement A handful of specifically designed customized condyle and fossa replacements are available. These should be reserved for severe symptomatic end-stage joint disease in the hands of those with a sub-specialist interest.

Major preprosthetic surgery

Minor procedures, 🕮 p. 388; implantology, 🕮 p. 390. The aim is to enable an edentulous patient to live comfortably with functioning dentures, therefore surgery without liaison with an understanding and competent prosthodontist is pointless. All procedures for improving the denture-bearing area of the jaws are dependent on the use of a denture with a modified fitting surface (stent), which is placed at operation and must be worn virtually permanently for up to 8 weeks post-op, the fitting surface being modified at intervals with a soft acrylic lining material. There are many who would claim these procedures do not work, and indeed there is little scientific support for them.

▶ Warn all patients undergoing lower jaw procedures about post-op mental nerve damage.

Epithelial inlay (vestibuloplasty) Basically a skin graft to the alveolar surface of the jaw, creating a deeper sulcus. Important points: excise all areas of scarred or hyperplastic tissue, dissect off any strands of mentalis in the lower jaw, ensure preservation of the alveolar periosteum, ensure the stent extends to the new sulcus depth, and ensure the skin–mucosa junction lies on the labial surface.

Combination mucosal flap and epithelial inlay Usually suffices in the maxilla due to its ↑ potential for denture retention.

Mental nerve repositioning Mental nerve compression by a denture flange following alveolar resorption is a common problem, producing a sensation like an electric shock but with a background ache which ↑ during the day and ↓ overnight. Leaving the -/F out for several days ↓ the pain. The mental nerve is repositioned by creating a new foramen under its present position or laterally transposing the entire nerve into the soft tissues in grossly atrophic mandibles.

Alveolar augmentation Problems with osseous donor site morbidity and length of procedure in elderly patients put these operations out of favour. The use of 'sandwich' procedures (where the augmenting material is literally sandwiched between horizontally osteotomized jaw), coupled with effective bone substitutes and tunnelling procedures (🕮 p. 388), have made augmentation, even in the comparatively frail elderly, a far better proposition. Younger, fit patients with severe jaw atrophy or those with incipient or actual pathological # may still benefit from split rib grafting.

Vertical distraction osteogenesis A preprosthetic component to this well-accepted technique for 'growing' bone by osteotomizing and gradually moving bone apart (1–2 mm/day) will probably replace all major augmentation procedures.

Sinus lift ↑ popular procedure combined with simultaneous or delayed implants. After raising subperiosteal buccal flaps a window is created to expose antral lining. Lining of the floor and walls is elevated intact and this space is filled with bone from the iliac crest, tibia, or chin to provide retention for implants.

Transmandibular implant A box frame construction placed in the mandible from a submental incision. Reputed to ↑ bone deposition. Rarely used.

Clefts and craniofacial anomalies

▶ 20% of cases of congenital facial malformation are accompanied by a 2nd or 3rd systemic malformation.

Cleft lip and palate (see also ☐ p. 170)

▶ The aim is to replace anatomical structures in their correct position; the price is scarring, which will restrict growth to some degree. It is important to recognize that the stigmata of surgery is due to growth of the patient. At least as much deformity has been caused in the past by poor surgery as has been caused by the cleft.

Lip closure Two main philosophies: **'Plastic' approach** Performed neonatally or up to 3 months; flaps transgress skin boundaries and use supraperiosteal dissection. Gives good early aesthetic results (e.g. Millard). **'Functional' approach** All skin boundaries are respected; uses subperiosteal dissection. Immediate aesthetics are less good due to pout caused by muscle repair but ↑ function and growth potential (e.g. Delaire). In the UK a trend is emerging to blend the techniques of these philosophies.

Palatal closure Extensive surgery restricts maxillary growth, therefore use minimal simple repair which recreates a functioning soft palate (e.g. Von Langenbeck or Delaire).

Alveolus Vomer flap to close anterior alveolus and gingivoperiosteoplasty are 1° procedures advocated by some and decried by others.

Ears Preschool audiology. Many will benefit from grommets.

Nasal deformity Perhaps the greatest surgical challenge. 1° functional lip/ nose repair may alter this.

Secondary surgery Lip revision (simple or complex). Sometimes required preschool or at time of alveolar bone graft.

Alveolar bone graft, ☐ p. 171.

Speech, nasendoscopy, and pharyngoplasty All cleft palate patients have impaired speech. Fibre-optic nasendoscopy allows visualization of the palate during speech and aids assessment. Pharyngoplasty narrows the velopharyngeal opening to ↓ hypernasal speech. Successful palate repair ↓ need for pharyngoplasty.

Orthognathic surgery, ☐ p. 474.

Craniofacial anomalies

A broad group of conditions involving the cranio-maxillofacial region. A simple classification is:

Congenital

- Orbital malformations (hypertelorism, orbital dystopia)
- Craniosynostoses (premature fusion of cranial sutures)
- Craniofacial synostoses (Apert syndromes, Crouzon, 📖 pp. 726, 727)
- Encephaloceles
- Others (Treacher–Collins, hemifacial microsomia, hemifacial hypertrophy and atrophy)

Acquired

- Tumours (benign or malignant)
- Dysplasias (fibro-osseous)
- Neurofibromatosis
- Post-trauma deformity

These patients need craniofacial teams (minimum: craniofacial surgeon, neurosurgeon, and anaesthetist). Coronal flaps to deglove the face are the mainstay of access, followed by craniotomy and osteotomy as required. Main risks are cerebral oedema, infection, damage to optic nerves and vessels; and, in neonates and children, paediatric fluid balance.

Orthognathic surgery

This is the surgery of facial skeletal deformity and merges with cleft and craniofacial surgery. Prime indications are functional: speech, eating. Secondary indications are aesthetic.

▶ Patients may not see these as quite such separate issues. Their reasons and motivation for seeking surgery must be understood and the limitations of surgery made absolutely clear before embarking on protracted and complex Rx.

Diagnosis and treatment planning, 📖 p. 168.

Mandibular procedures

Involve ramus, body, alveolus, or chin.

Intra-oral vertical subsigmoid osteotomy Used to push back the mandible. EO approach used when suitable equipment for IO not available. The IO procedure is straightforward, performed via an extended third-molar type incision. Bone cuts are made with a right-angled oscillating saw from sigmoid notch to lower border. Technique is very instrument-dependent.

Sagittal split osteotomy (Figure 10.5 and 10.6) Can move mandible backwards or forwards. IO incision similar to above. Bone cuts made from above lingula, across retromolar region, down buccal aspect to lower border. Split sagittally with osteotome followed by spreaders. Main complication is paraesthesia of IDN.

Inverted L- and C-shaped osteotomy Usually EO approach. Rarely used; can lengthen ramus if used with bone graft.

Body ostectomy Shortens body of mandible. Need to gain space orthodontically or remove tooth. Watch mental nerve.

Subapical osteotomy Used to move dento-alveolar segments. Technically more difficult than it looks. Risk to tooth vitality.

Genioplasty The tip of the chin can be moved pretty much anywhere; the secret is to keep a sliding contact with bone and a muscle pedicle. Fixation should be kept away from areas of muscle activity as this leads to bone resorption. Effective treatment for obstructive sleep apnoea.

Maxillary procedures

Segmental Can be single-tooth, or bone and tooth blocks, e.g. Wassmund procedure, which involves tunnelling incisions in buccal sulcus and palate to move premaxilla. Problems are finding space for bone cuts and avoiding damaging teeth.

Le Fort I Mainstay procedure. Standard approach is the 'down-fracture' with horseshoe buccal incision, bone cuts at Le Fort I level, and segment pedicled on the palate. The freed maxilla can be moved up, down, or forward. In cleft palate cases, concern over the adequacy of the palatal blood supply has led to some surgeons using tunnelled buccal incisions to make the bone cuts, thus preserving some of the buccal blood supply to the maxilla. Fixation is a problem when using this technique.

Le Fort II Usually used for mid-face advancement. Bilateral canthal and vestibular incisions allow bone cuts at the Le Fort II level.

Le Fort III Really a subcranial craniofacial operation using a coronal flap plus vestibular and orbital incisions to move the entire mid-face and malar complex.

Malar osteotomy Used for post-traumatic defects. Approach via coronal incisions. Risk to infra-orbital nerve from maxillary bone cut. Augmentation is an alternative (📖 p. 486).

Rhinoplasty The correction of isolated nasal deformity. Usually done intra-nasally, supplemented by tiny incisions over the nasal bones to allow bone cuts. 'Open rhinoplasty', which involves degloving the nasal skeleton via a collumella incision, is becoming popular.

Stability ↑ use of mini-plates in the fixation of the osteotomized segments has ↓ the reliance on bone grafts. Pre-surgical orthodontics (📖 p. 170) makes a significant contribution to ↓ rate of relapse. IMF &/or elastic traction remains vital for long-term success. Good dental interdigitation, and planning movements within the capacity of the soft tissues, are probably the best antirelapse measures.[1]

Distraction (📖 p. 170). The same principle coupled with conventional orthognathic osteotomies.

Fig. 10.5 A medial view of the bone cuts for the sagittal split osteotomy, note the position of the lingual.

1 D. Tuinzing 1993 *Surgical Orthodontics*, VU University Press.

Fig. 10.6 Lateral view of the bone cuts for the sagittal split osteotomy.

Salivary gland tumours

Diseases (see also 📖 pp. 420, 422)
Classified by WHO into epithelial tumours, non-epithelial tumours, and unclassified tumours.

Common benign tumours **Pleomorphic adenoma**, 📖 p. 422. **Monomorphic adenoma** Adenolymphoma (Warthin's tumour) affects M > F; rare <50yrs. Bilateral in 10%. Feels soft and cystic. Benign, very unlikely to recur despite being multifocal.

Carcinomas Rare. **Adenoid cystic carcinoma** Characteristic 'Swiss cheese' appearance histologically. Spreads locally, particularly along perineural spaces. Can be compatible with long-term survival despite propensity for 2° in lungs, although rarely cured. **Adenocarcinomas** There are a wide range of these malignant tumours, ranging from the highly aggressive to the relatively indolent, e.g. polymorphous low grade adenocarcinoma. It is essential that adequate histological Δ is made early (expert head and neck pathologist needed). Other carcinomas are rare, but may arise in a pre-existing pleomorphic adenoma or *de novo*. 5-yr survival ~30%.

Other epithelial tumours Include *acinic cell tumour* and *mucoepidermoid tumour*. Both have variable, unpredictable behaviour, can recur locally, and metastasize, and can occur at any age. On average, both compatible with ~80% survival.

Non-epithelial tumours Include haemangioma, lymphangioma, and neurofibroma. Account for 50% of salivary tumours in children.

Unclassified group Includes lymphomas, secondaries, lipomas, and chemodectomas.

Parotid History and examination are the prime diagnostic tools. Long history, no pain, and no facial nerve involvement suggest benign tumour. Facial palsy, pain, and rapid growth suggest malignancy. The feel of many tumours are characteristic. CT, FNAC, USS, MRI may help; however, Rx almost always involves parotidectomy and most investigations simply delay this.

Submandibular Less common tumours. Pleomorphic adenoma remains most common. Malignant tumours account for up to 30%. Rx of most is gland excision via a skin crease in the neck. Modified neck dissection for malignant or recurrent tumours.

Sublingual and minor glands >50% of tumours are malignant (mostly adenoid cystic) and require extensive surgery and reconstruction similar to floor of mouth cancer.

Surgery of the salivary glands

Surgery of the major salivary glands is primarily for tumours, obstruction, and, less commonly, inflammatory conditions. The minor glands are most commonly removed for mucoceles (📖 p. 376) and more rarely for tumours. With the exception of lymphomas *all* salivary gland tumours should have surgery initially, patient permitting.

Parotidectomy Principles are complete excision of tumour with margin of healthy tissue and preservation of facial nerve. Clinically benign tumours in superficial lobe have superficial parotidectomy; and in deep lobe, total conservative parotidectomy. Malignant tumours require radical excision &/ or radiotherapy. Whether or not to sacrifice the facial nerve adjacent to malignant parotid tumour is complex decision. Many would accept: *nerve clinically affected*, pre-op, sacrifice, and reconstruct; *nerve clinically intact*, pre-op, preserve, and rely on post-op radiotherapy.

Salivary duct calculi History is of recurrent pain and swelling in the obstructed gland, particularly before and during meals. Plain X-rays (lower occlusal for submandibular, cheek for parotid) reveal radio-opaque calculi, but do not exclude the radiolucent calculi and mucous plugs. Sialography reveals a stricture or obstruction. Commonest in the submandibular duct. Rx: *submandibular duct* for calculi lying anterior in duct—remove by passing a suture behind the calculus to prevent it slipping further down the duct, dissect the duct from an IO approach, and lift out stone; either marsupialize the duct or reconstruct. Posterior calculi—excise gland and duct. Rx: *parotid duct*—expose duct via IO approach for anterior stones or via a small skin flap onto a probe in the duct for more posterior calculi. Otherwise, selective superficial parotidectomy is the only safe approach.

Laser lithotripsy is available in some centres for proximal calculi in patients wishing to avoid gland excision and calculi <3mm.

Recurrent sialadenitis Severe recurrent infection of the parotid or submandibular glands leads to dilatation and ballooning of the ducts and alveoli called sialectasis. Sialography is the investigation of choice and often therapeutic, inducing long remissions between episodes of infection. *Conservative* Rx: massage and repeated antibiotics (amoxicillin if not allergic) or irrigation of gland with tetracycline solution. When remission periods are short or intolerable, or the patient requires *definitive* Rx: submandibular gland excision or total conservative parotidectomy with removal of 90% of the duct. Interventional sialography with specialized balloon/basket catheters is now being used to dilate or retrieve obstructions but has not replaced open surgery.

Surgery for drooling In severe cases it is possible to re-site the parotid ducts into the hypopharynx &/or perform bilateral submandibular gland excision to control drooling without impairing lubrication for swallowing and oral health (Wilkes procedure). A more physiological approach is to reposition submandibular ducts and excise sublingual glands, as these are major source of pooled saliva *at rest*. Intraglandular botulinum toxin can help.

Mucoceles, 📖 p. 376.

Facial skin cancer

Skin cancer, 🕮 p. 512.

The common facial skin cancers are BCC, SCC, and malignant melanoma. They may be preceded by actinic keratosis, carcinoma-*in-situ*, or lentigo maligna.

The 'best buy' Rx is usually excision with repair by 1° closure, skin graft, or local flap. Electron beam radiotherapy, topical photodynamic therapy and topical 5-FU cream are alternatives.

Margins A margin of normal skin around the cancer of 5mm for BCC, 10mm for SCC, and 10–30mm for melanoma, dependant on site.

Techniques Mark out the periphery of the tumour, line of excision, and any flap repair *before* injecting LA (if used). Cut at 90° to skin through dermis and excise at level of fat layer. *Always* obtain good haemostasis (bipolar diathermy). Mark specimen to orientate for pathologist.

Repair

1° closure Try to design excision in natural crease or resting skin tension line. Excise in an ellipse, undermine both sides, and close by halving the length of the wound. Use deep sutures to minimize tension. Excise any 'dog ears'.

Wedge excision Allows 1° closure of lip, eyelid, and helix.

Split skin grafts Are thin and take well, but tend to shrink and are a poor colour match. Taken with a Humby/Watson knife or a dermatome they leave a raw donor site. Useful for scalp defects.

No skin graft will take on bare bone, tendon, or cartilage. Grafts will fail if they move, develop haematoma, or become infected, as this prevents plasmatic imbibition and capillary ingrowth.

Full thickness skin grafts Thicker and more robust, they do not take as easily. They are taken with a scalpel and donor site is closed primarily. Better colour match.

Grafts are sutured to periphery of wound and immobilized with a bolster of antiseptic cotton or sponge and tie-over sutures for 7–10 days. The thicker the graft, the longer to take.

Local flaps

Have their own blood supply and work by a combination of geometry and widespread undermining.

Flap is marked out at same time as excision before LA. Held in new position by deep and skin sutures. Do not use pressure dressings. Haematoma is biggest cause of failure in adequately designed flaps: take sutures out to ↓ pressure and ↑ flap circulation with delayed resuture.

Common local flaps

Transposition flap Simple switch over of skin.

Rhomboid flap Very useful; relies on lax skin at donor site.

Bi-lobed flap Transfers circles 80% and 60% to created defect.

Subcutaneous advancement flap A teardrop of skin is advanced on a subcutaneous fat pedicle.

Oral cancer

Aetiology, epidemiology, Δ, and staging, 📖 p. 416; neck lumps, 📖 p. 442; salivary tumours, 📖 p. 477.

Various parameters affect the choice of Rx for patients with oral cancer; not least among these, but often forgotten, are the patients themselves, their general health, understanding of their disease, geographical location, and social and domestic commitments. Classically, broad Rx principles are based on tumour staging, using TNM classification, 📖 p. 416, and the patient's fitness for surgery (this tends to imply that if they can't cope with surgery they can cope with travelling for and side-effects of radiotherapy, which is not always the case). In many instances of oral cancer, combined surgery and radiotherapy constitutes optimal Rx.

Suggested management plan (this will vary according to the surgeon concerned).
1) Establish provisional Δ. History, examination, and get to know patient. FBC, ESR, U&Es, LFTs (including albumin), bone biochemistry, syphilis serology, blood group, CXR, ECG, DPT.
2) Arrange tissue Δ. By biopsy—usually under LA. Flexible nasendoscopy, head, neck, thorax, imaging (CT/MRI). This is to exclude synchronous 1° tumour in upper aerodigestive tract (present in, at most, 15% of cases). Palpate the neck for nodes. Stage tumour (TNM).
3) Unless patient has made it very obvious they do not want to know the Δ, first inform them, then relatives, fully.
   • T1-N0 Surgery or radiotherapy (often brachytherapy-radioactive implants) offer equal cure rate. Surgery often simpler and cheaper.
   • Tumour close to bone having radiotherapy: safest to remove associated teeth to prevent osteoradionecrosis.
   • T2 but imaging N0 have a 30% incidence of occult metastases; debate exists over watch and wait or selective neck dissection. Majority favour dissection.
   • T2 and T3 >50% of patients will have occult metastases; prophylactic radiotherapy (works for occult but not for obvious bulky nodes); or prophylactic selective neck dissection. In presence of imaging or palpable nodes latter usually best.
   • For large tumours, close or +ve margins, and extracapsular spread, radiotherapy given post-op.
   • Vastly ↑ access is obtained for resection by osteotomizing the mandible (position plate beforehand).
   • Anterior floor of mouth cancer may spread to bilateral lymph nodes; bilateral selective neck dissection is indicated.
   • Presence or absence of extracapsular spread in cervical lymph nodes is strongest prognostic indicator of poor outcome.

Simultaneous chemotherapy and radiotherapy can have a dramatic effect on poorly differentiated SCCs, especially those originating from post-nasal space, tonsil, and tongue base. This treatment has become increasingly popular and a little indiscriminate in some centres. The morbidity (osteo-radionecrosis, trismus, dysphagia, mucositis, neutropenia) and mortality of treatment has increased as a consequence.

5-year survival 90% for T1-N0, but 30% for T2/3-N1 and worse for T4; however, this does *not* mean that extensive combination therapy and reconstruction is pointless in those with advanced oral cancers. Death comes in many ways, and a fungating uncontrolled cancer of the head and neck is one of the less pleasant. Attempted surgical 'cure' which alleviates local disease and symptoms and allows the patient a few more years of life and a gradual demise due to carcinomatosis or another disease is still worthwhile from all viewpoints. (Palliative surgery with curative intent.)

Chemotherapy There is, as yet, no proven role for cytotoxics in oral cancer, other than in combination with radiotherapy or in palliation. Other oncocytic drugs are under investigation.

Photodynamic therapy Licenced for palliation in UK but treatment in other countries. This involves injection of a photosensitizing agent and illumination with a specific waveband non-thermal laser after a set time interval which causes tumour and tissue destruction by several different means. Defects heal surprisingly well by secondary intention.

Neck lumps

▶ Do not leave chronic cervical lymphadenopathy undiagnosed.
▶ A 1° head and neck malignancy must be excluded visually, by imaging or histology (or all three) before biopsy.

Children are an exception; inflammation is common and tumour is rare, so a watch and wait policy is reasonable.

Diagnosis Listen to the story, look at the patient and lump. Palpate it. If needed, carry out a full head and neck examination. Most diagnoses will be made by then.

Investigation Ultrasound, aspiration cytology, biopsy.

Causes Think (a) anatomy, (b) pathology, (c) oddity.

Skin Lesions lie superficially.

> *Sebaceous cyst* Look for punctum; is within skin. Excise.

> *Lipoma* Soft, often yellowish. Excise.

> *Sublingual dermoid cyst* Lies in floor of mouth, often under mylohyoid. Arises from trapped epithelium during embryonic fusion; contains keratin. Rx: total excision.

Lymph nodes Deep to platysma. Try to diagnose before biopsy. Opening of malignant nodes ↓ survival (📖 p. 480).

> *Infection* (📖 p. 442) Nodes are large and tender. Causes: viral (e.g. glandular fever, HIV), bacterial (e.g. mycobacterial (which can calcify), actinomycosis), or reactive to other head and neck infection.

> *Malignancy* Either metastatic from head and neck 1° (hard, rock-like nodes) or lymphoma/leukaemia (large rubbery), 📖 p. 442. FNAC unhelpful in lymphoma; biopsy needed.

Glandular Think anatomically.

> *Salivary* (📖 p. 477) Submandibular/lower pole of parotid: abscess, sialadenitis, obstruction, sarcoidosis, Sjögren syndrome. Sublingual: ranula, tumour.

> *Thyroid* Benign and malignant tumours, goitre, thyroglossal cyst (may lie anywhere between foramen caecum of tongue and thyroid, tract goes behind, around, or through hyoid bone, moves with swallowing).

Arterial Don't biopsy!

> *Carotid aneurysm* (pulsatile).

> *Carotid body tumour* Found around carotid bifurcation. Usually firm, not hormonally active, 5% malignant. Rx: excise if symptomatic.

> *Schwannoma/neurofibroma* All major nerves in neck can develop painless masses. Rx: subadvential excision, preserving healthy fibres if possible.

Pharynx

> *Diverticulum* (or pharyngeal pouch) Fills on swallowing. Evert endoscopically or excise.

Larynx

> *Laryngocele* Rare. Mainly M >60yrs. 80% unilateral. Excise.

Sternomastoid

'*Sternomastoid tumour*' (congenital ischaemic fibrosis causing torticollis).

True muscle tumours Rare.

Bone

Cervical rib, prominent hyoid bone

Infections (see also 📖 p. 370) Ludwig's angina, submasseteric abscess, retropharyngeal abscess, parapharyngeal cellulitis, collar stud abscess (TB), infected cysts or pouches.

Oddities

Branchial cyst Either a remnant from 2nd and 3rd branchial arches or degeneration of lymphoid tissue. Is an epithelial lined cyst which presents as a deep-seated swelling lying anterior to sternomastoid at or above the level of the hyoid. Prone to infection. Rx: total excision.

Branchial fistula A fistula from the tonsillar fossa to the skin overlying anterior lower ⅓ of sternomastoid. Present at birth; discharges intermittently. Rx: total excision of tract.

Cystic hygroma Presents in infancy and is a form of lymphangioma which appears as endothelium-lined multilocular cysts containing lymph. May be found anywhere in head–neck but classically behind lower end of sternomastoid. May suddenly ↑ in size if bled into or ruptured. Rx: total excision as soon as child is fit for operation. Cystic areas may be sclerosed using modified streptococcal antigen Picinabil. Macrocystic lymphangiomas are relatively easy to dissect, microcystic are almost impossible.

Flaps and grafts

A **graft** is transferred tissue dependent on the recipient site capillaries for its survival. A **flap** is transferred tissue independent, at least initially, of the recipient site capillaries for survival.

It is the possibility of functional reconstruction of the head and neck in conjunction with the potential for cure that justifies the mutilation of radical surgery for oral cancer; however, head and neck reconstruction is used in other aspects of maxillofacial surgery, particularly trauma.

Mucosal grafts, 📖 p. 212. **Mucosal flaps**, 📖 p. 212.

Skin grafts May be split thickness or full thickness. Split thickness (taken by knife or dermatome from thigh or inner arm) take quickly and become wettable in the mouth. They are 'quilted' in place with sutures or compressed with bolsters. Full thickness (supraclavicular, post-auricular, or abdominal) provide a mediocre colour match when repairing skin defects of the face. Full thickness donor sites are closed primarily.

Free bone grafts From rib, iliac crest, or calvarium. Rib, which is partially split at 1-cm intervals, can be bent to conform to the shape of the mandible. Iliac crest supplies cortical or cancellous bone and can be cut to a template, but ↑ risk of DVT. Various synthetic mesh containers as a mould for cancellous bone exist. Very few use cadaveric free bone grafts.

Nasolabial flap Random pattern pedicle flap based above and lateral to the upper lip; useful local flap. Requires division ~3 weeks later.

Tongue flaps Random pattern pedicle flap for lip and palate repair. Requires division and inset 3 weeks later.

Forehead flap Based on anterior branch of superficial temporal artery; very safe flap, rarely used because of the poor donor site defect. Requires division later.

Masseter muscle flap Limited in size; can be used intra-orally.

Temperoparietal fascial flap Pedicle or free flap based on superficial temporal vessels. Long flexible reconstruction. Difficult to raise.

Temporalis flap Inferiorly based on deep temporal branches of maxillary artery. Limited use due to size and tendency to fibrose.

Deltopectoral flap Based on perforating internal mammary vessels. Thin skin suitable for skin or mucosa repair. Usually divided and inset after 3 weeks.

Pectoralis major myocutaneous flap Also described with bone, but the bone is really a free rib graft. Based on acromiothoracic axis. Usually tunnelled after neck dissection. Very bulky flap; covers carotids after radical neck dissection. Workhorse head and neck pedicle flap.

Latissimus dorsi myocutaneous flap Bulky flap based on thoracodorsal vessels. Needs to be tunnelled through axilla if pedicled. More commonly used as a free flap.

Free tissue transfer by microvascular re-anastomosis has been the biggest advance in reconstruction. The following are useful and commonly used flaps.

Radial forearm flap A fasciocutaneous flap based on the radial artery. The skin available is thin and supple and can conform to the complex anatomy of the mouth (skin is often hairless, which is a big bonus). A thin segment of up to 10cm (length) 40% thickness of radius can also be transferred for bony reconstruction but the radius should be plated to prevent #.

Deep circumflex iliac artery flap Based on the deep circumflex iliac artery. This flap has potential for sufficient bone transfer to reconstruct the entire mandible. Internal oblique muscle usually transferred for soft tissue—good where non-mobile soft tissue repair needed. Skin transfer possible but less useful.

Free fibula flap 25cm of fibula can be excised within a muscle cuff supplied by the peroneal vessels. Excellent length and thickness of bone for mandibular reconstruction. Skin transfer for mobile soft tissue available.

Free rectus abdominus Bulky skin/muscle flap based on inferior epigastric vessels. Useful for massive facial defects but often limited by fat volume.

Anterolateral thigh free flap Soft tissue flap from thigh based on descending branch of lateral circumflex femoral artery. Skin thickness can limit usefulness infra-orally.

Subscapular system flaps Several skin, fat, and bone flaps can be harvested from these vessels; disadvantage is need to turn patient perioperatively.

Craniofacial implants Prosthetic eyes, ears, and noses can be securely fixed to the facial skeleton with implants using techniques similar to oral implants. Probably the best available ear reconstruction.

Aesthetic facial surgery

An increasingly popular area of surgery in the developed world. The mainstay procedures are described.

Browlift The older coronal excision is now rare being replaced by endoscopic browlift; approached through 3 vertical incisions using an arthroscope and suspension sutures. Aim is to reduce frown furrows and elevate brow.

Blepharoplasty Upper and lower eyelid surgery. Traditionally involved the removal of skin, fat and muscle, this often produced a sunken 'operated' appearance. Now the upper lid has skin and muscle excised but fat is simply cauterized producing shrinkage. The lower lid can be approached from the skin or the conjunctiva depending on whether skin excision is needed and fat may be removed, cauterized or repositioned.

Otoplasty Is the correction of external ear deformity, aims are to recreate the antihelix and reduce the angulation between the concha and the skull. Cartilage scoring and permanent sutures are the popular techniques.

Rhinoplasty The surgery of nasal deformity and function. Essential prerequisite is realistic expectations from the patient (beware young men seeking 'nosejobs'). Open rhinoplasty is performed through an incision in the columella skin, closed through nasal mucosa. Both aim to maintain or improve the airway and improve aesthetics by reshaping rather than removing constituent parts of the nose.

Rhytidectomy The facelift has several variants but the commonest is currently the Superficial MusculoAponeurotic System (SMAS) lift. This includes a diffuse layer of connective tissue which runs from the platysma in the neck to the temporoparietal fascia in the temple which is claimed to reduce relapse. The incision runs in the preauricular sulcus round the lobe and into the mastoid hairline. The jowl area is undermined, advanced up and back, excess removed, SMAS plicated and skin closed.

Liposculpture Is the selective removal of fat. The area to be reduced is infiltrated with a solution of normal saline, lidocaine 0.1%, adrenaline 1:1 000 000 and bicarbonate and suction performed with a blunt cannula under vacuum (0.5–1 atmosphere—can be generated by a syringe).

Botulinum toxin 4 different versions available 'Botox®' is actually the trade name of one of them (Vistabel®, Neurobloc® & Dysport® are others). It is a temporary (3–6 months) paralyzing agent which when injected into muscles of facial expression can remove 'dynamic' wrinkles particularly around the forehead, lateral eyes, upper lip and midline neck. Has therapeutic role in masseteric hypertrophy, blepharospasm, facial tics and some forms of trismus.

Fillers Temporary fillers made of collagen and hyaluronic acid and poly-L-lactic acid are popular to augment soft tissue of the face. They are injected into the lips, nasolabial folds, wrinkles, depressions or areas of fat atrophy (seen in HIV). Autologous fat can also be used. Avoid 'permanent' fillers.

Laser resurfacing, dermabrasion and chemical peels These are all ways of improving the surface texture of skin basically by removing the surface layers either by evaporation, mechanical abrasion or chemical burn. Risk of skin depigmentation and must avoid excessive sunlight afterwards.

Medicine relevant to dentistry

Contents

Medical theory

Emergencies

In-patients

Principal sources C. Scully 2005 *Medical Problems in Dentistry*, Wright (5th edn). M. Longmore et al. 2007 *Oxford Handbook of Clinical Medicine*, OUP. D. Mitchell 2006 *An Introduction to Oral and Maxillofacial Surgery*, OUP. M. Lubin et al. 2006 *Medical Management of the Surgical Patient*, Cambridge University Press (comprehensive but entirely North American perspective). Various 1995 *Procedures in Practice*, BMJ. BNF 54.

NB All drug doses relate to fit, adult patients ≅70kg in weight. Always check doses for children, the elderly, and those with other medical conditions.

Anaemia

Anaemia is a ↓ in the level of circulating haemoglobin to below the normal reference range for a patient's age and sex. It indicates an underlying problem and, as such, the cause of the anaemia should be diagnosed *before* instituting Rx.

▶ Never rush into transfusing patients presenting with a chronic anaemia. Perform basic blood investigations before giving iron or transfusing. Elective surgery in patients with an Hb <10g/dl is rarely appropriate.

Clinical features of anaemia are notoriously unreliable, but beloved of examiners and include: general fatigue, heart failure, angina on effort, pallor (look at conjunctivae and palmar creases, but unreliable), brittle nails &/or spoon-shaped nails (koilonychia), oral discomfort &/or ulceration, glossitis, and classically angular cheilitis.

Syndromes, 📖 p. 730.

Types of anaemia

Microcytic (MCV < 78fl) Iron-deficiency anaemia is by far the commonest cause. Causes: chronic blood loss (gastrointestinal or menstrual), inadequate diet. FBC and biochemistry show microcytic, hypochromic anaemia with a low serum iron and a high total iron binding capacity (TIBC). ↑ RBC zinc protoporphyrin is a fast and sensitive early test. Thalassaemia and sideroblastic anaemia are rare causes of microcytosis.

Normocytic Commonly, anaemia of chronic disease. Other causes: pregnancy, acute blood loss, haemolytic anaemia, and aplastic anaemia. Once pregnancy is excluded, the patient needs investigation by an expert. The TIBC is usually ↓.

Macrocytic (MCV > 100fl) Low B_{12} &/or low folate are the common causes. B_{12} is ↓ in pernicious anaemia (deficit of intrinsic factor), alcohol abuse, small gut disease, and chronic exposure to nitrous oxide. Low folate is usually dietary, but may be caused by illness (e.g. coeliac disease, skin disease) or drugs such as phenytoin, methotrexate, trimethoprim, and co-trimoxazole.

Management In all cases the cause must be sought; this may necessitate referral to a haematologist. Drugs used in iron deficiency: ferrous sulfate 200mg tds. Transfusion of packed cells covered with furosemide 40mg PO if elderly or ↓ cardiac function, indicated rarely for severe microcytic anaemia. Lifelong IM hydroxocobalamin 1mg 3-monthly is used to treat B_{12} deficiency, and folic acid 5mg od for folate deficiency.

▶ Never use folate alone to treat 'macrocytosis' unless it is proven to be the only deficiency. **NB** Folic acid is **not** the same as folinic acid.

Note on sickle cell anaemia A homozygous hereditary condition causing red cells to 'sickle' when exposed to low O_2 tensions, resulting in infarctions of bone and brain. In sickle cell trait (heterozygous form) the cells are less fragile and sickle only in severe hypoxia. Management: perform haemoglobin electrophoresis (or Sickledex if result needed urgently) on all Afro-Caribbean (and consider Mediterranean, Middle Eastern, and Indian) patients planned for GA.

Haematological malignancy

Leukaemias are a neoplastic proliferation of white blood cells. Acute leukaemias are characterized by the release of primitive blast cells into the peripheral blood and account for 50% of childhood malignancy. Acute lymphoblastic leukaemia, the commonest childhood leukaemia, now has up to 90% cure rate in favourable cases. May present as gingival hypertrophy and bleeding. Acute myeloblastic leukaemia is the commonest acute leukaemia of adults, but although an 80% remission rate is possible this is rarely maintained. Chronic leukaemias have cells that retain most of the appearance of normal white cells. Chronic lymphocytic leukaemia is the commonest and has a 5-yr survival of >50%. Chronic myeloid leukaemia is characterized by the presence of the Philadelphia chromosome, a fact beloved by examiners. Affects the >40s. Rx: interferon &/or bone marrow transplant (BMT) or stem cell transplantation. Remissions are common, although a terminal blast crisis usually supervenes at some stage.

Myeloproliferative disorders are proliferation of non-leukocyte marrow cells, with a wide range of behaviour and presentation, including anaemia, bleeding, and infections.

Monoclonal gammopathies such as multiple myeloma are B-lymphocyte disorders characterized by production of a specific immunoglobulin by plasma cells. Multiple myeloma is also a differential Δ of lytic lesions of bone, particularly the skull. Δ: monoclonal paraprotein band on plasma electrophoresis, Bence–Jones proteins in urine.

Lymphomas A group of solid tumours arising in lymphoid tissue; divided into Hodgkin's or non-Hodgkin's lymphomas, with the latter carrying a poorer prognosis. Lymphoma should always be considered in the differential Δ of neck swellings.

Cytotoxic chemotherapy Has been the mainstay of Rx for these diseases, with supplemental radiotherapy for masses or prior to BMT. It is essential to remember that any patient receiving these drugs will be both immunocompromised and liable to bleed.

Hints In haematological malignancy, anaemia, bleeding, and infection are the overwhelming risks. Look for and treat anaemia. Avoid aspirin, other NSAIDs, trauma, and IM injections. Prevent sepsis, and if it occurs treat very aggressively with the locally recommended broad-spectrum antibacterials and antifungals, e.g. piperacillin/tazobactam 2.25g and gentamicin 80mg IV tds plus fluconazole up to 100mg daily. Liaise with haematologist urgently.

Amyloidosis Characterized by deposits of fibrillar eosinophilic hyaline material in a wide range of organs and tissues. Two types: 1° *amyloidosis* (AL amyloid), a plasma cell dyscrasia. Signs and symptoms include peripheral neuropathy, renal involvement, cardiomyopathy, xerostomia, and macroglossia. Rx: immunosuppression (rarely helps). 2° *amyloidosis* (AA amyloid). It reflects an underlying chronic disease: infection, rheumatoid, neoplasia. May respond to Rx of underlying disease. Δ: biopsy of rectum or gingivae—stain with Congo red.

Other haematological disorders

For the practical management of a bleeding patient, 📖 see p. 348.

Bleeding disorders

Platelet disorders May present as nosebleeds, purpura, or post-extraction bleeding. Remember that aspirin is the most common acquired cause, its effect being irreversible for 1 week. Other causes include diseases such as Von Willebrand's disease; immune thrombocytopenic purpura (ITP); virally associated (especially HIV) thrombocytopenic purpura; thrombocytopenia secondary to leukaemia; cytotoxic drugs; or unwanted effects of drugs, notably aspirin and chloramphenicol. Management: ensure platelet levels of >50 x 10^9/l, preferably 75 x 10^9/l for anything more than simple extraction or LA. If actively bleeding, use a combination of local measures (📖 p. 348), tranexamic acid, and platelet transfusion. Platelet transfusions are short-lived and if used prophylactically must be given immediately prior to or during surgery. Liaise closely with the lab. The quality of preparation varies by locality. Tranexamic acid mouthwash may ↓ oral bleeding.

Coagulation defects Present as prolonged wound bleeding &/or haemarthroses. Causes include the haemophilias, anticoagulants, liver disease, and von Willebrand's disease.

Others Less common causes include: hereditary haemorrhagic telangectasia, aplastic anaemia, chronic renal failure, myeloma, SLE, disseminated intravascular coagulation, and isolated deficiency of clotting factors.

Haemophilia A (factor VIII deficiency) The commonest clotting defect. Inherited as a sex-linked recessive, it affects males predominantly, although female haemophiliacs can occur. All daughters of affected males are potential carriers. Usually presents in childhood as haemarthroses. Bleeding from the mouth is common. Following trauma, bleeding appears to stop, but an intractable general ooze starts after an hour or so. Severity of bleeding is dependent on the level of factor VIII activity and degree of trauma.

Haemophilia B (factor IX deficiency) Clinically identical to haemophilia A; also known as Christmas disease.

Von Willebrand's disease A combined platelet and factor VIII disorder affecting males and females. Mucosal purpurae are common, haemarthroses less so. Wide range of severity. May improve with age &/or pregnancy.

Management The haemophilias and Von Willebrand's disease should always be managed at specialist centres. Check the patient's warning card for the contact telephone number.

Anticoagulants

Heparin Given IV or high-dose SC for therapeutic anticoagulation. Its effect wears off in ~8h although it can be reversed by protamine sulfate in an emergency. Measure in activated partial thromboplastin time (APTT).

Warfarin Given orally; effects take 48h to be seen. Normal therapeutic range is an International Normalized Ratio (INR) of 2–4. Simple extractions are usually safe at a level within therapeutic range. Reverse the effects of warfarin with vitamin K +/or fresh frozen plasma if needed, but consider why the patient is anticoagulated in the first place. See p. 548.

Cardiovascular disease

This is the commonest cause of death in the UK.

Clinical conditions

Hypertension is a consistently raised BP (>140 systolic, >90 diastolic >3 months) and is a risk factor for ischaemic heart disease, cerebrovascular accidents, and renal failure. Up to 95% of hypertension has no definable cause: essential hypertension. 5% is secondary to another disease such as renal dysfunction or endocrine disorders.

Ischaemic heart disease is ↓ of the blood supply to part of the heart by narrowing of the coronary arteries, usually by atheroma, causing the pain of angina pectoris. If occluded, an MI occurs (📖 p. 522).

Heart failure is the end result of a variety of conditions, not all of them cardiovascular. Basically, the heart is unable to meet the circulatory needs of the body. In right heart failure, dependent oedema and venous engorgement are prominent. In left heart failure, breathlessness is the principal sign. The two often coexist. There is an ever-present risk of precipitating heart failure, even in treated patients, by ↑ the demands on the heart, e.g. by fluid overload or excessive exertion.

Hypovolaemic shock is collapse of the peripheral circulation due to a sudden ↓ in the circulating volume. If this is not corrected there can be failure of perfusion of the vital organs, resulting in heart failure, renal failure, and unconsciousness ending in death.

Murmurs are disturbances of blood flow which are audible through a stethoscope. They may be functional or signify structural disorders of the heart. Echocardiography will differentiate. They are of great relevance to dentists as their presence warns of the potential for colonization of damaged valves by blood-borne bacteria. Such a bacteraemia can be caused by dental procedures.

Dental implications

Patients with a PMH of rheumatic fever are very likely to have some damage to a heart valve, usually the mitral valve. Traditionally advice has been to provide antibiotic prophylaxis for invasive dental procedures, but recent guidance has advised against this.[1] The risk of precipitating heart failure or MI in patients with compromised cardiovascular systems is ever-present. Prevent by avoiding GA, especially within 3 months of an MI, using adequate LA with sedation if necessary, and avoid excessive adrenaline loads. Consider potential drug interactions (📖 p. 578) and remember some of these patients will be anticoagulated.

Exclusion of septic foci may be requested in patients at high risk from bacteraemia, e.g. heart transplant recipients, those with prosthetic valves or valvular damage, or those with a history of IE. It is prudent to err on the side of caution with these individuals and some will need dental clearances.

---

1 NICE Guidance 2008 ℘ www.nice.ork.uk

Respiratory disease

Disease of the chest is an everyday problem in developed countries. The principal symptoms are cough, which may or may not be productive of sputum, dyspnoea (breathlessness), and wheeze. The coughing of blood (haemoptysis) mandates that malignancy be excluded.

Clinical conditions

Upper respiratory tract infections Include the common cold, sinusitis, and pharyngitis/tonsillitis (which may be viral or bacterial), laryngotracheitis, and acute epiglottitis. *All* are C/I to elective GA in the acute phase. Sinusitis (🕮 p. 384). Penicillin is the drug of choice for a streptococcal sore throat. Avoid amoxicillin and ampicillin, as glandular fever may mimic this condition and these drugs will produce a rash, of varying severity, in such a patient. Epiglottitis is an emergency, and the larynx should NEVER be examined unless expert facilities for emergency intubation are to hand.

Lower respiratory tract infections Both viral and bacterial lower tract infections are debilitating and constitute a C/I to GA for elective surgery. Bear in mind TB and atypical bacteria, e.g. legionella, mycoplasma, and coxiella. Open TB is highly infectious and cross-infection precautions are mandatory (🕮 p. 718).

Chronic obstructive pulmonary disease (COPD) A very common condition usually caused by a combination of bronchitis (excessive mucus production, persistent productive cough >3 months per year for 3yrs) and emphysema (dilation and destruction of air spaces distal to the terminal bronchioles). Smoking is the prime cause and must be stopped for Rx to be of any value. Be aware of possible systemic steroid use.

Asthma Reversible bronchoconstriction causes wheezing and dyspnoea. Up to 8% of the population are affected; there is often an allergic component. Patients complain of the chest feeling tight. May be precipitated by NSAIDs. Penicillin and aspirin allergies are more common. Management of acute asthma, 🕮 p. 533.

Cystic fibrosis An inherited disorder whereby viscosity of mucus is ↑. Patients suffer pancreatic exocrine insufficiency and recurrent chest infections. Δ: by history and sweat sodium measurement.

Bronchial carcinoma Causes 27% of cancer deaths. Principal cause is smoking. ↓ incidence in females. Symptoms are persistent cough, haemoptysis, and recurrent infections. 2-yr survival is only 10%. Mesothelioma is an industrial disease caused by asbestos exposure.

Sarcoidosis Most commonly presents as hilar lymphadenopathy in young adults. Oral lesions can occur. Erythema nodosum common.

Dental implications

Avoid GA. Use analgesics and sedatives with caution; opioids and sedatives ↓ respiratory drive, NSAIDs may exacerbate asthma. Advise your patients to stop smoking (and if you are a smoker, stop). Refer if suspicious, especially in the presence of confirmed haemoptysis.

Gastrointestinal disease

The mouth and its mucosal disorders and disorders of the salivary glands are covered in Chapter 9.

Oesophagus Presents symptoms which can be confused with those originating from the mouth, the most important being *dysphagia*. Difficulty in swallowing may be caused by conditions within the mouth (e.g. ulceration), pharynx (e.g. FB), benign or malignant conditions within oesophagus, compression by surrounding structures (e.g. mediastinal lymph nodes), or neurological causes. It is a symptom which should be taken seriously and investigated by at least CXR, barium swallow, &/or endoscopy. Reflux oesophagitis is a common cause of dyspepsia, sore throat, cough, and bad taste.

Peptic ulceration and gastric carcinoma (duodenal malignancy rare) May present with epigastric pain, vomiting, haematemesis, or melaena.

Peptic ulceration Commonly due to infection with *Helicobacter pylori* and usually responds to *H. pylori* eradication therapy (combination of proton pump inhibitor/broad spectrum antibiotic/anaerobicidal, i.e. metronidazole). Other causes include stress ulceration in critically ill or major surgical patients, and elderly people on NSAIDs. Prophylaxis with sucralfate, a mucosal protectant, is more appropriate than H_2 antagonists as the gastric pH barrier is maintained but is a problem practically as it clogs fine bore NGT. Symptomatic relief of dyspepsia without significant ulceration is with antacids and alginates. Persisting epigastric pain or other symptoms *must* be investigated as gastric carcinoma requires early surgery and carries a poor prognosis. ▶ Endoscopic investigation of patients >40 with persisting epigastric symptoms is mandatory.

Non-malignant, *Helicobacter*-negative ulceration (oesophagitis, gastritis, duodenitis) clears with 1 month of proton pump inhibitor Rx (e.g. omeprazole 10–20mg od) and can often be maintained with H2 antagonists (ranitidine or cimetidine).

Small bowel This has a multitude of associated disorders which tend to present in a similar manner; namely, malabsorption syndromes, diarrhoea, steatorrhoea, abdominal pain, anaemia, and chronic deficiencies. Coeliac disease and Crohn's disease are the best known conditions. Coeliac disease is a hypersensitivity response of the small bowel to gluten and treated by strict avoidance. A number of oral complaints are related, typically 'cobblestoning' of the mucosa. Crohn's disease may affect any part of the gastrointestinal tract but has a preference for the ileo-caecal area. It is a chronic granulomatous disease affecting the full thickness of the mucosa and may result in fistula formation. Ulcerative colitis is often mistaken for Crohn's disease initially, but affects the colorectum only. Treatment with systemic steroids and other immunosuppresants is common.

Large bowel Diverticular disease is a condition with multiple outpouching of large bowel mucosa which can become inflamed, causing diverticulitis. The irritable bowel syndrome is a condition associated with ↑ colonic tone, causing recurrent abdominal pain; there may be some psychogenic overlay.

Colonic cancer is common in older patients; it may present as rectal bleeding, a change in bowel habit, intestinal obstruction, tenesmus (wanting to defecate but producing nothing), abdominal pain, or anaemia. It is treated surgically, with up to 90% 5-yr survival if diagnosed early (Duke's A). Familial polyposis coli is associated with the Gardener syndrome (📖 p. 728). Antibiotic-induced colitis results from overgrowth of toxigenic *Clostridium difficile* after use of antibiotics, commonly ampicillin and clindamycin. It responds to oral vancomycin or metronidazole.

The pancreas Malignancy has the worst prognosis of any cancer and most Rx is essentially palliative.

Acute pancreatitis Often a manifestation of alcohol abuse. Aetiology is not entirely clear. Causes acute abdominal pain. Amylase levels are a guide but not infallible. Patients need aggressive rehydration, maintenance of electrolyte balance, and analgesia, in high-dependency or ICU setting.

Hepatic disease

The main problems presented by patients with liver disease are: the potential for increased bleeding, inability to metabolize and excrete many commonly used drugs, and the possibility that they can transmit hepatitis B, C &/or D (Hep A and E are spread by faecal–oral route). The liver is also a site of metastatic spread of malignant tumours. Patients in liver failure needing surgery, especially under GA, are a high-risk group who should have specialist advice on their management.

Jaundice The prime symptom of liver disease. It is a widespread yellow discoloration of the skin (best seen in good light, in the sclera), caused by the inability of the liver to process bilirubin, the breakdown product of haemoglobin. This occurs either because it is presented with an overwhelming amount of bilirubin to conjugate (e.g. haemolytic anaemia), or it is unable to excrete bile (cholestatic jaundice). Cholestatic jaundice in turn may be either intrahepatic or extrahepatic. **Intrahepatic cholestasis** represents hepatocyte damage; this is reflected by ↑ aspartate transaminase levels on liver function tests, and results in impaired bile excretion, as indicated by ↑ plasma bilirubin. Causes include alcohol and other drugs, toxins, bacterial and viral infections. A degree of hepatitis is present with these causes, whereas primary biliary cirrhosis and anabolic steroids cause a specific intrahepatic cholestasis without hepatitis.

Extrahepatic cholestasis is caused by obstruction to the excretion of bile in the common bile duct by gallstones, tumour, clot, or stricture. Carcinoma of the head of the pancreas, or adjacent lymph nodes, may also compress the duct, and must be excluded.

Surgery in patients with liver disease
- Ascertain a Δ for the cause. Do hepatitis serology. Cross-infection precautions (🕮 p. 718).
- Do coagulation screen. May need correction with vitamin K or fresh-frozen plasma.
- **Always** warn the anaesthetist, as it will affect the choice of anaesthetic agents.
- If a jaundiced patient must undergo surgery correct fluid and electrolyte balance, and ensure a good peri-operative urine output by aggressive IV hydration with 5% dextrose and mannitol diuresis to avoid hepato-renal syndrome (see OHCM).
- Do not use IV saline in patients in fulminant hepatic failure, as there is a high risk of inducing encephalopathy.

Liver disease patients in dental practice
- Know which disease you are dealing with. If Hep B or C employ strict cross-infection control (🕮 p. 718).
- Be cautious in prescribing drugs (consult the BNF/DPF) and with administering LA.
- **Do not** administer GAs.
- Take additional local precautions against post-op bleeding following simple extractions (🕮 p. 348). A clotting screen should be obtained for anything more advanced, and in all patients with severe liver disease.

Renal disorders

The commonest urinary tract problems, infections, are of relevance only to those who manage in-patients. Rarer conditions such as renal failure and transplantation are, surprisingly, of more general relevance because these patients are at ↑ risk from infection, bleeding, and iatrogenic drug overdose during routine Rx.

Urine This is tested in all in-patients. 'Multistix' will test for glycosuria (diabetes, pregnancy, infection), proteinuria (diabetes, infection, nephrotic syndrome), ketones (diabetic ketoacidosis), haematuria (infection, tumour), and bile as bilirubin and urobilinogen (cholestatic jaundice).

Urinary tract infections A common cause of toxic confusion in elderly in-patients, especially females. Send a mid-stream urine (MSU) for culture and sensitivity, then start trimethoprim 200mg bd PO or ampicillin 250mg qds PO and ensure a high fluid intake. Minimal investigations of renal function are U&Es, creatinine, and ionized Ca^{2+}.

Nephrotic syndrome A syndrome of proteinuria (>3.6g/day), hypoalbuminaemia, and generalized oedema. Facial oedema is often prominent. Glomerulonephritis is the major precipitating cause and investigations should be carried out by a physician with an interest in renal medicine.

Acute renal failure (ARF) A medical emergency causing a rapid rise in serum creatinine, urea and K^+. It may follow surgery or major trauma and is usually marked by a failure to PU. *Remember* the commonest causes of failing to PU post-op are under-infusion of fluids and urinary retention. Rx: ↑ IV fluid input and catheterize (📖 p. 543). If ARF is suspected get urgent U&Es, ECG, and blood gases. Obtain aid from a physician. Control of hyperkalaemia, fluid balance, acidosis, and hypertension are the immediate necessities.

Chronic renal failure Basically the onset of uraemia after gradual, but progressive renal damage, commonly caused by glomerulonephritis (inflammation of the glomeruli following immune complex deposits), pyelonephritis (small scarred kidneys due to childhood infection, irradiation, or poisoning), or adult polycystic disease (congenital cysts within Bowman's capsule). It has protean manifestations, starting with nocturia and anorexia, progressing through hypertension and anaemia to multisystem failure. Continuous ambulatory peritoneal dialysis, haemodialysis, and transplants are the mainstays of Rx.

Main problems relevant to dentistry
- ↑ risk of infection, worsened by immunosuppression.
- ↑ bleeding tendency.
- ↓ ability to excrete drugs.
- Veins are sacrosanct; **never** use their A-V fistula.
- Bone lesions of the jaws (renal osteodystophy, 2° hyperparathyroidism).
- Generalized growth impairment in children.
- Potential carriage of Hep B, HIV.

Renal transplantation An increasingly common final Rx of renal failure, and when successful renal function may reach near normal levels. Kidneys are, however, immunosuppressed and at greatly ↑ risk from infection. They may share the problems associated with chronic renal failure depending on the level of function of the transplant.

Hints

- Take precautions against cross-infection (📖 p. 718).
- Treat all infections aggressively and consider prophylaxis.
- Use additional haemostatic measures (📖 p. 348).
- Be cautious with prescribing drugs (📖 p. 558).
- Never subject these patients to out-patient GA.
- Remember veins are precious.
- Try to perform Rx just after dialysis if possible.

Endocrine disease

Addison's disease 1° hypoadrenocorticism. Atrophy of the adrenal cortices causes failure of cortisol and aldosterone secretion. 2° hypoadrenocorticism is far commoner, due to steroid therapy or ACTH deficiency (🕮 p. 552). All need steroid cover.

Conn's syndrome Primary hyperaldosteronism causes hypokalaemia and hypernatraemia with hypertension.

Cushing's disease and Cushing syndrome These are due to excess corticosteroid production. The disease refers to 2° adrenal hyperplasia due to ↑ ACTH, whereas the syndrome is a 1° condition, usually due to therapeutic administration of synthetic steroid or adenoma. Classical features are obesity (moon face, buffalo hump) sparing the limbs, osteoporosis, skin thinning, and hypertension.

Diabetes insipidus Production of copious dilute urine due to ↓ ADH secretion or renal insensitivity to ADH. May occur temporarily after head injury.

Diabetes mellitus Persistent hyperglycaemia due to a relative deficiency of insulin (🕮 p. 550).

Gigantism/acromegaly Excess production of growth hormone, before and after fusion of the epiphyses, respectively.

Goitre A large thyroid gland, of whatever cause.

Hyperthyroidism Symptoms of heat intolerance, weight loss, and sweating occur. Signs are tachycardia (may have atrial fibrillation), lid lag, exopthalmos, and tremor. Commonest cause is Graves' disease (🕮 p. 728). Functioning adenomas are another cause.

Hypothyroidism Can be 1° due to thyroid disease, or 2° to hypothalamic or pituitary dysfunction. 1° disease is often an autoimmune condition. Symptoms are poor tolerance of cold, loss of hair, weight gain, loss of appetite, and poor memory. Signs are bradycardia and a hoarse voice.

Hyperparathyroidism 1° is caused by an adenoma. 2° is a response to low plasma Ca^{2+}, e.g. in renal failure, and 3° follows on from 2° when the parathyroids continue ↑ production, even if Ca^{2+} is normalized.

Hypoparathyroidism Usually 2° to thyroidectomy, when parathyroid glands inadvertently removed. Plasma Ca^{2+} ↓, resulting in tetany. Chvosteck's sign is +ve if spasm of facial muscles occurs after tapping over the facial nerve.

Hypopituitarism Can lead to 2° hypothyroidism or 2° hypoadrenocorticism.

Inappropriate ADH secretion Caused by certain tumours (e.g. bronchial carcinoma), head injury, and some drugs. Hyponatraemia, overhydration, and confusion occur.

Lingual thyroid May be the only functioning thyroid the patient has; do not excise lightly. Do pre-op isotope scan.

Phaeochromocytoma A very rare tumour of the adrenal medulla, secreting adrenaline and noradrenaline. Symptoms are recurring palpitations and headache with sweating. Simultaneous hypertension with a return to baseline on settling of symptoms, is a good marker.

Pituitary tumours May erode the pituitary fossa (seen on lateral skull X-ray) and can cause blindness via optic chiasma compression.

Endocrine-related problems

▶ Always ask yourself 'Is she, or can she be, pregnant?'

Pregnancy is a C/I to elective GA, the vast majority of drugs (📖 p. 558), and non-essential radiography (the most vulnerable period being in the first 3 months). Elective Rx is best performed in the mid-trimester.

Menopause The end of a woman's reproductive life and her periods. It is often associated with hot flushes and other relatively minor physical problems. Emotional disturbances may coexist, and the incidence of psychiatric disorders increases at this time.

Related problems

Suxamethonium sensitivity Around 1:3000 people have an inherited defect of plasma cholinesterase. These families are absolutely normal in every respect except in their ability to metabolize suxamethonium. This leaves them unable to destroy the drug which, normally wearing off in 2–4min, produces prolonged muscle paralysis. This paralysis requires ventilatory support until the drug wears off, which, in the homozygote, may take as long as 24h.

Malignant hyperpyrexia A rare, potentially lethal reaction to, usually, an anaesthetic agent. Characterized by ↑ pulse, muscle rigidity, and ↑ temperature. Dantrolene sodium and cooling may be life-saving.

Rare endocrine tumours

Glucagonoma Secretes glucagon causing hyperglycaemia.

Insulinomas Secrete insulin. Causes sporadic hypoglycaemic episodes.

Gastrinomas Secrete gastrin causing duodenal ulcers and diarrhoea (Zollinger–Ellison syndrome).

Multiple endocrine neoplasia (MEN) syndromes A rare group of endocrine tumours. MEN IIb is medullary thyroid cancer, phaeochromocytoma, and oral mucosal neuromas.

Bone disease

Pathology of the bones of the facial skeleton is covered in Chapter 8.

Osteogenesis imperfecta (brittle bone disease) An autosomal dominant type 1 collagen defect. Multiple # following slight trauma with rapid but distorted healing is characteristic. Associated with blue sclera, deafness, and dentinogenesis imperfecta (🕮 p. 67). The jaws are *not* particularly prone to # following extractions.

Osteopetrosis (marble bone disease) There is an ↑ in bone density and brittleness, and a ↓ in blood supply. Prone to infection which is difficult to eradicate. Bone pain, #, and compression neuropathies may occur. Anaemia can complicate severe disease. Facial characteristics are frontal bossing and hypertelorism.

Achondroplasia An inherited defect in cartilaginous bone formation, usually autosomal dominant. Causes a 'circus dwarf' appearance with skull bossing; many have no other problems.

Cleidocranial dysostosis An inherited defect of membranous bone formation, usually autosomal dominant. Skull and clavicles are affected. Multiple unerupted teeth with retention of 1° dentition is characteristic.

Disorders of bone metabolism

Rickets/osteomalacia Failure of bone mineralization in, respectively, children and adults. Can be caused by deficiency, failure of synthesis, malabsorption, or impaired metabolism of Vitamin D, and also hypophosphataemia or ↑ Ca^{2+} requirement in pregnancy.

Osteoporosis A lack of both bone matrix and mineralization. Important causes are steroid therapy, post-menopausal hormone changes, immobilization, and endocrine abnormalities. HRT in post-menopausal women appears helpful. Results in ↑ incidence of #, especially femoral neck and wrist. Bisphosphonates are being aggressively promoted in the treatment of osteoporosis resulting in some of the noted increase in BRON 🕮 p. 352.

Fibrous dysplasia Replacement of a part of a bone or bones by fibrous tissue with associated swelling. It usually starts in childhood and ceases with completion of skeletal growth. Termed monostotic if one bone is affected, polyostotic if more than one bone, and Albright syndrome if associated with precocious puberty and *café au lait* areas of skin hyperpigmentation.

Cherubism A bilateral variant of fibrous dysplasia.

Paget's disease of bone A common disorder of the elderly, where the normal, orderly replacement of bone is disrupted and replaced by a chaotic structure of new bone, causing enlargement and deformity. The hands and feet are spared. Complications include bone pain and cranial nerve compression, or, more rarely, high output cardiac failure or osteosarcoma. Another condition treated with bisphosphonates.

Diseases of connective tissue, muscle, and joints

Connective tissue diseases

These are mainly vasculitides (inflammation of vessels).

Cranial arteritis (temporal arteritis) Giant cell vasculitis of the craniofacial region. Presenting symptom is unilateral throbbing headache. Signs are high ESR with a tender, pulseless artery. Major complication of temporal arteritis is optic nerve ischaemia causing blindness, so start high-dose steroids (60mg prednisolone PO od) and monitor using ESR. Biopsy confirms.

Polymyalgia rheumatica More generalized vasculitis affecting proximal axial muscles. Accounts for 25% of cases of cranial arteritis. Responds to steroids; gradual improvement with time.

Disease of muscles

Muscular dystrophy A collection of inherited diseases characterized by muscle degeneration. Most are fatal in early adulthood.

Myotonic disorders Distinguished by delayed muscle relaxation after contraction. They are genetically determined in a complex fashion.

Polymyositis A generalized immune-mediated inflammatory disorder of muscle. If a characteristic rash is present the condition is known as **dermatomyositis** and has an association with occult malignancy.

Joint disease

Osteoarthritis 1° degeneration of articular cartilage, cervical and lumbar spine, hip and knee joints, commonly affected or 2° to trauma or other joint disease, resulting in pain and stiffness. Osteophyte formation and subchondral bone cysts, which collapse leading to deformity, are characteristic. Physiotherapy, weight loss, and analgesia are the mainstays of Rx. Joint replacement is definitive Rx.

Rheumatoid arthritis Immunologically mediated disease where joint pain and damage are the most prominent symptoms. Morning pain and stiffness in the hands and feet, usually symmetrical, is characteristic. There may be systemic upset and anaemia. Ulnar deviation of the fingers is pathognomonic. Rx includes NSAIDs, steroids, and physiotherapy. Second line or disease-modifying antirheumatic drugs (DMARDs) may favourably influence outcome at expense of unwanted effects, e.g. penicillamine, antimalarials, immunosuppressants (including TNFα chimeric monoclonal antibody—Infliximab). Dry eyes and mouth may be associated with rheumatoid arthritis (Sjögren syndrome, 🕮 p. 422). TMJ symptoms are rare in rheumatoid arthritis, although up to 15% of patients have radiographic changes in the joint.

Juvenile rheumatoid arthritis (Still's disease) Rarer form of the disease affecting children. It can be much more severe than the adult condition and can cause TMJ ankylosis.

Psoriatic arthritis Associated with the skin condition and affects the spine and pelvis. It is milder than rheumatoid arthritis and has no serological abnormalities. The TMJ can be affected, but symptoms are usually mild despite some isolated case reports to the contrary.

Gout Urates are deposited in joints, causing sudden severe joint pain, often in the great toe. Affected joints are red, swollen, and very tender. Gout 2° to drugs, radiotherapy, or haematological disease is commoner than that caused by an inborne error of metabolism.

Ankylosing spondylitis Affects the spine, usually in young men. Inflammation involves the insertion of ligaments and tendons. It is associated with HLA-B27. Later, kyphotic deformity and increased risk of cervical fractures.

Reiter syndrome Seronegative arthritis, urethritis, and conjunctivitis, usually in response to an infection. Oral lesions are often present. Genital and intestinal variants.

Perthes' disease Osteochondritis of the femoral head in, mainly, boys aged 3–11yrs. No systemic implications.

Neurological disorders

Cranial nerves

- **I Olfactory** Sense of smell is rarely tested, although damage is quite common following head &/or mid-face trauma.
- **II Optic** Examine the pupils for both direct and consensual reflex; assess the visual fields; check visual acuity and examine the fundus with an opthalmoscope (🕮 p. 9).
- **III Oculomotor** The motor supply to the extra-ocular muscles *except* lateral rectus and superior oblique. It supplies the ciliary muscle, the constrictor of the pupil, and levator palpebrae superioris. A defect therefore causes impairment of upward, downward, and inward movement of the eye, leading to diplopia, drooping of the upper eyelid (ptosis), and absent direct and consensual reflexes.
- **IV Trochlear** Supplies superior oblique, paralysis of which causes diplopia; worst on looking downward and inward.
- **V Trigeminal** The major sensory nerve to the face, oral, nasal, conjunctival, and sinus mucosa, and part of the tympanic membrane. It is motor to the muscles of mastication. Sensory abnormalities are mapped out using gentle touch and pin-prick. Motor weakness is best assessed on jaw opening and excursion.
- **VI Abducens** Supplies lateral rectus. A defect causes paralysis of abduction of the eye.
- **VII Facial** Motor to the muscles of facial expression. Supplies taste from the anterior ⅔ of tongue (via chorda tympani) and is secretomotor to the lacrimal, sublingual, and submandibular glands. It innervates the stapedius muscle in the middle ear. The lower face is innervated by the contralateral motor cortex, whereas the upper face has bilateral innervation. Assess by demonstrating facial movements.
- **XIII Vestibulocochlear** Is sensory for balance and hearing. Deafness, vertigo, and tinnitus are the main symptoms.
- **IX Glossopharyngeal** Supplies sensation and taste from the posterior ⅓ of the tongue, motor to stylopharyngeus, and secretomotor to the parotid. Lesions impair the gag reflex in conjunction with X
- **X Vagus** Has a motor input to the palatal, pharyngeal, and laryngeal muscles. Impaired gag reflex, hoarseness, and deviation of the soft palate to the unaffected side are seen if damaged. The vagus has a huge parasympathetic output to the viscera of the thorax and abdomen.
- **XI Accessory** Is motor to sternomastoid and trapezius, causing weakness on shoulder shrugging and on turning the head away from the affected side.
- **XII Hypoglossal** Motor supply to the tongue. Lesions cause dysarthria (impaired speech) and deviation towards the affected side on protrusion.

Headache

The vast majority of headaches are benign; the secret is to pick out those which are not. Read on.

Tension headache Commonest type. Due to muscle tension in occipito-frontalis. Usually worse as the day progresses; may feel 'band-like'. Responds to reassurance, anxiolytics, and analgesics.

Migraine A distinct entity characterized by a preceding visual aura (fortification spectra). Severe, usually unilateral headache with photophobia, nausea, and vomiting. Thought to be due to cerebral vasoconstriction, followed by reflex vasodilation (the latter is the cause of the pain). 5HT agonists, e.g. rizatriptan (C/I: ischaemic heart disease, cerebrovascular disease) abolish an attack if used early, and pizotifen is used prophylactically. F>M, the oral contraceptive being a contributing factor. There are many variants of classical migraine.

Migrainous neuralgia Rarer than migraine and causes localized pain, usually around the eye, with associated nasal stuffiness. M > F. There is a typical time of onset, often in early morning, which recurs for several weeks: 'clustering'. Alcohol is a common precipitant. 5HT agonists to treat and 5HT antagonists (e.g. pizotifen) for prophylaxis.

Raised intracranial pressure A cause of headache demanding urgent further investigation. Pointers are headache, worse on waking, irritation, ↓ level of consciousness, vomiting, sluggish or absent pupillary reflexes, bulging of the optic disc (papilloedema). **Rising BP and slowing pulse** are late premorbid signs of ↑ ICP.

Medication misuse headache Affects up to 1:50. Presents as daily headache due to excessive or regular use of OTC analgesics (especially codeine-containing) and some antimigraine preparations. Pain pathways may be altered and after withdrawal of the drug the headache may be slow to resolve.

Rare and wonderful headaches Ice-cream headache, post-coital headache, needle-through-eye headache, and many other distinctive and benign headaches are described.

More neurological disorders

CNS Infections

Bacterial meningitis Must be considered in the differential Δ of headache with photophobia and neck stiffness. Organisms are *Haemophilus influenzae*, *Neisseria meningitidis* (meningococcus), *N. gonorrhoeae*, and *Streptococcus pneumoniae*. In children, the meningococcus is especially important and classically associated with a non-blanching purpuric rash. This is one of the very few indications for instituting immediate blind antibiotic therapy (parenteral penicillin).

Viral meningitis Usually mild and self-limiting. Distinguished from bacterial meningitis by lumbar puncture.

Herpetic encephalitis A rare manifestation of infection with the herpes simplex virus. Can be distinguished from drunkenness or dementia by history and rapid onset. Parenteral aciclovir can be curative.

CNS tumours Most brain tumours are 2° deposits. Although both benign and malignant primary tumours are found, they are rare. Despite this, they are the commonest cause of cancer death in children after leukaemia.

Epilepsy An episodic outflow from the brain causing disturbances of consciousness, motor, and sensory function. Most causes are idiopathic but those with onset in adult life must be investigated for local or general cerebral disease. Major or *grand mal* epilepsy is characterized by an aura and loss of consciousness, and followed by tonic and clonic phases. Incontinence is a good guide to a genuine seizure. The fit rarely lasts >5min, if it does the patient has entered status epilepticus (🔲 p. 531).

Petit mal (absence attacks) Are epileptic attacks usually confined to children, taking the form of a short absence when movement, speech, and attention cease.

Temporal lobe epilepsy Characterized by hallucinations of the special senses.

Localized (Jacksonian) epilepsy Affects limbs in isolation. Patients with established epilepsy (once any treatable cause has been excluded) must be maintained on adequate levels of antiepileptic drugs.

Febrile convulsions Fits, usually in children >5yrs old, 2° to pyrexia.

Cerebrovascular accidents (strokes) A very common cause of death in the elderly. A stroke is basically death of part of the brain following cerebral ischaemia, either due to bleeding into the brain or occlusion of vessels. It is often clinically difficult to distinguish these different types of stroke. CT scanning is of value when Rx is to be attempted to decide if infarct or haemorrhage, but wait 24h after symptoms to allow infarct to become visible on scan. Cerebral angiography defines the source of subarachnoid bleeds.

Multiple (disseminated) sclerosis A disorder characterized by demyelination in multiple 'plaques' throughout the CNS. Symptoms are multiple and disseminated in both time and place. It is the commonest neurological disease of young adults. MRI helps in Δ but is not specific. No current cure; hyperbaric therapy and interferon remain controversial. Progress, although relentless, is widely variable.

Myasthenia gravis Muscle weakness due to inadequate response to, or levels of, acetylcholine. Extra-occular muscles are often first affected. Diagnosed using the 'tensilon' test.

Parkinson's disease A disease affecting the basal ganglia associated with a ↓ in the local levels of dopamine. Characterized by a 'pill-rolling' tremor, 'cog-wheel' rigidity, and bradykinesis with a shuffling gait.

Skin neoplasms

▶ The skin of the face is the commonest site of curable skin cancers, so look and think (📖 p. 479).

Basal Cell Carcinoma (epithelioma, rodent ulcer) An indolent skin cancer which very rarely metastasizes. If it kills it usually does so by local destruction. Chronic exposure to sunlight is a major aetiological factor. There are various forms, the commonest being an ulcerated nodule with raised pearly margins and a telangiectatic surface. Rx: excision (micrographic or conventional), radiotherapy (especially electron beam), cryotherapy, curettage, topical immune modulation, photodynamic therapy and electrodessication.

Squamous Cell Carcinoma of the skin is surprisingly indolent in comparison to SCC of mucosa but beware the external ear which can be aggressive in 40%. Presents as an ulcerated lesion with raised edges. Keratin horns may be present, and it may arise in areas of previously sun-damaged skin or in gravitational leg ulcers. Surgical excision or radiotherapy are Rx of choice.

Malignant melanoma This condition is being increasingly diagnosed, with a doubling of the incidence in the last 20yrs. The prognosis is dependent primarily on the depth of the tumour (Breslow thickness), as the thicker the lesion the poorer the prognosis. Early metastasis is common. Sunlight is a major aetiological factor, possibly due to burning at early age. Suspect if a pigmented lesion rapidly enlarges, bleeds, ulcerates, shows 'satellite' lesions or changes colour. Prompt referral for specialist management is needed. Lots of 'sun aware' campaigns emphasize prevention.

Naevi Areas of skin containing a disproportionate number of melanocytes.

Lentigo simplex A freckle.

Dysplastic naevi Premalignant lesions often found in patients with malignant melanoma. They should be excised and patients advised to use high-factor sunscreens.

Lentigo maligna A premalignant pigmented lesion of the elderly.

Carcinoma-in-situ (Bowen's disease) Presents as a scaly, red plaque. It is basically a squamous carcinoma which has not yet penetrated beyond the basal layer.

Actinic keratosis Persistently sun-damaged areas of skin in which cancer may arise.

Kaposi's sarcoma A purple, vascular, multifocal malignant tumour typically seen in AIDS and other immunocompromised patients. Also seen intraorally.

Metastatic deposits to the skin occur most frequently from breast, kidney, and lung, but skin secondaries from oral cancer are being seen increasingly.

Dermatology

Psoriasis A common, relapsing proliferative inflammatory skin disease. Appears as a red plaque with silvery scale, chiefly on extensor skin of knees and elbows, although any area can be affected. Can be associated with systemic disease, particularly arthropathy (📖 p. 506). Rx is mainly topical: steroids, coal tar, dithranol &/or UVB radiation, or psoralen-sensitized UVA radiation (PUVA). Rarely, methotrexate can be used.

Eczema Also called dermatitis. Has several variants according to aetiology.

Atopic eczema Starts in the 1st year of life with a red symmetrical scaly rash. Emulsifying ointments help prevent fissuring, although steroids are sometimes needed. Up to 90% grow out of it by age 12.

Exogenous eczema Can be produced in anyone exposed to a sufficient irritant. The hands are the usual target, with blistering, erythema, and cracking of skin.

Allergic contact eczema A genuine allergic response, e.g. to nickel.

Seborrhoeic eczema A fungal infection mainly affecting the scalp ('cradle cap') in neonates.

Skin infections Fungal infections are particularly common, causing angular cheilitis, athlete's foot, paronychia, vaginitis, etc. Furuncles are staphylococcal boils. Erysipelas is a streptococcal cellulitis. Viruses cause herpes zoster and simplex infections, molluscum contagiosum, and warts.

Infestations of the skin bring a shudder to most people, but they are also a hazard of working closely with patients! Head lice respond to malathion. Flea bites, as well as being unpleasant, can spread plague, among other serious diseases. Scabies is an infestation with a mite which creates a characteristic itchy burrow in the finger webs.

Acne Acne vulgaris is characterized by the blackhead (comedone), and is an inflammatory condition caused by increased sebum secretion. Hormone-dependent, although superinfection with the acne bacillus is a contributing factor. Tends to scar. After proprietary lotions, low-dose tetracyclines help. Dianette, a combined oral contraceptive, is a useful alternative in women. The teratogenic retinoid, isotretinoin, is particularly useful in severe and late onset acne unresponsive to other Rx.

The skin and internal disease

The skin, like the mouth, acts as an outside indicator for many internal diseases.

Erythema nodosum Painful, red, nodular lumps on the shins.

Erythema multiforme Circular target lesions.

Erythema marginatum Vanishing and recurring pink rings. These are all non-specific markers for a variety of diseases.

Vitiligo An autoimmune hypopigmentation, associated with other autoimmune conditions.

Pyoderma gangrenosum Blue-edged ulcers, especially on the legs; associated with ulcerative colitis and Crohn's disease.

Granuloma annulare Subcutaneous circular thickening and **necrobiosis lipoidica** (yellow plaques on the shins) are associated with diabetes.

Dermatitis herpetiformis Vesicular rash of knees, elbows, and scalp. Associated with coeliac disease.

Pretibial myxoedema Red swellings above the ankle. Associated with hyperthyroidism.

Skin diseases associated with malignancy are **acanthosis nigricans** (rough, pigmented, thickened areas of skin in axilla or groin) and **thrombophlebitis migrans** (tender nodules within blood vessels which move from site to site).

Psychiatry

One way of getting to grips with a new subject—and to virtually all dentists psychiatry as opposed to psychology is new—is to categorize. The major adult psychiatric diagnoses are listed in order of severity. This is known as the 'hierarchy of diagnosis'.

Organic brain syndromes

Acute organic reaction (delirium, toxic confusion) Clouding of consciousness and disorientation in time and place are major symptoms. Moodswings are common, and visual hallucinations, rare in other psychiatric conditions, can be present.

▶ There is an underlying, frequently treatable cause to this condition (infection, hypoxia, drugs, dehydration, alcohol withdrawal, etc.). Rx: find the cause and correct it, using sedation until the cause is identified and Rx has taken effect.

Chronic organic reaction (dementia) A global intellectual deterioration highlighted by a worsening short-term memory. *Never* label someone as demented until all other possible causes, including depression, have been excluded by a psychiatrist. Alzheimer's disease and multi-infarct dementia are the commonest causes. There is no cure, although effective support services and psychosocial interventions can improve the quality of life considerably. Anticholinesterase inhibitors, e.g. donepezil, and memantine may slow the rate of cognitive decline.

Mental disabilities, 📖 p. 46.

Psychosis

Contact with reality is lost and normal mental processes do not function. There is loss of insight. If an organic condition is excluded, the Δ is one of three.

Schizophrenia A disorder where the victims live in an incomprehensible world full of vivid personal significance. First-rank symptoms are a good guide to Δ: delusions, thought insertion, broadcasting and withdrawal, passivity feelings, visual and auditory hallucinations.

Affective disorders Mania, hypomania, manic-depressive psychosis, and depression. Mania and hypomania are characterized by euphoria, hyperactivity, overvalued ideas or grandiose delusions, and pressure of speech. They differ only in degree. Cyclical mania and depression is known as bipolar affective disorder. Rx is with major tranquillizers and prophylaxis with lithium carbonate.

Depression May be either psychotic or neurotic. Markers of major depressive illness are anhedonia (failure to find pleasure in things which once did please), anorexia, especially with weight loss, early morning wakening, tearfulness, inability to concentrate, feelings of guilt and worthlessness, and suicidal ideation.

Paranoid states are psychoses where paranoid symptoms predominate and, despite lack of insight, other diagnoses do not apply.

▶ The commonly abused drugs can all mimic or precipitate psychotic states, as can giving birth—puerperal psychosis.

Neuroses

A neurosis is a maladaptive psychological symptom in the absence of organic or psychotic causes of the symptom and after exclusion of a psychopathic personality. Insight is present.

Anxiety neurosis frequently coexists with depression. These patients often have physical symptoms for which there is no physical explanation.

Obsessional neurosis Intrusive thoughts or ideas which the subject recognizes as coming from within themselves, but resents and is unable to stop. May be associated with *compulsive behaviour* where repeated purposeless activity is carried out due to an inexplicable feeling that it must be done.

Phobia is the generation of fear or anxiety out of proportion to the stimulus. Numerous stimuli exist, including dentists.

Anorexia nervosa/bulimia nervosa

The development of weight reduction as an overvalued idea. Associated with weight ↓ of >25% of ideal body weight and obsessive food avoidance. Commonest in females, it is also associated with amenorrhea. Has a significant mortality rate; binge-eating followed by vomiting &/or laxative abuse can occur. Bingeing without weight loss is bulimia nervosa. Dental effects, 🕮 p. 268.

Personality disorders

These are not illnesses but extremes of normal personality traits, e.g. obsessional, histrionic, schizoid (cold, introspective). The most important is the psychopathic (sociopathic) individual who has no concept of affection, shame, or guilt, and is characterized by antisocial behaviour. They are often superficially personable, highly manipulative, and totally irresponsible. They have insight and are responsible for their own actions (bad not mad).

The immunocompromised patient

These are a group of individuals who present special problems because of defects in, or suppression of, their immune system. The condition with the highest profile among these is AIDS.

The chief effect of being immunocompromised is an ↑ susceptibility to infection, often due to opportunistic organisms. Anything which changes the host environment in favour of opportunistic pathogens (e.g. surgery, broad-spectrum antibiotics) can lead to potentially fatal infection with rare or otherwise innocuous organisms.

Drugs which suppress the immune response: corticosteroids, ciclosporin A, azathioprine, cytotoxics, etc., are now in common use therapeutically. Cross-infection, 📖 p. 718. Aggressive Rx of infections and antimicrobial prophylaxis are needed, 📖 p. 548.

Congenital immunodeficiency states There are at least 18 of these. The commonest is selective IgA deficiency, which affects ~1:600; it has a wide spectrum of severity but may remain asymptomatic.

Acquired immunodeficiency

Autoimmune disease, e.g. SLE, rheumatoid arthritis, carry a minor ↑ risk of infection.

Chronic renal failure (📖 p. 500) Moderately ↑ risk.

Deficiency states, e.g. anaemia. Carry a minor ↑ risk.

Diabetes mellitus is common and carries a moderate ↑ risk of infection.

Infections Severe viral infections, TB, AIDS (specific defect).

Neoplasia All haematological malignancies severely ↑ risk of infection.

AIDS

An increasingly common disease caused by the HIV (HIV-1, HIV-2). CD4 T-lymphocyte defect ensues with failure of (mostly) cell-mediated immunity. Although HIV exposure produces antibody response, the virus remains infective in the presence of antibody; it must therefore be regarded as a marker of infectivity. Absence of HIV antibody *does not*, however, guarantee that that person is not infected with HIV. HIV antibody +ve patients are at risk of developing AIDS, usually after a prolonged latent period during which CD4 cells ↓ in number. AIDS-related complex, which includes cervical lymphadenopathy, oropharyngeal candidiasis, and 'hairy leukoplakia', is precursor to full-blown AIDS. Infections characteristic of AIDS are *Pneumocystis carinii* pneumonia and disseminated mycobacterial infection. Kaposi's sarcoma is the tumour most often associated with the condition. The mode of transmission, for those visiting from another planet, is essentially, exchange of bodily fluids: unprotected sex, as a recipient of contaminated blood or blood products, or mother to fetus transmission. The main risk groups, in the developed world, are therefore male homosexuals, (transmission through the heterosexual population is variable depending on the part of the world), IV drug abusers. Transfusion recipients and haemophiliacs, who were at risk prior to screening of blood products, now have a minimal risk.

In the developing world, heterosexual spread is common and mother to fetus transmission is creating a huge ↑ in HIV +ve children. Antenatal testing for HIV is crucial as is avoiding breast-feeding. Highly Active AntiRetroviral Therapy (HAART) therapy and delivery by Caesarean section dramatically ↓ vertical transmission.[1] While there is no cure or vaccination, numerous symptom-reducing and life-prolonging Rx are available, with some promising results. HAART can prolong survival and delay disease progression.[2] Psychological and social support are the most helpful options after preventive advice. Prophylaxis consists of screening blood products, and avoidance of unprotected sexual activities and shared needles. Oral manifestations of AIDS, 📖 p. 400. Practical procedures for control of cross-infection, 📖 p. 718.

Prophylaxis after needlestick injury depends on estimation of the likely HIV exposure risk. Triple therapy guidelines in the USA. Local implementation via Genito-urinary consultant in UK.

1 Editor *BMJ* 1998 316.
2 *BNF* 2008 53 323-324.

Useful emergency kit

Every practice should possess apparatus for delivering O_2, or at least air. In addition, the facility to deliver nitrous oxide and O_2 mixture, e.g. via an anaesthetic or relative analgesia machine, can be invaluable.

The following should be readily available:
- Oral airway, preferably with a bag system, e.g. ambu-bag.
- High-vacuum suction.
- Disposable syringes (2, 5, and 10ml), needles (19 and 21G), and a tourniquet. Butterfly needles and IV canulae are great assets to those familiar with their use.
- Alcohol wipes.

Drugs
- Adrenaline, 1:1000 solution (1mg adrenalin in 1ml saline). EpiPee® (0.3mg) often held by high risk patients. Salbutalmol 0.5mg/ml injection.
- Hydrocortisone (as sodium succinate or sodium phosphate) (100mg and water for injection).
- Midazolam (5mg/ml 2ml ampoules).
- Glucose, as dextrose 20% or 50% solution and an oral glucose solution.
- Chlorphenamine 10mg injection.
- Flumazenil 100 µg/ml 5ml ampoule.
- Glucagon 1mg injection.

The above really is a **minimum** for any professional performing invasive Rx. Ideally, all public areas, let alone dental practices, should have access to an automatic defibrillator as this is the most valuable single piece of equipment in a cardiac arrest (📖 p. 524). Additional useful equipment include Clinistix/'BM' sticks, glyceryl trinitrate spray, salbutamol inhaler, one-way valve face mask, glucagon 1mg **IM** injection, atropine 3mg single-shot injection, IV fluids (crystalloid is cheaper and can be warmed). In hospital, check your 'crash cart' and be amazed at its contents.

▶ If you buy something learn how to use it!

Fainting

Fainting (vaso-vagal syncope) is innocuous providing it is recognized. It is easily the most common cause of sudden loss of consciousness, with up to 2% of patients fainting before or during dental Rx. The possibility of vaso-vagal syncope while under GA, and hence failure to recognize the condition and correct cerebral hypoxia, is the major reason for recommending the supine position.

Predisposing factors are pain, anxiety, fatigue, relative hyperthermia, and fasting. Characteristic signs and symptoms are: a feeling of dizziness and nausea; pale, cold, and clammy skin; a slow, thin, thready pulse which rebounds to become rapid, and loss of consciousness with collapse, if unsupported.

A faint may mimic far more serious conditions, most of which can be excluded by a familiarity with the patient's PMH. These include strokes, corticosteroid insufficiency, drug reactions and interactions, epileptic fit, heart block, hypoglycaemia, and MI.

Prevention
- Avoid predisposing factors.
- Treat patients in the supine position unless specifically contraindicated (e.g. heart failure, pulmonary oedema).

Management
- Lower the head to the level of, or below, the heart. Best achieved by laying the patient flat with legs slightly elevated.
- Loosen clothing (in the presence of a witness!).
- Monitor pulse. If recovery does not occur rapidly, then reconsider the Δ.
- Determine the precipitant and avoid in the future.
- If bradycardia persists with no evidence of recovery to rapid full pulse, try tiny dose of atropine (100µg IV). Dose may be repeated up to 600µg.

Acute chest pain

Severe, acute chest pain is usually the result of ischaemia of the myocardium. The principal differential Δ is between angina and MI. Both exhibit severe retrosternal pain described as heavy, crushing, or band-like. It is classically preceded by effort, emotion, or excitement, and may radiate to the arms, neck, jaw, and, occasionally, the back or abdomen. Angina is usually rapidly relieved by rest and glyceryl trinitrate (0.5mg) given sublingually, or GTN spray (400µg per spray), which most patients with a history of angina carry with them.

Failure of these methods to relieve the pain, and coexisting sweating, breathlessness, nausea, vomiting, or loss of consciousness with a weak or irregular pulse, suggest an infarct.

Management depends on your immediate environment, but always ensure the patient is placed in a supported *upright* position if conscious, as the supine position increases pulmonary oedema and hence breathlessness.

Management

In dental practice Summon help (ambulance). Administer analgesia; the most appropriate form available here will be nitrous oxide/O_2 mixture (50% O_2). Don't panic. Be prepared should cardiac arrest supervene. Give aspirin 150–300mg PO. Tell ambulance staff what you have done.

In hospital Nurse upright. Give O_2. Establish IV access and give an opioid analgesic if available (2.5–5mg of diamorphine is most useful). Get ECG, U&Es. Summon help; in units integrated into general or teaching hospitals this may best be achieved by contacting the medical on-call team via the switchboard urgently, as thrombolysis, if appropriate improves outcome.

Cardiorespiratory arrest

▶ Don't await 'expertise'. **ACT**.

Ninety percent of deaths from cardiac arrest occurring outside hospital are due to ventricular fibrillation (VF). This is also the commonest arrest pattern seen in hospital. It is potentially reversible by prompt (<90sec) defibrillation. The commonest underlying cause is ischaemic heart disease, but other causes may exist, especially in younger people. Acute asthma, anaesthesia, drug overdose, electrocution, immersion, or hypothermia often precipitate pulseless electrical activity (PEA) arrests. These are treatable conditions and potentially reversible.

In certain instances properly performed cardiopulmonary resuscitation (CPR) can sustain life for up to an hour while a precipitating condition is being treated.

Diagnosis and management These proceed simultaneously (see Figure. 11.1).

Approach and assess Protect yourself! Do not become another casualty, whether in the street, practice, or hospital environment. Gently 'shake and shout' to assess the person's level of consciousness. If there is no response, shout for help (and ask whoever goes for help to come back to tell you if help is coming). **Then:**

- In *witnessed* or monitored arrests a single sharp blow over the heart (precordial thump) is worthwhile.
- **Airway** Carry out a chin lift or jaw thrust, and clear oropharynx. Remove loose dentures, but retain if they are well fitting (it gives a better mouth seal).
- **Breathing** Look, listen, and feel for breathing for up to 10sec (if hypothermia suspected, up to 1min). If the person is breathing, place in recovery position. If not, get help even if this means leaving the patient yourself to do it. Move to:
- **Circulation** Feel for a carotid pulse. If it is present, provide 10 breaths per minute, checking the pulse for 10sec every 10 breaths. **If no pulse** commence chest compression, at the middle of the lower half of the sternum, delivering 30 compressions in the first instance, before providing 2 rescue breaths.
- Remember, statistically the patient's best chance at survival once absence of breathing is confirmed is defibrillation, therefore getting early help may be the most useful thing you can do. Children and victims of trauma or drowning are exceptions and may benefit from 1min of resuscitation before you leave to get help.

Rates of compression/ventilation:

- Ventilation only (good cardiac output) 10–15 breaths/min.
- CPR, single and two rescuer: 30 compressions to 2 ventilations.
- Aim for 100 compressions/min.

For those working in an environment where facilities for advanced life support (defibrillation, intubation/ventilation) exist, the 2005 UK Resuscitation Council/ILCoR Guidelines are reproduced in Figure 11.2.

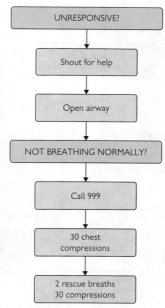

Fig. 11.1 Adult basic life support.
Reproduced from UK Resuscitation Council 2005 Guidelines/CoSTR

Fig. 11.2 Algorithm for advanced cardiac life support.
Resuscitation Council UK Guidelines 2005

Anaphylactic shock and other drug reactions

Penicillins are the commonest offender, but it is worth remembering that there is a 10% cross-over in allergic response between penicillins and cephalosporins.

An anaphylactic reaction is not an all-or-nothing response, and grades of severity are seen. Generally, the reaction starts a few minutes after a parenteral injection, and not immediately as does a simple faint. Some caution should be exercised, though, as the quicker the onset of an anaphylactic reaction the more severe it is likely to be. Some patients with known severe allergic reactions/previous anaphylaxis will carry an 'Epipen' (0.3mg adrenaline) to self-administer at the first sign of symptoms.

Principal symptoms are facial flushing, itching, numbness, cold extremities, nausea, and sometimes abdominal pain. Signs include wheezing, facial swelling and rash, and cold clammy skin with a thin thready pulse. Loss of consciousness may occur, with extreme pallor which progresses to cyanosis as respiratory failure develops.

It can be difficult to distinguish anaphylaxis from acute asthma in, e.g. an asthmatic given an NSAID they are allergic to. Don't panic, just go through management for acute asthma, then start on management for anaphylaxis (Figure 11.3). Adrenaline is a bronchodilator anyway. Befriend this drug!

Angio-oedema is sudden onset, with severe face and neck allergic swelling. The airway is at risk and therefore should be managed as for anaphylaxis.

Management
- Place patient supine with legs raised, if possible.
- Check ABCDE (Airway, Breathing, Circulation, Disability + Expose)
- 0.5ml of 1:1000 adrenaline IM or SC. Repeat after 15min, then every 15min until improved. Do not give IV in this concentration as it will induce ventricular fibrillation.
- Up to 500mg of hydrocortisone IV.
- Up to 20mg of chlorpheniramine slowly IV (if available).
- O$_2$ by mask.
- Salbutamol 0.5mg/ml (1ml) as IM or SC injection in patients on non-cardioselective beta-blockers if no response to adrenaline.

Other drug reactions and interactions

While there are a multitude of drug interactions which the dental surgeon should be aware of as a prescriber, the drugs most liable to present an emergency problem to the dentist are those which we administer as LAs.

Although it is possible to achieve toxic levels of lidocaine, adrenaline, prilocaine, or felypressin without intravascular injection, this generally requires a particularly cavalier attitude to the administration of LA. Commonly, this effect is due to intravascular injection of a substantial proportion of a cartridge of LA. Confusion, peri-oral tingling, drowsiness, agitation, fits, or loss of consciousness may occur. Do not use more than 10 x 2.2ml cartridges of lidocaine/adrenaline (440mg lidocaine). In practice, you will rarely consider coming near this amount.

Management

- Stop procedure! (They won't be numb.)
- Place supine.
- Maintain airway, give O_2.
- Await spontaneous recovery (in ~30min) unless tragically a serious event such as MI supervenes, in which case treat as indicated.

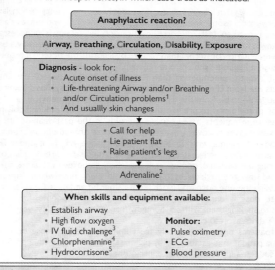

Fig. 11.3 Treatment for anaphylaxis algorithm.
Resuscitation Council UK Guidelines 2008

Collapse in a patient with a history of corticosteroid use

The use of corticosteroids therapeutically or otherwise for whatever cause may suppress the adrenal response to stress. The longer the course of Rx and the higher the dose used the more likely this is to occur. It is almost certain that a large number of people have unnecessary 'prophylaxis' with hydrocortisone and many would now argue that without evidence (short synacthen test) of adrenocortical insufficiency it is unnecessary. However, we take the view that you are less likely to cause harm by a brief supplementation of steroid than you are by ignoring the potential problem because it happens to be rare in reality.

It is worth remembering that virtually all serious steroid unwanted effects are from chronic usage (acute steroid induced psychosis being the exception—a risk from the high dose orthognathic regimens).

The prime aim is to prevent the occurrence of stress-induced collapse; therefore, if patients have received steroids in the past year or are on steroids at present, cover any stressful procedure, anaesthetic, infection, or episode of trauma with 25–50mg hydrocortisone IM (IV if under GA) 30min prior to elective stress. Seriously ill patients require IV qds doses covering the period of admission. It is a fallacy to believe you are ↓ risk of steroid unwanted effects by trying to avoid giving prophylactic steroids. Doubling the oral dose may work but is rather hit and miss. Calculating an 'exact' dose is unnecessarily complicated and risks people 'forgetting'. Stick to sticking them with 25–50mg hydrocortisone IM unless you have a very valid reason to change.

In patients presenting acutely, treat immediately. If collapse occurs in such a patient, Δ is established by pallor, rapid, thin pulse with a profound and sudden ↓ in BP, and loss of consciousness.

Management

- Place in supine position. Maintain airway. Give O_2. Obtain IV access.
- Up to 500mg hydrocortisone IV immediately.
- Ensure help (i.e. an ambulance) is requested.
- Exclude other causes of collapse.

Fits

The majority of epileptic fits do not require active intervention as the patient will usually recover spontaneously. All that is needed is sensible positioning to prevent the patient from damaging himself. Fits may be precipitated in a known epileptic by starvation, flickering lights, certain drugs such as methohexitone, tricyclics, alcohol, or menstruation. They may also follow a deep faint.

Diagnosis Many epileptics have a preceding aura followed by sudden loss of consciousness with a rigid extended appearance and generalized jerking movements. Frequently, they are incontinent of urine and may bite their tongue. There is a slow recovery with the patient feeling sleepy and dazed. There may be a *cause* for the fitting: trauma, tumour, and alcohol withdrawal are common. There are numerous others, any adult should have a first fit fully investigated by a neurologist.

▶ Should the fitting be repeated, the patient has entered the state of status epilepticus. This is an emergency and requires urgent control.

Management Get help. In a simple major fit the patient should be placed in the recovery position when practicable and allowed to recover. If they enter status epilepticus, 10mg midazolam IV usually aborts the fit, this dose can be given buccally or nasally if IV access cannot be obtained; beware respiratory depression. Assess cardiorespiratory function; clear and maintain airway, and give O₂ if available. It is worthwhile considering placing an IV cannula or a butterfly in any epileptic patient with less than perfect control, as stress is an important precipitant. Status epilepticus should not be allowed to continue for more than 20min as the mortality rate (up to 30%) and chance of permanent brain damage ↑ with the length of attack.

Management in hospital Get help. After giving IV benzodiazepines (lorazepam 4mg, midazolam or 10mg diazepam as emulsion 10–20 mg) and maintaining an airway, give an IV bolus of up to 50ml of 20–50% glucose unless certain blood glucose (BM stick) is >5mmol/l. Establish a 0.9% saline infusion and repeat the benzodiazepines if necessary. If the fits are not controlled it may be necessary to use a phenytoin infusion or induce anaesthesia with thiopentone, an intravenous barbiturate, paralyze and ventilate.

Hypoglycaemia

Hypoglycaemia is the diabetic emergency most likely to present to the dentist. It is an acute and dangerous complication of diabetes and may result from a missed meal, excess insulin, or increased calorific need due to exercise or stress. Most diabetics are expert in detecting the onset of hypoglycaemia themselves; however, a small number may lose this ability, particularly if changed to a new form of insulin. Recognition of this state is essential and an acutely collapsed diabetic should be assumed hypoglycaemic until proven otherwise, e.g. by 'BM' sticks or blood-glucose levels.

Diagnosis Disorientation, irritability, increasing drowsiness, excitability, or aggression in a known diabetic, suggest hypoglycaemia. They often appear to be drunk.

Treatment

- If conscious, give glucose orally in any available form. Get help.
- 1mg of IM glucagon.
- If unconscious, protect airway, place in recovery position, establish IV access and give up to 50ml of 20–50% dextrose.

Acute asthma

An acute asthmatic attack may be induced in a patient predisposed to bronchospasm by exposure to an allergen, infection, cold, exercise, or anxiety. Characteristically, the patient will complain of a **tight chest** and shortness of breath. Examination will reveal breathlessness, with widespread expiratory wheezing. The accessory muscles of respiration may be used to support breathing. If the patient is unable to talk, you are dealing with a potentially fatal episode.

Management Make use of the patient's own anti-asthmatic drugs, such as salbutamol inhalers. Ideally, this should be administered in the form of a nebulizer using 24% O_2 and nebulized salbutamol. A do-it-yourself nebulizer can be fabricated from the patient's own inhaler pushed through the base of a paper cup. Repeated depressions of inhaler plunger will create an aerosol inside the cup which the patient can inhale. This will relieve most reversible airways obstruction. Steroids should be administered either as oral prednisolone, if the patient carries these with them, or as IV hydrocortisone up to 200mg IV. This combination of salbutamol, steroids, and O_2 will often completely resolve an attack; however, in individuals who do not respond, an urgent hospital admission is required. Patients who are only partially responsive must have underlying irritants such as a chest infection either excluded or treated.

▶ Be aware of the possibility of anaphylaxis mimicking acute asthma. Remember adrenaline 0.5ml 1:1000 IM/SC.

Management in dental practice
- Keep the patient upright.
- Administer salbutamol either by inhaler or by DIY nebulizer.
- Give O_2.
- Give steroids.

If a complete response takes place it is reasonable to allow the patient to return home. If there is any doubt arrange for the patient to be seen at the nearest emergency department.

Management in hospital
- Nurse patient upright.
- Give nebulized salbutamol 5mg (with O_2) up to 2 hourly.
- Give nebulized ipratropium 500µg (with O_2).
- Establish IV access and give up to 200mg hydrocortisone IV or prednisolone 40mg PO.
- Monitor peak expiratory flow, arterial blood gases, and pulse oximetry.
- Obtain a CXR; exclude infection, pneumothorax.
- If incomplete response, obtain expert help rather than embarking on alternative Rx such as aminophylline.

Inhaled foreign bodies

The combination of delicate instruments and the supine position of patients for many dental procedures inevitably ↑ the risk of a patient inhaling a FB. Patients with facial trauma often have missing teeth—always think where could they be? Two basic scenarios are likely, depending on whether or not the item impacts in the upper or lower airway.

Upper airway This will stimulate the cough reflex, which may be sufficient to clear the obstruction. A choking subject should be bent forward to aid coughing. If the obstruction is complete or there are signs of cyanosis in:

1) *Conscious patient* Support chest with one hand, strike between the scapulae with the heel of your other hand. Repeat up to 5 times if needed. If this fails carry out abdominal thrusts (Heimlich manoeuvre) by encircling victim with your arms from behind and deliver sharp upward and inward squeeze to create sudden expulsion of air. Repeat up to 5 times. Alternate 5 back blows with the 5 abdominal thrusts. First attempt is most likely to succeed and they may vomit.

2) *Unconscious patient* Finger sweep to try to remove foreign body. CPR should be commenced; this will provide circulatory support as well as help dislodge the FB.[1]

If all else fails cricothyroid puncture may preserve life if the obstruction lies above this level.

Lower airway As only a segment of the lungs will be occluded this presents a less acute problem. It is also easier to miss. Classically, this involves a tooth or tooth fragment slipping from the forceps and being inhaled. With the patient in a semi-upright position the object ends up in the right posterior basal lobe. Should this happen, inform the patient and arrange to have a CXR taken ASAP. If the offending item is in the lungs (Figure 11.4), removal by a chest physician by fibre-optic bronchoscopy is indicated, as failure to remove the tooth is inevitably followed by collapse and infection distal to the obstruction. Rarely, lobectomy may be needed.

1 Resuscitation Council (UK) 2006 Guidelines.

Fig. 11.4 When a lost tooth cannot be located it must be searched for; ingestion is not a real problem but inhaled teeth must be removed.

If in doubt

When presented with a suddenly collapsed patient the first thing to assess is your own response. Don't panic.[1] You are only of value to the patient if you can function rationally. Always instigate a call for help—we are all useless without it. If presented with a case of sudden loss of consciousness, in the absence of an obvious Δ, the following steps should be followed.

- **Maintain the airway** and provide O_2 if available.
- **Place in supine position.** If the patient has simply fainted they will recover virtually immediately.
- **Are they breathing?** If not begin artificial respiration, 📖 p. 524.
- **Feel for the pulse.** If it is absent, there has been a cardiac arrest (📖 p. 524). If it is present:
- Establish IV access and give up to 20ml 20–50% dextrose IV.
- Give hydrocortisone up to 200mg IV.
- If unable to get access, use glucagon 1mg IM.

These measures will usually resolve most cases of sudden, non-traumatic loss of consciousness.

If the patient is acutely distressed and breathless they should be treated in an upright position and given O_2 while you try to differentiate between an acute asthmatic attack, anaphylaxis, and heart failure, and treat as indicated.

Always ensure that someone has requested assistance in the form of an ambulance or, if in hospital, that the appropriate staff have been contacted. If at all possible, try to speak to the receiving doctor **yourself**.

Immediately after resolution of an emergency there tends to be a period of numb inactivity amongst the staff involved. Use this period to review your management of the situation and carefully document what happened. If the patient has been transferred to hospital or another department a brief, legible account of proceedings must accompany them. Include drugs used, their dosages, and when they were given. Try to ensure that a friend or relation of the patient is aware of the situation.

---

1 Thank you Douglas Adams!

Management of the dental in-patient

The vast majority of in-patients will experience considerable anxiety on being admitted for operation, including about those procedures which are in themselves 'routine'. In addition, as dentists have little training in medical clerking and ward work, there is a substantial risk of compounding an already stressful situation by being overly stressed yourself. Minimize this by preparation. Learn about the ward(s) you will work on before taking up a post. Never be afraid to ask nursing staff if you are unsure, and try to know a day in advance what cases are coming in.

Pre-operation

All patients attending as in-patients for operation must (i) be examined and 'clerked', and (ii) have consented to surgery. In addition, many will require a variety of pre-op investigations; these vary widely from consultant to consultant, so get to know the local variations. Common investigations and their indications are listed below. Sampling techniques, 📖 p. 540; samples, 📖 p. 12.

(i) Clerking This basically consists of taking a complete medical and dental history from the patient, including any drugs they are taking at present (which you must remember to continue while in hospital by writing up in the drug 'kardex'), a family history for inherited disease, and a social history for problems related to smoking, alcohol, drug abuse, and ability to cope at home post-op. This is followed by a systematic clinical examination (📖 p. 8). Any special investigations are then arranged, and the results of these should be seen before the patient goes to theatre. Any problems uncovered should be relayed to the anaesthetist, who is the only person capable of saying whether or not the patient is 'fit for anaesthesia'. Any required pre-, peri-, or post-op drugs are written up, 📖 p. 558.

(ii) Consent All patients undergoing GA or sedation must give written, informed consent. It is advised that patients receiving interventions under LA also do so. Every hospital has its own surgical consent form which you complete. After having the procedure and its likely potential risks explained, the patient also signs. It is essential that you are happy in your own mind that you understand what the operation entails, current UK regulations suggest the surgeon who will operate or someone who is capable of doing the operation should take the consent. Obtain consent only for procedures with which you are familiar.

Investigations (📖 p. 12)

Full blood count Elderly patients. Any suspicion of anaemia.

Sickle cell test All Afro-Caribbeans for GA. Consider also those of Mediteranean, Arabic, or Indian origin. There may be a local policy but usually not. Ask your anaesthetist.

Urea and electrolytes All patients needing IV fluids, on diuretics, diabetics, or with renal disease. Have a low threshold for doing this test.

Coagulation screen All major surgery, any past history of bleeding disorders, liver disease, or history of ↑ alcohol, anticoagulants.

Liver function tests Liver disease, alcohol, major surgery.

Group and save/cross-match Major surgery, trauma, shock, anaemia.

ECG Heart disease, all major surgery, most patients >50.

CXR Trauma, active chest disease, possible metastases.

Hepatitis B and C, and HIV markers Varies; usually at-risk groups only; pre-test counselling now considered mandatory. Check local hospital policy.

Post-operation

Immediately post-op, patients are resuscitated in a recovery room adjacent to theatre, with a nurse monitoring cardiorespiratory function. Once recovered, unless they are to be monitored in the ICU/HDU they will be returned to the ward. In all patients, ensure a patent airway and consider:

Analgesia may take the form of LA (should be given post-anaesthetic/pre-surgery), oral or parenteral NSAIDs, or oral or parenteral opioids. Immediately post-op, analgesia is best given parenterally. Antiemetics such as cyclizine 50mg oral, IM, or IV, or ondansetron 4mg IM or IV should be given if nausea or vomiting is present. Many anaesthetists consider this their responsibility—ask.

Antimicrobials are given in accordance with the selected regimen (📖 p. 548). Certain patients may benefit from corticosteroids pre- and post-op to ↓ oedema; regimens vary.

Nutrition is a problem principally for patients undergoing major head and neck cancer surgery (📖 p. 480), who should have had a dietetic assessment preop and a decision made about postop feeding (NGT, gastrostomy) but it is worthwhile reminding nursing staff to order soft diets for all oral surgery patients who can feed by mouth and to have liquidizers available for patients in IMF.

Fluid balance is covered on 📖 p. 541.

Postoperative airway Special consideration needs to be given to patients in IMF and those with tracheostomies. Immediate post-op rigid IMF is now rare however post-op elastic IMF is common. These patients need to be specially attended by a nurse looking after that patient only, for the first 12–24h ('specialed'). Lighting, suction, and the ability to place the patient head-down if they vomit, is mandatory. Other techniques include tongue suture, prolonged retention of a nasopharyngeal airway, elective prolonged intubation, and tracheostomy. Avoiding this situation, 📖 see p. 464. Tracheostomy is a great aid to secure airway management, but enormously inconvenient for patients and has its own complications. If indicated it is essential to care for the tube by suction and humidification to ensure patency.

Venepuncture and arterial puncture

Venepuncture To become proficient in the skills of venepuncture you must practise the art in all its forms. To develop the skill of placing IV cannulae, cultivate a sympathetic anaesthetist, as anaesthetized patients are venodilated and will not feel pain! When carrying out cannulations and arterial punctures on patients in the ward, a drop or two of 2% plain lignocaine deposited SC with a fine needle will aid both your peace of mind and the patient's comfort. While most hospitals have phlebotomy services you will be asked to get blood and cannulate out of hours and when the phlebotomists fail so learn as soon as you can.

Tools of the trade Tourniquet, alcohol wipes, cotton wool. Green (21G) needles and butterflies are commonly used. Many hospitals have adopted sealed 'vacutainer' systems which are convenient but fiddly to use. Learn the basics first, then your hospital's system. Sometimes finer needles or butterflies are needed, e.g. blue (23G). Many hospitals now have sealed sterile 'cannulation packs' for bedside use. Patients who are difficult to cannulate can have fluids and certain drugs through fine (20G) or even 22G IV cannulae; most have 18G. Shocked patients or those needing blood should have at least a 16G and preferably a 14G cannula inserted. Note that gauges and colours are not consistent between needles and cannulae.

Sites of puncture

For sampling First choice is the cubital fossa. Inspect and palpate; veins you can feel are better than those you can only see. Insert the needle at a 30–40° angle to the skin and along the line of the vein. If no veins are found in the cubital fossa try the back of the hand with a butterfly and use a similar approach. The veins of the dorsum of the foot are a last resort before the femoral vein lying just medial to the femoral artery in the groin.

For infusion Single bolus injections; use a 21G butterfly in a vein on the back of the hand.

- For IV fluids or multiple IV injections place a 18G IV cannula in a straight segment of vein in the forearm, hand, or just proximal to 'anatomical snuffbox'. Try to avoid crossing a joint as the cannula tissues more quickly if subjected to repeated movements. When inserting the cannula ensure the skin overlying the vein is fixed by finger pressure; pierce the skin, and move the stilette along the line of the vein until it enters the vein and blood flows into the cannula. As soon as you enter the vein, pull the stilette back into the cannula to minimize the risk of going through the vein. Insert the full length of the cannula into the vein and secure. Keep patent with saline flush.

Arterial puncture Whenever possible, obtain an arterial sampling syringe. Use LA unless patient anaesthetized. The syringe and needle must be flushed with heparin. Use radial, brachial, or femoral arteries. Palpate, prepare area with alcohol wipe, and insert needle at 30–60° to skin. When the needle enters the artery, blood pulsates into the syringe. Only 1–2ml are needed. All ITUs have a blood gas analyzer and some other areas of your hospital will have one too, find out where it is and how to use it. If not the specimen goes in a chilled bag to the biochemist. The puncture site needs to be firmly pressed on for 2–3min to prevent formation of a painful haematoma.

Intravenous fluids

Principles The maintenance of daily fluid requirements plus replacement of any abnormal loss by infusion of (usually) isotonic solutions. Normal requirements are ~2.5–3l in 24h. This is lost via urine (normal renal function needs an absolute minimum of 30ml/h, but aim for 60ml/h), faecal loss, and sweating. Where possible replace with oral fluids; IV fluids are a second best.

Common IV regimens 1l normal saline (0.9%) and 2l 5% dextrose in 24h, or 3l dextrose/saline solution in 24h. Add 20mmol potassium chloride per litre after 36h, unless U&Es suggest otherwise. Hartmann's solution is more expensive but most physiological crystalloid (aka Ringer's lactate).

Increase the above in the presence of abnormal losses, burns, fever, dehydration, polyuria, and in the event of haemorrhage or shock.

Special needs
- For burns, start with Hartmann's and be guided by the Burns Centre.
- For fever, use saline.
- For dehydration or polyuria, use 5% dextrose, unless hyponatraemic. Exception is ketoacidosis: use saline.
- Haemorrhage demands replacement whole blood if available (rarely is); packed cells are what you will be offered in most hospitals in most countries. Shock needs, crystalloid challenge, blood and control of haemorrhage. Be guided by the pulse, BP, urine output, haemoglobin, the haematocrit, and the U&Es.

↓ the above in heart failure, and avoid saline. Shock and dehydration are rare complications of maxillofacial trauma or any other condition principally presenting in their presence consider damage to other body systems and seek appropriate advice.

Polyuria Post-op, is usually due to over-transfusion. Review anaesthetic notes, and if this is the case simply catheterize and observe.

Oliguria Post-op, is usually due to under-transfusion or dehydration pre- or perioperatively. First, palpate abdomen for ↑ bladder and listen to chest to exclude pulmonary oedema. Then catheterize the patient to exclude urinary retention and allow close monitoring of fluid balance. Then ↑ rate of infusion of fluid (**max** 1l/h) **unless** the patient is in heart failure or bleeding. The former needs specialist advice, the latter needs blood or an operation. In an otherwise healthy post-op patient, if this does not produce a minimum of 30ml/h of urine, a diuretic (20–40mg furosemide PO/IV) may be tried. Take care when using fluid challenges, as if failure to PU is renal it is possible to fluid overload the patient quickly. Review the fluid balance, U&Es, over several days for an overview.

Blood transfusion

▶ Group and save—you won't get blood; group and cross-match—you will get blood in ~1hr; type specific group—you will get blood urgently.

Blood may be required for patients in an acute (e.g. traumatized) situation, electively (e.g. peri-operatively) during major surgery, or to correct a chronic anaemia (🕮 p. 490). In practice, the former two are much more commonly encountered by junior dental staff.

Whole blood is indicated in patients who have lost >20% blood volume, exhibit signs of hypovolaemic shock, or in whom this appears inevitable.

▶ Remember maxillofacial injuries **alone** only rarely result in this degree of blood loss (🕮 p. 454).

Always take blood for grouping in severely traumatized patients, and proceed to cross-match as indicated by the clinical signs. Always use cross-matched blood, except in utter extremis when O Rhesus −ve blood can be used. Massive transfusions create problems with hyperkalaemia, thrombocytopenia, and low levels of clotting factors; therefore in patients with severe haemorrhage, simultaneous fresh frozen plasma (4–6 units) and platelets (6 units) will be needed. Most labs only provide packed cells.

Autologous blood is blood donated by a patient prior to elective surgery for use only on themselves. It avoids risks of cross-infection but requires a specially interested haematology department, so check locally. Autotransfusion is sometimes used in vascular surgery.

Packed cells are used for the correction of anaemia if too severe for correction with iron, or if needed prior to urgent surgery. This ↓ the fluid load to the patient, but elderly individuals and those in heart failure should have their transfusion covered with 40mg frusemide PO or IV.

Useful tips
- Cross-match one patient at a time and be sure you are familiar with local procedures.
- Nurse will perform regular observations of temperature, pulse, respiration, and urine output during transfusion—look at them!
- Don't use a giving set which has contained dextrose, as the blood will clog.
- Except in shock, transfuse slowly (1 unit over 2–4h; >4h the cannulae start to clog).
- 1 unit of blood raises the Hb by 1g/dl = 3% haematocrit.

Complications
- ABO incompatibility. Causes anaphylaxis; manage accordingly (🕮 p. 528).
- Cross-infection.
- Heart failure can be induced by over-rapid transfusion.
- Milder allergic transfusion reactions are the commonest problem; Rx by slowing the transfusion. If progressive or temperature >40°C stop transfusion and inform lab to check cross-matching. IV hydrocortisone 100mg and chlorphenamine 10mg are useful standbys.
- Citrate toxicity is a hazard of very large transfusions and can be countered by 10ml of calcium gluconate with alternate units.

Catheterization

This is not a topic normally covered by the dental syllabus, but the dental graduate may find him or herself confronted with a patient needing urethral catheterization if working on an oral and maxillofacial surgical ward. The only procedure they are likely to need to be able to perform is temporary urethral catheterization. This is indicated for urinary retention (almost always post-op), for precise measurement of fluid balance, or, rarely, to avoid use of bedpan or bottle. Avoid catheterization if a history of pelvic trauma is present, as an expert is needed. Catheters are associated with a high incidence of UTIs, and presence of a UTI is a relative C/I.

Equipment Most wards have their own; ask for it and ensure you have an assistant available. It should contain a tube of local anaesthetic gel, a dish with some aqueous chlorhexidine, swabs, a waterproof sheet with a hole in the middle, sterile gloves, a 10-ml syringe filled with sterile water, and a drainage bag. In most cases a 14–16 French gauge Foley catheter will suffice. Use a silicone catheter if you anticipate it being *in situ* for more than a few days.

Procedure Explain what you are going to do and why. If catheterizing for post-op fluid balance, do it in the anaesthetic room after intubation (ask the anaesthetist first!). The operating theatre is the best place to learn. The procedure can be made both aseptic and aesthetic by wearing two pairs of disposable gloves; one pair is discarded after achieving analgesia, which is done by instillation of lignocaine gel (also acts as a lubricant). Find the urethral opening and, using the nozzle supplied, squeeze in the contents of the tube. In the female, finding the opening is the only significant problem and most women are catheterized by female nursing staff. In the male, it is necessary to massage the gel along the length of the penis and leave *in situ* for several minutes before progressing. Once analgesia is obtained, the female urethra is easily catheterized; if you have been unable to find the meatus to instil LA you should not proceed but get help. In the male, hold the penis upright and insert the tip of the catheter; pass it gently down the urethra until it reaches the penoscrotal junction, pull the penis down so that it lies between the patient's thighs, thereby straightening out the curves of the urethra, and advance the tip into the bladder until urine flows.

Once urine flows, the catheter balloon can be inflated with sterile water. In the conscious patient it should be painless; if not, deflate the balloon and reposition the catheter. In the anaesthetized patient, insert the catheter all the way, inflate, then pull back. Connect the drainage bag and remember to replace the foreskin over the glans to avoid a paraphimosis.

▶ If, in the presence of adequate analgesia, you are unable to pass the catheter **do not** persist, but get expert assistance.

Enteral and parenteral feeding

The main role for this type of feeding, as far as dental staff are concerned, is in the care of debilitated patients and those undergoing surgery for head and neck cancers. In view of the latter, it is worthwhile having a basic understanding of the subject.

Enteral feeding is providing liquid, low-residue foods either by mouth, by fine-bore nasogastric tube or gastrostomy. A range of proprietary products are available for these feeds. Be guided by the local dietitian, who has expertise in this area which you will lack. The major problem is osmotic diarrhoea, which can be ↓ by starting with dilute solutions.

Fine-bore nasogastric tubes are the mainstay in enteral nutrition for patients undergoing major oropharyngeal surgery. In many institutions, nurses are not allowed to pass these tubes, although they are allowed to pass standard nasogastric tubes for aspirating stomach contents. You can therefore find yourself asked to pass such a tube by someone who is more proficient but forbidden to do so. Gastrostomy tubes are placed by the relevant specialists (and have higher complication rates).

Technique Wear gloves. Explain the procedure to the patient and have them at 50–60° upright with neck in neutral position. Place a small amount of lidocaine gel in the chosen nostril after ensuring it is patent. Keep a small drink of water handy. Select a tube; check the guidewire is lubricated and does not protrude. If a tracheostomy tube is present the cuff should be deflated to allow passage of the tube. Lubricate the tube and introduce it into the nostril; pass it horizontally along the nasal floor. There is usually a little resistance as the tube reaches the nasopharynx; press past this and ask the patient to swallow (use the water if this helps). The tube should now pass easily down the oesophagus, entering the stomach at 40cm. Secure the tube to the forehead with sticky tape and only now remove the guidewire, being careful to shield the patient's eyes. Inject air into the tube and listen for bubbling over the stomach. Confirm position with a CXR. (Some systems require leaving a radio-opaque guidewire in prior to X-ray: check the tube you are using).

Problems
- *Nasal patency* Select the least narrow nostril, use a lubricant, and, if necessary, a smaller tube and topical vasoconstrictor.
- *Gagging/vomiting* Press ahead; all sphincters are open.
- *Tube coiling into mouth* Cooling the tube makes it more rigid and often helps. As a last resort, topical anaesthesia and direct visualization with a laryngoscope or nasendoscope, while an assistant passes the tube, may be necessary.
- *Tube pulled out by patient* If they must have the tube, consider a nasogastric tube 'bridle' designed for this problem or a stitch to the septum or soft tissue of the nose.

Parenteral feeding Hazardous and expensive. Central or peripheral lines are required and need to be maintained. Neither as safe nor efficient as enteral feeding. Avoid if at all possible.

Refeeding syndrome Patients who have been starved for more than 5 days and are then fed eneterally or parenterally risk this electrolyte and fluid imbalance characterized by severe hypophosphataemia with other biochemical disturbances. Avoid by supplementation with B vitamins and gradated biochemical correction.[1]

Percutaneous endoscopic gastrostomy *(PEG)* Feeding tube placed directly in stomach through abdominal wall at endoscopy.

Radiologically inserted gastrostomy *(RIG)* Ultrasound version of PEG. Needs NGT in place to inflate stomach.

1 H. Melena 2008 *BMJ* **336** 1495.

Pain control

LA (📖 p. 584); RA (📖 p. 590); IV sedation (📖 p. 592); cryoanalgesia (📖 p. 374); and TENS (📖 p. 587).

Pain control aims to relieve symptoms while identifying and removing the cause; the exception is when the cause is not treatable, as in palliative and terminal care. Then, the approach is to deal with the symptoms to enable the patient to have a quality to their life.

Acute and post-op pain May often be well controlled by LA (📖 p. 584), but it is often necessary to use systemic analgesics. Useful analgesics in this situation include paracetamol (1000mg PO/PR/IV 4 hourly) and ibuprofen (400–600mg 8 hourly). Both these can be combined with codeine (8–30mg). NSAIDs such as diclofenac (50mg PO 8 hourly or 75mg IM perioperatively, followed by one further dose of 75mg IM). These drugs are all simple analgesics and, with the exception of paracetamol, have the advantage of an anti-inflammatory action which is at least as important as their central analgesic effect. In *post-op* pain, opioid analgesics are helpful when used parenterally and short term. Morphine 10mg 3–4 hourly combined with an antiemetic such as metoclopramide (10mg IM/IV) is useful in the immediate post-op period. PCA systems (see below) after major surgery are commonly used. They are set up by the anaesthetists.

Pain following maxillofacial trauma is a problem, as these patients must be assessed neurologically for evidence of head injury which C/I opioids. The addition of codeine phosphate (60mg IM) to a NSAID is often effective and does not significantly interfere with neurological observations. Alternatively, PR or IM diclofenac sodium may suffice. There is often a hospital acute pain team who will be happy to advise in difficult cases.

Facial pain not of dental or iatrogenic origin is covered on 📖 p. 426. These conditions often require the use of co-analgesics such as antidepressants, antiepileptics, and anxiolytics.

Pain control in terminal disease An important subject in its own right. Points to note include: aim for continuous control using oral analgesia; use regular, not on demand, analgesia titrated to the individual; diagnose the cause of each pain and prescribe appropriately (e.g. steroids for liver secondaries or ↑ intracranial pressure, NSAIDs &/or radiotherapy for bone metastases, co-analgesics for nerve root pain, etc.). Remember that psychological dependence is very rare in advanced cancer patients using long-term opioids, and analgesic tolerance slow to develop. When starting patients on opioid analgesia, always consider using an antiemetic (📖 p. 567) and a laxative. OH may be incredibly difficult for patients with oral cancer or following head and neck surgery. Use of chlorhexidine gluconate (Corsodyl®) and metronidazole (200mg bd) ↓ the smell associated with wound infection or tumour fungation even when there is no prospect of eliminating it entirely. Patients rarely develop the disulfiram reaction to metronidazole on this regimen that occurs with higher doses.

Pre-emptive analgesia Surgery is painful. Providing LA (consider the long-acting agent bupivocaine/levobupivocaine) or systemic analgesia before surgery begins may ↓ overall requirements for analgesia.

Patient-controlled analgesia The optimal technique for severe post-op pain. Small machine delivers a bolus (1–2mg morphine) when patient presses a button. Can be repeated as needed.

Two variables: (i) bolus dose; (ii) 'lock out time' time during which machine will not respond (allows time for opioid to achieve maximum effect and prevents overdosage).

Prophylaxis

Prophylaxis is the prevention of an occurrence. In surgery this is usually infection or thromboembolism. Prophylaxis used to prevent the occurrence of bacterial infection is quite different from treating an established infection. There are two broad categories of patients requiring antibiotic prophylaxis: (i) those who have it to prevent a minor local bacteraemia causing a serious infection out of all proportion to the procedure, e.g. the immunocompromised; (ii) those who receive it to prevent local septic complications of the procedure, e.g. wisdom-tooth removal.

Principles of antibiotic prophylaxis The regimen should be short, high dose, and appropriate to the potential infecting organisms. The aim is to prevent pathogens establishing themselves in surgically traumatized or otherwise at-risk tissues, therefore the antimicrobial must be in those tissues prior to damage or exposure to the pathogen. It must not, however, be present too long before this, as there is then a risk of pathogen resistance and damage to commensal organisms. The regimen should therefore start immediately pre-op (i.e. <6h) or perioperatively (e.g. with anaesthetic induction) and should be continued for 24–48h maximum. When practicable, select an antimicrobial as specific to the common pathogens for that procedure as possible, except in the immunocompromised, where broad-spectrum prophylaxis is appropriate.

Prophylaxis against infective endocarditis is no longer indicated on a routine basis.[1]

Examples
- *Immunocompromised* (e.g. severe leukopenia) 2.25g piperacillin/tazobactam plus 120mg gentamicin IV pre-op. Repeat qds for 24h.
- *Dento-alveolar surgery* Simple extractions need not be covered but third-molar surgery often is. Regimens: metronidazole 400mg PO (500mg IV) pre-op followed by 400mg tds for 24h, amoxicillin 1g PO/IV followed by 500mg tds for 24h.

Prophylactic anticoagulation[2] Prevention of DVT &/or pulmonary embolus in susceptible patients (e.g. women on the pill, prolonged surgery, iliac crest grafts) can be achieved using daily low-molecular weight heparin SC od (various types available—check which one your hospital favours). Thromboembolic antiembolism (TED) stockings will also ↓ DVT. Rx of pulmonary embolus, 🕮 p. 554.

1 NICE Guidance 2008 (ℜ www.nice.org.uk).
2 J. Hill 2007 *BMJ* **334** 1053.

Management of the diabetic patient undergoing surgery

▶ Many hospitals have a diabetic team who will advise on the management of these patients. Find out if this happens in your locality and make use of them. Type 2 diabetics are an increasing group in the developed world and have a plethora of health problems.[1]

Guidelines

- Know the type and severity of the diabetes you are dealing with.
- Inform the anaesthetist (and diabetic team if available).
- Remember these patients are more likely to have occult heart disease, renal impairment, and ↓ resistance to infection, so get an ECG, U&Es, and use antibiotics prophylactically.
- If nursing staff are experienced with blood glucose estimation using blood monitoring (BM) sticks or similar, 2–4 hourly BMs will suffice for monitoring control. Otherwise pre-, peri-, and post-op blood glucose estimation is needed.
- If in doubt and you are on your own (although you never should be) use a GKI (see below).
- Always have diabetics first on the operating list, in the morning if possible. Admit to hospital the day before surgery if insulin regimen is to be used.

Management: non-insulin-dependent

If anything other than a minor, short procedure, treat as insulin-dependent. If random blood glucose is >15mmol/l treat as insulin-dependent.

Patients being treated under LA, or LA and sedation should maintain their carbohydrate intake and any oral hypoglycaemic drugs as normal. Plan surgery to fit their regular mealtimes. Have carbohydrate readily to hand if needed, and ensure adequate post-op analgesia, as pain or trismus can easily interfere with their usual intake. Remember antibiotic prophylaxis.

Patients for GA Halve the dose of oral hypoglycaemic 24h prior to surgery and omit on day of surgery. Do BM sticks or blood glucose pre- and post-op (if >15 go to GKI). Halve normal dose of oral hypoglycaemic until able to take normal diet, then back to normal dose. Keep an eye on the K^+ concentration (U&Es pre- and post-op) and keep well hydrated. If in doubt, manage as for insulin dependant.

Management: insulin-dependent

Admit 24–48h pre-op to optimize control. If glycaemic control poor, involve diabetic team *early*. Examine the patient carefully. Get an ECG, FBC, U&Es, and random blood glucose. Look for heart and respiratory disease, leucocytosis indicating infection, anaemia, hypo- or hyperkalaemia, and renal impairment. If these are acceptable, normal insulin/carbohydrate intake up to and including evening meal the day before surgery. Omit long-acting insulin on the day before surgery. Starve following this, and place on an IV infusion of *glucose* (dextrose 5–10% 500ml), *potassium* (10mmol K^+ injected into bag of dextrose) infused via

1 P. Home 2008 *BMJ* **336** 1306.

a controlled rate device over 5h, i.e. 100ml/h. This is infused via three-way tap into a peripheral cannula. Simultaneously, *insulin* (short acting e.g. actrapid) is infused via a pump through the three-way tap into the same cannula at a rate indicated by the sliding scale. The insulin is normally made up as 49ml N saline with 50IU of actrapid giving 50ml = 50IU insulin, but always check your local nurses' policy.

The original GKI had a fixed amount of insulin injected into the 500ml of dextrose but the flexibility of sliding scale delivery has made this technique the most frequently used.

Sliding scale

BM	Insulin IU/h
>22	8
18–22	6
14–18	4
10–14	3 Target zone
6–10	2
2–6	1
<2	Stop and give glucose/dextrose

The scale details will vary according to the type of fingerprick glucose tests available in your locality; numbers are *not* absolute but the principle will always work. Choice of crystalloid is variable; 10% dextrose ↑ carbohydrate and anabolism but tends to tissue veins quickly.

Once the patient can eat and drink, resume normal insulin regimen and discontinue infusion as BMs normalize.

Management of patients requiring steroid supplementation

Principle These patients are unable to respond to the stress of surgery due to depletion or absence of their endogenous corticosteroid response.

Groups Patients with Addison's disease, patients prescribed corticosteroids for modulation of the immune system, and steroid abusers from various 'sports'.

Addison's disease The rarest of these groups but requires the most aggressive supplementation as sufferers are entirely reliant on prescribed steroids. Minor surgery can safely be covered with IM hydrocortisone sodium succinate 100mg qds the day of surgery. Major surgery should be covered for 3 days using the same regimen. IV administration is kinder over the longer period.

Patients prescribed steroids Do you know why they are on these drugs? Consider the underlying disease and whether it has any bearing on your Rx plan; e.g. a patient receiving steroids as part of a cytotoxic regimen will also be at risk from bleeding and infection. In an uncomplicated case before minor surgery, all that is needed is a single IM injection of hydrocortisone 50mg 30min prior to the procedure. Alternatives are an IV injection immediately pre-op followed by double the normal oral dose of steroid. Another way is to ask the patient to take a double dose on the day of the operation, normal dose plus 50% the day after, and normal plus 25% on the third day, thereafter returning to their usual dose. Those undergoing major surgery should have the IM/IV regimen over 24h or longer.

Steroid abusers Unfortunately these are a real and ↑ problem.[1] Although these drugs are taken for their androgenic effect, few 'sportspersons' have access to appropriate advice or drugs and many users will have a degree of suppressed steroid response. It is probably safest to cover procedures using the IM regimen as for those on prescribed steroids, although this could be considered overkill. Remember the risk of shared needles.

---

1 HMSO, *Drugs and Therapeutics Bulletin*, January 2004.

Common post-operative problems

General

Pain Use appropriate analgesia (📖 p. 652).

Pyrexia A small physiological ↑ in temperature occurs post-op. Other causes: atelectasis, infection (wound, chest, urine), DVT, incompatible transfusion, allergic reactions.

Nausea and vomiting Antiemetics, e.g. IM/IV cyclizine 50mg. Prochlorperazine 12.5mg or metoclopramide 10mg. Ondansetron for the recalcitrant (4mg IV/IM, 8mg PO).

Sore throat Common after intubation; needs reassurance and simple analgesia. Cold water ↓.

Muscle pain Often follows suxamethonium use in anaesthetic induction. Again, reassurance and simple analgesics.

Hypotension Usually caused by autonomic suppression by a GA. Treat by placing 'head-down'. If necessary, speed up IV infusion for a short while.

Chest infection CXR, culture sputum, and start on ampicillin or cefuroxime until culture results available.

Confusion A symptom, therefore look for the cause, e.g. infection, electrolyte imbalance, alcohol withdrawal, hypoxia, or dehydration, and correct. Only consider sedation, e.g. haloperidol 1–5mg (care in the elderly), after action has been taken to deal with the cause and the patient constitutes a threat to themselves or others.

Rarer general complications

Urinary retention Comparatively rare, even after major maxillofacial surgery. Early mobilization and adequate analgesia helps; if not, use temporary catheterization (📖 p. 543).

Superficial vein thrombosis Follows 'tissued' cannulae or irritant IV injections. Observe for infection, treat pain, and consider supportive strapping.

DVT Signs are painful, shiny, red, swollen calf, usually unilaterally but may be bilaterally. 'At risk' are immobile patients especially following pelvic surgery, patients with cancer, women on the pill, the elderly, and the obese. Confirm by doppler US or ascending venography. Prevent by using a low molecular weight heparin (dalteparin, enoxaparin) pre-op and 5 days post-op &/or pressure stockings, and ensure early mobilization. Stop the pill prior to any major surgery. Rx: bed rest, leg strapping and elevation, analgesia and heparinization (give 5000 units stat IV followed by 50 000 units in 50ml normal saline by syringe driver infusion starting at 1000 units/h (1ml/h) and adjust according to the KCT/APTT, keep between 1.5–2.5 times the control values). The major risk of DVT is the development of pulmonary embolus. This classically presents 10 days post-op when the patient has been straining at stool and may occur despite no apparent DVT. Symptoms are pleuritic chest pain, dyspnoea, cyanosis, haemoptysis, and a ↑ jugular venous pressure. Signs of shock are often present, ranging from very little in the young who can compensate, to cardiac arrest!

Usually a clinical Δ, confirmed after heparinization, analgesia, and O_2 have been instituted, by CXR, blood gases, spiral CT, or lung ventilation—perfusion scan &/or pulmonary angiography. ECG will sometimes show deep S waves in I, pathological Q waves in III, and inverted T waves in III (SI, QIII, TIII). Must be followed up by 3–6 months anticoagulation with warfarin, so involve a haematologist.

Less serious but more common are post-phlebitic limb, varicose veins, limb swelling, and skin discoloration. May lead to varicose eczema.

Local complications following oral surgery

Local pain, swelling, infection, and trismus are the commonest. Antral complications may follow maxillary surgery. These are considered in the relevant chapters.

Therapeutics

Contents

Principal sources BMA/RPSGB March 2008 BNF 55. Consumers Association *Drugs and Therapeutics Bulletin*

NB Although available on the Internet BNF.org is **NOT** recommended for use in clinically critical situations. British National Formulary now has an amalgamated BNF/Dental Practitioners Formulary.

Relevant pages in other chapters Chapter 11: Medicine relevant to dentistry; Chapter 13: Analgesia, anaesthesia, and sedation; asepsis and antisepsis, 🕮 p. 342; antiseptics and antibiotics in periodontal disease, 🕮 p. 202; fluorides, 🕮 p. 28; sugar-free medications, 🕮 p. 116.

Generic: pharmaceutical name.
Proprietary: trade name.
Depending on patents, a generic drug may have more than one proprietary name.

Poisons information
UK National Poisons Information Service: 0870 600 6266
Drugs in sport: 🕉 www.uksport.gov.uk/did 0800 5280004 drug-free @uksport.gov.uk
Medicines information services

Birmingham	0121 311 1974	Southampton	0238 079 6908/9
Bristol	0117 928 2867	Cardiff	0292 074 2979
Ipswich	0147 370 44331	Aberdeen	0122 455 2316
Leeds	0113 3923547	Dundee	0138 263 2351
Leicester	0116 255 5779	Edinburgh	0131 242 2920
Liverpool	0151 7948113/4/5/7	Glasgow	0141 211 4407
London	0207 18 83849	Belfast	0289 063 2032
	0208 869 3973	Dublin	00 3531 473 0589
Newcastle	0191 232 1925		

UK medicines information pharmacists' group: 🕉 www.ukmi.nhs.uk
Drug therapy in relation to dental treatment 0151 7948206
Paediatric Drug Information Advisory Line (DIAL) 0151 2525837, info@dial.org.uk 🕉 www.dial.org.uk

Prescribing

The following pages are a brief guide to the clinical use of some of the more commonly used and useful drugs in hospital and general dental practice. Doses are for healthy adults.

Prescribing in general dental practice Extremely useful information is available in the BNF, which is updated every 6 months. Use this as the first line of enquiry when unsure about any topic concerning drugs. Drugs listed in the DPF (found at the back of the BNF) can be prescribed in the UK within the NHS on form FP10 D (GP14 in Scotland, WP10 D in Wales, HS47 in Northern Ireland). Any other required drugs must be prescribed privately or via the patient's GMP. Many are available more cheaply OTC at pharmacies.

Prescribing in hospital The BNF is the definitive reference and should always be available for consultation. Use this to check dose alterations in children (BNF for Children) and the elderly, and for more detailed tables of drug interactions, C/I, and unwanted effects. Any drug in the hospital pharmacy may be prescribed by a hospital dentist for in-patients, patients being discharged, and out-patients. The only exception is controlled drugs for addicts, which must be prescribed by specially licensed doctors, usually a psychiatrist.

In hospitals, there are three methods of prescribing: (i) A hospital prescription chart recording both prescriptions and dispensing, kept on the ward for in-patients. (ii) A take-home prescription form redeemable only at the hospital pharmacy for patients being discharged from the ward. (iii) Hospital out-patient prescriptions, used in emergency departments and some out-patient clinics, redeemable at outside pharmacies.

Good prescribing Avoid abbreviations and write drug names legibly, using the generic whenever possible. Always describe the strength and quantity to be dispensed. When describing doses, use the units micrograms, milligrams, or millilitres when possible. Do not abbreviate the term microgram or unit (when prescribing insulin) as these are easily misinterpreted.

Controlled drugs Each prescription must show, in the prescriber's own handwriting in ink: the name and address of the patient, the form, strength, dose, and total quantity of the drug to be dispensed, in both words and figures. When writing in general practice the prescription must also incorporate the phrase 'for dental treatment only'.

Prescribing in the elderly Doses may need adjustment and are often substantially lower than for adults (often 50% lower).

Prescribing for children Children differ markedly from adults in their response to drugs, especially in the neonatal period when all doses should be calculated in relation to body weight. Older children can usually be prescribed for in age ranges, usually up to 1yr, 1–6yrs, and 6–12yrs. All details of dosages should be checked in the BNF or BNF for Children.

Prescribing in liver disease (📖 p. 498) As most drugs rely on hepatic metabolism, it is prudent to seek medical advice before prescribing for patients with severe liver disease.

Prescribing in renal impairment (📖 p. 500) Doses almost always need to be
↓ and some drugs are C/I completely. Medical advice should be sought.

Prescribing in pregnancy (📖 p. 504) Avoid if possible.

Prescribing in terminal care, 📖 p. 546.

Dose and route abbreviations:

Dose	Route
od once a day	**IM** intramuscular
mane in the morning	**INH** inhalation
nocte at night	**IV** intravenous
bd twice daily	**NEB** nebulization
tds three times daily	**PO** by mouth
qds four time daily	**PR** per rectum
prn as required	**PV** per vagina
	SC subcutaneous
	SUB sublingual
	TOP topical

Analgesics in general dental practice

▶ Consult BNF for dosages in children. See also 📖 p. 558. Most dental pain is inflammatory in origin and hence most responsive to drugs with an anti-inflammatory component, e.g. aspirin and the NSAIDs.

Of the peripherally acting analgesics in the DPF, aspirin, paracetamol, and ibuprofen are available cheaper direct to the public from pharmacies.

Aspirin Used in mild to moderate pain, it is also a potent antipyretic, which should **not** be used in children <12yrs (due to the rare but serious risk of Reye syndrome). Avoid in bleeding diathesis, gastrointestinal ulceration, and concurrent anticoagulant therapy. Ask about aspirin allergy, particularly in asthmatics. Often causes transient gut irritation (as do all NSAIDs). *Dose:* 600–900mg 4 hourly PO. Topical sakylate gels are now C/1<16.

Ibuprofen Popularly used for mild to moderate pain; has a moderate antipyretic action. Risks and side-effects are similar to those of aspirin but less irritant to the gut. *Dose:* 400–600mg 8 hourly PO.

Paracetamol Similar in analgesic efficacy to aspirin but has no anti-inflammatory action and is a moderate antipyretic. Does not cause gastric irritation or interfere with bleeding times. Overdosage can lead to liver failure. *Dose:* 1000mg 6 hourly PO (maximum dose 4g/24 hours in adults).

Diflunisal A prescription-only drug available on the DPF, with similar properties and problems to aspirin. *Dose:* 250–500mg bd with food PO.

The addition of **codeine** to the minor analgesics, while never being proven to be of advantage, may have marginal benefits in some cases. No combination analgesics are currently prescribable on the DPF.

There are very few indications for the use of opioid analgesics in general dental practice. Although **dihydrocodeine** remains in the DPF it has been demonstrated to be hyperalgesic in certain types of dental pain.[1]

Pethidine In tablet form (the only form in the DPF), is worse than dihydrocodeine in terms of side-effects.

Carbamezipine (📖 p. 576) Prescribable in the DPF.

NB While all NSAIDs *may* exacerbate asthma and there is a higher incidence of NSAID allergy in asthmatics, the CSM recognizes that this *does not* constitute a C/I for the use of these valuable analgesics. Frank allergy to NSAIDs or proven exacerbation of asthma *is* a C/I.

1 R. A. Seymour 1982 *Lancet* 1425.

Analgesics in hospital practice

In addition to those available in the DPF, some drugs available only within hospitals are of considerable value.

Diclofenac sodium is available in tablet, IM injection, suppository, and in once-daily, slow-release form. It is a mid-potency NSAID, and a useful alternative to high-dose lower potency NSAIDs or an opioid which has no anti-inflammatory effect. *Dose for tablets*: 50mg tds after food; IM injection: 75mg bd for no more than 2 days (it's a painful injection); suppositories: 100mg PR od. Soluble tablets are available.

Ketorolac trometamol 30mg/ml injection has advantage of small volume of injection. However ↑ unwanted effects have been noted and it is no longer recommended for general use.

Opioid analgesics

The opioids act centrally to alter the perception of pain, but have no anti-inflammatory properties. They are of value for severe pain of visceral origin, post-op (acting partly by sedation), and in terminal care. However, they all depress respiratory function and interfere with the pupillary response, and are C/I in head injury. All opioids cause cough suppression, urinary retention, nausea, constipation by a ↓ in gut motility, 'and tolerance and dependence. The risk of addiction is, however, greatly overstated when these drugs are used for short-term post-op analgesia and in the terminal care context. Fear of creating addicts should **never** cause you to withhold adequate analgesia.

Codeine phosphate A moderate opioid analgesic useful for short-term analgesia and less likely to mask a head injury; 30–60mg 4 hourly IM/PO. May be some advantage when used in combination (8/15/30mg) with simple analgesics or NSAIDs.

Morphine In oral form (tablets, elixir, or slow-release tablets MST), the drug of choice in the management of terminal pain. Always prescribe a laxative (macrogols are currently in favour: see BNF). *Dose*: dependent on previous analgesia, but often starts at 10mg morphine 4 hourly or 30mg MST bd. When used IM or IV for acute or post-op pain: 10–20mg 2–4 hourly; give an antiemetic.

Papaveretum A mixed opium alkaloid, frequently prescribed, but appearing to have no advantage over morphine. The presence of noscapine created a C/I in women of childbearing age. Noscapine-free equivalent (Omnopon® 10 + 20). Neither of these is in general use currently in UK.

Buprenorphine A mixed agonist/antagonist with similar problems to pethidine and pentazocine. Unique in that it can be given sublingually. *Dose*: 200–400µg 8 hourly. This is often used in opioid withdrawal.

Diamorphine (heroin) A very potent opioid which should be reserved for severe pain in an in-patient setting. Like morphine it is reversed by naloxone. Dose 1–2mg IV with appropriate patient monitoring.

Tramadol An opioid which acts by two central methods. Lower side-effect profile. 50–100mg PO 4 hourly. *Slow* IV 50–100mg 4–6 hourly.

▶ Chronic and post-op pain require *regular*, not as-required, analgesia, given in adequate amounts and within the therapeutic half-life of the drug.

PCA (📖 p. 546) A computerized system for post-op pain control allowing patients to deliver small regular doses of IV/SC morphine/diamorphine. Gold standard post-op analgesia for severe pain.

Anti-inflammatory drugs

These are among the groups of drugs that may be either analgesics or co-analgesics (drugs which are not analgesic in themselves but may aid pain relief either directly or indirectly). The two major groups are the NSAIDs (📖 p. 560) and the corticosteroids.

Steroids are used in various forms, topical, oral, intralesional, and parenteral, and all have uses in dentistry.

Topical steroids

Hydrocortisone lozenges 2.5mg lozenges dissolved in the mouth qds.

Triamcinolone in carboxymethylcellulose paste 0.1% paste applied in a thin layer qds. Sticks only to dry mucosa and is rapidly rubbed off the palate and tip of tongue. Both these preparations are available in the DPF and are of use in the management of recurrent apthous ulcers, lichen planus, etc. They are low-potency steroids and unlikely to have any of the systemic side-effects of steroids, such as ↑ of diabetes, osteoporosis, psychosis, euphoria, peptic ulceration, immunosuppression, Cushing syndrome (📖 p. 502), or adrenocortical suppression.

Benzydamine A topically active NSAID. Used as spray or mouthwash to ↓ pain from inflammatory mucosal conditions.

Betamethasone phosphate tablets Prepared as a 0.5mg soluble tablet (Betnesol®) made into a 1mg in 10ml mouthwash rinsed qds, or a *betamethasone* inhaler designed for use in asthma, but can be used to spray on aphthae (1 spray = 100µg). Repeatable to a maximum of 800µg. Currently difficult to obtain in the UK, predisolone dispersible tablets 5mg are an alternative.

Hydrocortisone 1% and oxytetracycline 3% Ointment or spray (hydrocortisone 50mg oxytetracycline 150mg per aerosol unit) qds, are useful Rx for aphthae and related conditions seen in hospital. Hydrocortisone 1% cream is also available with miconazole 2% in DPF.

Intralesional steroids

Triamcinolone acetonide 1ml (40mg) injected into lesion. Needs LA. Used in granulomatous cheilitis, intractable lichen planus, keloid scars and painful postsurgical trigger spots.

Intra-articular steroids

These can be used to induce a chemical arthroplasty in arthrosis of the TMJ (📖 p. 468).

Hydrocortisone acetate 5–10mg single injection.

Triamincinolone (40mg/ml) can be used intra-articularly.

Systemic steroids

Main indication is prophylaxis in those with actual or potential adrenocortical suppression. Occasionally used in erosive lichen planus, severe aphthae, e.g. Behçet syndrome (📖 p. 404) or arteritis (📖 p. 506).

Hydrocortisone sodium succinate used for prophylaxis; dose 100mg IM 30min pre-op. Doubts exist about the need for this unless the patient has demonstrated adrenocortical insufficiency (short synacthen test).

Prednisolone 10–20mg PO as enteric-coated tablets given with food in ↓ dose. Regimen dependent on the condition treated.

Methylprednisolone 40mg/ml. Various regimens described for control of oedema, post major surgery.

Dexamethasone 4mg/ml. Various regimens described for control of oedema, post surgery.

Other immunosuppressants

Azathioprine and **thalidomide** are sometimes used in specialist centres. Topical tacrolimus in carboxymethylcellulose base is used for erosive lichen planus.

Antidepressants

Another group of drugs which can be used as co-analgesics. In conditions such as atypical facial pain they may be used as the sole 'analgesic'. However, there are no antidepressants prescribable in the DPF.

In the past, there has been considerable debate about the potential interactions between the commonest antidepressants, the tricyclics, and the monoamine oxidase inhibitors (MAOIs), and adrenaline contained in LA (which constitutes the most commonly professionally administered drug anywhere). To date, there is *no clinical evidence* of dangerous interactions between the adrenaline in LA preparations commonly used in dentistry and the tricyclics or the MAOIs.[1] In hospital practice, the two most commonly used antidepressants are amitriptylne (a sedative tricyclic antidepressant) and dosulepin (a related compound).

Amitriptyline also used for neuropathic pain. Use with caution in patients with cardiac disease (as arrhythmias may follow the use of tricyclics) and avoid in diabetics, epileptics, and pregnant or breast-feeding women. It can precipitate glaucoma, ↑ the effect of alcohol, and cause drowsiness (which can impair driving). In common with other tricyclics it can cause sedation, blurred vision, xerostomia, constipation, nausea, and difficulty with micturition, although tolerance to these side-effects tends to develop as Rx progresses. There is often an interval of 2–4 weeks before these drugs reach a level that exhibits a clinically evident antidepressant effect. *Dose:* 50–75mg either as a single dose nocte or in divided doses, maximum 150–200mg daily. Children and elderly, half-dose.

Dosulepin has similar properties and unwanted effects to amitryptiline. It has, however, been demonstrated to be of value in the Rx of 'facial arthromyalgia' (a composite group of TMPDS and atypical facial-pain patients).[2] *Dose:* initially 75mg nocte, increasing to 150mg daily if needed. Half-dose in elderly.

Nortriptyline A less sedating tricyclic. *Dose:* 10–30mg nocte; can be increased.

Tranylcypromine A MAOI that may be of value in treating facial pain unresponsive to tricyclics. *Dose:* 10mg tds before 16.00 hours.[3]

MAOIs can precipitate a hypertensive crisis induced by dietary and drug interactions (sympathomimetics, opioids, especially pethidine, and foods containing tyramine, e.g. cheese, meat, or yeast extracts). LA is, however, safe.

Selective serotonin re-uptake inhibitors (SSRIs) Much less-sedative antidepressants, given as single dose a.m. Fluoxetine (Prozac®) is best known (20mg daily) and also abused (overprescribing and used to prolong effects of MDMA or Ecstasy). Paroxetine 20mg mane, sertraline 50mg mane and citalopram 20 mg mane (available as oral drops—8mg/4drops = 10mg tablet) are similar.

---

1 DPF 2000–02. In BNF **40** 2000.

2 C. Feinmann 1984 *BDJ* **156** 205.

3 M. Harris 1993 *BDJ* **174** 129.

Antiemetics

There are no antiemetics prescribable in the DPF; however, they form an essential part of in-patient hospital prescribing. The common indication is the control of post-op nausea and vomiting, which may be due to the procedure, anaesthetic, post-op analgesia, or blood in the stomach.

Prochlorperazine A phenothiazine antiemetic which acts as a dopamine antagonist and acts at the chemoreceptor trigger zone. Avoid in small children as the drug's major side-effect, the production of extrapyramidal symptoms, is especially common in this group. *Dose*: 12.5mg IM 8 hourly, 20mg initially followed by 10mg tds PO. Buccal absorption 3–6mg bd. Not licensed for IV use.

Metoclopramide has both peripheral and central modes of action. It ↑ gut motility, thus emptying the stomach. Acute dystonic reactions may occur, especially in young women and children; a bizarre acute trismus is sometimes seen as one of the manifestations. *Dose*: 10mg tds PO, 10mg IM 8 hourly. High-dose intermittent and continuous IV regimens are used for antiemesis in centres using cytotoxic chemotherapy.

Domperidone is less likely to cause central unwanted effects such as sedation and dystonia, as it does not cross the blood–brain barrier. Acts on the chemoreceptor trigger zone and is particularly useful for chemotherapy patients. *Dose*: 10mg 4 hourly. May be used as part of a combination regimen, e.g. domperidone, prednisolone, and nabilone (a synthetic cannabinoid).

Ondansetron A selective 5-HT$_3$ receptor antagonist very effective in prevention and Rx of post-op nausea and vomiting. *Dose*: 4mg single IV dose or 8mg PO. Granisetron and tropisetron are similar 5-HT$_3$ receptor antagonists.

Hyoscine, antihistamines, and major tranquillizers all have antiemetic properties but are rarely indicated. If unable to control emesis with one agent use two, acting at separate sites *after* excluding intestinal obstruction, e.g. due to opioid constipation.

Cyclizine is an antihistamine and is often combined with opioid preparations as an antiemetic—however, it can aggravate heart failure. Cheap. *Dose*: 50mg tds IM or PO.

Do not forget the benefits of a nasogastric tube in preventing nausea and vomiting from a distended or irritated stomach. Constipation can also cause nausea—remember to exclude it as a cause.

Anxiolytics, sedatives, hypnotics, and tranquillizers

The short-term control of fear and anxiety associated with dental Rx is an entirely appropriate use of the benzodiazepines. It should not be confused with the long-term control of anxiety which is rife with problems of dependence and drug withdrawal. A benzodiazepine may also be a valuable adjunct in the management of TMPDS, where it acts as both a muscle relaxant and an anxiolytic ([ ] p. 446). IV and oral sedative techniques prior to surgery, [ ] p. 594.

Diazepam Has long half-life and is cumulative on repeated dosing. Like all benzodiazepines, can cause respiratory depression, therefore patients should be warned not to drive or operate machinery while on this drug. *Dose for anxiety/TMPDS*: 2mg tds, maximum 30mg in divided daily doses. Paradoxical disinhibition may occur in children and its use in the <16s is not advised. Diazepam in lipid emulsion (Diazemuls®) is the IV Rx of choice in status epilepticus ([ ] p. 531). A rectal preparation is popular for paediatric sedation in some countries ([ ] p. 592).

Midazolam water-soluble benzodiazepine of about double the potency of diazepam. Its main use is in IV sedation ([ ] p. 592). Also popular as a paediatric sedative for suture removal.

Nitrazepam A long-acting hypnotic which tends to cause a hangover effect. *Dose*: 5–10mg nocte.

Temazepam Shorter-acting hypnotic. *Dose*: 10–30mg nocte. Main indication is pre-op or as pre-medication. An OP sedation technique is described, [ ] p. 594. Gelatine capsule preparations should no longer be used as they can be melted down for IV abuse.

In hospital practice

The following may also be prescribed:

Chlordiazepoxide Sometimes used instead of diazepam in TMPDS. It has the same side-effect profile. *Dose*: 10mg tds, ↑ to maximum of 100mg daily, in divided doses. It is drug of choice in the stabilization of alcohol-dependent in-patients.

Lorazepam Sometimes used as a pre-med by anaesthetists. *Dose*: 2mg nocte, 2mg 1h pre-op. Alternative to diazepam in epileptics.

Chlormethiazole A hypnotic sometimes used to ↓ severe insomnia in the elderly. *Dose*: 1–2 capsules nocte (each cap = 192mg). Main indication is in management of alcohol withdrawal. Regimen: day 1: 3 caps qds; day 2: 2 caps qds; day 3: 1 cap qds. Acute withdrawal is sometimes managed by IV infusion; however, this is a dangerous technique, not to be undertaken lightly.

Zopiclone A non-benzodiazepine hypnotic. *Dose*: 7.5mg nocte. Problems similar to benzodiazepines. May be of practical help when local policy controls use of temazepam.

Haloperidol Very useful in control of acute psychosis, in a dose of 10–20mg stat IM. Less painful than, and does the same job as chlorpromazine, but main problem is extrapyramidal side-effects.

Flumazenil A specific benzodiazepine reversal agent (📖 p. 592). Dosages should be ↓ in elderly. Avoid in children.

Trimeprazine (alimemazine) An antihistamine; a useful sedative for children. *Dose*: 2–3mg/kg 1–2h pre-op.

Chloral hydrate (Chloral Elixir, paediatric) 5ml used as a sedative for removing facial sutures. Oral midazolam is an alternative.

Antibiotics—1

Principles of antibiotic use

When prescribing, consider: (i) the patient; (ii) the likely organisms; (iii) the best drug. Patients influence choice, in that they may be allergic to various drugs, have hepatic or renal impairment, be immunocompromised, be unable to swallow, be pregnant or breast-feeding, or taking an oral contraceptive; consider also age and severity of the infection. The infecting organism should ideally be isolated, cultured, and its sensitivity to antibiotics determined, but this is only feasible in hospital practice. In reality, most infections are treated blind, therefore it is essential to know the common infecting organisms in your field, and their sensitivities. You also need to know the drugs' modes of action, absorption, unwanted effects, development of resistance, interactions, and techniques available for delivery. The best drug is the one which is safe in that patient, specific to the infecting organism, and can be given in a reliable convenient form. Remember prophylaxis (☐ p. 548) differs from Rx with antibiotics, and antibiotics do not replace the drainage of pus in abscesses.

Benzylpenicillin Inactive orally and only used IM or IV. *Dose:* 600–1200mg IV/IM qds. Drug of choice in streptococcal infections. Like all penicillins is bactericidal: it interferes with cell-wall synthesis. Good tissue penetration except for CSF. Most important unwanted effect is hypersensitivity, which is usually manifested as a rash, rarely as fatal anaphylaxis. Patients allergic to one penicillin will be allergic to all; theoretically 10% will be allergic to cephalosporins as well. A history of atopy (e.g. asthma) ↑ risk.

DPF prescribable antibiotics

Phenoxymethyl penicillin Oral equivalent of above. *Dose:* 250–500mg qds PO. Has a narrow spectrum, but is now largely superseded by

Amoxicillin Has a broad spectrum similar to **ampicillin**, but is better absorbed and achieves higher tissue concentrations. *Dose:* 250–500mg tds PO. Both ampicillin and amoxicillin cause a maculopapular rash in patients with glandular fever, lymphatic leukaemia, or possibly HIV infection (this is **not** true penicillin allergy). Amoxicillin was drug of choice in prophylaxis against infective endocarditis (☐ p. 548). May interfere with the action of oral contraceptives. All penicillins decrease excretion of methotrexate, therefore ↑ risk of toxicity.

Tetracycline One of a group of broad-spectrum antibiotics with a problem of ↑ bacterial resistance. It is likely to promote opportunistic infection with *Candida albicans*, particularly when used topically, as has been recommended for the Rx of aphthae. Other problems are the deposition of tetracyclines in growing bone and teeth, causing staining and hypoplasia (therefore avoid in children <12yrs and pregnancy) and erythema multiforme. It is also particularly likely to render the oral contraceptive ineffective. *Dose:* 250–500mg qds PO. Absorption inhibited by chelation with milk, etc., therefore should be taken well before food. May be of value in periodontal disease (☐ p. 202). Doxycycline 200mg day 1, then 100mg od PO and oxytetracycline 250–5000mg qds PO are prescribable.

Erythromycin A similar spectrum to penicillin, but bacteriostatic. Active against penicillinase-producing organisms. Formerly an alternative to amoxicillin for endocarditis prophylaxis (superseded by clindamycin). Nausea is a major problem. *Dose:* 250–500mg qds PO/IV.

Oral cephalosporins Of little value in dental practice, but cefalexin 250–500mg bd or tds PO and cefradine 250–500mg qds PO are prescribable. Clindamycin and metronidazole are also in DPF (see p. 572).

Antibiotics—2

Clindamycin Should be used cautiously in the management of dental infections, due to the risk of antibiotic-induced colitis. Useful in staphylococcal osteomyelitis in conjunction with metronidazole (which inhibits overgrowth with *Clostridium difficile*). Has replaced erythromycin for single-dose prophylaxis of infective endocarditis (📖 p. 548) when indicated.

Metronidazole An anaerobicidal drug, and as such effective in many acute dental and oral infections. Classical dose for NUG is 200mg tds PO 3 days. For other anaerobic infections is more often used as 400mg bd/tds (depending on severity) PO. Available in tablets, IV infusion, or suppository. Main problem is severe nausea and vomiting if taken in conjunction with alcohol (disulfiram reaction). Remember, it is NOT effective against aerobic bacteria.

Antibiotics of use in hospital practice
(in addition to the aforementioned)

Flucloxacillin A penicillin active against penicillinase-producing bacteria. Dose: 250–500mg qds PO/IV. Can be combined with ampicillin as co-fluampicil.

Co-amoxiclav Is amoxicillin plus clauvulanic acid. The latter destroys beta-lactamase (penicillinase) and hence widens the range of amoxicillin to include the commonest cause of resistance in infections of the head and neck. Dose: 1–2 tabs tds PO or 600–1200mg tds IV. Problems as for amoxicillin.

Cefuroxime A parenteral broad-spectrum cephalosporin often used in combination with metronidazole for surgical prophylaxis in contaminated head and neck procedures. Dose: 750–1500mg tds IV (500mg bd PO).

Gentamicin A bactericidal aminoglycoside antibiotic, active mainly against Gram –ve organisms. Complementary to the penicillins and available as a topical (ear use) or parenteral preparation. Major problem is dose-related ototoxicity and nephrotoxicity (monitor levels if used for >24h). Dose: up to 5mg/kg monitored use local guidelines. Endocarditis prophylaxis, 📖 p. 548.

Co-trimoxazole Has few indications in the head and neck which have not been replaced by trimethoprim alone (200mg bd). It is used, however, in ear, sinus, and urinary infections, but C/I in pregnancy and folate deficiency (as it is a folate antagonist).

Chloramphenicol Useful topically in bacterial conjunctivitis (0.5% eye drops, 1% eye ointment, apply 3 hourly). Systemic use is strictly limited due to toxicity. Ointment is an excellent wound dressing.

Vancomycin A unique bactericidal antibiotic. Two main uses are orally in the Rx of antibiotic-induced colitis (125mg qds 10 days PO), and for prophylaxis of patients at high risk from infective endocarditis (📖 p. 548). Ototoxic, nephrotoxic, prone to cause phlebitis at infusion sites, and makes people feel generally unwell, therefore not to be used lightly.

Teicoplanin Similar to vancomycin. Lasts longer. Can be given IV or IM. Fewer unwanted effects and kinder on patient, but more expensive.

Antifungal and antiviral drugs

Antifungals

The main fungal pathogen in the mouth is *Candida albicans* (🕮 p. 400).

Amphotericin Best used as lozenges 10mg dissolved slowly in the mouth qds 10–15 days. Double dose if needed.

Nystatin Available as pastilles or mixture. *Dose:* 100 000 units qds either by sucking a pastille qds or using 1ml of the mixture and holding it in the mouth before swallowing.

Miconazole Useful drug, particularly in management of angular cheilitis, as it is active against streptococci, staphylococci, and candida. Miconazole oral gel 24mg/ml is of use in chronic mucocutaneous and chronic hyperplastic candidosis. *Dose:* place 5–10ml in the mouth and hold near the lesions before swallowing, qds. Miconazole cream is used topically for angular cheilitis.

Fluconazole Available in both oral and IV formulations for severe mucosal candidosis in both normal and immunocompromised patients as a second line to topical preparations. Avoid in pregnancy. *Dose:* 50mg od PO 7–14 days, 200–400mg IV od. Itraconazole, posaconazole and voriconazole are other new antifungal drugs.

There are recognized potentially serious interactions between miconazole, fluconazole, and related drugs and: antibacterials, anticoagulants, antidiabetics, antiepileptics, antihistamines, anxiolytics, cisapride, ciclosporin, and theophylline. Check what your patient is currently taking. Candidal resistance to fluconazole is now recognized—get C&S if Rx not working.

Antivirals

Most viral infections are treated symptomatically. Herpes labialis is the viral condition most often seen and treated by dentists.

Aciclovir Active against herpes simplex and zoster; relatively non-toxic and can be given systemically or topically. *Dose:* herpes labialis: apply aciclovir cream to site of prodromal or early lesion 4 hourly for 5 days; herpetic stomatitis: 200mg (400mg in immunocompromised) PO 5 times daily for 5 days; herpes zoster: 800mg PO 5 times daily for 7 days.

Penciclovir as a 1% cream applied 2 hourly for 4 days is prescribable on the DPF for herpes labialis.

Idoxuridine Available as idoxuridine 5% in dimethyl sulfoxide. Regarded as being of little value nowadays. Other anti-herpes drugs include: **famciclovir** and **valaciclovir** (both pro-drugs). **Ganciclovir** Active against all herpesviruses, EBV, and CMV; however, it is very toxic and therefore has no indications in dentistry. HIV infection, there is no known cure but combinations of drugs slow or halt disease progression. 19 different antiretrovirals were in use in 2007. These can be used (unlicensed) for post exposure prophylaxis. Get immediate expert advice if in this situation. Lipodystrophy syndrome is associated with antiretroviral therapy. **Inosine pranobex** is licensed for use in treating mucocutaneous herpes simplex in conjunction with podophyllin. **Interferon** is an interesting drug, with no indications in dentistry.

Antihistamines and decongestants

Antihistamines

Rarely used in the usual range of dental practice. Sometimes indicated in the management of allergy, especially hayfever, for pre-medication and sedation in children, occasionally as antiemetics, possibly in the management of over-active gag reflex, and as part of the emergency Rx of angio-oedema and anaphylaxis (🕮 p. 528). Main differences between the antihistamines are duration of action and degree of accompanying sedation and antimuscarinic effects.

Chlorphenamine A sedative antihistamine. Dose: 4mg qds PO.

Promethazine Also a sedative antihistamine. Dose: 10–20mg 2–3 times bd/tds PO or 20–30mg nocte when used as a hypnotic. On sale to the public as a hypnotic.

The sedative effects of these drugs potentiate alcohol and ability to drive or operate machinery safely. They should be used with caution in glaucoma, prostatic hypertrophy, and epilepsy.

Although these drugs are available in the DPF, probably the most useful antihistamines are not. These include:

A wide range of non-sedating antihistamines; e.g. cetirizine, loratadine are available as OTC generics to the public, largely replacing terfenadine due to its greater unwanted effects.

Trimeprazine (alimemazine) A sedative antihistamine which may be of some value in the itching of uraemia, and occasionally used by anaesthetists as a pre-med in children. Adult dose: 10mg bd/tds; paediatric pre-med: 5–10mg, dependent on age.

Decongestants

Valuable in the management of sinusitis and particularly in the closure of oro-antral fistulae.

Ephedrine nasal drops Produce vasoconstriction of mucosal blood vessels and ↓ the thickness of nasal mucosa, thus relieving obstruction. Avoid in patients taking MAOIs. Other problems: prolonged use leads to a rebound vasodilatation and a recurrence of nasal congestion, and long-term use results in tolerance and damage to nasal cilia. Dose: ephedrine nasal drops 0.5–1%, 1–2 drops into the relevant nostril qds for 7–10 days. For symptomatic nasal decongestion and as an adjunct to the management of oro-antral fistulae (🕮 p. 384) inhalation of menthol and eucalyptus is valuable. Dose: 1 teaspoonful of menthol and eucalyptus inhalation BP is added to a pint of hot water, and the warm, moist air is inhaled with a towel over the head.

Xylometazoline and oxymetazoline nasal drops and spray 0.1% are a more potent alternative to ephedrine, but more likely to cause a rebound effect. Systemic decongestants are of dubious value and contain sympathomimetics. They do not, however, cause rebound. For prescribed, short-term use, thereby avoiding risk of rebound, xylometazoline or oxymetazoline are drugs of choice; spray into relevant nostril tds.

Miscellaneous

A number of drugs not fitting into any specific category are important in managing oral and dental disease. These include:

Carbamazepine Primarily an antiepileptic drug which is of considerable value in the management of trigeminal and glosso-pharyngeal neuralgia. C/I in those sensitive to the drug, patients with atrioventricular conduction defects, porphyria, and should be used with extreme caution in patients on MAOIs, who are pregnant, or who have liver failure. May interfere with the oral contraceptive. Common unwanted effects are gastrointestinal disturbances, dizziness, and visual disturbances. Rarely, rashes may occur, as can leukopenia. Do a FBC soon after starting carbamezipine: blood dyscrasias usually occur in the first 3 months. *Dose:* 100–200mg bd; can be ↑ gradually to 200mg tds/ qds. Maximum 1600mg daily in divided doses. Important to be sure of your diagnosis before starting patients on long-term carbamezipine (🕮 p. 426). A slow-release preparation with fewer unwanted effects is available.

Vitamins There is no indication for first-line Rx with vitamins in dental practice. Deficiency due to inadequate dietary intake in the UK is exceedingly rare. Although it can occur in the elderly and alcoholics, these people should be fully investigated and not treated empirically. Severe gingival swelling, stomatitis, glossitis, or pain should be fully investigated before using vitamin supplements. The only preparations available in the DPF are:

- Vitamin B compound tablets, strong A combination of nicotinamide 20mg, pyridoxine 2mg, riboflavin 2mg, thiamine 5mg. *Dose:* 1–2 tablets tds.
- Ascorbic acid tablets BP (vitamin C) ↑ iron absorption and prevents scurvy.

Artificial saliva Valuable adjunct in the management of xerostomia, especially after radiotherapy and in Sjögren syndrome. A slightly viscous, inert fluid which may have a number of additives, such as antimicrobial preservatives, fluoride, flavouring, etc. Useful preparations are Glandosane® and Saliva Orthana®, aerosol sprays sprayed sublingually 4–6 times per day. The latter contains fluoride. Saliva Natura® is an 'organic' alternative. Regular sips of water may be of more practical long-term help. DPF has Artificial Saliva DPF 60ml unit. Use: all should be sprayed into the floor of mouth area to act as a 'puddle' for redistribution. Do not spray all over mucosa. Use qds.

Topical anaesthetics Two main uses:
1 For preparation of a site prior to injection, e.g. of LA. Lidocaine 5% ointment or spray is the most useful. Flavoured benzocaine pastes are available in some countries (not UK).
2 EMLA and amethocaine (Ametop®) can be used on mucosa. Carmellose gelatin paste acting as a mechanical barrier is useful in areas where it will adhere. Many OTC agents are available; few are of great potency. To ↓ pain from minor oral lesions (e.g. for HSV 1 or aphthae). Benzydamine rinse is a mainstay.

Fluorides Fluoride supplementation is discussed on 📖 p. 28. It is important when using rinses, and particularly gels, that the fluid is not swallowed, since there is a risk of toxicity (📖 p. 30).

Retinoids Used in some centres to manage erosive lichen planus and leuko-plakia; have proved disappointing.

Alarm bells

When prescribing any drug for patients already compromised by concomitant disease or drug therapy, it is essential to exclude possible interactions. This can be achieved fairly quickly by consulting the comprehensive BNF.

Interactions with the most commonly given drug (LA) are covered on p. 584.

Common drugs with relative contraindications in renal disease	Common drugs with relative contraindications in liver failure
Aspirin	Aciclovir (↓ dose)
All benzodiazepines	All penicillins (↓ dose)
All opioids	All opioids
All sedatives	Amphotericin
All antihistamines	Cephalosporins (↓ dose)
All NSAIDs	Co-trimoxazole (↓ dose)
Erythromycin	Benzodiazepines (↓ dose)
Metronidazole (↓ dose)	NSAIDs
Paracetamol	Tetracyclines
Tetracyclines	
Fexofenadine	

Common drugs with relative contraindications in pregnancy	Common drugs with relative contraindications in breast-feeding
Aspirin	Antihistamines
Benzodiazepines	Aspirin
Carbamezipine	Benzodiazepines
All opioids	Carbamezepine
Co-trimoxazole	Co-trimoxazole
NSAIDs	Metronidazole
Metronidazole	Tetracyclines
Tetracyclines	

These lists are not comprehensive and some of the drugs mentioned can be used in suitably modified dose or under specific circumstances. These tables are designed to ring alarm bells, and encourage you to both think and consult the BNF.

Adverse reactions

Almost any drug can produce these, and many are missed. Try to avoid polypharmacy, and never prescribe without being aware of a patient's full medical history. Always enquire about drugs, including self-prescribed medication.

Report suspected adverse reactions to Medicines and Healthcare products Regulatory Agency (MHRA): email: info@mhra.gsi.gov.uk, phone: 0800 731 6789, or in writing to:

CSM Freepost, London SW8 5BR
CSM West Midlands SW 2991, Freepost, Birmingham B18 7BR
CSM Mersey, Freepost, Liverpool L3 3AB
CSM Northern, Freepost, Newcastle NE1 1BR
CSM Wales, Freepost, Cardiff CF4 1ZZs

Report • **all** serious adverse reactions;
• **any** reactions to 'black triangled' drugs in the BNF/DPF.

Emergency drugs

Oxygen	Cylinder size D (3401) or E (6801) plus reducing valve, flow-meter, tubing, and oxygen mask
Adrenaline	1mg in 1ml (1:1000) solution (IM injection)
Hydrocortisone sodium succinate	100mg powder, plus 2ml water for injection (IM injection)
Chlorphenamine maleate	10mg in 1ml solution (IM injection)
Glucagon	1mg powder, plus 1ml water for injection (IM injection)
Glucose or sugar	Drink, tablets, or gel (PO administration)
Salbutamol inhaler	0.1mg per dose (INH administration)
Glyceryl trinitrate	0.5mg tablets or 0.4mg per dose spray (SUB administration)
Aspirin	300mg tablets (PO administration)
Midazolam	10mg in 2ml solution (IV/IM injection)

Drugs influencing dental treatment

Warfarin Although many patients are taking anticoagulants (aspirin, clopidogrel) warfarin is the drug which excites most concern. Although an evidence base exists suggesting that there is no significant increase in post-extraction bleeding in patients with an INR within the reference range (2–4) and many regions' oral & maxillofacial surgery units routine practice is to perform extractions as normal for patients on warfarin with an INR of <4, some controversy still exists. BNF 53 recommends this practice only if the INR <3 but gives no reason for this.

In general there is no greater risk if performing small numbers of extractions in patients anticoagulated with warfarin if the INR<4. Local measures such as packing the socket with oxidized cellulose and suturing gingivae with local pressure will achieve haemostasis. Patients with an INR >4 should be referred to their anticoagulant clinic or physician. Patients requiring multiple extractions or with other significant co-morbidities should be seen in an area which can provide a higher level of care.

Bisphosphonates

These are a range of drugs which act on osteoclasts and reduce the rate of bone turnover. They bind to hydroxyapatite and their effect is therefore extremely long term (possibly up to 10 years). They are an important group of drugs in the prophylaxis and treatment of osteoporosis, steroid-induced osteoporosis, Paget's disease, bone metastases (particularly breast, myeloma and prostate) and hypercalcaemia of malignancy.

They come in differing degrees of potency, non-nitrogen containing oral preparations being the least potent and nitrogen containing IV preparations being the most. Osteoporosis tends to be managed with less potent drugs and hypercalcaemia and bone metastases with the most.

Bisphosphonate Related Osteonecrosis of the Jaws (BRON) is a condition where alveolar bone is exposed in the mouth in patients taking these drugs. The condition appears to be progressive and there is no established effective treatment although several are being investigated. Bone necrosis without mucosal beach is also now being described. The incidence is variable but is probably less than 1% for patients treated with low potency drugs for osteoporosis up to 30% for myeloma survivors at 10 years who have received highly potent drugs and who have had extractions.

Prevention is the most useful management strategy and all patients prior to starting bisphosphonates should have optimum dental health established such that it is highly unlikely they will ever need to have a tooth removed in the future. This is a shift away from the 'benefit of the doubt' approach most dentists are currently trained in. The nearest comparable approach is in the prevention of osteoradionecrosis.

Management of established BRON 📖 p. 352.

Bisphosphonate preparations currently available and their relative potency

	Primary indication	Nitrogen containing	Dose	
Etidronate (Didronel®)	Paget's Disease	No	5mg/kg Daily for 6 months	1
Sodium clodronate (Bonefos®/ Loron®)	Myeloma Bone mets (breast)	No	1600mg daily	10
Tiludronate (Skelid®)	Paget's Disease	No	400mg daily For 3 months	50
Alendronate (Fosamax®)	Osteoporosis	Yes	10mg/day 70mg/week	1000
Risedronate (Actonel®)	Osteoporosis	Yes	5mg/day 35mg/week	1000
Ibandronate (Bonviva®/ Bondronat)	Osteoporosis Bone metastases	Yes	150mg po/month 3mg iv/3 monthly 50mg po od 6mg iv/3 weekly	1000
Pamidronate (Aredia®)	Bone metastases	Yes	90mg/3week	1000–5000
Zoledronate (Zometa®)	Bone metastases	Yes	4mg/3 weeks	10 000+

Analgesia, anaesthesia, and sedation

Contents

NB Since the report of the GDC in 2001[1] the status of general anaesthesia in dental practice, and inevitably the medico-legal aspects of anaesthesia and sedation in the UK have altered considerably. This varies widely from country to country. General principles, however, remain the same.

Relevant pages in other chapters LA for children, 📖 p. 78; emergencies in dental practice, 📖 p. 520.

Principal sources D.A. Mitchell 2006 *An Introduction to Oral & Maxillofacial Surgery* (Chapter 4), OUP. Standing Committee on Sedation in Dentistry 2007 Standards *for conscious sedation in dentistry: alternative techniques* ℘ www.rcseng.ac.uk/fds/docs/SCSDAT%202007.pdf

Definitions
General anaesthesia (GA) A state of unrousable unconsciousness to which analgesia and muscle relaxation is added to produce 'balanced anaesthesia'.
Analgesia The absence of pain.
Sedation An altered level of consciousness in which the patient, although awake, has a ↓ level of fear and anxiety.

---

1 GDC *Maintaining Standards: General Anaesthesia and Resuscitation* (Amendment November 2001).

Indications, contraindications, and common sense

When dealing with LA, GA, and sedative techniques, indications, and contraindications are often relative, and the following should be thought of as guidelines rather than immutable laws.

LA

The technique of choice for simple procedures or when a GA is C/I. LA is C/I in:

- uncooperative patients (of any description)
- infection around the injection site
- patients with a major bleeding diathesis
- most major surgery

Adverse reaction to LA is a C/I, but in reality once allergy to preservatives in the solution is excluded, LA allergy probably does not exist.

Conscious sedation

This is an extension of LA technique using drugs and patient-management techniques. It is of benefit to anxious or mildly uncooperative patients and is a kind supplement to apicectomy or third-molar removal. C/I include:

- Cardiorespiratory, renal, liver, or psychiatric pathology.
- An unescorted patient or one unable or unwilling to conform to the requirements of conscious sedation (🕮 p. 594).
- A demonstrated adverse reaction to sedative agents.
- Pregnancy, during which benzodiazepines should be avoided.

GA

Indicated when LA or LA and sedation is ineffective or inappropriate (as above). C/I include:

- All those for conscious sedation.
- Presence of food or fluid in the stomach (most anaesthetists require at least 6h fasting after food and 4h after fluid).

The anaesthetist usually prefers hospital admission for patients with the following:

- Cardiovascular or respiratory disease (especially MI <6 months ago).
- Uncorrected anaemia, sickle cell trait or disease.
- Severe liver or renal impairment.
- Uncontrolled thyrotoxicosis or hypothyroidism.
- Poorly controlled diabetes, adrenocortical suppression.
- Porphyria.
- Pregnancy.
- Neurological disorders, e.g. myopathy or multiple sclerosis.
- Cervical spine pathology such as rheumatoid arthritis or cervical spondylosis.
- Certain drugs, e.g. steroids, antihypertensives, MAOIs, anti-coagulants, narcotic analgesics, antiepileptics (need to avoid using methohexitone), lithium, alcohol. Malignant hyperpyrexia, scoline apnoea, and other unwanted reactions to anaesthetic agents.

- Causes of upper airway obstruction such as angio-oedema, submandibular cellulitis, Ludwig's angina, and bleeding diathesis affecting the neck. (In fact, these are indications to secure the upper airway).
- Previous problems with anaesthesia.

Ask about previous GA and any problems.

While all these conditions create problems with anaesthesia they may not preclude it absolutely within the hospital setting. They do, however, indicate the need for careful assessment and early prior consultation with the anaesthetist.

Local analgesia—tools of the trade

While any disposable needle and syringe system can be used to give LA, the vast number of LAs given in dental practice (>50 000/dentist/lifetime) has led to some very useful modifications.

LA cartridges Two sizes, 1.8 and 2.2ml, come pre-sterilized. Commonest solution used is lidocaine 2% with adrenaline 1:80 000. A latex-free version is available for patients with latex allergy.[1]

Cartridge syringes Use with above, resterilizable. Used with ultra-fine disposable needles. Major advantage is the ability to perform controlled aspiration during LA injection (although the consistency with which this is achieved has been questioned).

Lidocaine/adrenaline Most commonly used preparation (2% lidocaine 1:80 000 adrenaline), gives effective pulpal analgesia for 1.5h and altered soft-tissue sensation for up to 3h. Extremely safe; maximum dose (adult) 500mg (10 x 2.2ml cartridges). Also available in ampoules 1% + 2% lidocaine plain or 1:200 000 adrenaline. There are theoretical criticisms that the maximum dose is too high but these have not been borne out in practice.

Prilocaine/octapressin Similar but slightly less duration and effect compared to lidocaine/adrenaline. May cause methaemoglobinaemia in excess. Maximum safe dose (adult) 600mg (8 x 2.2ml cartridges). In reality, there are few hard indications for the use of prilocaine over lidocaine.

Mepivacaine Short-acting LA advocated for restorative work but has not really caught on. Maximum safe dose 400mg.

Bupivacaine Long-acting LA (6h plain, 8h with adrenaline); useful as a post-op analgesic. Maximum safe dose 2mg/kg. Only available in ampoules. Levobupivacaine is a similar drug.

Articaine At least as effective as lidocaine; said to diffuse through bone better. No hard evidence of superiority however not recommended for IDB due to cases of permanent altered sensation after its use.

Topical analgesics Lidocaine is the only really useful topical analgesic among the above. It is available as a spray or a paste which is applied to mucosa several minutes prior to injecting. There is a high incidence of contact eczema in people frequently exposed to these preparations, so do not apply with bare fingers. Benzocaine in lozenge or paste form is used for mucosal analgesia. Amethocaine is a topical analgesic for use on mucous membranes. Cocaine 4% solution is used as a nasal mucosal analgesic and vasoconstrictor.

1 Astra Pharmaceuticals.

EMLA® cream, a eutectic mix of lidocaine and prilocaine, is an invaluable skin topical analgesic, used prior to venepuncture in children. Apply to puncture site and cover with 'Opsite' or equivalent dressing for at least 30min. Amethocaine (Ametop) is similar and has a quicker onset of action.

Handling equipment One cartridge and needle per patient. Discard cartridge if a precipitant is seen in the solution or if air bubbles are present. Store in a cool dark place and use before expiry date. Warm cartridge to ↓ discomfort and load into the syringe immediately prior to use. Aspirate before injecting. The ↑ risk associated with needlestick injuries has spawned a number of devices to aid resheathing the needle. It is simpler to hold the cover in a pair of artery forceps.

Local analgesia—techniques

The inferior dental block and local infiltrations are the mainstay of LA technique; however, numerous others are available as alternatives, supplements, and fallbacks.

IDB (inferior alveolar block) Technique of choice for mandibular molars; also effective for premolars, canines, and incisors (the latter if supplemented by infiltration). Aim is to deposit solution around the inferior alveolar nerve as it enters the mandibular foramen underneath the lingula. The patient's mouth must be widely open. Palpate the landmarks of external and internal oblique ridges and note the line of the ptyerygomandibular raphe. With the palpating thumb lying in the retromolar fossa, the needle should be inserted at the midpoint of the tip of the thumb slightly above the occlusal plane lateral to the ptyerygomandibular raphe. The needle is inserted ~0.5cm and if a *lingual nerve block* is required 0.5ml of LA is injected at this point. The syringe is then moved horizontally ~40° across the dorsum of the tongue and advanced to make contact with the lingula. Once bony contact is made the needle is withdrawn slightly and the remainder of the LA injected. It should never be necessary to insert the needle up to the hub. Note that the mandibular foramen varies in position with age (children, 📖 see p. 78). In the edentulous, the foramen, and hence the point of needle insertion, is relatively higher than in the dentate.

Gow–Gates technique Blocks sensation in Vc by depositing LA at head of condyle.[1] Akinosi approach: LA deposited above lingula.[2]

Long buccal block The long buccal nerve is anaesthetized by injecting 0.5–1ml of LA posterior and buccal to the last molar tooth.

Mental nerve block The mental nerve emerges from the mental foramen lying apical to and between the first and second mandibular premolars. LA injected in this region will diffuse in through the mental foramen and provide limited analgesia of premolars and canine, and to a lesser degree, incisors on that side. It will provide effective soft-tissue analgesia. Place the lip on tension and insert the needle parallel to the long axis of the premolars angling towards bone, and deposit the LA. **Do not** attempt to inject into the mental foramen as this may traumatize the nerve. LA can be encouraged in by massage.

Sublingual nerve block An anterior extension of the lingual nerve can be blocked by placing the needle just submucosally lingual to the premolars, use 0.5ml of LA.

Posterior superior alveolar block A rarely indicated technique. Needle is inserted distal to the upper second molar and advanced inwards, backwards, and upwards close to bone for ~2cm. LA is deposited high above the tuberosity after aspirating to avoid the ptyerygoid plexus.

1 Gow–Gates 1973 *OS, OM, OP* **36** 321.
2 Akinosi 1977 *BJOS* **15** 83.

Nasopalatine block Profound anaesthesia can be achieved by passing the needle through the incisive papilla and injecting a small amount of solution. This is extremely painful (hints on how to overcome pain on palatal injections below).

Infra-orbital block Rarely indicated. Palpate the inferior margin of the orbit as the infra-orbital foramen lies ~1cm below the deepest point of the orbital margin. Hold the index finger at this point while the upper lip is lifted with the thumb. Inject in the depth of the buccal sulcus towards your finger, avoid your finger, and deposit LA around the infra-orbital nerve.

Infiltrations The aim is to deposit LA supraperiosteally in as close proximity as possible to the apex of the tooth to be anaesthetized. The LA will diffuse through periosteum and bone to bathe the nerves entering the apex. Reflect the lip or cheek to place mucosa on tension and insert the needle along the long axis of the tooth aiming towards bone. At approximate apex of tooth, withdraw slightly and deposit LA slowly. For palatal infiltrations, achieve buccal analgesia first and infiltrate interdental papillae; then penetrate palatal mucosa and deposit small amount of LA under force.

Intraligamentary analgesia Individual teeth can be rendered pain free by injecting small amounts of LA along the periodontal membrane via a specially designed system (high-pressure syringe and ultra-fine needles). Has the advantage of rapid onset and specific analgesia to isolated teeth; it is a useful adjunct to conventional LA and in some hands may replace it for minor procedures. Disadvantages include post-injection discomfort due to temporary extrusion and an apparent ↑ incidence in 'dry socket'.

Intraosseous analgesia A recently reintroduced technique which produces profound single-tooth analgesia. Needs specialized equipment and technique.

▶ When developing LA technique there is no alternative to seeing, doing, and doing again.

Local analgesia—problems and hints

Failure of anaesthesia

There are enormous differences in individual response to a standard dose of LA, both in the speed of onset, duration of action, and the depth. Soft-tissue analgesia is more easily obtained, needing a lower degree of penetration of solution into nerve bundles, than does analgesia from pulpal stimulation. A numb lip does not therefore indicate pulpal anaesthesia.

Causes of failure are:

- Poor technique and inadequate volume of LA.
- Injection into a muscle (will result in trismus which resolves spontaneously).
- Injection into an infected area (which should not be done anyway as this risks spreading the infection).
- Intravascular injection; clearly of no analgesic benefit. Small amounts of intravascular LA cause few problems. Toxicity, 📖 p. 528.
- Dense compact bone can prevent a properly given infiltration from working. Counter by using intraligamentary or regional LA.
- Infrequently, anastomosis from either aberrant or normal nerve fibres not transmitted with a blocked nerve bundle.

Pain on injection

This is to a certain degree inevitable, but can be ↓ by patient relaxation; application of topical LA; stretching the mucosa; and slow, skilful, accurate injection of slightly warmed solution in reasonable quantities. Causes of pain include:

- Touching the nerve when giving blocks, resulting in 'electric shock' sensation and followed by rapid analgesia (it is extremely rare for any permanent damage to occur).
- Injection of contaminated solutions (particularly by copper ions from a pre-loaded cartridge). Avoid by loading the cartridge immediately prior to use.
- Subperiosteal injections are painful and unnecessary, therefore avoid.

Other problems with administration

Lacerated artery May be followed by an area of ischaemia in the region supplied, or painful haematoma. Rare.

Lacerated vein Followed by a haematoma which resolves fairly quickly.

Facial palsy Can be caused by incorrect distal placement of the needle tip, allowing LA to permeate the parotid gland. The palsy lasts for the duration of the LA.

Post-injection problems

Lip and cheek trauma Tell patient to avoid smoking, drinking hot liquids, biting lip or cheek. Assure them the sensation will pass in a few hours and that their face is not swollen (whether adult or child). If the advice goes unheeded and they return with traumatized mucosa, Rx: antiseptics/antibiotics and simple analgesia.

Needle-tract infection Rare. Broad-spectrum antibiotic if needed.

General points

Thick nerve trunks require more time for penetration of solution and more volume of LA. In nerve trunks autonomic functions are blocked first, then sensitivity to temperature, followed by pain, touch, pressure, and motor function. Concentration of analgesic ↑ rapidly around the nerve at first and provides soft tissue analgesia; however, this is reached substantially before the levels needed for pulpal analgesia, which takes several minutes and will wear off first (usually within an hour of a standard lidocaine/adrenaline LA). Disinfection of mucosa prior to LA is not required in reality; however, sterile disposable needles are absolutely mandatory due to risks of cross-infection. LA for children, 📖 see p. 78. Faints, 📖 p. 521.

Sedation—relative analgesia

RA is the most commonly used and safest form of sedation in dentistry. It has two aspects: (i) the delivery of a mixture of nitrous oxide and O_2; (ii) a semi-hypnotic patter from the sedationist. In dentistry, two different techniques of nitrous oxide sedation have been described: (i) inhalational sedation with a fixed concentration of nitrous oxide; (ii) RA in which nitrous oxide is titrated to the patient. In the authors' view RA is the most useful.

Nitrous oxide

Has both sedative and analgesic properties; the former is the most useful. The analgesic effect requires high levels of nitrous oxide. It is an inert gas which does not enter any of the body's metabolic pathways and is distributed as a poorly soluble solution. This allows very rapid distribution; peak saturation is reached within 5min and is similarly eliminated (90% in 10min). Usually administered as a 50% mixture with oxygen (Entonox®) by paramedics, for analgesia the technique was modified for dentistry using one of 2 techniques; Relative Analgesia (RA) and Inhalational Sedation.

Indications It is of particular value in anxious patients undergoing relatively atraumatic procedures and in children, for whom the benzodiazepines are less suitable.

Contraindications Few, but upper airway obstruction, e.g. a cold. Pregnancy, first trimester makes the procedure difficult and pre-existing vitamin B_{12} deficiency would C/I its use. Other C/I, e.g. complex medical history, are relative and may limit nitrous oxide use in practice but not in hospital.

Nitrous oxide pollution The major problem associated with RA. It is essential to have a scavenging system in place as nitrous oxide accumulation can lead to B_{12} deficiency and demyelination syndromes. There is a real potential hazard to pregnant staff working in confined conditions with this gas.

Aim

To produce a comfortable, relaxed, AWAKE, patient who is able to open their mouth on request with no loss of consciousness or the laryngeal reflex. During the procedure patients will experience general relaxation, a tingling sensation often in the fingers or toes, and describe feeling mildly drunk. There is often a sense of detachment and distortion of the sense of time. Rarely, patients may dream despite being awake, and these can be sexual fantasies, which is another reason for always having a second person in the surgery.

Technique

An RA machine will not deliver less than 30% O_2. Start by delivering 100% O_2 via a nasal mask and set flow control to match their tidal volume (flow rates 6–8 L/min for adult, 4 L/min for child). Then give 10% nitrous oxide for 1min, ↑ (if needed) to 20% for 1min, ↑ to 30% (if needed) for 1min, and so on. Most patients achieve adequate levels of sedation at 20–30%; some may require less, a few rather more. Remember that RA relies on the reassuring banter of the operator more than any of the other sedation techniques, and many view this as hypnosedation. Give LA and carry out Rx. To discontinue, turn flow to 100% O_2 and oxygenate patient for 2min. Then remove mask and get the patient to sit in a recovery room for 10min, by which time 90% of nitrous oxide will have been blown off and they will be safe to leave the surgery.

Sedation—benzodiazepines

General pointers, problems, and hints

Benzodiazepines are both sedative and hypnotic drugs which are useful for sedation of patients. Two techniques are generally used: oral and IV.

Elderly patients tend to be very sensitive to benzodiazepines and doses are best halved in the >60-yr age group initially. Interestingly, children show not only resistance to these drugs but sometimes paradoxical stimulation, and benzodiazepine sedation is not recommended for the <16s.

Post-op drowsiness is perhaps the biggest problem, as patients may be influenced by, e.g. diazepam for up to 24 h after administration (this time is ↓ with midazolam). There is also a re-sedation effect caused by enterohepatic recirculation.

Poswillo Committee Its report redefined 'sedation' as the 'single injection of a single drug'. In terms of IV sedation in an out-patient setting this is the surest way to avoid problems provided the 'single injection' is titrated and incremental.

IV sedation The most efficient and effective method of extending the use of LA in dental Rx; however, it requires substantial skill and confidence in venepuncture and administration of the drugs; therefore an inexperienced operator, or a patient with needle phobia, form relative C/I. As do inability to be accompanied, the need to be in a responsible position within 24h of sedation (e.g. looking after young children on own, driving, etc.), patients with liver or renal impairment, glaucoma, psychoses, pregnancy, or a demonstrated allergy to the benzodiazepines.

Certain drugs interact including cimetidine, disulfiram, anti-parkinsonian drugs, other sedatives, narcotic analgesics, antiepileptic drugs, antihistamines, and antihypertensives. Patients on these may be best treated (and then cautiously) in a hospital environment. Patients addicted to alcohol or other drugs may require a substantial dose modification; usually a big ↑. Those being sedated need to give written informed consent. Always provide written post-op instructions because the patients will not remember verbal ones. The role of operator sedationist is a perfectly sound and legal occupation, but note that a second appropriate person, i.e. one trained in CPR, must be present. At no time should the patient lose consciousness during IV sedation. There is no need to starve patients prior to being sedated, although many local policies dictate this and oral medication should be continued. Rectal sedation is popular in some countries using a prepackaged solution of diazepam (Stesolid®) given PR dose 2–10mg. Nasal inhalation techniques are also being introduced.

Alternative techniques In many countries multiple drug techniques are only carried out by trained anaesthetists although in the USA oral surgeons are trained in these techniques. These techniques include:
- Any form of conscious sedation for patients <12yrs (other than RA).
- Benzodiazepine & any other IV agent e.g. opioid, propofol, ketamine.
- Propofol alone or with any other agent.
- Inhalational sedation using any agent other than Nitrous Oxide.
- Combined routes (IV/Inh) except using NO for cannulation.

American oral surgeons recognize these techniques which are now the subject of a prospective new training program in conscious sedation in dentistry.[1, 2]

Flumazenil A specific benzodiazepine reversal agent. *Dose:* 200 µg IV over 15sec followed by 100µg at 60-sec intervals until reversal occurs. **NB** This drug has a shorter half-life than the drugs it will reverse, therefore multiple doses may be required. Patients **should never** be reversed, then left unsupervised. This is an essential emergency drug for IV sedationists.

1 Conscious sedation for dentistry: an update ℘ www.nature.com/bdj/journal/v203/n11/ful/bdj.2007.1105.html

2 DoH and FGDP(UK) 2008 Guidelines for the appointment of dentists with a special interest in conscious sedation. ℘ www.fgdp.org.uk/dwsi/docs/dwsiconssed.pdf

Benzodiazepines—techniques

Oral sedation

This is of use for managing moderately anxious patients. There are problems, however, with absorption time and the risk of sedation occurring too early or too late. There is again a risk of patients having sexual fantasies under the influence of these drugs. Two drugs are used:

Temazepam 30mg, 1h pre-Rx produces a degree of sedation similar to that seen with IV techniques.

Diazepam, either divided regimen, 5mg night before, 5mg morning of Rx, and 5mg 1h pre-Rx; *or* as 10–15mg 1h prior to Rx. Both drug and technique are highly variable in consistency and quality of sedation achieved. Both doses may have to be modified depending on the size and age of the patient.

IV techniques

A far greater control of the duration and depth of sedation can be consistently achieved with this approach. Gives excellent sedation with detachment for ~30min with amnesia for the duration of Rx. The major disadvantage is a potential for respiratory depression, post-Rx drowsiness, and amnesia (a reversal agent is available but not suitable for routine reversal of conventional sedation, 🕮 p. 592). Skill with venepuncture is a prerequisite of the technique. Diazepam has been entirely superseded by diazepam in lipid emulsion (diazemuls) as diazepam is not water-soluble and is very irritant.

Midazolam A water-soluble benzodiazepine of roughly double the strength of diazepam. Has a much shorter half-life, with no significant metabolites, creating a quicker and smoother recovery, and it is more amnesic than diazepam. It is supplied in both 2ml and 5ml ampoules, both containing 10mg midazolam (5ml ampoule is preferable, as it is easier to control the increments, given at 1mg/increment). Drug of choice.

Diazepam in lipid emulsion Diazepam is metabolized to desmethyldiazepam, which has a long half-life. It is presented in a 2-ml ampoule containing 10mg diazepam, given in slow IV increments (usually 2.5mg via a butterfly) until signs of sedation are observed. Suggested maximum dose 20mg.

IV Technique Relax the patient and have them sitting in the chair. Place a tourniquet around the most convenient arm and ask them to dangle the arm at their side. Any useful veins on the dorsum of the hand will become quickly evident. While this is happening, get your equipment ready: sticky tape, spirit wipe, butterfly, and drug in syringe. Look at the hand; is there a reasonable straight segment of vein? (If not, cut your losses and look elsewhere.) If there is, secure the hand with your non-dominant hand, palmar surface to palmar surface, with your thumb in a position to tense the skin overlying the selected vein. Stroke the back of the hand and tap the vein to engorge it. Prepare the skin with spirit wipe; get your 'second appropriate person' to help remove the needle cover and inform the patient there will be a slight scratch. Introduce the butterfly tip at a shallow angle through skin, then ↓ the angle further and move along the line of the vein until it has entered, as revealed by a flashback into the extension tubing.

Then introduce the length of the needle along the vein carefully, so as to avoid cutting through, and secure with tape. Remove air by aspirating blood into the tubing and release tourniquet. Place the patient in the supine position and give a small bolus (2–3mg diazepam, 1–2mg midazolam). Wait for 1min and then give further increments until adequate level of sedation is achieved. Leave the butterfly in to maintain venous access. Loss of laryngeal reflex constitutes oversedation and means you must stop and ensure the airway is patent, only proceeding if there is no respiratory depression and the airway can be protected.

Monitoring A 'second appropriate person' must be present. Pulse and BP should be monitored. Pulse oximetry is mandatory. An itchy nose is an early sign of 'complete' sedation. Hiccups constitute oversedation.

Post-sedation Allow time for recovery (30–60min) in calm surroundings. The patient must be accompanied home and forbidden to drive or assume a responsible position for 24h.

Anaesthesia—drugs and definitions

Anaesthesia is a triad of unconsciousness, muscle relaxation, and analgesia.

IV anaesthetic agents

Thiopentone (dose 4mg/kg) Although an ultra-short-acting barbiturate anaesthetic, its half-life is 6–12h. It is a poor analgesic and relatively sparing to the laryngeal reflexes, requiring a greater depth of anaesthesia to prevent laryngospasm. Highly irritant on injection but cheap and very popular as an in-patient induction agent. It will abolish epileptic seizures in induction doses.

Propofol (dose 2.5mg/kg) A true ultra-short-acting anaesthetic and is completely metabolized within 5h. Less irritant than the others and the drug of choice for day-case anaesthesia.

Etomidate (dose 0.3mg/kg) An IV induction agent often used for patients with compromised cardiovascular systems as its hypotensive side-effect is less than other agents. Can be associated with involuntary movements, cough, and hiccup.

Ketamine (dose 1–2mg/kg) Can be given IM at higher doses (unique among anaesthetic agents for this). Tends to maintain the airway and causes little respiratory depression. It is a good anaesthetic agent for use in the 'field' where there is limited equipment. Its use is limited by a high incidence of severe nightmare hallucinations in adults, which are eased by midazolam.

Inhalational anaesthetics

Nitrous oxide Excellent analgesic but weak anaesthetic, mainly used to supplement other inhalational anaesthetics or in RA. Problem created by its rapid excretion if used for perianaesthetic analgesia; wears off rapidly so no post-op analgesic benefits.

Halothane Largely superseded by newer agents. Weak analgesic. Causes hypotension and dysrhythmias. The concomitant use of injected adrenaline should be avoided in non-ventilated patients breathing halothane as it ↑ risk of VF. Very rarely hepatotoxic after repeated anaesthetics in adults. Extremely rarely *de novo*.

Enflurane Weaker anaesthetic than halothane but less likely to produce dysrhythmias or hepatitis. Avoid in epileptics.

Isoflurane Close relation of enflurane but more potent. Causes less cardiac problems than halothane. Commonly used hospital agent may cause coughing with inhalational induction.

Sevoflurane Newer agent with rapid onset and recovery. Good for inhalation induction and becoming increasingly inhalational agent of choice.

Desflurane Another rapid onset inhalational agent. Can cause coughing.

All inhalational agents cause muscle relaxation.

Muscle relaxants

Used to create laryngeal relaxation for intubation; this stops patients breathing, and they must then be ventilated until the agent wears off or is reversed.

Suxamethonium Used for emergency cases for rapidly securing airway. Short-acting depolarizing muscle relaxant; quick, good recovery but cannot be reversed. Main problems for the patient are muscle pains, which arise 24–48h after administration. These can be very severe and are more likely in the ambulant. It can also cause severe bradycardia, especially on repeat dose in children. Metabolized by plasma cholinestese, absence of which can lead to suxamethonium sensitivity, 🕮 p. 504. Causes an ↑ in K^+, therefore know U&Es in all but very routine cases.

Pancuronium, atracurium, vecuronium, and rocuronium All non-depolarizing muscle relaxants; slower acting and longer lasting, but can be reversed using neostigmine.

Mivacurium A short-acting non-depolarizing agent which, it was hoped, would fill the role of suxamethonium. Disappointing in practice.

Analgesics Opioids are mainstay and include:
- Morphine—long acting, mainly used for post-op analgesia.
- Fentanyl—first of the short-acting opioids.
- Alfentanil—purely used as anaesthetic opioid due to short duration.
- Remifentanil—continuous infusion needed because of ultra-short duration; ideal for anaesthesia but not post-op pain relief.

Anaesthesia and the patient on medication

Certain drugs should ring alarm bells when patients require a GA. These include:

Monoamine oxidase inhibitors Should be stopped 2 weeks prior to GA.

Antiepileptic drugs Must be continued up to, during, and after GA; however, methohexitone should be avoided.

Antihypertensives Should be continued, but ensure the anaesthetist is aware they are being taken.

Bronchodilators Should be continued. Give inhaler with pre-medication and ensure nebulizer is available post-op.

Cardioactive drugs Should all be continued. Warn the anaesthetist, as these patients often benefit from a pre-op anaesthetic assessment.

Cytotoxics Patients on these rarely need GA, but if they do they need FBC, U&Es, LFTs. Suxamethonium should be avoided.

Diabetic drugs For management, see p. 550.

Lithium Measure levels. Omit prior to major surgery.

Oral contraceptives Think about DVT prophylaxis, although experience suggests the risk is remote. BNF recommends discontinuing 4 weeks prior to major elective surgery; this is generally unnecessary for maxillofacial/ oral surgery. Be guided by local policy. HRT does *not* need to be stopped.

Sedatives and tranquillizers If the patient takes a regular dose these can be maintained, but warn the anaesthetist.

Corticosteroids Patients on long-term steroids require supplementation, pp. 504, 530, 552.

Oral anticoagulants Stop and heparinize for all major surgery. Monitor clotting. INR for warfarin. KCT for heparin.

Anaesthesia—hospital setting

With the exception of the out-patient GA service provided by some hospitals, GA in a hospital setting is similar to that for any other surgical service. The provision for, and the care of the patient immediately prior to, during, and after the anaesthetic is the domain of the trained anaesthetist. The input from the hospital junior is the same, whether in a dental or surgical specialty, and is mainly covered on 🕮 p. 538. The fundamental problem for any dental, oral, or maxillofacial anaesthetic is that the surgeon and anaesthetist both need to have access to the same anatomical site: the shared airway. The means by which this is overcome in hospital practice is by endotracheal, particularly nasendotracheal intubation, muscle relaxation, and ventilation.

Endotracheal intubation Secures the airway by placing a tube into the trachea via the nose, mouth, or a tracheostomy. This tube has an inflatable cuff which prevents aspiration of debris and is connected to an anaesthetic machine to allow delivery of O_2, nitrous oxide or air, and an inhalational anaesthetic. Most anaesthetists also use a throat pack to supplement the cuff, **which must be removed at the end of the operation**. Intubation is a specialist skill and must be learned by practice; skilled practitioners can perform blind nasendotracheal intubation, which is of enormous value in cases with trismus; most cases are, however, performed by direct vision of the vocal cords using a laryngoscope with the patient's neck fully extended. The major risk of intubation is intubating the oesophagus **and not recognizing it.** Other complications include: traumatizing teeth; vocal cord granulomata; minor trauma to the adenoids; rarely, pressure necrosis of tracheal mucosa and laryngeal stenosis.

The laryngeal mask airway The LMA has become an acceptable method of maintaining the airway. Structurally, it is a curved tube with a large cuff at its end. It is a device which is inserted orally without direct vision following the normal curve of the pharynx. Its onward progression is stopped by the upper end of the oesophagus and at this point the cuff is inflated, forming a seal around the entrance to the larynx. Patients must be starved as it does not protect against aspiration. It occupies a substantial volume in the mouth. The necessity of movement of the LMA to allow surgical access may displace the cuff, possibly causing laryngeal obstruction. Expensive, but autoclavable up to 40 times. It requires quite deep anaesthesia both to pass and maintain the LMA, which may prolong anaesthesia inappropriately.

The LMA should only be used by those trained in intubation.

Muscle relaxation Essential for successful intubation in elective patients. These drugs are covered on 🕮 p. 596. For most oral surgery, once intubated ventilation is aided by small doses of non-depolarizing muscle relaxant. An alternative is a continuous infusion of a very short-acting opioid (e.g. remifentanil).

Ventilation May be hand or mechanical. The latter is more precise and convenient for the anaesthetist. It involves a machine providing intermittent +ve pressure ventilation.

Monitoring There are increasingly sophisticated non-invasive techniques available: pulse oximetry to measure the percutaneous saturation of haemoglobin with O_2 (a normal person breathing air will have a saturation >95%); capnograph to measure end-tidal $PetCO_2$ (normal: 5.2kPa or 40mmHg); ECG and automatic BP machines. It must be stressed, however, that these machines do not replace, only ↑, the ability of the anaesthetist to use clinical observation of pulse, colour, skin changes, and ventilatory pattern. Minimum standard of monitoring set by Royal College of Anaesthestists is: BP, ECG, SaO_2, end-tidal CO_2.

Malignant hyperpyrexia, 📖 p. 504.

Anaesthesia—practice setting

Since the GDC's 2001 amendment to *Maintaining Standards: General Anaesthesia and Resuscitation*, the administration of GAs in dental practice setting has been effectively abolished in the UK. This has seen a huge pressure to ↑ the number of specialist (particularly) paediatric day units concentrating on paediatric exodontia and minor oral surgical work. This is often integrated with the community service for special-needs dentistry patients out-patient (ambulatory) setting.

The ideal team to provide exodontia under GA is a small skilled group, e.g. anaesthetist, dentist, and nurse, who have received appropriate post-graduate training and have suitable facilities.

Out-patient anaesthesia is given to healthy patients; the majority of anaesthetics, from induction to recovery, are a few minutes. The LMA is frequently used as an airway adjunct for day-case extraction, avoiding the need for muscle relaxation and intubation.

Controversial points

Pollution with anaesthetic gases In the hospital environment it is possible to scavenge the majority of gases as patients are either intubated, or have an LMA or a relatively leak-proof face mask. This is not the case in a dental surgery, as the patients are breathing through a nasal mask and, invariably, through their mouths.

Hazards of inhaling anaesthetic gases These are not well established. It is true that patients continuously breathing nitrous oxide for 24h or so begin to have suppression of the bone marrow and that chronic recreational abuse can cause subacute combined degeneration of the spinal cord. The short-term and intermittent long-term effects of exposure to nitrous oxide, halothane, enflurane, and isoflurane are, however, simply not known. It remains common sense that no one should work in a polluted atmosphere. The current guidelines are HC (76) 38.

Selected principal recommendations of the Poswillo Committee

Sedation

- Sedation be used in preference to GA whenever possible.
- For sedation by inhalation, the minimum concentration of O_2 be fixed at 30%.
- Flumazenil be reserved for emergency use.
- Intravenous sedation be limited to the use of one drug with a single titrated dose to an endpoint remote from anaesthesia.
- The use of IV sedation in children be approached with caution.
- Dentists must be aware of the significance of pulse oximetry readings.
- All patients treated with the aid of sedative techniques be accompanied by a responsible person.
- Undergraduates should have experience of managing at least 5 cases of IV sedation and 10 cases of inhalation sedation, and be proficient in venepuncture.
- Interested dentists should complete a recognized course in IV sedation within 2 years of qualification.

2001 GDC recommendations on GA and dentistry

These reinforce and extend the Poswillo recommendations. A *referring* or treating practitioner who breaches these recommendations will now be liable to a charge of serious professional misconduct.

Points to note

Referring

- A full PMH must be taken.
- A full explanation of risks and alternatives must occur before referral.
- Justification for the use of GA must be made in the referral letter.
- A copy of the letter must be retained.

Facilities to treat

- Access to critical care.
- Written protocol and training in ALS.
- Anaesthetist must be on GMC Specialist Register or working under supervision of same.
- Is supported by an Operating Department Practitioner.

Treatment

- Rx must only be provided if the treating dentist believes it is appropriate.
- The dentist should be supported by a dental nurse or equivalent.

The likely outcome should be a ↓ in numbers of GAs for dental procedures, and safer GAs but with a vast ↑ in cost and a major ↑ in hospital workload.

Dental materials

Contents

Principal sources J. F. McCabe 2008 *Applied Dental Materials*, Blackwell Publishing.

Properties of dental materials

Definitions

Coefficient of thermal expansion The fractional ↑ in length for each degree of temperature ↑.

Creep The slow plastic deformation that occurs with the application of a static or dynamic force over time.

Elastic modulus A measure of the rigidity of a material, defined by the ratio of stress to strain (below elastic limit).

Fatigue When cyclic forces are applied, a crack may nucleate and ↑ by small increments each time the force is applied. In time the crack will ↑ to a length at which the force results in # through the remaining material.

Hardness Resistance to penetration. A number of hardness scales are in use (e.g. Vickers, Rockwell). Between these scales hardness values are not interchangeable.

Resilience The energy absorbed by a material undergoing elastic deformation up to its elastic limit.

Stiffness An indication of how easy it is to bend a piece of material without causing permanent deformation or #. It is dependent upon the elastic modulus, size, and shape of the specimen.

Strain Change in size of a material that occurs in response to a force. It is the change in length divided by the original length.

Stress Internal force per unit cross-sectional area acting on the material. Can be classified according to the direction of the force: tensile (stretching), compressive, or shear.

Wear The abrasion (mechanical or chemical) resistance of a substance.

Thermal conductivity Ability of a material to transmit heat.

Thermal diffusivity Rate at which temperature changes spread through a material.

Toughness The amount of energy absorbed up to the point of #. A function of the resilience of the material and its ability to undergo plastic deformation rather than #.

Wettability Ability of one material to flow across the surface of another, determined by the contact angle between the two materials and influenced by surface roughness and contamination. The contact angle is the angle between solid/liquid and liquid/air interfaces measured through the liquid.

Yield strength (or elastic limit) The stress beyond which a material is permanently deformed when a force is applied.

Evaluation of a new material

Before it reaches the dental supply companies a new material should have undergone the following tests:

- *Standard specifications* (i.e. physical properties), e.g. compressive strength, hardness, etc. The actual values obtained are mainly of value in comparing the new material with those already in use and which are performing satisfactorily. Compliance with an international (ISO) standard indicates fitness for dental use.
- *Laboratory evaluation* Should be relevant to the clinical situation, but this is easier said than done!

- *Clinical trials* Usually conducted under optimal conditions. Many materials have been less successful under the conditions imposed by clinical practice, particularly those with demanding placement techniques.

Clinically, the important questions to ask the rep include:
- Details of the chemical constituents.
- Handling characteristics, e.g. presentation, mixing, working time, setting time, and dimensional changes on setting.
- Performance in service.
- Cost.
- Shelf-life.
- Does the material meet the relevant ISO standard?

Then decide whether this new material has any significant advantages over the material you are familiar with. Help can be sought from user ratings bodies such as Reality (℗ www.realityesthetics.com).
'Be not the first by whom the new are tried, nor yet the last to lay the old aside.' Alexander Pope.

Restoration of teeth

When restoring or replacing teeth it should be remembered that the teeth themselves are composed of enamel, dentine and pulpal tissues each with quite different properties that must be taken into account when selecting a material with which to restore them. In addition the teeth emerge from a complex dentogingival junction and are supported in alveolar bone by the viscoelastic periodontal ligament. All of these features are difficult to reproduce with current dental materials and most likely will not be until teeth themselves are able to be bioengineered.

Amalgam

An amalgam is a mixture of Hg and another metal. Dental amalgam is made by mixing together Hg with a powdered silver–tin alloy (mercury around 50% by weight) to produce a plastic mass that can be packed into a preparation before setting. Despite toxicity scares and the introduction of posterior composites, amalgam is still widely used, mainly because of its ease of handling. In Norway, Denmark and Sweden dental amalgam is banned for environmental reasons.

Types of amalgam

There are two ways of classifying amalgam:

Particle shape Can be lathe-cut (irregular), spheroidal, or a mixture of the two. Spheroidal particles give a more fluid mix which is easy to condense, can be carved immediately, and take 3h to reach occlusal strength (compared to >6h for lathe-cut amalgams). Spheroidal amalgams are preferable for pinned restorations.

Particle composition The first (conventional) alloys introduced had a low copper content (5%). The weakest (Sn–Hg or γ-2) phase of the set amalgam could be eliminated by ↑ the proportion of copper, so a variety of high copper (10–30%) amalgams have been introduced that react to eliminate it. These are more expensive, but superior in terms of corrosion resistance, creep, strength, and durability of marginal integrity. There are two types of high-copper alloy: (1) a single composition alloy of silver–tin–copper; (2) a blended (dispersion) mix of silver–tin and copper–silver alloys. Of these, (1) is the most resistant to tarnishing.

Handling characteristics

Mixing or trituration This is carried out mechanically, in one of two ways:
1) Pre-encapsulated by manufacturer, with automatic vibrator. The preferred method.
2) Using an amalgamator which dispenses Hg and alloy in correct proportions and mixes them. However, the amalgamator requires re-filling by hand which ↑ likelihood of Hg spillage occurring. The duration of trituration varies from 5 to 20sec.

Condensation Carry out incrementally by hand instruments (lathe-cut or spheroidal). Preparations should be overfilled so that the Hg-rich surface layer is removed by carving.

Carving With spherical alloys this can be commenced immediately, but with lathe-cut a delay of a few minutes is advisable. Burnishing is now back in vogue.

Polishing Polished amalgams look good, but whether polishing is necessary is still the subject of debate. **NB** Maximum strength takes 24h to develop.

Marginal leakage

Whilst amalgam corrosion products will form a marginal seal in time, microleakage can be ↓ by the use of either a conventional cavity varnish (e.g. Copalite®) or a bonding agent (e.g. Amalgambond® or Panavia-21™).

The latter (an anaerobic resin adhesive) also bonds to set amalgam.[1] Alternatively, sealing over the completed restoration with a fissure sealant has been suggested, and this is a possible solution to the 'ditched', but caries-free amalgam.

Toxicity

'There is insufficient evidence to justify the claim that Hg from dental amalgam has an adverse effect on the vast majority of patients'.[2] However, current advice includes avoiding the placement of amalgam fillings during pregnancy.[3] In addition there does seem to be a link between allergy to constituents of dental amalgam and lichenoid eruptions in the oral cavity.

The greatest risk appears to be related to the inhalation of Hg vapour and as such the dental team as well as patients is theoretically at risk; Attention should be paid to the following:

- Avoid spilling Hg.
- Waste amalgam should be stored in a screw-top bottle under old radiograph (X-ray) fixing solution.
- When removing old amalgams, safety glasses, masks, and high-volume aspiration are a wise precaution.
- Amalgam separation devices in use as per Hazardous Waste Directive (91/689/EEC).

Types of amalgam currently available

Conventional lathe-cut, conventional spherical, high-copper dispersion lathe + spherical, high-copper single spheroidal, high-copper single lathe-cut.

Average composition (%)	Silver	Tin	Copper	Zinc
Conventional	68	28	4	0–2
High copper	60	27	13	0

1 D. C. Watts 1992 *J Dent* **20** 245.

2 B. M. Eley 1993 *BDJ* **175** 161.

3 Department of Health 1998 Letter no. PL/CDO(98).

Composite resins—constituents and properties

The modern composite resin is a mixture of resin and particulate filler, the handling characteristics of which are determined largely by the size of the filler particles and method of cure.

Constituents

Resin Most composite resins are based on either Bis-GMA (addition product of bisphenol A and glycidylmethacrylate) or urethane dimethacrylate plus a diluent monomer, triethylene glycol dimethacrylate (TEGMA).

Filler (e.g. quartz, fused silica, glasses such as aluminosilicate and borosilicate). Confers the following benefits on the composite resin:
- compressive length, abrasion resistance, modulus of elasticity, and # toughness.
- thermal expansion and setting contraction.
- aesthetic qualities.

Composite resins can be subdivided according to particle size:

Macrofilled (or conventional) Contains particles of radio-opaque barium or strontium glass 2.5–5µm in size, to give 75–80% by weight of filler. Good mechanical properties, but hard to polish and soon roughens.

Microfilled Contains colloidal silica particles 0.04µm in size and 30–60% by weight. Retains a good surface polish, but is unsuitable for load-bearing situations, has poor wear resistance, and ↑ contraction shrinkage.

Nanofilled By combining nanometric particles and nanoclusters in a conventional resin matrix manufacturers claim to offer ↑ wear resistance as well as polishability and lustre.

Hybrid Contains a mixture of conventional and microfine particles designed to optimize both mechanical and surface properties. Contains 75–85% by weight of filler, of which the bulk is conventional (1–50µm). Some manufacturers achieve up to 90% filler loadings by using blended sizes of filler particles.

Initiator/activator
1) Chemically cured: benzoyl peroxide (or sulfinic acid) initiator + tertiary amine activator.
2) Light-cured: amine + diketone activated by blue light (460–70nm).

Other constituents include pigments, stabilizers, and silane coupler to produce bond between particles and filler.

Composites may also be classified as:
- microfilled
- posterior composite
- all-purpose
- flowable
- condensable/packable

Important properties of composites
- Polymerization shrinkage of 1–4%.
- Thermal expansion is significantly greater than enamel or dentine, and without acid-etch bond can result in marginal leakage.

- Elastic modulus should be high to resist occlusal forces. Modulus of hybrid type is greater than other composite resins, amalgam, or dentine. However, composite resins are still brittle and # if used in thin section.
- Wear resistance is greatest in hybrids.
- Radio-opacity is particularly useful, especially for posterior resin composites.
- ? toxicity. Resins have been found to be toxic in cell culture. Also controversy surrounding the oestrogenicity of composite resins.

Newer developments include hydroxyl ion releasing composite resin to counteract demineralization during periods of low pH in the restoration. Also use of fibre reinforcement to fabricate posts and cores as well as bridges/splints.

Composite resins—practical points

Method of polymerization

Chemical (self-cure) No additional equipment required, but mixing of two components introduces porosity and the working time is limited.

Light activation Provides long working time, command set, and better colour stability, but requires a light source, has a limited depth of cure, and the temperature ↑ during setting can be as high as 40°C. Three types of light source are currently available: quartz tungsten halogen (QTH), plasma arc light (PAC), and light-emitting diode (LED). QTH is the most widely used although the newer PAC and LED lights confer theoretical advantages in e.g. speed and depth of cure, portability, lifetime and reliability of light source. Ramping of intensity of light emission confers the theoretical benefit of less polymerization shrinkage.

Dual-cure Curing is initiated by a conventional light source, but continues chemically to help ensure polymerization throughout the restoration.

Practical tips for light activation
- Replace bulbs every 6–12 months. Some lights correct for the effects of bulb ageing.
- Air attenuates light beam, ∴ position as close to tooth as possible.
- Preparations >2mm depth should be cured incrementally.
- Precautions are necessary to protect eyes from glare, ∴ use safety shield, get the patient to close their eyes, and the DN to look away.
- Efficiency of light source can be tested by curing a block of composite. Practical depth of cure is half thickness of set material.
- The greater the intensity of the light source the greater the depth of cure.

Finishing Ideally, a mylar strip to produce the contour of the restoration. Then refine with microfine diamond or multi-bladed tungsten carbide finishing burs (under water spray), finishing strips, and then polish with aluminium oxide-coated discs (Shofu, Soflex). Shofu points or finishing pastes are useful for inaccessible concave surfaces.

Problems with composite resins
1) Difficult to obtain satisfactory contact points and occlusal stops. Modern placement techniques have largely overcome this.
2) Post-op sensitivity.
3) Polymerization shrinkage.
4) Depth of cure of light-cured materials is limited. This is a particular problem in posterior teeth.

Indirect composite inlays may circumvent the last two problems (📖 p. 232).

Fissure sealants Composite resins containing little or no filler, which are either self- or light-cured. Clear or opaque types are available, the former having better flow characteristics (whether this is an advantage depends upon the position of the tooth). Success depends upon being able to achieve good moisture control for the acid-etch bond.

Flowable composite resins are now available. They are predominately resin with a reduced percentage of filler particles, and consequently shrink considerably on curing. Some advocate using them as liners or in the bottom of proximal preparations, but the high shrinkage precludes this. RMGIC is preferable in proximal preparations, which are below the cemento-enamel junction (bonded-base approach); however, they have a place in the marginal repair of restorations and some advocate their use for facial cervical margin restorations.

Acid-etch technique

Recent research would suggest that:
- Success depends upon adequate moisture control, as contact with saliva for as little as 0.5sec will contaminate etch pattern.
- A prophylaxis prior to etching is not required unless abundant plaque deposits are present.
- 30–50% buffered phosphoric acid provides the best etch pattern.
- An etching time of 15–20sec is adequate for both primary and permanent enamel, and 15sec for dentine is recommended.
- The etch pattern is easily damaged, using a probe to aid etchant penetration of pits and fissures, or applying etchant by rubbing vigorously with a pledget of cotton wool, is C/I.
- There is no difference in bond strength whether an etchant solution or gel is used. Gels take twice as long to rinse away but have the advantage of greater viscosity and colour contrast.
- Rinse for at least 15sec.
- Remineralization of etched enamel occurs from the saliva, and after 24h it is indistinguishable from untreated enamel.
- Etched enamel is porous and has a high surface energy. The etch pattern consists of three zones (from surface inwards):

Etched zone (enamel removed)	10µm
Qualitative porous zone	20µm
Quantitative porous zone	20µm

Composite resin tags may penetrate up to 50µm into enamel to give micromechanical retention.

NB Many of the newer dentine adhesive systems do not have a separate acid-etch stage. These systems use a combination of acidic primers and bonding resins, either as a single stage or applied separately (Adper™ Prompt™ L-Pop™, iBond®, Xeno IV®). (See *dentine bonding section*, 🕮 p. 616)

Dentine-adhesive systems (dentine bonding agents)

The advantages of bonding to dentine (e.g. preservation of tooth tissue) have fuelled considerable research effort. The problems that have had to be overcome include the high water and organic content of dentine; the presence of a 'smear layer' after dentine is cut; and the need for adequate strength immediately following placement, to withstand the polymerization contraction of composite resin. These difficulties have been approached in a number of ways, making the topic of dentine bonding confusing, a situation which has been exacerbated by the pace of new developments and by the claims of the manufacturers.

Indications
- Marginal seal where preparation margin in dentine or cementum, e.g. cervical (Class V), proximal (Class II) box.
- Retention and seal of direct resin-composite restorations.
- Retention and seal of indirect porcelain and composite inlays.
- Dentine adhesives have also been used for repairing # teeth, cementing ceramic crowns and veneers, and as an endodontic sealer.

The smear layer consists of an amorphous layer of organic and inorganic debris, produced by cutting dentine. It ↓ sensitivity by occluding the dentine tubules and prevents loss of dentinal fluid. The smear layer is partially or completely removed &/or modified during dentine bonding.

Mechanism of dentine bonding

Most dentine adhesive systems aim to modify and partially remove the smear layer, by the application of an acidic primer. This demineralizes the underlying surface, exposing the collagen and opening up the dentinal tubules. It is important to keep this surface moist to prevent the collagen becoming flattened (**not** with saliva, though!). This layer is then infiltrated using a resin with bi-functional ends: one hydrophilic end, which is able to bond to wet dentine and one hydrophobic end capable of bonding to the composite resin. In this infiltrated hybrid layer molecular entanglement of the collagen and resin occurs, providing the basis for the bonding system.

Practical points
- Follow manufacturer's instructions.
- For better results use a matched resin-composite and adhesive system.
- When a dentine adhesive is used polymerization shrinkage of composite resin is more likely to result in cuspal deformation and post-op pain. An incremental filling and curing technique will help to solve this problem.
- Pre-curing the adhesive bonding agent before placing the composite ↑ bond strength.[1]
- No technique produces zero microleakage.

1 J. F. McCabe 1994 *BDJ* **176** 333.

Techniques

Total Etch 37% phosphoric acid usually used to remove the smear layer and demineralize the surface dentine. A primer is then used often containing a solvent such as acetone to eliminate water in the dentine that is then filled by resin tags. Another method is to use an aqueous primer solution. Benefit of ease of use as well as stronger acid etching of the enamel.

Self-etching primer A weaker acid is used to solubilize the smear layer and at the same time act as the difunctional primer (hydrophilic and hydrophobic ends).

One bottle systems The resin bonding agent is mixed in the same liquid as the etch and primer. Often unidose presentation and coupled with the one step technique theoretically less room for problems with technique sensitivity and evaporation of contents/cross infection.

Bonding to metals and ceramics

The above bonding systems may be used in conjunction with preparation of metal or ceramic surfaces to allow bonding of materials other than composite resin to the tooth surface. Metal surfaces are usually sandblasted to provide roughness for micromechanical retention then prepared with a 4-META derived conditioner before application of a composite luting cement. Ceramic surfaces are usually etched then silanated before luting. This allows for a great variety of clinical uses including orthodontics as well as fixed prosthodontics.

Glass ionomers—properties and types

Glass ionomer (polyalkenoate)

Setting reaction

Alumino-silicate glass + polyalkenoic acid → calcium + aluminium polyalkenoates (base + polyacid → polysalt + water).

The set material consists of unreacted spheres of glass surrounded by a silicaeous gel, embedded in metal polyalkenoates. Fluoride is uptaken and released from the cement to give theoretical cariostatic properties.

Presentation

1 Powder + liquid.
2 Powder (with anhydrous acid) + water.
3 Encapsulated.

Tartaric acid is added to lengthen working time. In some products polymaleic acid replaces polyacrylic and one newer material is glass polyphosphonate (Diamond Carve™).

Properties

Adhesion To enamel and dentine by: **1** ionic displacement of calcium and phosphate with polyacrylate ions; **2** possible absorption of polyalkenoic acid onto collagen. Some authors recommend pre-conditioning the dentine, e.g. with 10% polyalkenoic acid (GC Dentin Conditioner™) for 30sec. Whether this ↑ adhesion is controversial. GI cement also bonds to the oxide layer on SS and tin.

Cariostatic Due to fluoride release throughout the lifetime of the restoration. GI are also able to take up fluoride when the IO concentration is raised, the 'reservoir effect'. However, the therapeutic benefit of fluoride release has yet to be shown to be effective.

Thermal expansion Similar to enamel and dentine.

Strength Brittle material. Tensile strength is only 40% of composite resin.

Radiolucent Except for the cermets, which are rarely used.

Abrasion/erosion resistance Poor, but ↑ all the time, especially with the high-viscosity versions.

Biocompatibility This is being questioned following reports of pulpal inflammation when used as a luting cement, but this is not a problem clinically.[1]

Applications

GIs are unable to match the aesthetics and abrasion resistance of the composite resins, and brittleness limits their use to non-load-bearing situations. However, their adhesive and fluoride-releasing properties have resulted in a range of applications and matching formulations.

1 R. van Noort (ed.) 1994 *J Dent* **22** 8.

Type I Luting cements for crowns, bridges, and orthodontic bands.

Type II Restorative cements. There are two subtypes: (a) aesthetic; (b) reinforced. Can also be used as a fissure sealant, for the restoration of deciduous teeth (📖 p. 80) and for repairing defective restorations.

Type III Fast-setting lining materials. Defer placement of amalgam for at least 15min and composite for 4min. In load-bearing situations or where lining is exposed to the oral environment (e.g. in sandwich technique), use of a type II reinforced cement or RMGIC is preferable.

Type IV Includes the light-cure and dual-cure GI (use of a light source optimizes the properties of the dual-cure materials, although they will self-polymerize without). It has been suggested that the light-cured GI have higher bond strengths than self-cure GI.[1]

1 C. G. Plant 1988 *BDJ* **165** 54.

Glass ionomers—practical points

Practical tips

- A dry field is essential.
- Encapsulated systems ensure optimal mixing and allow placement via syringe tip, e.g. Ketac-Fil™.
- Cement should be inserted before its sheen is lost.
- GI sticks to instruments, ∴ use powder as a separator.
- Cellulose or soft metal strips provide the best finish.
- Water balance during setting is critical. Absorption of water results in dissolution, and dehydration leads to crazing, ∴ cement must be protected with waterproof material e.g. light-cured bonding resin, which acts as a lubricant for finishing and can then be cured.
- Although most manufacturers claim that trimming can be started 10–15min after placement, it is better to defer for >24h.

Other glass ionomer/composite based products

The following is a quick run through for those who don't know their ormocers from their ceromers or their giomers from their compomers!

Resin modified glass ionomers

These allow 'command' setting and help overcome the moisture sensitivity and low early mechanical strength associated with conventional GI. The acid–base reaction of GI is supplemented by the addition of ~5% resin (HEMA Bis-GMA). The initial set of the material is due to the formation of a polymerization matrix, which is strengthened by the acid–base reaction. They are easier to handle than conventional GI and may be polished immediately after light-curing. Aesthetics approach those of resin-based materials, plus the advantage of fluoride release.[1] These materials can be used in conjunction with composite resin for placement in deep proximal preparation where the deepest parts of the preparation are below the cemento-enamel junction. This type of open sandwich restoration fell into disrepute when restorations were placed with traditional GI cement. The development of RMGICs has improved the technique, with good results reported at 7yrs.[2] Widely used as lining materials and luting cements.

Compomer

Another hybrid material. It combines the adhesive and fluoride-releasing properties of GI with the abrasion resistance of composite resin and is called, with a touch of originality, 'compomer'. Composed of a single hydrophobic resin filled with acid-leachable glass particles. Bonded with a bi-functional primer and light-cured. It is claimed that the chemical reaction takes place through uptake of water from saliva leading to fluoride ions leaching out. Popular in general practice due to ease of technique and especially useful for restoration of deciduous teeth.

Giomers/modified composites

This group of materials is more correctly described as composite resins with active filler particles. The filler particles are based on pre-reacted surface or fully reacted GI filler particles (Giomers) whereas the acid–base reaction process occurs after initial setting in acid-modified composites. Have been shown to be capable of sustained fluoride release and uptake. Possibly useful for high-caries risk individuals.

Ormocers

Organically modified ceramics e.g. Admira®
Made up of three components; organic polymers, ceramic glasses and poly-vinylsiloxane. Claimed to confer less polymerization shrinkage, good handling, marginal integrity and biocompatibility (less free diluent monomer). Lack of clinical trials to date.

1 S. K. Sidhu 1995 *Dental Update* **10** 429.

2 J. W. van Dijken 1999 **78** 1319.

Cermets

These are similar to GI, except that the ion-leachable glass is fused with fine silver powder. Mixing with a polymeric acid gives a cement consisting of unreacted glass particles to which silver is fused, held together by a metal–salt matrix with the benefit of increased wear resistance. Cermets have been largely superseded by the RMGICs.

Ceromers

Ceromers are second generation **indirect** composite resins. Their main components are silanized microhybrid inorganic fillers embedded in a light-curing organic matrix. Ceromers have high filler content and so improved mechanical properties compared to traditional composites. It is, however, less wear resistant than enamel with potential problems in the long term in high loading sites. The material may be used as indirect onlays with benefits over porcelain in 'camouflaging' of shade as well as a fire-reinforced crown or bridge material (Targis Vectris®) with variable success.

Cements

Based on zinc oxide eugenol (ZOE)

Powder of pure zinc oxide is mixed (in a ratio of 3:1) with eugenol liquid to give zinc eugenolate and unreacted powder. Setting time is 24h. This is the weakest cement, but the eugenol acts as an obtundent and analgesic, ∴ used as a sedative dressing. The following modifications change the properties for various indications.

Accelerated ZOE, e.g. Sedanol®. Addition of zinc acetate to the powder ↑ setting time to 5min.

Resin-bonded ZOE, e.g. Kalzinol®. Addition of 10% hydrogenated resin to the powder ↑ strength.

EBA, e.g. Staline, Opotow®. Addition of ortho-ethoxybenzoic acid (62%) to the liquid ↑ strength.

Zinc phosphate

e.g. De Trey® Zinc. The powder consists of zinc and magnesium oxides, and the liquid 50% aqueous phosphoric acid. The working time is ↑ by adding the powder in small increments. Popular in the past because of its strength. Although its low setting pH theoretically C/I its use for vital teeth, in practice this does not seem to be a problem.

Zinc polycarboxylate

e.g. Poly-F®, Durelon™. The powder is a mixture of zinc and magnesium oxides and the liquid is 40% aqueous polyacrylic acid. Recently, anhydrous acid formulations have been introduced, which are mixed with water. The powder should be added quickly to the liquid. The temptation to remove excess cement should be resisted until it has reached a rubbery stage. Adheres to dentine, enamel, tin, and SS. Often used as temporary cement where ↑ adherence required.

Calcium hydroxide

Chemically curing types comprise two pastes which are mixed together in equal quantities. One paste contains the calcium hydroxide plus fillers in a non-reacting carrier, and the other polysalicylate fluid. The set material consists of an amorphous calcium disalicylate complex plus calcium hydroxide and has a pH of 11. In addition to being bacteriostatic, calcium hydroxide can induce mineralization of adjacent pulp. Light-cured formulations which are resin-based are available. Have ↓ bactericidal properties, but ↑ strength.

RMGIC

Is a popular luting cement used for cast indirect restorations and for cavity lining.

Strength Phosphate>EBA or polycarboxylate>resin-bonded ZOE> accelerated ZOE>calcium hydroxide.

Practical points

- Generally, the thicker the mix, the greater the strength.
- Heat ↓ setting time, ∴ a cooled slab is advisable.

- To stop cement sticking to the instruments during placement, dip in cement powder (except calcium hydroxide) or use non-stick instruments.
- When luting, apply cement to crown or inlay before tooth.

Choice of cement

Temporary restorations Choice depends upon how long the dressing needs to last and whether any therapeutic qualities are required. Pure ZOE is useful for a tooth with a reversibly inflamed pulp, but resin-bonded ZOE is stronger. GI is preferable for semi-permanent dressings and endo provisionalization because it seals the preparation margins.

Luting cement Zinc phosphate, GI, and polycarboxylate are all popular as luting cements. EBA cement is C/I because of ↑ solubility. Composite-based luting systems are available, which are often used in conjunction with dentine adhesive systems. Mandatory for cementing ceramic or porcelain inlays/onlays and ceramic veneers. Now available as one-step luting cements with no etching or bonding required.

Lining cement Choice of lining depends upon the depth of the preparation and the material being used to restore it.

   Amalgam Minimal: preparation sealer (Gluma® Desensitiser); moderate: RMGIC (Vitrebond™); deep: use a sub-lining of calcium hydroxide (direct or indirect pulp capping) and any of the cements listed above. Typically RMGIC is recommended as it seals as well as lines the preparation.

   Composite resin Dentine adhesive system with direct or indirect pulp capping as indicated.

Pulp capping Hard-setting calcium hydroxide or MTA.

Sedative dressing ZOE &/or calcium hydroxide.

Bacteriostatic dressing Calcium hydroxide plus GI (stepwise excavation).

Impression materials

Classification

Non-elastic		Elastic
	Elastomers	*Hydrocolloid*
Compound	Silicone	Reversible
ZOE paste	Polysulfide	Irreversible
Wax	Polyether	

Elastomers

Indicated when accuracy is paramount, e.g. crown and bridge work, and implants.

Condensation-cured silicone These materials are relatively cheap compared with other elastomers, but prone to some shrinkage and should be cast immediately. Addition-cured silicones are preferred.

Addition-cured silicone, e.g. Aquasil®, President, Express 2™. This type of silicone is very stable, which means that impressions can be posted or stored prior to casting. A perforated tray or rim lock tray is advisable as the adhesives supplied are not very effective. Up to five viscosities are manufactured, allowing a range of impression techniques. **NB** Powdered latex gloves (now rarely used) can retard setting of putty materials.[1]

Polysulfide, e.g. Permlastic®. Messy to handle, but useful when a long working time is required. Use with a special tray and, although stable, cast within 24h. Not recommended except in complete denture cases.

Polyether, e.g. Impregum™. Popular because it uses a single mix and a stock tray. The set material is stiff, although newer products (e.g. Penta Soft™) have addressed this and removal can be stressful in cases with deep undercuts or advanced periodontitis. Absorbs water; ∴ do not store with alginate impressions. Can cause allergic reactions. Routinely used for implant cases and crown and bridge work, especially when there are multiple preps.

Hydrocolloids

Reversible hydrocolloid is accurate, but liable to tear. Requires the purchase of a water bath and not cross-infection friendly.

Irreversible hydrocolloid (alginate) Setting is a double decomposition reaction between sodium alginate and calcium sulfate. Popular because it is cheap and can be used with a stock tray. However, it is not sufficiently accurate for crown and bridge work. Impressions must be kept damp and cast within 24h. Alginate can retard the setting of gypsum and affect the surface of the model.

1 W. W. L. Chee 1992 *J Prosthet Dent* **68** 728.

Impression compound

Available in either sheet form for recording preliminary impressions, or in stick form for modifying trays. The sheet material is softened in a water-bath with warm water (55–60° C) and used in a stock tray to record edentulous ridges. The viscosity of compound results in a well-extended impression, but limited detail. Admix impression material (mix of green-stick and impression compound) is useful for denture cases with severe resorption.

Zinc oxide pastes

Dispensed 1:1 and mixed to an even colour. Used for recording edentu-lous ridges in a special tray or the patient's existing dentures, but C/I for undercuts. Setting time is ↓ by warmth and humidity.

Impression techniques

(For crown and bridge work)
Time spent recording a good impression is an investment, as repeating lab work is costly.

Special trays Help the adaptation of impression material and ↓ the amount required, i.e. ↑ accuracy and ↓ cost. Can be made in cold-cure acrylic or light-activated tray resin. Special trays are rarely used for crown and bridge work impressions, with stock trays used routinely.

For crown and bridge work an accurate impression of the prepared teeth is required. Usually the palate does not need to be included, so design the special tray accordingly or use a lower stock tray. For the opposing arch, alginate in a stock tray will suffice.

Monophase technique (e.g. polyether) The same mix of medium-viscosity material is used for both a stock tray and syringe. Although less accurate than other methods, it is adequate for most tasks.

Double-mix technique (e.g. polysulfide, addition-cured silicone) A single-stage technique necessitating the mixing of heavy- and light-bodied materials at the same time, and use of a special or stock tray.

- Apply adhesive to tray.
- Mix light- and heavy-bodied viscosities simultaneously for 45–60sec.
- Remove retraction cord or preferably leave in place and dry preparation, while nurse loads syringe with light-bodied material.
- Syringe light-bodied mix around prep. A gentle stream of air helps to direct material into crevice.
- Position tray containing heavy-bodied material.
- Support tray with light pressure until 2min after apparent set.

Putty and wash technique (e.g. silicone) The putty and light-bodied viscosities can be used with a stock tray, either:

1) *Single-stage* Similar to the double-mix technique above, or
2) *Two-stage* This involves taking an impression of the prep with the putty, using a polythene sheet as a spacer. This is then relined with the light-bodied material, which is also syringed around the prep. The trend is, however, away from putty wash towards monophase or a double-mix technique.

Cost In decreasing order:

- addition-cured silicone using putty/reline;
- polyether with special tray;
- addition-cured silicone using double mix and special tray;
- polysulfide with special tray;
- condensation-cured silicone using putty/reline;
- hydrocolloid.

Automixing dispensers This double-cartridge presentation is exceptionally popular. The two pastes are extruded and mixed in the nozzle when the trigger is pressed. Appears expensive, but ↓ waste and the mixture is void free. Many manufacturers are now producing their materials in this format.

Disinfection of impressions

Impressions should be rinsed to remove debris and then immersed in a solution of sodium hypochlorite (1000ppm available chlorine) or a gluter-aldehyde-free proprietary disinfectant such as Perform for 10min. In general dimensional stability of impressions seems unaffected by current protocols.[1]

1 E. Kotsiomiti 2008 *J Oral Rehab* **35** 291.

Casting alloys

An alloy is a mixture of two or more metallic elements. The chemistry of alloys is too complicated for this book chapter (and its author), so for a fuller understanding the reader is referred to the source text.

The properties of an alloy depend upon:
- The thermal treatments applied to the alloy (including cooling).
- The mechanical manipulation of the alloy.
- The composition of the alloy.

NB The properties of an alloy may differ significantly from that of its constituents.

The main examples of alloys in dentistry include amalgam (p. 608), steel burs and instruments, metallic denture bases, inlays, crowns and bridges, Nickel Titanium endodontic instruments and orthodontic wires.

Casting alloys

A warm moist mouth provides the ideal environment for corrosion. To overcome this problem, dental casting alloys comprise an essentially corrosion-resistant metal (usually gold), with the addition of other constituents to enhance its properties. However, with the possible exception of titanium all have the potential to affect hypersensitive individuals.

Additions to gold alloys

Copper ↑ strength and hardness, but ↓ ductility.

Silver ↑ hardness and strength, but ↑ tarnishing and ↑ porosity.

Platinum/palladium (as in Type III/IV gold alloys) ↑ melting point (which confers advantage for soldering).

Zinc or indium Scavenger, preventing oxidation of other metals during melting and casting.

Traditional dental casting gold alloys

ISO standard is that the noble metal (gold, platinum, palladium, iridium, ruthenium, rhodium) content must >75% up with no less than 65% gold. Four types are defined by proof stress (*stress required to cause a permanent deformation of a particular value (e.g. 0.2%)—similar to elastic limit*) and elongation (ductility) values from Type I (low strength for castings subject to low stress) to Type IV (extra-high strength).

Clinically this means the Type I and II alloys are used in low load-bearing situations such as inlays, Type III where demands are higher such as full cuspal coverage onlays, crowns and bridges and Type IV where rigidity is required for removable partial denture bases or clasps.

Dental casting semi-precious alloys

Have 25–74% noble metal content.

Low gold alloys Similar to the traditional gold alloys, four types are defined by proof stress and elongation properties. High palladium content imparts 'whiteness'. Popularity ↑ with ↑ cost of gold.

Silver palladium Palladium (generally >25%), silver, gold, indium, and zinc. Cheaper than gold alloys and of equivalent hardness, but less ductile, more difficult to cast, and prone to porosity.

Base metal casting alloys

Contain no gold, platinum or palladium.

Nickel chromium 75% nickel, 20% chromium. Used in crowns and bridge work. In latter ↑ rigidity compared to gold alloys is an advantage. However, castings are less accurate than gold, and nickel sensitivity can C/I its use.

Cobalt chromium 35–65% cobalt, No less than 25% chromium. Modulus of elasticity (rigidity) twice that of Type IV gold alloys ∴ good for denture base but not as good for clasps. Proportional limit (ability to withstand stress without permanent deformation) high. A good polish is difficult to achieve, but durable. Used mainly for P/-.

Titanium

Good biocompatibility; used for implants and their superstructure and in patients with allergies to other materials as a denture base material. In its use for implants the titanium can be subjected to post-manufacture heat treatment to optimize the grain structure (small α grain size and well-dispersed β phase with a small α–β interfacial zone. This improves the properties with regard to cyclic fatigue and crack propagation. (Also see Chapter 6).

Alloys for porcelain bonding

Requirements:
- Higher melting point than porcelain.
- Similar coefficient of thermal expansion to porcelain (leucite used in the porcelain to bring it closer to that of the metal).
- Will not discolour the porcelain.
- High modulus of elasticity (rigidity) to avoid flexure and # of porcelain.
- Ability to bond to the porcelain to avoid detachment.

Indium is usually added to facilitate bonding to porcelain. Copper is C/I as it discolours the porcelain. A matched alloy and porcelain should be used.

High gold ↑ palladium or platinum content (to ↑ melting point) compared to non-porcelain alloys but need thick copings for strength ∴ bulkiness. Also costly.

Medium gold 50% gold, 30% palladium. Good properties and economical. Widely used.

Silver palladium Cheap, but care required to avoid casting defects.

Nickel chromium Very high melting point and modulus of elasticity, but casting more difficult due to shrinkage, voids. Also bond strength to porcelain via ceramic oxide weak. **NB** Some patients are sensitive to nickel.

Casting

For gold (melting point <950°C)
- Wax pattern and sprue are invested in gypsum bonded material.
- Wax burnt out by slowly heating investment mould to 450°C.
- Alloy melted either by gas/air torch or electric induction heating and cast with centrifugal force.
- Casting allowed to cool to below red-heat.
- Quenched. Some alloys are used as cast and others heat-hardened.
- Cleaned with ultrasonics and acid immersion.

For nickel chromium and cobalt chromium alloys (melting points 1200–1500°C), need silica or phosphate bonded investment and either oxyacetylene torch or electric induction heating.

Casting faults

A casting may be:

- dimensionally inaccurate (depends on balancing out of casting contraction and investment expansion on setting);
- display finning (due to overheated and cracked investment material) and bubbling (due to surface porosities in the investment material);
- be porous/contaminated (broken pieces of investment or dirt falling down the sprue) or incomplete (sprue problem, premature solidification of the molten metal, insufficient centrifugal force, back pressure effects from poor escape of gases, cooling shrinkage).

Wrought alloys

Wrought alloys are hammered, rolled, drawn, or bent into the desired shape when they are solid.

Stainless steel

Steel is an alloy of iron and carbon. The addition of chromium (>12%) produces a passive surface oxide layer which gives SS its name. The SS used in dentistry is also known as austenitic steel (because the crystals are arranged in a face-centred cubic structure) or 18:8 steel (due to the chromium and nickel content). Available as:

1 Pre-formed sheets for denture bases. The SS is swaged onto the model by explosive or hydraulic pressure. This produces a thin (0.1mm), light denture base resistant to #. Rarely used today.
2 Wires are produced by drawing the SS through dies of ↓ diameter until the desired size is achieved. This work-hardens the wire, but heat treatments are carried out to give soft, hard, or extra-hard forms. Manipulation of SS wire also work-hardens the wire in the plane of bending, ∴ trying to correct a bend is more likely to result in #. Main applications are orthodontics and partial denture clasps. SS can be welded and soldered.

Soldering SS Requires use of a flux (e.g. Easy-flo™ flux) to remove the passive oxide layer (this reforms after soldering). Do not overheat as this can anneal and soften the components.

- Melt a small bead of low fusing silver solder (e.g. Easy-flo™ solder) onto the wire.
- Mix up the flux with water to a thick paste and apply to the item to be added.
- Heat up the solder so that wire underneath is a cherry red.
- Bring the fluxed wire into the molten solder and remove the flame at the same time.

This is not easy and requires practice, which explains the popularity of electrical soldering.

Cobalt chromium

Has a similar composition to the cast form (□ p. 630).
Cobalt chromium alloys Used in orthodontics as an archwire material (Elgiloy®). It has the advantage that it can be hardened by heat treatment after being formed. Also used for post fabrication in post and core crowns (Wiptam wire).

Titanium alloys

Nickel and titanium alloy (nitinol) is useful in orthodontics as it is flexible, has good springback, and is capable of applying small forces over a long period of time. However, it is not easy to bend without #. Titanium molybdenum alloy (TMA) is also used for archwires and has properties midway between SS and nitinol.

Gold

Expense limits the application of wrought gold alloys to partial denture clasp fabrication.

Alloys for dentures

Cast cobalt chromium is the material of choice for partial denture connectors because of its high proof stress and modulus of elasticity: thin castings are strong, rigid, and lightweight. Although wrought gold alloys are more suitable for clasps, the advantage of being able to cast connector and clasps in one means that cobalt chromium is more commonly used (📖 p.298). Be aware of nickel allergy.

Ceramics—dental porcelain

Ceramics are simple compounds of both metallic and non-metallic oxides. Although many of the materials used in dentistry are ceramics, the term is commonly used to refer to porcelain and its derivatives. Dental porcelain actually more closely resembles a glass and is basically an oxide based glass–ceramic system. Its main constituents are feldspar, quartz (for strength and translucency), and in some types kaolin (for strength and colour), plus pigments. Most dental porcelain is reinforced with alumina particles (40–50% by mass) to provide greater strength. Unfortunately, this ↑ the opacity, ∴ the proportion of alumina in enamel porcelains is ↓.

Dental porcelain has three basic requirements; function (durability, strength and biocompatibility), form (ability to form complex shapes) and aesthetics (colour, translucency and transmission of light).

The main types used currently are
- Feldspathic
- Leucite reinforced
- Pressable e.g. Empress®
- Castable e.g. Dicor®
- Aluminous e.g. In-Ceram®, Procera®
- Zirconium-based

Conventional PJC construction During construction of a PJC a platinum matrix is laid down on the die produced from the impression of the prepared tooth to act as a base. The porcelain powder is mixed with water to form a slurry, which is built-up in layers onto the foil until the desired shape is achieved. The porcelain is compacted by removing water from the preparation by blotting with absorbent paper or by flicking with a brush. This compaction against the platinum foil ↓ firing shrinkage. The crown is then fired to ↓ porosity, which ↑ strength and ↑ translucency. Glazing produces a glossy outer skin which resists cracking and plaque accumulation. It can be added as a separate layer or by firing at a higher temperature after the addition of surface glazes. The platinum foil lining is unaffected by the firing and so should maintain accuracy of fit throughout. It is removed prior to cementation to give space for the cement lute (~25μm).

Other ceramic crowns are built-up on a refractory die (dentine-bonded crowns), heat-processed core (Empress), or Computer Aided Design/Computer Aided Manufacture (CAD/CAM) sintered core (Procera®).

Properties
- Firing shrinkage 30–40%, ∴ crown must be overbuilt.
- Chemically inert provided the surface layer is intact.
- Low thermal conductivity.
- Good aesthetic properties.
- Brittle. The main cause of failure is crack propagation which almost invariably emanates from the unglazed inner surface. This can be ↓ by
  (1) fusion of the inner surface to metal, as in the platinum foil and metal-bonded techniques;
  (2) by the use of an aluminous porcelain core
- High resistance to wear.
- Glazed surface resists plaque accumulation.

CAD/CAM[1]

Relies on a 3-D representation of either the prepared tooth or wax-up. Ceramics may be;

- Directly machined fully-dense ceramics e.g. Empress® CAD
- Constructed on an enlarged die upon which ceramic powder is packed e.g. Procera®
- Machined from an oversized part for firing by machining blocks of partially fired ceramic powder e.g. Lava®

Survival rates appear relatively high with the most studied Cerec system and Vita MkI and MkII ceramics, often over 90% survival over 4–10 years, outshining laboratory constructed ceramic inlays. Similarly high survival rates have been reported for CAD/CAM crown construction (Procera®, In-Ceram® Alumina).

1 J. R. Kelly 2007 *Clin Oral Impl Res* **18** 205.

Dental ceramics—practical applications

Porcelain jacket crown Now considered somewhat old-fashioned. A core of aluminous porcelain is laid down first, onto which 'dentine' and then 'enamel' porcelains are built up. For strength a minimum porcelain thickness of 0.8mm is required and a 90° butt joint at the margin.

Porcelain fused to metal crown The porcelains used for bonding to a metal substructure have additional leucite added to ↑ the coefficient of thermal expansion to almost match the alloys used. Also, a porcelain which fuses below the melting point of the alloy is required. Bonding to the metal occurs by a combination of:
- mechanical retention;
- chemical bonding to the metal oxide layer on the surface of the alloy.

The ↑ strength of porcelain bonded to metal crowns is due to:
- the metal substructure supporting the porcelain;
- ↓ crack propagation by bonding the inner surface of the porcelain to metal;
- the outer surface of porcelain being under tension, thus ↓ crack propagation.

Glass ceramic or castable ceramics Semi-crystalline glasses, e.g. tetrasilicic fluormica glass (Dicor), produced by adding a nucleating agent onto which the glass crystals precipitate during cooling. This structure resists crack propagation, having a similar strength to core aluminous porcelain. An additional advantage is that the lost wax process can be used, so compensation for firing shrinkage is not required. A wax pattern is built-up by the technician and invested and cast. Following cooling, the casting is reheated to allow crystal growth to occur. The castable ceramics have ↑ translucency compared to porcelain, but dentine colour has to be created with surface glazes, which requires time and skill. Glass ceramic crowns are more expensive than PJC, but useful for young translucent teeth. Hot-pressed (IPS-Empress I and II) and glass infiltrated (Inceram) ceramics do not match the strength of porcelain fused to metal.

All ceramic systems now also include flame-sprayed (Techceram) or CAD-CAM (Procera) alumina cores onto which conventional porcelains are fired. Also zirconium oxide cores can be fabricated by CAD-CAM technology to produce anything up to full arch fixed restorations (Lava/Etkon).

Porcelain veneers A thin shell of porcelain or castable ceramic ~0.5–0.8mm thick (🕮 p. 250). Their thin section limits their ability to hide underlying tooth discoloration. Amenable to CAD-CAM fabrication.

Porcelain inlays Promising alternative to conventional treatment procedures. Only limited long-term studies available. Also amenable to CAD-CAM fabrication.

Porcelain repairs Can be carried out using composite and a silane coupling agent. A number of proprietary kits (Cojet) are available.

Denture materials—1

Acrylic resin

Acrylic is the most commonly used polymer for denture bases. Not only can it be re-lined, repaired, and added to comparatively easily, but it is also aesthetic and lightweight. Acrylic is composed of a chain of methacrylate molecules linked together to give PMMA.

Presentation Usually comprises a liquid and a powder mixed together. The liquid is stored in a dark bottle to ↑ shelf-life.

Powder	Liquid
PMMA beads (<100mm)	Methylmethacrylate monomer
Initiator, e.g. benzoyl peroxide	Cross-linking agent
Pigments &/or fibres	Inhibitor, e.g. hydroquinone activator (self-cure only)

Manipulation The powder and liquid should be mixed in a ratio of ~2.5:1 by weight. The mix passes through several distinct stages: sandy–string–dough–rubbery–hard (set). The dough stage is the best for handling and packing.

In denture fabrication the wax pattern and teeth are invested in plaster. The wax is then boiled out and the plaster coated with sodium alginate as a separator. The resultant space is then filled to excess (to allow for con-traction shrinkage of 7%) with acrylic dough under pressure. The acrylic is then polymerized.

Mode of activation

Self-cure acrylics show less setting contraction, but more water absorp-tion than heat-cure. This may result in the final item being slightly over-sized, thus ↓ retention. Self-cure acrylics are more porous, only 80% as strong, less resistant to abrasion, and contain a greater level of unreacted monomer compared to heat-cure. The main applications of self-cure acryl-ics are for denture repairs and re-lines, and orthodontic appliances, al-though for the latter the greater strength of heat-cure is preferable.

Heat-cure Conventionally polymerization requires heating in a hot-water bath for 7h at 70°C, then 3h at 100°C. The flask should be cooled slowly to minimize stresses within the acrylic. However, resins with differ-ent curing cycles (fast heat-cure) are now available. Microwave energy can be used to cure acrylic resin, but (apart from lunchtime) has no advantage over a water bath.

Light-cure resins are supplied as mouldable sheets. Used for denture bases or special trays.

Properties

- The glass transition (or softening) temperature of self-cure acrylic is 90°C, and for heat-cure 105°C.
- Poor impact strength and low resistance to fatigue #.
- Abrasion resistance not very good, but usually adequate.

- Good thermal insulator—undesirable as it can lead to the patient swallowing foods which are too hot.
- Low specific gravity (i.e. not too heavy).
- Radiolucent. Attempts to ↑ radio-opacity have not been very successful.
- Absorbs water, resulting in expansion. Drying out of acrylic should be avoided.
- Residual monomer (due to inadequate curing) weakens acrylic and can cause sensitivity reaction.
- Good aesthetics.

The strength of a denture depends upon:
1) Design, e.g. adequate thickness, avoidance of notches.
2) Strength of the acrylic, i.e. low monomer content, ↓ porosity, adequate curing. Can be ↑ by using high-impact resin.

Researchers are still evaluating methods of ↑ strength of denture resins. The addition of high-performance fibres (e.g. glass fibres) appears promising (Stick Tech).

Denture materials—2

Rebasing

Rebasing a denture base involves replacement of the fitting surface. Rebases can be either:

- Hard: heat or self-cure.
- Soft:
  - permanent: heat, self-cure, or light-cure.
  - temporary
    - —tissue conditioner: self-cure.
    - —functional impression material: self-cure.

The properties of self-cure materials are generally inferior, ∴ should only be used as a temporary measure.

Hard rebases Heat-cure PMMA is preferred, but requires the patient to do without the denture while it is being added. A self-cure material has obvious advantages, but even the higher acrylics, e.g. butylmethacrylate should only be used as a temporary measure as they are weaker than PMMA and discolour.

Soft liners require a material with a glass transition temperature below or at that of the mouth so that it is soft and resilient. The majority of soft liners are either based on silicone or acrylic (polyethylmethacrylate or PMMA powder plus alkyl methacrylate monomer and a plasticizer) or polyphosphazene fluoroelastomer.[1]

Plasticized acrylic	Silicone polymers
Good bond to denture	Bond with denture base not reliable
Harden over time	Maintain resilience
More readily distorted	Absorb water: candida colonization
	More elastic

Heat, light, or self-cure types are available. The self-cure materials have inferior properties, but all require replacement during the lifetime of the denture.[2]

Tissue conditioners usually comprise powdered polyethylmethacrylate to which a plasticizing mix of esters and alcohol is added. No chemical reaction takes place, the liquids merely soften the powder to form a gel and leach out over time, resulting in hardening. To ensure maximum tissue recovery the lining should be a minimum thickness of 2mm and replaced every few days. E.g. Coe-Soft®, Coe-Comfort™, Viscogel®. May be used when relining denture after implant placement for minimal loading during osseointegration.

Functional impression materials The tissue-conditioning materials are usually used for this purpose, an impression being cast of the fitting surface after a few days of wear.

1 F. Kawano 1992 *J Prosthet Dent* **68** 368.
2 E. R. Dootz 1993 *J Prosthet Dent* **69** 114.

Biocompatibility of dental materials

Before a new material can be marketed it must successfully pass both laboratory and clinical trials to evaluate its biocompatibility. Yet, some adverse effects only become apparent after the material has been in clinical use. Unless used with care many materials may prove a hazard to the patient or the dentist and his/her staff.

Hazards to the patient

Systemic effects

Allergic reactions

- *Amalgam* Although genuine cases of amalgam allergy exist, these are rarer than the tabloid press would suggest. For proven cases composite resin or cast restorations should be used.
- *Nickel* Constituent of some alloys can cause contact eczema. Sensitive patients often have a history of allergy to jewellery or watch casings. Alternative alloys are available.
- *Acrylic monomer* Can cause an allergic reaction and should be considered in a patient complaining of a 'burning mouth'. The concentration of monomer is ↑ in poorly cured acrylic and greater in self- than heat-cure. Extended curing, e.g. 24h, may ↓ concentration of monomer to an acceptable level; if not a cobalt chrome or SS denture base will be required.
- *Epimine* In polyether impression material.

If an allergy is suspected, refer to a dermatologist.

Directly toxic

- Beryllium, present in some nickel alloys, is known to be a carcinogen. Provided the alloy is not ground any risks are confined to the production laboratory. Beryllium-free alloys are becoming ↑ available.
- Fluoride in excess can be toxic (📖 p. 28).

Ingestion or inhalation of air-borne dust must be avoided.

Local effects

Eye damage Curing lamps can cause eye damage due to the glare. The simplest solution is to ask the patient to close their eyes and use a shield.
Thermal injury Can result: **1** to the pulp, e.g. caused by exothermic setting reactions; **2** to the mucosa, e.g. caused by dentures which are thermal insulators, as the patient may swallow drink/food that is too hot, or by the setting reaction of self-cure denture re-line materials; **3** to the soft tissues, e.g. by hot instruments.
Chemical injury Can be caused by noxious chemicals (e.g. etchant, hydrogen peroxide) being allowed to come into direct contact with the tissues.
Hypersensitivity reactions Can occur in response to the materials that cause systemic allergy.

Hazards to staff

In the surgery

- Allergic reactions, e.g. topical anaesthetics, latex gloves, methyl methacrylate monomer, dentine adhesive systems.
- Eye damage from light sources. Use eye protection or shielding.

- Alginate dust.
- Mercury vapour.
- Nitrous oxide.

In the laboratory

- Cyanide solution for electroplating.
- Vapours from low-fusing metal dies.
- Silicaeous particles in investment materials.
- Fluxes containing fluoride.
- Hydrofluoric acid used for etching porcelain veneers.
- Beryllium in some alloys.
- PMMA powders.
- Methyl methacrylate monomer.
- Casting machines.

Law and ethics

Contents

Relevant pages in other chapters Hiring and firing staff, 📖 p. 694.

Principal sources and further reading BDA 2000 Advice sheet *Ethics in Dentistry*. GDC 2005 *Standards for Dental Professionals*. P. Heasman 2008 *Master Dentistry Volume 2*, Churchill Livingstone. P. Lambden 2002 *Dental Law and Ethics* Radcliffe Medical Press. R. Rattan and J. Tiernan 2004 *Risk Management in General Dental Practice* Quintessence.

Definitions

Claimant (or in Scotland, *pursuer*) The claimant in a civil action.
Defendant (or *defender*) The person against whom a claim is made.
Legislation A country's written law. In the UK laid down in Acts of Parliament.
Secondary legislation The precise implementation of the general rules laid down in the Act (often published as Statutory Instruments).
Litigation An action brought in a court of law.
Claim form A document setting out the details of a proposed action, which is served to the defendant.
Affidavit A written statement on oath.

On qualification

Register with the GDC (📖 p. 662)
Get professional indemnity cover (📖 p. 660)
Consider taking out sickness and accident insurance.

Legal processes

England, Wales and Northern Ireland

Civil law

Civil cases involve claims made by individuals against other individuals/organizations for a breach of civil rules e.g. breach of contract, negligence, unpaid debt. Civil cases are decided on the balance of probabilities and the only remedy is financial recompense. The losing party is liable for the costs of both sides.

Depending upon financial value, cases are allocated to:
- Small claims track: claims with value of <£5000 (<£2000 in NI) or personal injury <£1000
- Fast track
- Multi track
- County Court
- High Court

Appeals are referred to the Court of Appeal (civil division) and, occasionally, to the House of Lords.

Criminal law

Criminal prosecutions are undertaken when the 'law' has been broken, e.g. speeding, fraud, assault. The decision to proceed with a prosecution is made by the Crown Prosecution Service (CPS). In criminal law, the case must be proved beyond reasonable doubt. Depending upon the severity of the crime, cases are heard in:
- Magistrates' court. Appeals to Crown Court.
- Crown Court (with a judge and jury). Appeals go to the Court of Appeal (criminal division).

Scotland

Civil law

The Sheriff court is the lowest civil court with appeal going to the Inner House of the Court of Session which sits at Parliament House in Edinburgh. The final court of appeal for civil cases is the House of Lords.

Criminal law

The decision to proceed with a criminal prosecution is made by the office of the Procurator Fiscal (PF). The PF is a qualified advocate/solicitor appointed by the Lord Advocate.

Depending upon the severity of the crime, criminal cases are heard in:
- Justice of Peace Courts (replacing former district courts)
- Sheriffs Court (cases heard by sheriff +/− jury)
- High Court of Justiciary (cases heard by judge + jury) and the final appeal court for criminal cases.

Coroners Court

This straddles the two systems and meets to consider unnatural and unexpected deaths, e.g. a death in the dental chair. The process is investigative (as opposed to the claimant versus defendant stance taken in the other courts).

Any unexpected death should be reported to the Coroner in England, Wales, and N. Ireland, or to the Procurator Fiscal in Scotland, either directly or through the police (the Registrar of Deaths will notify the authorities if this has not already been done).

Jury service

Dentists are no longer automatically exempt from jury service. It is possible to apply for discretionary exemption or deferral of service using the form sent with the summons. Jury service can only be deferred once. Where a person has attended for jury service in the previous 2 years they have a right to be excused service.

Complaints[1]

A complaint is any expression of dissatisfaction about any aspect of a dental service or treatment that requires a response. It may be spoken or written in nature. It is part of the responsibility of a dental professional to deal with complaints properly and professionally.[2] All providers of dental services should have a complaints procedure with an appointed responsible person for dealing with complaints. All members of the team should be familiar with the complaints procedure. A written record of all complaints received should be retained and an annual report produced.

Stages

Local resolution

A complaint may be made either to the practice or direct to the PCT. Once a complaint is received:

- Acknowledge receipt/respond to the complaint within 2 working days. If the complaint is made in person, provide the patient with a copy of the complaints procedure. Advise in writing of the estimated response timetable (normally a full response should be provided within 10 working days for a practice or 20 working days hospital/trust).
- Fully investigate the complaint. Contact defence society for advice if required.
- Phone or arrange a meeting to discuss the complaint with the patient, if appropriate.
- Provide a full written response to the complainant, ensuring all points raised by the complaint are addressed along with a solution where appropriate. Resolution may include refund/replacement of work as a 'gesture of goodwill', an explanation or an apology.
- If the patient is still not satisfied, inform the patient of additional options for resolution:
  - PALS (Patient Advice and Liaison Service)/Local Health Councils (Scotland)/Health and Social Services Councils (NI)
  - Ombudsman/Health Board
  - Dental Complaints Service (private patients)
- Co-operate fully with any formal enquiry into the treatment of a patient.

Time limits Complaints must be made ≤12 months after the event or <6 months after the complainant realises there was a problem. Where a good case can be made, this latter time bar may be extended.

PALS/Local Health Councils Although not part of the complaints procedure, they can give advice about the process and may be able to resolve concerns informally.

PCT/Health Board Can deal with a complaint direct, or with the patient's consent refer the complaint to the practice/provider. Where a complaint is difficult to resolve it can:

---

1 BDA Advice Sheet (B10) 2007 Handling complaints.
2 GDC Principles of Complaints Handling 2006.

- Offer mediation—a confidential, voluntary process which seeks to assist complaint resolution in a non-confrontational manner
- Advise patient of their right to approach the Independent Review Secretariat (Wales/NI)/referral direct to the Ombudsman (Wales/Scotland/England)

Independent Review Secretariat: A Convener is appointed by the Board/Trust to decide whether a panel should be convened. Following investigation by a review panel, a written report is sent to both parties and the Board/Trust will decide whether service improvements are recommended.

NHS Ombudsman: The ombudsman is independent of the NHS and investigates complaints relating to NHS services within hospitals/trusts/health authorities/practice. The ombudsman may not become involved in complaints where legal action is intended or has commenced, and will only deal with complaints that have failed to be resolved through local resolution/independent review. Can investigate the complaint and make recommendations where appropriate, e.g.
- apology
- explanation of what went wrong
- change of decision made
- repayment of costs incurred as result of incident
- change in procedure
- improvement in facilities

Dental Complaints Service: The DCS is an independent complaints service funded by the GDC which aids in the resolution of complaints regarding private dental treatment in the UK. Where a patient contacts the service, they will encourage the complainant to try and resolve the issue with the practitioner directly through their complaints procedure. Where this has been tried, they will contact the practitioner and provide assistance to both parties to try and reach a fair resolution.

Care Quality Commission (CQC): The CQC regulates the quality of health and social care. Although it has no direct role in the complaints process the CQC requires registered provides of services to investigate complaints effectively and learn lessons from them. It is a legal requirement for all Trusts providing services for patients to register with the CQC from April 2009 and it is planned that regulation of primary care services will commence in 2011.

Disciplinary procedures

A PCT/Health Board has the right to investigate and instigate disciplinary proceedings. The decision to investigate may occur
- following a report from an Independent Review Panel/CQC
- where a complaint raises concerns regarding performance indicating the dentist was in breach of their terms of service/contract
- where a dentist is under investigation by a statutory body.

A PCT/Health Board has the power to suspend a dentist to protect the interests of patients, staff and the practitioner. The decision to suspend a dentist may be made whilst awaiting a decision from a statutory body or whilst investigation is ongoing. Throughout the process, a practitioner may elect to receive support from a colleague or member of their local dental committee (LDC).

Complaint by GDP against GDP The Local Dental Committee may be asked to arbitrate. Advice can also be sought from the defence organizations.

Consent

Consent is the voluntary and continuous permission of a competent patient to receive a particular treatment based on the patient being informed regarding the purpose, nature and likely risks of the treatment, including the likelihood of its success and any alternatives to it. Permission given under any unfair or undue pressure is not consent.

Treatment without any consent = assault/battery

Treatment with general consent, but without explanation of what is involved may = negligence.

Consent should always be obtained by the clinician in immediate charge of the treatment. Consultants must ensure that junior staff are appropriately trained and qualified to obtain consent.

Consent can be given in writing, verbally, or be implied.

Written consent preferable, especially when extensive treatment is planned and essential before a GA is given. A written consent form provides evidence that the patient has consented but not necessarily proof that the consent is valid.

Verbal consent should be the minimum obtained for treatment. The benefits of having a third party present at all times are obvious.

Implied consent to a dental examination is given by attending an appointment and sitting in the dental chair, however this does not cover provision of treatment.

Consent for children

Those aged 16 and 17yrs are presumed to have the competence to give consent for themselves. Younger children who understand fully what is involved in the proposed procedure can also give consent (although their parents will ideally be involved). In other cases, someone with parental responsibility must give consent on the child's behalf, unless they cannot be reached in an emergency. If a competent child consents to treatment, a parent cannot override that consent (the 'Gillick competence' principle). Legally, a parent can consent if a competent child refuses, but it is likely that taking such a serious step will be rare. For children in care consult an authorized representative of the local authority.

Consent for adults who are not competent to give consent

A patient is unable to make a decision for themselves if they are unable:
- To understand information relevant to that decision
- To retain that information
- To use or weigh that information as part of the process of making the decision
- To communicate the decision (whether by talking, using sign language or by any other means).

- Under common law, no person can consent for a patient who lacks mental capacity, however, The Mental Capacity Act 2005[1] enables an individual with capacity to give another individual a lasting power of attorney (LPA) to make medical decisions on their behalf should their capacity become impaired. Where no LPA exists, a patient lacking capacity may receive treatment necessary to preserve life, health or well-being provided that the treatment is in the best interests of the patient and no valid 'advance refusal' exists. Treatment of patients lacking capacity must take into account the MCA Code of Practice.[2]

Some specific problems

- Treatment of an unconscious patient is valid under the legal doctrine of 'necessity', but is limited to emergency care.
- If a patient's photographs are to be used for a lecture or presentation, written consent should be obtained.

1 The Mental Capacity Act 2005 🔊 http://www.opsi.gov.uk/ACTS/acts2005/ukpga_20050009_en_1
2 The Mental Capacity Act Code of Practice 2007.

Contracts

A contract is a legally binding agreement between parties and can be verbal, written or implied. In law, they are equally binding, but as the parties may have differing recollections of what was said, the advantages of a written agreement are apparent.

Between dentist and patient Although in the past the majority of contracts were made verbally, GDC guidance is that whenever a patient is returning for treatment following an examination, a written treatment plan and cost estimate should be given. Dentists providing NHS dental services are required to provide a written treatment plan advising of any NHS charges +/− alternative options for private treatment under the terms of their contract. The treatment plan and estimate should be signed by the patient if they wish to proceed with treatment, and ideally should advise patients of the need to attend booked appointments, payment policy and practice procedure for failed or missed appointments. As treatment progresses patients should be informed of any changes to the original treatment plan and any effect on costs. In the event of any dispute over treatment or costs, the signed plan can be referred to.

Legally, the dentist is expected to exercise a reasonable degree of care, while the patient also has a duty to keep appointments and pay the agreed fee.

Where fees are not paid and no response to written accounts is received, the options for recovery of fees are: (1) issue a County Court Summons (the Citizen's Advice Bureau have an explanatory leaflet), or (2) employ a debt-collection agency. The latter is considerably easier.

Between dentist (provider) and PCT/Health Board. A dentist working within GDS/PDS in England/Wales has a contract agreement to provide NHS dental services. The level of service provided is measured against an allocated number of 'units of dental activity (UDA)', or 'units of orthodontic activity (UOA)'. Compliance with clinical governance/quality assurance requirements is an integral part of the contract. In Scotland, provision of NHS services is remunerated on a fee per item basis in compliance with NHS Terms of Service. Breach of either contract or terms of service may lead to disciplinary action.

Between principals/providers and associates/performers, or partners Because of their importance these should be written with the help of a solicitor. The BDA has sample agreements for partnerships, assistantships, associateships, performers and for expense-sharing arrangements, and in cases of dispute can arrange arbitration. A barring-out clause is a common inclusion designed to prevent unfair competition by a rival practice being set up in the near vicinity. However, these need to be fair (e.g. 1 mile radius in a busy suburban area for 1yr) to be enforceable. Arrangements for payment of fees for any remedial or replacement work also need to be agreed and included. Careful consideration should be given to include safeguards in case the practice runs into financial difficulties. For performers, the contract should include details of how many UDAs/UOAs are allocated to the performer, how payment will be made and how UDAs performed will be assessed and any discrepancy addressed.

Between dentist and staff Terms and Conditions of employment should include a job description, pay, holiday entitlements and arrangements, bonuses for additional qualifications and loyalty, sickness allowances, pensions, disciplinary rules, and termination procedures with details of notice required by each party. Advice sheets are available from the BDA.

Negligence

Professional negligence is defined as a failure to exercise reasonable care, in one's professional capacity.

Often negligence cases hinge on what constitutes 'reasonable care'. If a dentist can show that his actions were in line with those of a large number of his colleagues, he is unlikely to be held negligent (Bolam test).

For a negligence case to win, the onus is on the claimant's or pursuer's lawyer to prove the following:
- The dentist owed a duty of care to the patient.
- There was a breach of that duty.
- Damage occurred to the patient as a result of that breach.

Where no demonstrable loss has occurred a patient has no recourse in the law and can only voice his complaint to the PCT or Health Board. The ploy of attempting to shift the onus of proof onto the defendant by pleading *res ipsa loquitur* (the facts speak for themselves) is rarely successful. If the case is proved, financial compensation will be awarded by the court, taking into account the damage that occurred and the steps necessary to put it right.

Criminal negligence For criminal proceedings to be started the negligent action must be very serious and have some accentuating factor, e.g. the dentist was drunk or drugged, or disregarded well-known safety principles.

Contributory negligence When the actions of a patient have been partially (or completely) to blame for the damage that occurred, then contributory negligence can be pleaded; e.g. failure to follow post-op instructions.

Vicarious liability An employer can be held responsible for any negligence by an employee that occurs during his employ. This means that a dentist is responsible for the actions or omissions of his staff; e.g. dental nurse, receptionist, technician. However, as every individual is responsible for his own acts, a charge of negligence could be brought against both employee and employer.

Time bar Usually 3yrs; this does not begin to run until the patient knows, or ought to have known, of the damage that is said to have been done. For children the time bar does not start until 18yrs of age; there is no time bar in the case of mental disability. A patient may petition the Court to set aside the time bar if they can show reasonable grounds for this to be done.

The steps involved in a civil action for damages

- Usually the first intimation of trouble is a solicitor's letter (known as a letter before action). This should be dealt with only after consultation with a defence society. Notification of a Legal Aid application should also be passed on.
- If the patient's solicitor proceeds, a letter of claim or summons will be served. As there is a time bar (usually 14–21 days) within which notification of a defence to the claim must be given to the court, it is important to respond quickly via a defence organization.
- The defence society will then make their own investigation into the claim and if necessary seek the advice of an 'expert'. Should the case appear not to be defensible, then the society will try to settle the

matter out of court. Where there is no evidence of negligence, the case may proceed to a full hearing.

- Prior to the trial, counsel for the defence will need to establish the full facts of the case. This can be time-consuming.
- At the end of the trial the verdict will be given on the balance of probability, and the level of compensation set as appropriate.

There but for the grace of God go I?

It must be remembered that doctors and dentists are human beings and not infallible. The law does realize that unforeseen accidents can happen. The defence organizations advise: 'In circumstances where complications and errors arise it is proper that objective, factual information, with appropriate clinical reassurance is provided. Adequate explanations assist in reducing fear and uncertainty which may give rise to complaints and claims.'[1]

The importance of clear, concise, and contemporaneous notes cannot be over-emphasized. Good quality record cards, X-rays, and study models (where appropriate) are invaluable.

---

1 Medical Protection Society, *Annual Report 1986* and *1987*.

Professional indemnity and defence organizations

All GDC registrants are required to have adequate and appropriate indemnity cover to ensure that patients can claim compensation if they are entitled to it. The GDC presently recognizes arrangements provided by:
- Dental defence organizations
- Professional indemnity insurance
- NHS indemnity

The GDC standards committee is presently considering issuing guidance regarding the minimal acceptable requirements of an insurance only indemnity approach.

Dental defence organizations

In the UK there are three non-profit-making, mutual organizations:
- Dental Protection (part of Medical Protection Society) (DPL)
- Medical and Dental Defence Union of Scotland (MDDUS)
- Medical Defence Union (MDU)

Their addresses are given on 📖 p. 746.

As well as providing professional indemnity cover they provide their members with advice, information and support in proceedings involving professional matters e.g. GDC disciplinary hearings, PCT investigations. They also contribute significantly to the social life of medical and dental students.

Indemnity insurance

Provided by commercial insurance companies, cover is provided according to the conditions and terms of the insurance policy. Some professional organizations e.g. British Association of Dental Nurses and Dental Practitioners Association include some degree of indemnity insurance as part of their membership subscription. Insurance based indemnity provides cover for claims arising during the period that the policy is in force. 'Run-off' cover may need to be purchased to cover claims arising outside of the insurance term if changing indemnity provider or retiring.

NHS indemnity

Crown/NHS indemnity provides cover relating to acts or omissions of doctors and dentists working in NHS hospitals and Salaried Primary Care. Crown/NHS indemnity covers work undertaken within the NHS contract; it does not provide assistance for private treatment, disciplinary issues (GDC/GMC), fatal accident enquiries or coroner's inquest. It is recommended that additional professional indemnity is taken out to cover involvement in such situations.

It is important to ensure that indemnity cover is sufficient to cover all aspects of work being undertaken e.g. implants, maxillofacial surgery, cosmetic procedures.

Professional standards and ethics[1]

Do as you would be done by.

Although not imposed by legislation, ethical behaviour is necessary, to maintain the standing of the profession in the eyes of the public. Clinicians who behave unethically may have to account for their actions to the GDC. The GDC expects dental professionals to abide by the following principles:

- Put the patients' interests first and act to protect them.
- Respect the patient's dignity and choices.
- Treat information about patients as confidential and only use it for the purpose for which it is given. Breach of confidentiality may be justified only in exceptional circumstances if in the patient's or public interest.
- Co-operate with other team members and colleagues in the interests of the patient and respect their role in caring for patients.
- Do not make claims which could mislead patients. Be trustworthy.
- Maintain appropriate standards of personal behaviour in all walks of life so that patients have confidence in you and the public have confidence in the dental profession.
- Do not solicit patients from other dentists.
- When consulted for emergency treatment by a colleague's patient: treat as necessary to alleviate pain and refer the patient back with an explanation of what was done.
- Refer to suitably qualified colleagues, cases which are beyond your competence and require specialist advice and/or treatment.
- Although the restrictions on advertising have now been lifted, all adverts must still be legal, decent, truthful, and have regard for professional propriety.

See also Chapter 16.

---

1 GDC 2005 *Standards for Dental Professionals*.

The General Dental Council and Registration

The GDC is a statutory regulatory body set up by the Dentists Act to regulate dental professionals in the UK. Anyone wishing to work in the UK as a dentist, therapist, dental hygienist, clinical dental technician, orthodontic therapist, dental technician or dental nurse must be registered with the GDC or be 'in training' on an approved training scheme. The Council comprises 29 members comprising 15 dentists and 4 dental care professionals (DCPs) elected by the profession and 10 appointed lay members

Functions of the GDC

- *Maintain a register of qualified dental professionals*
- *Set standards of dental practice/conduct*
- *Assure quality of dental education*
- *Protect patients and assist with complaints*

In addition to the Dentists and DCP registers, the GDC maintains 12 Specialist Lists covering oral surgery, paediatric dentistry, prosthodontics, oral medicine, dental and maxillofacial radiology, endodontics, restorative dentistry, oral microbiology, orthodontics, periodontics, dental public health and oral pathology. A special care dentistry list is to open in the near future. In addition to having the required qualifications, to be included on the register an applicant must pay the annual retention fee and complete the necessary CPD requirement (📖 p. 714). Failure to complete CPD or pay the retention fee can lead to erasure from the list.

A dentist or DCP shall be liable to have his name erased from the Register if, either before or after he is registered, he has been convicted of a criminal offence or has been found that their fitness to practice is impaired. If a registrant enters a plea of guilty in a criminal matter or accepts a caution for a charge, even where the professional has a defence, this will be taken as an admission of guilt by the GDC.

Fitness to Practise proceedings

If the GDC receives information that raises questions about a registrant's fitness to practice it can investigate and where necessary impose conditions on an individual's registration. Fitness to practice may be alleged to be impaired due to:

- Misconduct either professional or personal including convictions/cautions received in UK or elsewhere
- Deficient professional performance
- Adverse health

The GDC has a set procedure to investigate concerns about fitness to practice.

1. Caseworker considers information to assess if issues are raised regarding a registrants fitness to practice. If yes, the case is reviewed by the GDC registrar and where appropriate referred to the *Investigating Committee*. A letter is sent to the professional advising them of the investigation and inviting them to respond to the allegations. The registrar can also refer the case to an *Interim Orders Committee* where it is felt that interim suspension of the registration may be necessary.

2. Investigating Committee (IC) meets in private and assesses all information relating to allegation including the professional's response. The IC can decide to:

- Take no further action
- Issue advice or warning either privately or public (attached to register entry)
- Refer to Practice Committee

3. Practice Committee (PC) The IC may refer the case onwards to:

The Professional Performance Committee for allegations relating to deficient performance.

The Health Committee for allegations relating to physical or mental health problems e.g. drug/alcohol dependency, depression.

The Professional Conduct Committee for criminal convictions or gross misconduct.

When the PC decides that 'on the balance of probability', fitness to practise has been impaired it may impose the following sanctions:

- Erasure from the register for 5 years (except for grounds of adverse health)
- Suspension from the register for up to 12 months
- Conditions applied to registration for a period of up to 3 years
- Reprimand

Hempsons Solicitors produce an excellent GDC Fitness to Practise Guide. Email: dental@hempsons.co.uk

Wise precautions or how to avoid litigation

When in doubt contact your defence organization

- Good records are invaluable and should be concise, factual, and objective. They should contain details of treatment and advice given and especially any that the patient declines. All appointments made and failed should be noted. Do not record anything that you would not wish a patient to read (e.g. personal comments about a patient's behaviour). The Data Protection Act 1998 allows patients access to manual and electronic records (📖 p. 708).
- Take adequate radiographs whenever clinically necessary. Record justification and X-ray findings in the clinical records.
- Clinical records (including X-rays and models) should be kept for at least 11yrs. For children, they should be retained until age 25yrs, or for 11yrs, whichever is the longer. Where extensive work has been carried out or problems occurred it is wise to retain records indefinitely.
- Protect the patient's eyes and airway.
- Update the medical history at every recall.
- Keep up to date. Comply with CPD requirements. Continuing with outmoded techniques could render a dentist liable to a charge of professional misconduct. Similarly, be wary of using controversial or unproven procedures or materials. Have a personal development plan to ensure structured learning.
- Always have a third person present during treatment to act as a chaperone. This is of extreme importance if using sedation, as reports of patients having erotic fantasies under the influence of nitrous oxide, diazepam, or midazolam can no longer be regarded as amusing anecdotes.[1]
- Obtain written consent for any expensive or complicated procedures.
- Refer a patient when it is their best interests.
- Ensure cross-infection policies are adhered to. (📖 p. 718).
- Where a GA is being administered this must be by a medically qualified anaesthetist, with a written protocol for referral and management of the patient. This must include appropriate arrangements for immediate transfer of the patient to a critical care facility.
- Read and comply with current guidance issued by the GDC (🖰 www.gdc-uk.org).
- Comply with the Ionizing Radiation Guidelines. (📖 p. 720).

If you are sued, immediately contact your defence society. Never alter records under the threat of litigation. Alterations to records, made at any time, should be dated and initialled.

Advice lines

Dental Protection: 0207 7399 1400/0113 2436436.
Dental Defence Union: 020 7202 1500.
Medical and Dental Defence Union of Scotland: 0845 270 2034.

---

1 M. Fields 1990 *BDJ* **169** 4.

Forensic dentistry

Theoretically forensic dentistry encompasses all aspects of dentistry and the law, but here we will confine ourselves to the application of dental science to criminal investigations.[1]

Identification

Dental tissues survive the effects of fire, water and time well; information from the surviving dentition may be helpful in identification where other means of distinguishing a person have been lost. Teeth can be used to indicate the approximate age of a victim and may be compared to dental records to aid identification. Examination of the skull and jaw may also provide information relating to age, sex, racial origin, and time elapsed since death.

When comparing dental records with post mortem records it must be remembered that dental treatment may have been carried out subsequent to the last dental chart and that missing teeth or additional restorations do not necessarily exclude identification. Comparative radiographs may be as individual as fingerprints. From a forensic point of view the value of accurate up-to-date records, and identification marks in dentures, are self-evident. Notes regarding intra-oral piercing and tattooing may also prove valuable.

Occasionally, a practitioner may be requested by the police to reveal the dental records of a live, but missing person. The advice of a defence society should be sought, as legally a patient's confidential records should not be revealed without a Court Order.

Bite marks

Bite marks in inanimate objects left at the site of a crime have on occasion contributed to the conviction of the perpetrator. If the 'evidence' is a perishable foodstuff, a permanent record can be made either by casting in stone or rubber base material, following photography with a linear scale.

Bite marks may be found on human skin both on a victim of assault as well as on the perpetrator where a victim has bitten their assailant. Additionally they may be seen in children who have been the victim of abuse. Good photographs, including a linear scale, are essential. If the victim/suspect is alive, photographs need to be repeated 24 hourly as the clarity of the bite may improve with time. A swab of the bite mark may provide a saliva sample which can be compared to a suspect's saliva.

---

1 K. Whittaker 1989 *A Colour Atlas of Forensic Dentistry*, Wolfe.

Chapter 16

Professionalism and communication

Contents

Relevant pages in other chapters Complaints, ☐ p.650; Consent, ☐ p.654; Professional standards and ethics; ☐ p.661; The GDC, ☐ p. 662; Management skills, ☐ p.692; Hiring and firing staff, ☐ p.694; Clinical governance, ☐ p.714; CPD, ☐ p.714; Clinical audit and peer review, ☐ p.714.

Principal sources GDC guidance on standards in dentistry (updated) ℘ http://www.gdc-uk.org/; RCS Eng Good Surgical Practice ℘ http://www.rcseng.ac.uk/standards/good-surgical-practice/overview; Various at ℘ www.rcseng.ac.uk/publications/docs.

What is professionalism?

A dictionary definition of 'professionalism':

'The occupation which one professes to be skilled in and to follow. A vocation in which a professed knowledge of some department of learning or science is used in its application to the affairs of others or in the practice of an art founded upon it. In a wider sense, any calling or occupation by which a person habitually earns his living'.

How different from this broad definition is medical and dental professionalism? Do we individually profess special skill and knowledge? No—that is transparently defined by our peers by assessment, qualification and registration to effectively prove that we have these properties. In the UK the GDC holds registration lists for all dentists and certain specialists (GMC for oral & maxillofacial surgeons) and similar legal structures exist throughout the world. Royal Colleges, Faculties and Specialist Associations all see a major part of their role as 'standard setting' for their areas of expertise. Again, this is repeated throughout the world. It is this concept of a universal sense of commitment to a role that defines medical and dental professionalism, not any individual country's legal definition of it (which is why professions often constitute the major opposition to dictatorships or other extreme political systems).

A useful definition of medical and dental professionalism for our purposes is international and based on the work of Swick.[1] They

- show altruism (subordinate their interests to the interests of those in need);
- adhere to high ethical standards;
- respond to the needs of society, behaviours reflect a social contract with their communities;
- show the values of probity, compassion, empathy and respect for themselves, patients and colleagues (not just peers);
- exercise accountability for themselves and colleagues;
- recognize and act appropriately on conflicts of interest;
- reflect critically on their practice and strive for improvement;
- show a commitment to continuing professional development (in its widest sense);
- can deal effectively with high levels of complexity and uncertainty;
- respond positively to appropriate suggestions for improvement whatever the source;
- demonstrate an appreciation of diversity;
- adhere to the principles of 'duty of care'.

Individual and collective professional self regulation lies at the heart of the concept of medical and dental professionalism. That is based on the precept that society trusts us with certain privileges by virtue of the job (in all its aspects) that we do and we maintain that trust by individual high standards of behaviour and collective regulation and remediation or censure of those who fail to live up to those standards. I suspect for many of you this concept is self evident although you may not have considered it in quite these terms. Why does 'professionalism' now need to be transparently and didactically taught?

1 H. M. Swick 2000 *Academ Med* **75** 612.

Although the concept of the doctor (and latterly the dentist) as a 'healer' goes back into antiquity, the concept of a dual role 'healer' and 'professional' is relatively new with the emergence of the 'learned professions' in the middle ages. Until the 1960s the role and commitment of the healing professional was largely implicit, evolving and supported by the majority of society. During the next 20 years an increasingly critical view of the professions developed among the social sciences, managerial echelons and politicians, documenting failures and questioning its relevance to society. In the 1980s and onward an increasing dominance of either state or corporate sector employers and a diminishing influence of the medical professional is seen. This tended to increase the value of systems to state or corporate sector over the values of healthcare professionalism. However, more recently it has been widely recognized that 'neither economic incentives, nor technology, nor administrative control has proved an effective surrogate for the commitment to integrity evoked in the ideal of professionalism'.[1] We therefore give more 'bang for their buck' by committing to being professional than any externally imposed system. Given that we, as healthcare professionals, have been disrespected and disenfranchised by these influential groups why should we adhere to the notion of professionalism? Clearly the great and good of the medical and dental political world see it as important—is this just to protect their own status?

Probably not. Individually or collectively we cannot do our jobs without a functioning system to work within. The best way to influence that is to wield the power that comes with the trust afforded by society in general in an organized, unified and responsible fashion. Society needs healers, we are still far and away the most trusted of groups in society. The general public is not happy with their leaders. The bureaucrats (state or corporate) control the marketplace and are blamed for defects in the system. Being a professional is the best way to improve the system and genuinely being professional is what makes you want to improve it—for the betterment of all.

Therefore a better definition might read 'An occupation whose core element is work based on the mastery of a complex body of knowledge and skills. It is a vocation in which knowledge of some aspect of science or learning or the practice of an art founded upon it is used in the service of others. Its members are governed by codes of ethics and profess a commitment to competence, integrity and morality, altruism, and to the promotion of the public good within their domain. These commitments form the basis of a social contract between the profession and society, which in return grants the profession a monopoly over the use of its knowledge base, the right to considerable autonomy in practice and the privilege of self-regulation. Professions and their members are accountable to those served and to society'.[2]

1 W. Sullivan 1999 Hastings Centre Report **7**.
2 S. Cruess *et al.* 1999 *Academ Med* **74** 878.

Politics and the public

Social contract this is a term derived from Gough[1] 'the rights and duties of the state and its citizens are reciprocal and the recognition of this reciprocity constitutes a relationship which by analogy can be called a social contract'. It is a complex mix of the explicit; written, legal or paralegal codes, rules and regulations and the implicit; unwritten, individual and collective senses of obligation and purpose reflecting personal and group codes of ethics and morals. It can have universal and local components (i.e. those applicable internationally and those that are country or locality specific). Importantly it is constantly evolving and seeks to balance society's expectations of medicine with medicine's expectations of society.

Professionalism is the basis of dentistry's contract with society. In common with medicine it requires placing the interests of patients above those of ourselves (within reason), setting and maintaining standards of competence and integrity and providing expert advice to society on matters of health.

For professionalism to have any effective basis in reality the public must trust in us individually and collectively, this depends on our integrity both individually and collectively. The fact that annual polls consistently place doctors and dentists at the very top of lists in which the public place their trust bears out the fact that this has been the case since the origin of our professions.

This in itself can create problems.

The patient, individual or as a community, is *not* the customer who is always right. Politicians elected or unelected do *not* always have the best interests of the population at heart. In situations where we as professionals see this to be the case we are obliged to speak out. This can carry with it accusations of paternalism or politicization.

Political implication it is illogical to believe that health is not a political issue—it affects the public good and is a right in most civilizations. It is therefore part of being a professional to express both concerns and potential solutions at systems that fail to deliver what they should for patients. What is counterproductive is the descent into party or partisan politics which is the rightful quagmire of the politician.

Equally a desperate avoidance of the appearance of being paternalistic in the name of political correctness becomes counterproductive if we fail to advise patients what we feel is in their best interests. They are entitled to ignore that advice (providing they are competent to do so) and go elsewhere but they are not entitled to demand that we provide a treatment we genuinely believe is not in their best interest.

The fact remains that, as healthcare professionals, we are trusted and society needs us. The continuing commitment to the role of the healthcare professional is key to that.

1 J. Gough 1957 *The Social Contract*. New York. OUP.

Standards

The principle standard setting bodies in the UK for dentistry are the GDC, the Specialist Dental Education and Training Board, the Conference of Postgraduate Dental Deans, the Dental Faculties of the Royal Colleges of Surgeons, the Speciality Associations, the British Dental Association and the dental degree awarding Universities. Each of these has a different and sometimes conflicting role and each can be influenced to a greater or lesser degree by government. Each country has its own bodies with variations on the same functions.

Principles All these bodies claim to seek to uphold standards and all to a greater or lesser degree speak for a constituent group. This has the inevitable problem of creating a potential conflict of roles. Each organization has to manage the conflict between altruism and self-interest, professional representation and state or corporate control, public good and a union function.

Self-regulation It has been mentioned that self-regulation is a key principle of professionalism and one which is regularly attacked by state and corporate bodies. The preservation of collective self-regulation carries with it certain obligations on the individual; maintenance of competence, participation in the process of self-regulation, support for the relevant bodies and behaviour that reflects integrity. The collective must demonstrate that individuals falling short of their obligations are corrected.

Re-establishing the primacy of the healthcare professional will require a renegotiation of the social contract. There are legitimate worries on both sides and advantage is taken of serious failures in professional behaviour to disproportionately undermine the healthcare professional's viewpoint. The repeated use of Shipman (a GP serial killer), or Karadzic (a psychiatrist mass murderer) as examples reinforces this even though these individuals' monstrous personality disorders could not have been contained by conventional medical self-regulation.

Balancing needs and wants Society wants (and needs) healers with a professional mindset. It has to have healthcare professionals using their knowledge and skill to heal, cure and relieve suffering. It wants individual's competence in discrete areas guaranteed. People want to be involved as patients. They want to see that those they trust behave to high ethical (and arguably moral) standards. It also needs accountability. Professionals want (and need) trust and respect and the acknowledgement that some failings are inevitable. Their expertise should be recognized and made appropriate use of. They should be sufficiently autonomous to act in the best interests of patients (politicians dictating and lawyers second guessing helps no-one). They need reasonable, reliable, validated and trusted regulatory and training processes which they have ownership of. They need adequate resources to care optimally for patients. They need to work in a system which transparently promotes the values society wishes to see in its healthcare professionals; caring, altruism, courtesy and competence.

The best way forward Is to ensure the balanced role of competent healer and caring professional in all training and practicing dentists.

CanMEDS[1]

The Royal College of Physicians and Surgeons of Canada have been involved for many years in a project designed to describe the competencies required of a physician. As you can see these include the role of 'professional' although their definition is narrower than that already used as it overlaps with the other CanMEDS roles. This descriptive system has been used extensively by the Royal Colleges in the UK in designing higher training curricula, the Modernising Medical Careers group and the equivalent group for basic postgraduate training in dentistry in the UK.

It comprises:

- Medical expert—the central role based on clinical knowledge and skills but integrating with the other described 'competencies'.
- Communicator—valuing and being effective in the doctor–patient relationship including the continuous dynamic exchanges that occur before, during and after the encounter.
- Collaborator—the idea being recognition of and respectful working within a healthcare team to achieve optimal patient outcome.
- Manager—accepting that we are all part of whichever healthcare organization we work in and the development and maintenance of sustainable practice, allocation of resources and effectiveness of the system are part of our responsibility.
- Health advocate—using your professional status to improve the health and well-being of individuals, communities and populations.
- Scholar—the demonstration of a lifelong commitment to reflective learning and the creation, dissemination, application and translation of clinical knowledge and skills.
- Professional—a commitment to the health and well-being of individuals and society through ethical practice, profession-led regulation, and high personal standards of behaviour.

1 Based on the CanMEDS 2005 framework which was sourced from Frank J. R. *et al. Report of the CanMEDS Phase IV Working Groups.* Ottawa: Royal College of Physicians and Surgeons of Canada. March 2005.

Commitments

Most of us never actually took a Hippocratic Oath although many think we did. The statement you read out at graduation will have been a modern day version outlining your commitment to professionalism. It was none the worse for that because at the time it was a marker of how you felt about the profession you were entering. The genuinely wonderful OHCM ed. 7 includes both the old and a new version (📖 pp. 0 & 1) so rather than repeat it (go and buy the book) I've included a synopsis of principles and commitments based on a physicians charter.

Principles

- *Primacy of patient welfare* We serve the interests of our patient(s).
- *Patient autonomy* We must empower patients to make informed decisions about their treatment.
- *Social justice* Discrimination has no place in healthcare. Resources should be fairly allocated.

Commitments

- *Professional competence* Commitment to lifelong learning and maintenance of all relevant knowledge and skills.
- *Honesty* With patients and peers in relation to consent and medical error.
- *Confidentiality* Well recognized but of even greater significance in the electronic age.
- *Probity with patients* Avoidance of any misuse of the relationship between professional and patient; for sexual, financial or any personal advantage.
- *Improving quality of care* Including working collaboratively with others to reduce error, increase patient safety, optimize use of resources and patient outcome.
- *Improve access to care* All healthcare systems should aim to have a uniform and adequate standard of care.
- *Scientific knowledge* Demonstrate integrity in the creation and use of scientific knowledge.
- *Avoid conflicts of interest* Be honest. Recognize and disclose conflicts of interest in practice, teaching or research.
- *Professional responsibilities* Set and maintain standards, show due respect and work collaboratively in educating, assessing and remediation of colleagues.

It should by now be becoming obvious that many groups are saying similar things about both the nature of professionalism and the perception of professionalism. The primacy of 'doing the right thing' for your patients, your colleagues, your society and yourself is the key principle that shines through.

Understanding (and overcoming) systems

Introduction as we all work in systems of greater or lesser complexity we need to learn how to cope with, redesign or overcome systems that prevent optimum outcome for our patients. In a general dental practice (a very small system) considerable power and autonomy is placed with the dentist and system design is important. In huge environments like hospitals many aspects of the system may be out of our control so learning how to overcome or adapt existing systems becomes crucial.

Process describes the individual steps that constitute each point in a journey through a system from start to finish. The easiest way to understand this is to imagine a patient's journey in great detail. This is the process view and it is essential when implementing an error avoidance strategy. The first step is to identify the high level view; an overall stepwise progression of the journey that highlights 15–20 key steps. Next, detailed process mapping takes place inviting the views of all the staff involved in the process (remember it is looking at the system first and individuals only if there is a defined problem with one individual's behaviour). Avoid rarities and personal anecdote. Look for waste in the process: of time, money, effort, goodwill etc.

Process pathology this includes: bottlenecks which may be real (a step performed by one person, at one time that takes longest) or functional (trying to do multiple non-consecutive tasks which wastes time between each task). *Demand/capacity mismatch*, the failure to understand these terms are a root cause of much of the mismanagement of the UK health service. Demand is the need plus want for the service i.e. all requests for the service, *activity* is what has been done (always retrospective), *capacity* is what the system could do under optimal conditions, *backlog* is cumulative unmet demand. *Carve-out* is where overall capacity is reserved for particular demands (e.g. fast track cancer referrals).

Responsibility/authority mismatch is a core underlying problem in most systems and the major source of stress in most hospital environments— the person held responsible (i.e. blamed when things go wrong) does not have the necessary authority to prevent them from going wrong.

Understanding that a patient's journey is a system allows you to improve it and use the techniques for error avoidance outlined in the next page. In the microcosm of a dental practice the most difficult thing may be simply accepting this concept. In the huge, highly complex externally interfered with hierarchical systems within hospitals the emphasis has to be on adapting the aspects of the overall system so that you have authority over it to improve it even if this effectively subverts imposed aspects of that system.

Human factors

Introduction Sometimes referred to as 'ergonomics' this consists of a group of subjects concerned with human–human and human–system interaction with a particular relevance to the prevention of error. Popular over the last 20 years or so in so-called 'high risk industries': aviation, nuclear, petrochemical and military they have recently become recognized as being of potential value in healthcare, particularly in the Anglophone world.[1]

The blame culture A longstanding tradition of managing when things go wrong is to find out who is to blame and punish them. That's it. It is astonishing that it has taken so long to accept that this is not the most useful way of going about things.

Error and error avoidance We all make mistakes, this is inevitable and inescapable. What is important is that the potential for serious harm coming from those mistakes is minimized and that we and others learn from those mistakes. In order to do that a move away from the blame culture has to take place. In some industry this has been achieved to a large extent (aviation). In healthcare there have been some notable attempts. These have been successful where the system is trusted, usually anonymized and reliable feedback is given. They have largely failed where a system has been imposed by an outside body which is not trusted (government or corporate body), league tables devised and feedback has been minimal or useless.

System failure The recognition that humans make mistakes (that are usually non malicious) but that things go disastrously wrong only when these mistakes are compounded, led to an approach where the system was analysed for failure rather than an individual being blamed.

Swiss cheese This is an analogy for systems failure and error occurrence.[2] For something to go seriously wrong (e.g. a patient dies from taking the wrongly prescribed drug) multiple failings have to happen. Think of trying to thread a straw through multiple layers of Swiss cheese. It will only pass through if all the holes, which are in different places on each slice line up. One slice out of place and it won't pass (i.e. the error won't happen). In the patient analogy, the wrong drug might be prescribed, but the dispensing pharmacist might recognize this or the patient might realize they were allergic to it.

Red flags This is the term given to the signs and symptoms of an error in progress. Recognition of a 'red flag', e.g. a change in the order of an operating list, should make everyone more aware of the potential for an error to occur.

1 J. Reason 2000 *BMJ* 320 768.

2 J. Reason 1990 *Human Error*, New York, Cambridge University Press.

Situational awareness This is our capacity to be aware of multiple aspects of our immediate environment, a simple example would be driving behind a car which is travelling slower than you in the inside lane of a 3-lane motorway at the point of a junction which has another car travelling at the same speed coming on the motorway. The calculation you make to position yourself safely without losing speed is your situational awareness. Stress massively reduces this and effectively blinkers you to potentially important outside influences.

Root Cause Analysis (aka Critical Event Analysis) Is the post mortem and coroner's report of the events around a significant event. This is supposed to happen after 'clinical incident' reporting, the idea being the areas of system failure are identified and measures put in place to prevent failure at that point in the future. Obviously this requires feedback and resource for change going to the people and places affected.

Effects of stress and personality As mentioned before individual personalities and learning techniques exist for all of us. If we are put in a position where we have to work or learn in a way that is at odds with our preferred approach we become to a greater or lesser extent stressed. The effect of stress on situational awareness is described. If situational awareness is decreased the potential for error increases. This is one logical reason why certain types of professions have to be assessed under stress, we have to be competent and able to function under levels of stress that would cripple others.

Crisis intervention techniques If you are working in a hierarchy how do you tell the boss he is doing something wrong? One excellent technique is the PACE approach.

Probe 'is it me? I don't understand why we are doing (the wrong thing) this'. This is usually enough and saves face all round.

Assert 'I'm sorry but I don't think this is right. I'm not happy'. The ante has been raised but it is still non confrontational. It takes real bull-headedness to press on in the face of this.

Confront 'Look this isn't right. I know you're the boss but I am sure this is not what should be happening'. This is a point of no return but you are doing the right thing.

Emergency 'Stop. I am not going to let this happen'. An extreme situation where you intervene (possibly even physically) to prevent harm to a patient.

Leadership and followership The concept of leadership is often that of someone who is always in control, always knows what to do, is always right and carries all the responsibility. Just reading that should make everyone realize it is nonsense. True leadership is about keeping things together, using the right people in the right place at the right time to achieve an agreed goal. Followership is acknowledging this and the leader who gives way (and becomes a 'follower' temporarily) to allow someone with a more appropriate skill set to lead is enabling that to happen.

Understanding personalities

We are all different. That seems self evident but the fact that different personality types exist and that they have a direct bearing on the way we learn and act does not seem to have permeated training structures or workplace management.

While no human being is completely stereotyped into a category with regard to both personality and learning preferences most of us show tendencies towards various behaviour types. It is important to realize that no one type is better than another but that certain types are more suited to certain roles in life and certain ways of learning new information, skills or behaviours and that being forced to act outwith that type can lead to significant stress. We might not be able to change the environment we work, teach or learn in but understanding that someone may be of a personality type where that environment produces counterproductive stress may help us modify the situation or them to accept that this is not a role they are suitable for.

Myers–Briggs type inventory This is one (there are others) way of assessing personality types. This is a quite lengthy questionnaire which categorizes 'preferences' in 4 main categories:

Introversion/extraversion—essentially this reflects the extent to which you engage the world in your head or the 'real world'.

Sensing/intuiting—this is about how you gain information; do you rely on the 5 senses (are heavily factual) or have a 6th sense feel for things.

Thinking/feeling—do you prefer a critical/analytical approach to decision making or rely on instinct more heavily?

Judging/perceiving—do you seek order, sense and predictability or are you happier to take things as they come?

This is a gross simplification of the process but gives you an idea of how people can differ, no one 'type' (indicated by the letters allocated to the different sections) is better than another but certain types cope better in certain situations, jobs, roles and in interpersonal relationships. Just going through the process aids in personal insight and reflective capability.

Learning types Just as there are 4 distinct personality traits which flow into each other so there are equivalent learning types. These also match the stages of learning and reflection and development of what has already been learned. The distinction between people is that they tend to prefer one stage more than another and can feel uncomfortable or even stressed if forced into an area they are less comfortable in.

Stage 1 reflective observation (thinking about buying a computer, reading all the magazines).

Stage 2 abstract conceptualization (reading the manual after buying it).

Stage 3 active experimentation (bought it, chucked the manual away, plug it in and start pressing buttons).

Stage 4 concrete experience (got one that works and going to stick with it).

Change management

Ownership is the key.

Change Is an inevitable and ongoing process in our everyday lives and the workplace and is certainly no bad thing in itself. The intense resentment felt by most professionals towards change has come about by imposed change, with no or facile consultation, no evidence base and no internal motivation for that change. The fact that most of these imposed changes fail, often due to the incredible power of healthcare professionals' inertia even in the absence of tacit opposition is a lesson that those who would impose change continually fail to learn.

Change management Is a useful concept both because we may wish to change practices, systems or treatments within our control for good reasons and because we may wish to oppose change where we feel it is potentially harmful, wasteful, lacking in evidence or just plain wrong. To do that, it helps to understand a little of the processes.

What can change? In terms of our professional environment three basic groups: individuals (ourselves, patients, colleagues), groups of individuals (nurses, trainees, those who are sharing a common experience) and organizations and systems.

Approaches There are 2 which are not mutually exclusive but tend to have different emphasis: changing attitudes in the relevant individuals and hoping that behavioural change will follow ('hearts and minds') and a more punitive approach emphasizing the legal and business reasons for change. While the latter has become increasingly popular it is unsurprisingly less effective with highly motivated and educated healthcare professionals.

Helpful concepts There is an unfortunate tendency for many trying to implement change to stick with conventional management theory which looks on organizations as machines with staff as components of that machine. This leads to the folly that a detailed plan for change can be worked out in advance (often by outsiders) people are told what to do and will both do it and do it consistently and that this process will be automatically replicable from one area to another. A much more useful concept is that organizations are complex evolving ecosystems functioning on a series of interdependent nested systems.[1] This concept believes guidance from a few simple rules will allow permanent effective change generated by internal motivation. It is the theory behind 'brainstorming' and 'post it note' exercises—although all too often these are corrupted by those 'in charge' falling back on conventional practice.

Groups of individuals need leaders but leaders do not have to be the font of all knowledge (📖 p. 679) acting as enablers or facilitators they can earn the support of the group by active listening, designing a plan of action, facilitating that plan (rather than doing it themselves, seeing what happens and giving feedback (📖 p. 689).

---

1 Mitleton-Kelly 2003 *Complex systems and Evolutionary Perspectives on Organisations*, Elsevier.

Individuals to function effectively with change need to develop emotional intelligence 'the capacity for recognizing our own feelings and those of others, for motivating ourselves and for managing emotions well in ourselves and in our relationships'.[1] Discovering what motivates ourselves and others is the key technique in ensuring people feel they 'own' the change and the change process, the key aspect of successful change management.

---

1 Goleman 1996 *Emotional Intelligence*, Bloomsbury.

Verbal and non verbal communication

'God gave us two ears and one mouth, but they are rarely used in those proportions'

Learning to listen Hard to do but hugely rewarding. Try to cultivate an active listening style, don't interrupt unless it is essential and if you do always give the opportunity to come back to a point that may be vital to them at some time in the future.

Time is needed to learn these skills, to use them in imparting news (especially bad news) to people and to allow people to absorb that news. Allocate it, allow it and stick to it.

Preparation When communicating, it is helpful to be sure of the information you are imparting and that you want to impart it. Prepare what you want or have to say as well as how you will say it.

Words have power Saying 'sorry' can be taken as an admission of guilt or as a sincere form of empathy. Timing, intonation and body language influence how the same word is understood by the person hearing it.

Honesty is best but does not mean burdening someone with extraneous detail which clears your conscience but unnecessarily harms someone else.

Questions People will have questions but may need time to refocus to ask them—suggest they write them down for next time. They will also have a legitimate need to have some answered—if you can do so, but don't be afraid to admit you don't know. If you can't, but know someone who can, then that is a fair response. Equally you may ask questions; the most useful after breaking bad news, perhaps surprisingly, is 'how do you feel about that?' The number of different response will astonish you and it is of huge importance to let people express themselves at this point.

Consistency Few things are more disorientating than being told different things by different people about the same subject, especially if that subject is your personal health or that of a loved one. Be sure of what has been said before—ask the person you are talking to as it is what they remember or understand that is important to the conversation. Try to ensure all team members do this before launching into some detailed explanation which may be at odds with what has gone before. If previous information is incorrect it must be corrected but include an explanation of how that 'misunderstanding' arose.

Empathy and compassion are important components of communication but this does not mean you are a limitless source nor does it mean you are an emotional punch bag for upset individuals. Having boundaries in your role as a professional communicator is essential to prevent burn out.

Principles of neurolinguistic programming

Neurolinguistic programming (NLP) was first developed by a psychologist, Richard Bandler and John Grinder, a linguist, in the 1970s. NLP is often referred to as the 'art and science of personal excellence'.

What is neurolinguistic programming (NLP)?

It is a set of interpersonal skill techniques to improve the impact and effectiveness of communication.

- **Neuro** is associated with the brain and what happens in your mind. We all use our senses, Visual, Auditory, Kinaesthetic, Olfactory, and Gustatory (VAKOG) to interpret the world around us. In other words what you see, hear, feel/touch, smell and taste all impact on your thought processes, interpretation of that information and subsequent behaviour or response.
- **Linguistic** is associated with language and how you communicate and influence others. What you say, how you say it and what you mean by it!
- **Programming** relates to patterns of behaviour which you learn and repeat (a learned behaviour). Internal thoughts and previous experiences have an influence on patterns of behaviour. Those patterns may help you make sense of situations, solve problems and help make decisions.

Four key principles of NLP

1. Rapport: When communicating with others build rapport, this can be done through matching body language, eye contact, tone of voice (pace and leading) and active listening. Understand the situation from the other person's perspective, 'Seek first to understand, then to be understood'.[1]

2. Outcomes: Know the outcome you want, 'begin with the end in mind'.[1]
- Frameworks such as SWOT and SMART can assist in developing a 'well formed outcome'
- SWOT (Strengths, Weakness, Opportunities and Threats)
- SMART (Specific, Measurable, Achievable, Realistic and defined Time frame)

3. Senses: Use all your senses VAKOG to interpret and make sense of the world around you. Be aware we all see, hear and feel things differently.*

4. Flexibility: Be flexible in your approach. Others may interpret situations/ the world differently. The more flexible you can be the more options you create.*

*NB We all live in our own unique worlds, and have our own 'map of the world', check out the world of others before presuming/interpreting you are talking about the same experience/thing! You maybe surprised!

1 Covey S. R. 1994 *The Seven Habits of Highly Effective People*, Simon & Schuster. London.

Presentation skills

Presenting is not teaching, but it can be a useful tool in teaching. It can also be a nerve wracking chore (job interview presentations) or a rite of passage exercise in survival at a national scientific conference. Regardless of its intended purpose it can be made better and more pleasant (for you and your audience) by following some simple rules that are based around preparation, planning and delivery.

Preparation What are you trying to say—this is essential, if you don't know what you want to say how can you say it? No-one wants to listen to you work it out on the spot—that is boring and embarrassing. It is also vital that you understand whether what you want to say agrees with what the audience wants to hear and what the organizers want you to say. It is not always the same thing. Why do they want you—do you have or have promised some special expertise or are you a replacement? Who are you speaking to and who has asked you to speak, are their agendas the same (some attendances are 'mandatory' which tends to produce a hostile audience which needs to be defused), what are their backgrounds, ages, degree of knowledge of the subject you are asked to speak on. What would they like to get out of it? How many people will be there? This has obvious implications for the choice of media—PowerPoint to 5 people is dull and ineffective, a flipchart to 100 is impossible. What is the context of your presentation, is it a 10-minute talk with 5-minute questions wedged into a plethora of others; part of a structured course with experts before and after you; or just you with relative flexibility? This is essential for timing considerations; if you are allocated a finite time you must stick to it which means starting and finishing to the minute. If you are allocated a vague time ('40 minutes to an hour') set yourself a specific time and break it into 20-minute chunks (the attention span of most people for listening). Work out how you get to the venue, a backup plan and who to contact if things go wrong, get there early and ensure all audiovisuals are working before the audience arrives (getting your presentation to work while the audience sits there growing restless is a cardinal sin).

Planning Now you have an idea of what is going to happen you can plan the presentation. It is crucial you know your subject and are up to date for the level of your prospective audience. Once you have a good idea of the relevant content work out what is feasible to deliver (in the allocated time and to that particular audience). More really is often less in presentations. What sort of language are you going to use? What sort of dress style will be right for that occasion? What technique are you going to use to deliver the presentation?

The message not the media is the defining aspect of your presentation. Media include: blackboards, whiteboard, flip chart, overhead projector, visualizer, 3-D objects (for smaller groups) and microphones, computers/LCD projectors for larger groups. Video and handouts can be used for both. Be familiar with what you are actually going to use (it often won't be your own computer, many a video clip disaster has stemmed from this). Mastery of the older presentation techniques, which are often more suitable for smaller groups requires greater skill and confidence than slide based approaches which explains their popularity and overuse. Many presentations will use PowerPoint, while this has many advantages the mis-use of the technology has created the well recognized condition of 'death by PowerPoint'—too many flamboyant slides, rushing through multiple slides that contribute nothing and give the impression of bad preparation and freezing of the system if multiple lines and pictures are added to the slide. Do not become obsessed with the media, it can distract the audience from what is important—your message. Design this like a story, know what the end is going to be then work out a way to get there. Now you know where you are going work out the start—an interesting title and an outcomes slide coupled with a short friendly introduction helps. Build into the bulk of your talk avoiding abbreviations, keeping it short and simple and re-emphasizing important points and why they are relevant to the audience. If your talk is longer than 20 minutes build in 'energisers' these can be liter-ally breaks where people move about and do things (for the brave and experienced) or interjecting questions into the audience.

Delivery using the set, dialogue, closure approach for teaching helps structure every presentation (📖 p. 688). Start on time, ensure your non-verbal communication (📖 p. 684) is positive and open. Engage the audience and introduce yourself in a way that gains credibility, tell them what you are going to talk about and why it is important to them (or why they might enjoy it). Ensure text slides or OHPs are clear and legible with no more than 7 words per line and 5 lines per slide. Do not read your slides to the audience, it's insulting, they can read too! It takes a minute to read a text slide. Use good quality pictures and diagrams that are relevant, don't just show off. Avoid extra logos and pictures on a slide that will simply distract the audience. Ensure you have a summary slide at the end. Practice so that you know which slides are where and how far into the presentation you are by which slide you are using.

When allowed by the structure of the environment try to ask questions at the end before you summarize what you've talked about. This enables you to check the audience has understood you and to build anything missing into your summary and creates an opportunity for a definitive termination of the presentation (which prevents things dragging on and the audience remembering some daft question rather than your summary).

Remember: perfect practice prevents piss poor performance.

Teaching, learning, and assessing professionalism

Teaching In order to teach effectively you have to ensure others are enabled to learn.

Learning In order to learn you have to participate actively in different styles of teaching.

Domains of learning This is the term given to what can be learned. Usually three are described—cognitive (knowledge) psychomotor (skills) affective (attitude). Some would argue (and I agree) that a 4th domain exists—interpersonal as this is a group of abilities (verbal and non verbal) that can be used for good and bad reasons. Each of these domains has more appropriate ways of teaching, learning and assessing them (e.g. you don't assess operative skill with an MCQ).

Learning outcomes The current term for aims and objectives. Basically this is working out what you are trying to learn or teach before you start trying to do it. From a teacher's perspective it is useless to start trying to teach something unless it can be feasibly learned in that episode. It helps to state what you are going to do in whatever period of time and with whatever learner(s) you have. From that you can work out how to do it. Think of it as knowing where you want to go then working out the best way to get there on any given day and in any set of circumstances.

Structure of a learning episode Set, Dialogue and Closure. This structure allows the efficient construction of any high quality teaching episode.

Set is the initial preparation of the episode, ensuring the environment is the best it can be, introducing yourself, discovering your audience and agreeing your roles. Establish what you are going to do and how you are going to do it.

Dialogue this is the bulk of the teaching, the information imparted or the skill taught. Interactivity with your learners is crucial and achieved by questions, eye contact and direct involvement. Skills teaching involves a 4-stage procedure during this phase.
- a silent demonstration
- a talked stepwise demonstration
- an opportunity for the learner to talk the skill through by directing the teacher to do the skill
- a demonstration of the skill by the learner saying what they are going to do before they do it.

Closure the end is important as it is often the aspect best remembered by the learner. An effective closure consists of questions with explanations followed by a summary followed by a termination. A definitive stop prevents the process from becoming messy and the last (strongest) memory of the learners from being something irrelevant.

Teaching knowledge Books, journals, lectures and the internet are all sources of knowledge. Retention is improved by repetition and application. Simple acquisition of facts is only the first step in possessing useful knowledge. It is the integration of data and its application to variable information i.e. working out a treatment plan from a series of signs and symptoms that is essential in a dentist.

Teaching skills The 4-stage technique works but has specific challenges in carrying out procedures on conscious patients (need to agree code words) and in long complex procedures (which have to be broken down into smaller steps).

Teaching interpersonal skills The ability to relate effectively to other people can be taught and learned in a variety of ways although the most effective is watching people in action and analysing what they are doing and what impact their words and actions are having on the people around them.

Teaching attitudes Attitudes are the essence of professionalism, they govern what drives us and are defined by what we do (not what we say). The only really effective way of teaching appropriate attitudes is by acting them out as role models who are valued by those who are learning.

Feedback use 'Pendleton's rules': ask what went well, if they struggle tell them or if in a group ask others, then ask them how they would improve or do things differently the next time, ensure they are told about any significant points for improvement if they miss them (either personally or using others in a group).

In workplace assessment tools

In workplace assessment tools Given that what we do is the most crucial aspect of assessment and the workplace is the most real life environment these tools have been created to get as close to real life as possible.

Current popular tools These consist of 2 observational tools; Mini clinical examination exercise (Mini-CEX) and Direct Observation of Procedures (DOPS) or Procedure based Assessment (PBA) (the names will change again but the principles are valid), an interactive tool, Case base Discussion (CbD) and a peer assessment tool (Mini-PAT).

Mini-CEX. This assesses an interaction with a patient using either a checklist or a global rating scale (depending on level of the assessment) and can assess, knowledge, interpersonal skills, examination skills and, to a certain extent, attitude.

DOPS/PBA The latter is a similar idea but intended to assess technical skills. There is a generic checklist built into the proforma but it is important to understand that this tool was primarily intended to assess physicians carry out relatively simple technical skills (it originated from the Royal College of Physicians). The PBA adapted from DOPS by the Royal College of Surgeons of England is designed to assess more complex technical skills however the checklist approach is less appropriate in assessing higher skill levels than a Global rating scale.

CbD is an interactive discussion between assessor and assessee around case notes picked by the assessee, designed to assess a wide range of hard and soft thought process and skills (i.e. from technical quality of note keeping to ability to reflect on a mistake).

Mini-PAT (aka 360 degree appraisal, Multisource feedback, etc). Assessee chooses 8–15 relevant people to complete a structured questionnaire. Statistically valid results achieved if at least 8 completed returns. Sceptics should try this one and it can be extremely useful in helping self reflection and improvement on a range of subjects. Originally developed by the Royal College of Physicians and Surgeons of Canada (see CanMEDS).

LEPS an in workplace tool for general dental practice developed by NHS Education Scotland, being replaced by the tools described above.

Assessing the healthcare professional Clearly all the domains of learning or the subdivisions of these described in the CanMEDS document have to be assessed and a range of techniques are needed for this. While basic facts can be tested by rigid, simple tools like single best answer MCQs, assessing the higher levels of function demanded of a healthcare professional needs much more. A combination of the in workplace assessment tools and externally validated conventional examinations (incorporating rigid but reliable assessments like MCQs and OSCE as well as the more flexible and valid interactive techniques like structured vivas, moulages and scenario based assessments) are clearly necessary to ensure what both dentistry and society need—the competent healthcare professional.

Practice management

Contents

Relevant pages in other chapters Contracts, 📖 p. 656; biocompatibility of dental materials, 📖 p. 644.

Principal sources and further reading The BDA have an excellent range of leaflets covering many of the topics in this chapter. GDC 2005 *Standards for Dental Professionals*; J. O. Forrest 1984 *A Guide to Successful Dental Practice*, Butterworth Heinemann; K. J. Lewis 1989 *Practice Management for Dentists*, Butterworth Heinemann; R. Rattan 1996 *Making Sense of Dental Practice Management*, Radcliffe Medical Press.

Management skills

Management courses are now big business and certainly worth investing in. They can help in developing systems leading to ↑ efficiency, ↓ stress, and ↑ job satisfaction—for the whole dental team. A happy practice environment is not only more pleasant to work in, but the bonhomie will also be transmitted to patients.

Keys to successful management

Good communication: Good communication skills are essential not only when relating to patients but equally between team members to ensure smooth running of the practice. Joking about the receptionist's latest boyfriend (strange though he may be) is not communication. It should be remembered, good communication involves the ability to listen as well as talk. An effective complaints/feedback procedure should allow patients to be able to raise concerns openly (however minor) thereby enabling the practice to learn from the issues raised and improve their service.

Staff meetings: For teamwork to be successful the opportunity for team members to discuss problems and ideas for improvements needs to be created. Regular structured staff meetings should be planned with an agenda prepared in advance to which all team members should be encouraged to contribute. Patient feedback, complaints, changes in guidance/policies should be discussed. Minutes of the meeting should be kept, recording date of meeting, members present, matters discussed and actions taken. The minutes should be accessible to all team members for future reference.

Delegate: Delegate tasks that do not require your training and expertise. In addition to ↓ stress and freeing time to concentrate of tasks that do require your skills, this also ↑ job satisfaction for ancillary staff, provided they are given the training and time to cope with new responsibilities; e.g. getting the hygienist to do the fieldwork involved in deciding which new ultrasonic scaler to buy.

Teamwork: The importance of building a mutually supportive team can readily be appreciated by trying to work in an environment where everyone has been forced to protect their corner. Successful leadership involves encouraging staff to develop their potential both as an individual and as a valued member of the team, and encouraging discussion as to what the goals are to be and how to achieve them. Motivation to work as a team can be fostered by monetary incentives linked to the performance of the practice (see below), but it is wise to find out what motivates individual members of the practice as money may not be the most important factor for all employees.

Staff training: All new staff members should undergo training in practice procedures and policies. A record of training should be kept. Review of all staff training should be carried out annually and development of further skills encouraged allowing delegation of additional tasks where appropriate. To comply with GDC requirements, all dentists and DCPs must carry out CPD (📖 p. 714). Practice owners should ensure reasonable opportunity is given to staff members to undertake CPD and ensure that skills and knowledge are being updated.

A manual of practice procedures, routines and policies should be kept which is freely available to all staff. All members of staff should be involved in reviewing and updating this information. In-house training days with speakers either from within the practice, or invited, are useful especially in areas such as dealing with emergencies and cross infection.

Dentist and DCPs involved in the taking and development of radiographs should have received appropriate training and have this training updated (p. 720). Documented evidence of appropriate training should be kept.

Pay: Motivation can often be enhanced by financial incentives.[1] Therefore by structuring payment to comprise: **1** a fixed hourly rate; **2** an individual bonus, which is related to attendance, sickness record, and productivity paid as a percentage of the hourly rate; and **3** a group bonus which is a fixed proportion of the profits of the practice; all staff have an inducement to reduce overheads and improve efficiency in the practice.

1 C. M. Scola 1990 *BDJ* **169** 334.

Hiring and firing staff

Hiring

1) Define what tasks the practice team would like the new member of staff to perform (do not limit possible applications only to Superman). Decide on the criteria for an ideal candidate, as this will aid selection later.

2) Draw up a job description and person specification. Consider including details of the practice, role of the new member in the team, required skills, in-job training to be provided, hours of work, pay, and other benefits. Check with local colleges for availability on dental nurse training courses should this be applicable.

3) Advertise post. Use local press/hospitals/internet/professional magazines. Remember to include a realistic closing date for applications.

4) Short-list candidates.

5) Interview, preferably with two or three people on the panel. This should be structured so that candidates are asked the same questions, to aid comparison. Notes should be made, because after several interviews the candidates may begin to merge! Hopefully a suitable person will be found and they should be offered the job in writing, subject to references, and where applicable occupational health screening including proof of Hep B inoculation, proof of registration and professional indemnity. If no-one is acceptable, go back to **1** and reassess requirements.

6) Draw up provisional terms/conditions of employment; include length of any trial period and how assessment is to be carried out at the end of the trial period (usually 6–8 weeks is long enough). Both employee and employer should retain a signed copy. For non-registered dental nurses apply for a place on a training program.

7) Orientate and train the new member of staff, giving plenty of time for feedback in both directions. Both employer and employee should keep a record of training given.

8) Towards end of trial period reassess. If progress is satisfactory draw up formal terms/conditions of employment (📖 p. 656).

9) Do not discriminate on grounds of disability, sex, race, religion, marital situation, or whether they have children or not.

Always put all matters regarding employment in writing.

The BDA have an excellent advice sheet on recruitment.

Firing

The BDA have advice sheets on dismissal and redundancy and the Advisory, Conciliation and Arbitration Service (ACAS) will also give guidance. Both from a practical and emotional point of view, dismissal of staff is not easy and if taken to tribunal, can be expensive. The Trade Union and Labour Relations Acts allows for dismissal relating to capability, conduct, contravention of the law, retirement, and redundancy.

To prevent a claim of unfair dismissal the practice should follow a set disciplinary procedure:

- Investigate any allegations re performance/conduct to determine whether a formal disciplinary procedure is indicated.
- Notify the employee in writing of a formal hearing to discuss their conduct advising them of the allegation. The employee should be

allowed to bring a fellow employee or union representative to the interview.

- At the formal meeting, allow the employee opportunity to give an explanation (e.g. inadequate training) and consider this explanation.
- Decide on what action to take:

Oral warning A note of the oral warning should be recorded. The reasons for the oral warning should be given in writing to the employee. Give the employee a timetable for improvement and advise that this is the first stage of the disciplinary procedure.

Written warning (first/second/final written warning) that if there is no improvement, dismissal will follow.

Written notice if the employee fails to meet the requirements stated in the written warnings. The amount of notice should concord with that agreed in the employment contract. The minimum statutory notice required depends upon length of service: <1 month = no notice; 1 month to 2yrs = 1 week; 2–12yrs = 1 week for each complete year worked. >12yrs = 12 weeks.

Instant dismissal Instant dismissal is acceptable where an action is deemed to amount to gross misconduct. Examples of gross misconduct include theft, breach of confidentiality, breach of Health and Safety regulations and alcohol/drug related incapacity.

Redundancy is dismissal for reasons other than the personal behaviour of the employee. Statutory redundancy payments are required for staff who have been employed continuously for >2yrs (full or part-time). The amount paid depends upon pay, length of service, and age. Staff facing redundancy are also entitled to paid time-off to look for a new job or undergo training.

Health and safety[1]

Hazard Anything with the potential to cause harm.

Risk The likelihood that someone will be harmed by a hazard.

Risk assessment A systematic evaluation of what could cause harm (e.g. equipment, chemicals, work activities) in the workplace and ensuring precautions are in place to minimize these risks.

Health and Safety at Work Act 1974

The HSW Act aims to protect employers, employees, self-employed contractors and public within the work environment. Failure to comply with the Act could lead to investigation and prosecution by the Health and Safety Executive (HSE), a statutory body responsible for enforcing the HSW act. The HSE has the power to enter premises (with or without notice) and carry out an inspection. If required they can issue an improvement notice (advising of a time by which compliance must be achieved) or a prohibition notice (closing the premises until compliance is achieved) +/− prosecution. Employees are also expected to take reasonable care for their own and other people's safety—refusal to comply is grounds for dismissal.

Compliance with the HSW Act requires
- Equipment and systems of work to be safe and instruction, training, and supervision to be provided.
- Maintenance of practice premises, including entrances/exits, in a safe condition.
- Safe handling and storage of potentially harmful and dangerous substances.
- All practices employing >5 members of staff to have a written Health and Safety policy.

COSHH

The Control of Substances Hazardous to Health regulations 2002 requires employers to identify all substances (e.g. vapours, microorganisms) in the workplace which are potentially hazardous, and take steps to prevent or ↓ any risks to health. The following procedure is recommended:
- Assess the risks to health from hazardous substances. Identify who might be harmed by their use and how.
- Identify precautions needed e.g. eye/skin protection, ventilation.
- Prevent exposure (e.g. don't use substance) or control exposure (if preventing use is not practicable).
- If >5 employees, make and keep a record of the findings of the assessment.
- Ensure that measures to control exposure are used and safety procedures followed.
- Monitor exposure and carry out health monitoring when indicated by the initial risk assessment.
- Prepare a plan to deal with accidents/emergencies involving hazardous substances.
- Ensure all employees are properly trained and supervised.

---

1 BDA Advice Sheet, *Health and Safety Law for Dental Practice*. Feb. 2008.

Mercury (Hg) Encapsulated amalgam should be used in preference to non-encapsulated. Use should be confined to impervious surfaces where any spillage will be limited, ideally a lipped tray lined with foil. Staff should wear gloves when handling Hg-containing substances. Waste should be stored in a sealed, labelled container containing solution to suppress mercury. Disposal of amalgam/mercury and capsules should be by a licensed person. Documentation/contract relating to waste disposal needs to be kept.

Amalgam separators are a legal requirement for all dental practices to ensure amalgam is filtered out of the main water drainage.

Lead from radiographic packets can be used for absorbing small spillages along with a paste of equal parts calcium hydroxide and flowers of sulfur and water, or a proprietary spillage kit can be purchased.

Latex allergy Affects ~1% of the population and 10% of health-care workers. The range of latex-free products is ↑.[1]

RIDDOR

The Reporting of Injuries, Diseases and Dangerous Occurrences Regulations (1995) places a legal duty upon employers, self employed and people in control of premises to report

- Work-related deaths
- Major injuries including any injury resulting in admission to hospital >24hrs unless for observation only
- Injuries causing individual being unable to work >3days
- Work-related diseases
- Dangerous occurrences including explosion of e.g. compressor, inhalation/ingestion substance requiring medical treatment

Reporting of such incidents should be carried out immediately to allow the HSE and local authorities to investigate. For injuries leading to >3days off work a report must be made within 10 days. Reports can be made online at ⅋ www.hse.gov.uk/riddor/online.htm, by post on standard form (from HMSO bookshops), or by phone. A written record should be kept of all accidents in the practice documenting date and time of accident, name person affected and their occupation, nature of injury and how accident occurred.

Cross-infection control— 📖 see p. 718.

Hepatitis B/C: Dentists are responsible for ensuring that any of their staff who carry out procedures that could bring them into contact with blood (e.g. assistants, hygienists, dental nurses) should be immunized against Hepatitis B. Any health-care worker who becomes e-antigen +ve is obliged to cease practising.

Blood/body fluid spillage The management of this requires written protocols.— 📖 see p.719.

---

1 E. A. Field 1998 *BDJ* **185** 65.

Display screen equipment— 📖 see p. 708.

Disposal of waste

Under the Environmental Protection Act, dentists are responsible for segregating waste, storing it safely, and arranging for its disposal. Practices should have a policy relating to classification and disposal of waste. Clinical waste for incineration should be stored in yellow containers and disposed of by a registered collector. Non-clinical waste should be stored in black containers.

Employers' liability

A certificate of insurance must be displayed on the premises. PCTs/Health Boards are now empowered to carry out practice inspections—the above issues are likely to be high on the agenda of any such inspection.

First-aid

The Health and Safety (First-Aid) Regulations 1981 require all workplaces to have first-aid provisions. The practice should be assessed to ensure compliance based on number of people employed and the risks associated with the work. Practices <20 employees should have an appointed person in attendance during practice hours. Practices >20 employees must have a qualified 'first-aider'. First-aid boxes should be appropriate for the number of employees and level of risk.

Medical Devices Directive

A dental prosthesis or orthodontic appliance is now viewed as a custom-made device requiring a written prescription from the dentist. All dental labs need to register with Medical Devices Agency.

Smoking

Practices should display a 'no-smoking' sign at the entrance to the premises. The sign should advise that 'it is against the law to smoke in these premises'.

X-rays/radiography 📖 see p. 720.

Financial management

Find a good accountant and a friendly bank manager, preferably on the recommendation of another practitioner.

It is advisable to develop a structured system for dealing with fees and estimates, tailored to the individual practice, which is understood and adhered to by all staff.

Delegating many aspects of calculating and collecting fees, to appropriately trained and motivated staff should make the practice more cost-effective. However, failure to monitor the situation adequately can, at best, result in a false sense of security.

Book-keeping is time-consuming but necessary. Many book-keeping tasks can be performed by computer, either with an integrated practice management system or stand-alone software. Suggested minimum:
- Fees due and fees received.
- Bank deposits.
- Patient lists.
- Record units of activity performed compared to monthly targets. Monitor practice and individual performance and address any imbalance early.
- Income/expenditure. Every month compile an income/expenditure record to develop a feel for the financial situation. Suitable ledgers (e.g. Admor) can be purchased from stationers. It is wise to seek the advice of your accountant as to the methodology—accurate accounts will make his job easier (and ∴ cheaper).
- Petty cash transactions should be recorded, together with all relevant receipts. The money (<£50) is best stored in a separate locked box. For larger sums a practice cheque can be cashed.
- Wages.
- Staff absences and sickness records.

Banking: It is helpful to bank all monies at the end of each day, as the bank statement then indicates the daily takings. To encourage settlement of fees, it is wise to accept payment in any form, i.e. cash, cheque, or credit card. Although credit cards incur a commission, patients with cash-flow problems may be happy to accept this form of payment as a face-saver; then their lack of funds becomes the credit company's problem. It is good policy to negotiate overdraft facilities in advance to cover those occasions where cash-flow problems arise.

Budgeting: An annual forecast and budget should be prepared jointly with the accountant.

Bad debts: These can often be prevented by having a definite Practice Payment Policy which is widely advertised to patients and adhered to; e.g. payment in part at the beginning of Rx and the balance on completion; or payment in full, up front. At the examination appointment patients should be given a written estimate and reminded when payment is due. If a patient forgets, at the last visit they should be asked to sign a form confirming that the Rx has been satisfactorily completed and that they agree to pay (£x) within 7 days. If payment is still not forthcoming, reminders should be sent out at 7, 14, and 28 days. If there is still no joy, consider using debt collectors, but beware of a counter claim of negligence.

Tax: This is really where a good accountant comes in. By providing him with information on income and expenditure on a monthly basis, he will be able to provide advice on what to do before the end of the financial year to minimize the taxman's percentage.

Insurance: Essential for property, contents, equipment, indemnity, staff, loss of income, and personal insurance.

Consumer Credit Act 1974 (reformed in 2006) requires those extending credit to the public by allowing them to pay for goods/service in instalments to obtain a licence. A licence is not required if the business only accepts credit cards provided by another company, or allows customers to pay bills in <4 installments within 1 yr. For further details, contact the Office of Fair Trading and/or obtain legal advice to assess whether a license is required.

Running late

Running late happens occasionally to everyone, usually when you were hoping to finish early and rush off to do something else. A common reaction is to cut corners, a strategy which can misfire and as a result waste even more time.

If running late is becoming a habit, stop and re-assess/audit your working practices. Assess reasons why the clinic runs late; ?unplanned emergencies, ?insufficient appointment length ?incorrect appointment booking ?patients attending late ?clinic not starting on time. Once identified, ensure steps are taken to deal with causes of delays.

Some additional hints to ↓ everyday stress:

- Have an appointment book, divided into 5min blocks to provide flexibility.
- Ensure appointment times are realistic and allow time for setting and clearing up.
- Within reason do not try to carry out treatment that wasn't planned for that appointment.
- Ensure patients in reception are fully informed of any delays and given opportunity to rearrange their appointments if they wish.
- If another member of staff is free, e.g. hygienist or dental nurse, you may be able to delegate some simple tasks.
- A working day comprising a longer morning and a shorter afternoon is more productive.
- If you are so busy that longer procedures have to be booked well in advance, designate some specific sessions for them each month (thus ↓ the temptation to squeeze them in).
- For busy sessions, try and utilize two surgeries.
- Schedule more complex work for the morning and less stressful work (e.g. check-ups) for the end of sessions.
- For last-minute cancellations, have a list of patients who are willing to come in at short notice.
- Define the working day and try not to extend beyond this.
- Coffee-breaks and lunchtime should not always be used to catch up on other work; have a rest occasionally.
- After holidays, book out extra time for dealing with more urgent treatments/emergencies. Then you will be able to cope with fitting in urgent patients on your return and not feel stressed.
- Allocate time each day for 'emergency appointments'.

Emergencies can be defined as the patients who are willing to attend at any time. The patient who tries to stipulate when they are seen is not a true emergency. If buffer zones are built into your timetable, fitting in emergencies should not be a problem. For emergencies out-of-hours there should be a number to contact for advice and treatment if appropriate. Ensure staff understand which conditions need to be seen as an emergency and should not be delayed.

Marketing

The general public are consumers of health care and have a choice as to where they go for their treatment. Whether NHS, private, or independent, the success or otherwise of a practice is going to depend on its ability to attract and keep patients. Marketing involves identifying and defining needs/desires of potential clients. Advertising is the means by which we communicate with these potential and existing clients.

Advertising: Relaxation of the GDC restrictions on advertising has opened up a range of opportunities. Advertising does not need to be brash; after all, it is merely a means of letting the public know about the existence of a practice and the services that are available. Apart from the 'yellow pages', this information can be disseminated via:

- Practice Information Leaflets (📖 see p. 706) these can be distributed to existing patients and possible sources of new recruits, e.g. nurseries, doctors' waiting rooms.
- Open days. These allow apprehensive patients to find out more about painless dentistry without the need to have an examination or Rx.
- Practice website. With the increasing popularity of the internet this can be an efficient and dynamic medium for practice promotion. The practice website can additionally be linked to other sites e.g. 'find a dentist' 'local services'.
- Adverts in local publications: but follow the GDC guidelines.
- The best advert is a satisfied patient who will recommend you by word of mouth.

First appearances count: This starts before the patient arrives at the surgery as most patients will make their initial enquiry by phone. So the phone should always be answered promptly, in person (not by an answer machine), with a friendly and welcoming greeting. When the prospective patient arrives at the surgery the external and internal decor, together with the welcome they receive, will play a role in determining a patient's impression of the professionalism of the practice. Ensure non-dental areas are well maintained and that the exterior of the premises looks well cared-for, with a professional-looking plate. The reception should be relaxing and inviting with comfortable seating to add to the ambience. A small area for children to play in with toys and some books, or if possible a crèche, are good practice-builders. A range of interesting magazines (look at the range available at your optician's, rather than the doctors' waiting room) and practice leaflets on different aspects of dental care/health should be available.

Staff: The receptionist must be friendly and helpful (even on Monday mornings). It is worth spending some time with the receptionist, deciding on stock responses to some of the more common problems that arise (e.g. dealing with the angry patient) and to ↑ their knowledge of dental techniques available so that patients' queries can be answered correctly.

It is also helpful if the receptionist can ask new patients how they heard about the practice, so as to better target future marketing strategies. The presentation and attitude of all the staff is of vital importance. An attractive and functional uniform in the practice colour or bearing the practice logo is bound to impress.

Emergencies: Although it is tempting to exclude non-registered patients from receiving out-of-hours emergency Rx, it is a good practice-builder to see anybody in pain, as some of them will become regular patients.

Market research: It is vital to know your patient base. Is there a significant group which may need special attention (e.g. elderly or young families)? What extra services would your patients like to see (e.g. implants; a crèche)? What do they feel about your opening times—is there another group of patients who might attend if the opening times were amended?

Remember, the most important marketing aid is without doubt the personal touch.

Practice leaflets

What information to include?

Dentists providing services under the new NHS dental contract must ensure that a practice information leaflet is available and is reviewed every 12 months. The contract requires specific information to be included, which is a useful starting point for all practices whether private or NHS:

- The name of the contractor/partners (providers), or for corporate practices the names of directors.
- Full name of each person performing services under the terms of the contract.
- Professional qualification of each performer.
- Whether any teaching/training is carried out or likely to be carried out by the contractor.
- Address of each of the practice premises.
- Contactors phone/fax/website details (if applicable).
- Details of how to request services and what services are available.
- The rights of the patient to express a preference for which practitioner they wish to see.
- Whether the practice premises have disabled access and alternative arrangements where this is not the case.
- Normal surgery hours and days of opening.
- Arrangements for out of hours care—if not provided by the contractor it should advise that the PCT is responsible for commissioning the care.
- Telephone number/web address of NHS direct.
- Complaints Procedure details.
- Rights/responsibilities of the patient e.g. to keep appointments.
- How the practice deals with violent/abusive patients.
- Information regarding who has access to patient information and patient rights regarding disclosure of information.
- Name, address, phone, website of PCT.

Further *optional* information can be included in the leaflet:

- Practice philosophy.
- Map showing location of practice.
- Further information on the special interests of the dentists, both dental and non-dental.
- Illustrations of the practice, and photos of staff and facilities.
- Details of charges for broken private appointments if applicable.
- Methods of payment accepted.
- Special facilities and Rx available, e.g. sedation, crèche.

How to set about producing a leaflet Broadly speaking there are two approaches: either get professional help (e.g. designer, photographer, printer) or DIY, using a desk-top printing package on the practice computer. However, the two are not mutually exclusive and all practices should, at least, consider taking advice from a designer. Before seeking help it is important to have some idea of what you want.

- What is your potential market (young families with small children, older professionals and their families)?
- Black/white or two or more colours?
- Glossy booklet or a folded A4 sheet?

- How much money do you want to spend?
- How many copies do you need (avoid being lead astray by the bulk discounts)?
- How is the leaflet to be distributed?

It is wise to shop around and examine the work of several professionals before choosing.

Design and layout The leaflet aims to create the impression of a caring practice, and to inform. The key to success is simplicity. One helpful tip is to have a practice logo &/or house style (or colours), replicated in other items of practice stationery. This idea of a corporate image is not new, but has worked well in the business world. A designer will be able to suggest styles and layouts best suited to your projected market, as well as help with the text wording. Photos and illustrations will ↑ the cost, but also the impact, as will using more than one colour.

Points to watch

- Don't say that a dentist has specialist expertise unless registered on a specialist list with the GDC.
- Don't advertise other services or goods.
- Be legal, decent, honest, and truthful.

Computers and dental practice

The use of computers in practice is well established, whether used solely for practice administration or as a fully integrated reception and in-surgery system. It is important to ensure that a back-up of all information is carried out daily and the back-up data stored off-site in a fire proof container. An audit trail must be present within the software to allow any alterations made to clinical records to be identified.

Computers and visual display units (VDUs)

The Health and Safety (Display Screen Equipment) Regulations 1992 require employers to minimize risks arising from working with VDUs/monitors/display screen equipment. Employers should assess the work area, furniture and equipment, the nature of the work being carried out and any special needs of individual staff. The following should be addressed:
- Chairs should be adjustable so comfortable working height is achieved.
- Workspace should be sufficient to allow keyboard/mouse and screen to be positioned and used comfortably.
- Lighting should be optimal for working with VDU with minimal reflection. Brightness of the VDU should be adjustable.
- Breaks/change of activity should be allowed to prevent long periods of VDU work.
- Eye tests should be provided and paid for by the employer if requested by an employee. If glasses are prescribed specifically for working with the VDU (and normal glasses cannot be used) the employer must also pay for these.
- Training should be given to ensure employees use the VDU and workstation comfortably and safely to minimize health risks.

Data Protection Act[1]

The Data Protection Act 1988 covers use of manual as well as computerized records. A dentist storing personal data on a computer system must register with the Data Protection Commissioner. The practice should have a data protection policy.

Under the terms of the Act, data must be:
- obtained fairly and used only for a specific and lawful purpose
- should not be excessive but adequate and relevant
- only disclosed to certain recipients
- protected and held securely
- accessible to patients on request
- not kept for longer than necessary

---

1 BDA Advice Sheet, *Data Protection*.

Independent and private practice

'Independent' is the term preferred by many for private practice, as it sounds less avaricious. An ↑ proportion of dentists are turning to other methods of remuneration than the NHS; indeed the pace of change is so fast that it is difficult to provide information that will necessarily be relevant in the future ∴ these pages are limited to discussing general principles.

Researching the market

To develop the potential of a practice it is necessary first to fully evaluate its present position. An appreciation of the existing patient base can be gained simply by going through the manual or computer records and looking at the geographical spread and socio-economic groups. If most patients are part of a family group, then future developments need to provide advantages for parents and children; e.g. if changing to independent practice, then a family-based capitation scheme might be more applicable.

Also, the potential for attracting new patients to the practice, and the competition from other practices in the area for those and existing patients, should be assessed.

It is also important to research and take into consideration staff views about any changes to be made to the practice. Ensure staff are informed about the reasons and advantages these changes will bring.

Business planning

If the financial basis of a practice is to be changed a business plan will need to be drawn up and discussed with the practice's accountants and bankers. Two fashionable business planning tools are:

- The planning cycle is shown in Figure 17.1:

Fig. 17.1 The planning cycle.

- A SWOT analysis is a consideration of the Strengths, Weaknesses, Opportunities, and Threats, to and of a business.

Fee setting

This difficult exercise should be carried out in conjunction with the advice of the practice accountant. The following will need to be calculated:
- Practice overheads.
- Profit desired (realistically!).
- Inflation.
- Number of sessions worked per week.

From this the target hourly rate can be calculated. Local market conditions need to be considered, which may necessitate a little rounding down of the profits desired, or a ↓ in overheads if that is possible. Once a realistic hourly rate has been calculated, *either* fees can then be determined for each procedure by the average amount of time taken, to give a set price list, *or* patients charged according to the time taken. Laboratory charges and hygienist fees, as indicated, should be additional.

Types of independent practice

There are basically four different approaches:

- A combination of independent and NHS practice. For example, exempt patients are seen on the NHS, whereas other adults are seen privately. In practice, this two-tier system can cause difficulties and friction. The option of having 'child/exempt' only NHS contracts varies between different PCTs/Health Boards and is likely to change in future. Practices with such contracts must accept all child patients not just restrict their NHS contract to children of private adult patients.
- Low-cost independent practice.
- Traditional 'private' practice.
- Insurance-based schemes.

Private dental schemes

This is one of the real growth areas in modern dentistry. At present there are five types:

- **Capitation-based** (e.g. Denplan) Patients pay a monthly fee to the company (which is passed on to the GDP minus an administration fee), usually determined by their dental status and the practice's overheads. The dentist then provides Rx as indicated, but certain items, e.g. orthodontics and laboratory fees, may be excluded.
- **Insurance schemes** Rx costs are reimbursed.
- **Corporate dental schemes**
- **Savings schemes** At present these are restricted to orthodontics.
- **Maintenance schemes** Prevention and diagnosis covered by a monthly payment. Fees paid for item of service Rx. Insurance for trauma, out-of-hours emergency Rx, etc.

Prescribing for private and independent patients

When a private patient requires medicines as part of their Rx, a private prescription should be provided. Dentists can also supply or sell medicines to any patient, but are bound by pricing and other dispensing rules. Alternatively, common drugs can be given as required and their cost included in the overall fee.

Complaints

If patients are paying more for their Rx they are likely to have ↑ expectations of the service provided. In a large proportion of cases, a potential problem can be dealt with by good communication. If patients are provided with the means to voice any complaints within the practice setting, an opportunity is given to resolve the situation early. It is now mandatory to have a written practice complaints procedure.

If having followed the practice complaints procedure, a complaint cannot be resolved, the practice should advise the patient to contact the Dental Complaints Service (see p. 650).

Vocational training

Vocational training (VT) is designed to give a supervised and mentored introduction into general dental practice and is an obligatory requirement for new graduates working within NHS general practice.

Trainees: work as salaried performers thereby reducing pressure to achieve a high-volume turnover. In England/Wales, a notional allocation of 1820 UDAs is attached to a VT practice contract. Each region organizes a day-release scheme (30 days or more per year), which should cover the clinical and administrative aspects of NHS practice, as well as patient and financial management. Each trainee will also receive on-the-job training and supervision from their trainer, as well as tutorials on a weekly basis. Trainees are members of the NHS superannuation scheme and their contribution is deducted at source. On completion of VT a vocational training number and certificate is awarded which enables a dentist to apply to provide NHS dental services in their own right.

Trainers: To be accepted, a practice needs to satisfy the criteria set by the VT Committee and the trainer needs to be present not less than 3 days a week. Trainers are themselves trained for their roles in teaching and assessment. A grant is paid and the trainees' salary is reimbursed in full.

Procedure: GDPs with >4yrs experience are eligible to become trainers. They are selected after a visit to the practice to check suitability as a training environment, and its compliance with Clinical Governance requirements and wider legislation. They are also required to attend an interview. Details of each regional scheme are advertised to final-year students or are available from the Regional VT Adviser. Potential trainees are responsible for contacting practices on the approved list and arranging visits and interviews.

Contract: A standard contract, which both parties are required to sign, is available from the BDA and course organizers. The contract runs for 12 months, at the end of which each party is free to make their own arrangements. It includes a binding-out clause which prevents the trainee subsequently accepting as a patient someone he has treated at the practice, should they move to another practice.

Community vocational training: This is also compulsory, and extends over 2yrs. Each region has a nominated trainer. There is often some tie-in with the GDS VT course.

General professional training (GPT): Is defined as 'the structured further development of knowledge, skills and attitudes common to all branches of the dental profession, which will provide a basis for informed career choice and improved dental care.' At present GPT is a voluntary scheme run by several deaneries, comprising a 2-yr period of post-basic training in two or more disciplines. There are several modes of GPT available. The least structured is to complete VT and then apply for CDS or SHO posts. At the other extreme is a scheme that integrates general dental practice VT and house officer posts in the hospital service into a seamless 2-yr period of training. It is expected that it will become compulsory for all graduates in the near future.

Clinical governance, continuing professional development, clinical audit, and peer review[1]

These are the buzzwords in terms of quality assurance and good clinical practice.

Clinical governance

Part of the NHS drive to ↑ the quality of health care and to make providers accountable for delivering a consistent standard of care. A practice with an NHS contract must comply with clinical governance arrangements established by the PCT including:

- Having a nominated person responsible for operating the quality-assurance system.
- Displaying a written statement relating to the quality assurance system.
- Having effective cross-infection control measures.
- Satisfying legal requirements relating to health and safety and radiological protection.
- Complying with requirements of the GDC in respect of continuing professional development.

Continuing professional development (CPD)

CPD is now a mandatory requirement for registration with the GDC.

Dentists
- Recertification every 5yrs.
- 250 hours of CPD in every 5-yr cycle (average 50h/yr).
  - Minimum 75h verifiable, e.g. approved courses.
  - Remaining hours non-verifiable/general CPD; e.g. reading professional journals, books.
- From 1 Jan 2007 new recommendations for CPD in 'core subjects' applies to each 5-yr cycle:
  - Medical emergencies (10hrs)
  - Disinfection/Decontamination (5hrs)
  - Radiography/Radiation Protection (5hrs)
  - For dentists working within a clinical environment, CPD in legal/ethical issues and handling complaints should be carried out (verifiable or non-verifiable)
- All dentists must maintain their own records, keep certificates, etc. and submit records to the GDC if requested.
- Failure to comply can result in erasure from the Register.

DCPs
- Compulsory CPD starts on 1 Aug 2008 for all DCPs on the register at this date.
- 150 hours of CPD over 5-yr cycle with minimum 50 hours verifiable.

Clinical audit

What it is: A systematic critical analysis of the quality of care, covering procedures used for Δ and Rx, use of resources, and the outcome for

1 BDA Advice Sheet, *CPD Clinical Governance, Audit and Peer Review.*

the patient. The aim of clinical audit in dentistry is to encourage dentists to self-assess different aspects of their practice, implement changes, and monitor them with a view to improving service and patient care.

What it is not: Clinical audit is not the same as its commercial equivalent, which is the assessment of an institution's financial status against best practice. It is not a management tool for dictating clinical policy to clinicians. It is non-judgemental, and should not be used for disciplinary measures.

Aims and objectives: Improvement of the quality of care provided. This is achieved by identifying less-than-adequate care and raising it to the standard of the agreed best.

General principles The basis is frank and open discussion without fear of criticism. Identify agreed standards against which the quality of care provided can be compared. These standards should not be fixed and immutable, so as to allow evolutionary change. It is imperative that the results of such discussion should lead to changes in practice when indicated. Confidentiality is an absolute prerequisite. Other crucial elements are genuine motivation and interest amongst the participating staff, honesty, and adequate data. Appropriate information technology, while of undoubted benefit, is not essential. An 'audit cycle' is illustrated below. Possible topics include cross-infection control, appointment systems, and clinical methodology.[1]

Audit cycle

Meeting to agree a 'gold standard' of care for a specific condition.

↓

Prospective analysis of care for that condition.

↓

Meeting to compare actual standard with 'gold standard'. Identify areas where deficiencies exist and make recommendations.
Agree to implement recommendations for improvement.

↓

Prospective analysis of care following implementation of new recommendations.

↓

Meeting to compare actual standard with 'gold standard'.
'Gold standard' not met → re-enter cycle.
'Gold standard' met → is 'gold standard' good enough?
If yes—recognize, and periodic review only.
If no—agree new standard and re-enter cycle.

Peer review The aim of peer review is to improve the quality of care provided in dental practice by encouraging communication between dentists and to identify areas in which change can be made.

British Standards 5750 BS5750 can be gained by any manufacturer or service sector organization that can demonstrate quality management systems. A number of dental practices have successfully achieved this standard.

---

1 K. A. Eaton 1998 *BDJ* **184** 178.

Evidence-based medicine/dentistry[1]

EBM/D involves making clinical decisions based on the best available evidence, which should include sound research, epidemiology, basic science, and clinical experience. EBM is essentially the same as:

Clinical effectiveness This involves using those clinical interventions which have been shown to be effective both by research and audit.

Hierarchy of evidence:
1) Systematic review and meta-analysis
2) Randomized controlled clinical trial
3) Cohort studies
4) Case control studies
5) Cross-sectional surveys
6) Case series or case reports
7) Expert opinion

The 'gold standard' for clinical studies is a well-planned RCCT, but in many areas of clinical practice evidence from such trials is yet not available. In the meantime clinicians should continue to evaluate carefully the techniques they use and the results of studies reported in the literature, although the sheer volume of scientific literature makes keeping up to date a difficult task.

Systematic review A method of collating and assessing the results of research on a particular topic. This implies that a thorough search for suitable articles and indeed unpublished work has been made, and explicit criteria used to decide whether an article should be included or rejected.

Meta-analysis A systemic review which uses special statistical methods to combine the results of several studies. Only RCCTs should be included. By considering a number of studies the effects (and side-effects) of a Rx are magnified as the sum total of subjects is effectively ↑. Whether the findings are consistent for different population groups or Rx variations can also be evaluated. For example, if this technique had been used to evaluate the results of research into the use of streptokinase in the treatment of myocardial infarction a positive benefit would have been demonstrated almost 20yrs before it became apparent from the individual studies.

The Cochrane collaboration This aims to collate the results of systematic reviews in all areas of health care and ensure that the findings are kept up to date. The results can be accessed electronically via the Cochrane library, which is available quarterly on computer disc, CD-ROM, and the Internet (📖 p. 744).

Clinical guidelines Another fashionable topic. They are defined as 'systematically developed statements which assist clinicians and patients in making decisions about appropriate treatment for specific conditions'.[2] They may be developed nationally or locally, but should always be seen as guidance and are not a substitute for, clinical judgement. To be effective, clinical

---

1 D. L. Sackett 1997 *Evidence-Based Medicine*, Churchill Livingstone.
2 T. Mann 1996 *Clinical Guidelines*, NHS Executive.

guidelines should be brief, practical, and based on the results of sound research. They should be reviewed regularly in the light of new research and their effectiveness audited.

Clinical guidelines can be drawn up by any group of clinicians; in dentistry this approach is mainly being coordinated nationally by the Royal Colleges &/or specialist societies.

The National Institute for Clinical Excellence (NICE) is a government based body that also investigates the effectiveness of different Rx modalities. See their guidelines relating to the removal of wisdom teeth, dental recall interval, and antibiotic prophylaxis.

Prevention of cross-infection[1]

Cross-infection is the transmission of infectious agents between patients and staff within the clinical environment. Potential risks include not only hepatitis and HIV, but also other viruses (e.g. herpes) and bacteria (e.g. *Streptococcus pyogenes*). Transmission can occur by inoculation or inhalation by direct or indirect contact. The BDA recommends:

- Universal precautions: a standard cross-infection control policy for all patients. This is advisable because it is not possible to identify the healthy carrier. An effective policy will ↓ the risks to the dentist and his staff, as well as being a practice-builder.
- Carriers of blood-borne viruses (hepatitis, HIV) can be treated in general dental practice, provided routine procedures are implemented rigorously.
- Patients with manifestations of immunosuppression should be referred for specialist hospital care.
- All staff should have documented training in cross-infection control and every practice must have a written infection control policy displayed in every surgery to ensure uniformity of procedures.
- It is unethical to refuse dental care on the grounds that it could expose the dentist to personal risk.

Immunization All clinical staff must be immunized against Hepatitis B with a single booster 5yrs after the primary course. Protection is indicated by HbsAb >100mIU/ml. Antibody levels <10mIU/ml indicate a non-responder. Poor responders have antibody levels of 10–100mIU; it is not clear what protection is afforded by this level of response so consultation with occupational health services is required to determine need for additional blood tests/ boosters. You must keep documentary evidence of immunization and response for all staff. Staff should also be immunized against common illnesses.

Medical and social history Tact and discretion are required if truthful answers are to be obtained to sensitive questions.

Personal Protective Equipment (PPE) and hand hygiene[2] Disposable gloves, eye protection and face protection are necessary for clinical procedures. Hand washing/disinfection should occur at the start and end of each session, before and after removing PPE, after washing instruments, completion of decontamination procedures and before handling sterilised instruments. In addition, when carrying out decontamination procedures PPE should include heavy duty gloves and disposable aprons. To prevent skin drying out a water-based cream should be used at the end of each session.

Surgery design and equipment[3] New and existing surgeries should include separate areas for dentist and DN, within which are designated 'clean' zones. Layout and equipment must be planned to allow easy cleaning, and to minimize the number of surfaces touched; e.g. taps or lights that can be turned on with infrared light switches or foot controls.

---

1 BDA Advice Sheet, *Infection Control in Dentistry*.
2 Health Technical Memorandum 01–05. DH publications.
3 L. S. Worthington 1988 *BDJ* **165** 226.

Cleaning and sterilizing instruments Disposable instruments and cleaning materials should be used wherever possible, especially instruments that are difficult to clean. Reusable items must be cleaned and sterilized after use according to the manufacturers' decontamination instructions. A washer-disinfector is preferable to manual washing of instruments prior to sterilization. *Endodontic files/reamers* must be disposed of after single use.

Treatment of work surfaces During use, instruments should only be placed on a sterilizable tray or impervious disposable covering. Care is required to avoid contamination of areas which are difficult to disinfect. A system of zoning increases efficiency as only those areas which are likely to be contaminated need to be cleaned and disinfected with a suitable viricidal disinfectant. Equipment handles, controls, and tubing should be covered by plastic sheeting.

Aerosols Minimize these by high-volume suction. Wear gloves, eye protection, and masks. Flush aspirators and tubing through daily with a recommended disinfecting agent. Use of rubber dam reduces splatter and aerosols.

Blood spillages Immediately cover with disposable towels; treat with 10 000ppm sodium hypochlorite solution. After 5mins dispose of in clinical waste. Use protective clothing and heavy duty gloves.

Disposal of sharps Care is required to prevent needlestick injuries, and preferably a re-sheathing device should be used. Sharps must be placed in a rigid sharps container and not filled to more than ⅔ full. Disposal can be arranged via PCT/Health Board.

Needlestick injuries (📖 see p. 343) Allow wound to bleed, and wash under warm water. Get advice from occupational health services. If a risk of infection, serological tests of staff and patient may be indicated.

Laboratory items Rinse and disinfect all impressions and appliances according to the manufacturer's recommendations prior to dispatch to the lab. Proprietary products are available for impression disinfection. Ensure lab sheet is marked to show appropriate disinfection of laboratory items has been carried out.

Transmissible spongiform encephalopathies These include Creutzfeldt–Jakob disease (CJD) and variant CJD (VCJD/BSE). Patients with a known history of one of these conditions or those at risk (growth hormone Rx before 1985; recipients of dura mater grafts; or family history of this disease) are best treated in a specialist environment as routine autoclaving does not destroy the causative agent: prions.

Current advice is available at 🖱 www.dh.gov.uk

X-rays—the statutory regulations[1]

The Ionizing Radiation Regulations 1999 (IRR99)
The Ionizing Radiation (Medical Exposure) Regulations 2000 (IRMER)

Terminology

The **legal person** is responsible for implementing the regulations and good working practice. Usually the practice owner.

The **radiation protection supervisor (RPS)** is appointed by the legal person and is responsible for implementing the local rules. Can be an appropriately trained dentist or DCP.

An **IRMER practitioner** is the dentist responsible for justifying an exposure, and ensuring the benefits outweigh the risks.

A **referrer** is a dentist who refers a patient to an IRMER practitioner for radiological examination.

An **operator** is any person who carries out all or part of the practical aspects associated with a radiological examination, including taking the X-ray, developing films, identifying the patient, etc.

A **radiation protection adviser (RPA)** must be appointed in writing to provide advice on complying with legal obligations, e.g. testing of equipment, staff training, risk assessment, quality assurance program, etc.

With the introduction of these regulations to the statute books, the dentist (legal person) must:

- Complete an inventory of X-ray equipment (including age, manufacturer, model, and serial number) and notify Health and Safety Executive.
- Complete a risk assessment in consultation with the RPA to exposure of staff and patients. It should be documented and reviewed at least every 5yrs.
- Ensure every IRMER practitioner and operator has appropriate training and undertakes continuing education. Update every 5yrs and keep records of training for inspection.
- Appoint a RPS.
- Complete a radiation protection file. This should include the local rules and other documentation relating to radiation protection within the practice, e.g. written procedures for patient protection, guidelines for referral for radiological examination, quality assurance programs, records of training, etc.
- Have a set of local rules, which must include name and contact details for RPA, operating instructions, details of controlled areas, and a contingency plan in the event of an equipment malfunction.
- Identify designated controlled areas. This is usually within a radius of 1.5m, except in the direction of the beam, where it extends until the beam is attenuated.
- Ensure that all equipment is regularly serviced and a radiation safety assessment carried out at least every 3yrs (this can be done by post by the National Radiological Protection Board).

---

1 BDA Advice Sheet, *Radiation in Dentistry* 2003.

- Keep radiation dose As Low As Reasonably Practicable (ALARP). This has several aspects:
  - Be able to justify taking every radiograph.
  - There must be written guidance for exposure settings for all types of radiograph.
  - A clinical evaluation and report in patient's records for all films.
  - Avoiding repetition by recording all X-rays taken in the patient's records; send X-rays with patient for referrals.
  - Rectangular collimation, with minimum skin-to-focus distances as follows:<60kV = 10cm; >60kV = 20cm.
  - A quality assurance program to ↑ diagnostic yield and ↓ need for repeat X-rays.
  - Use of fastest film consistent with good diagnostic quality (ISO speed E or faster).
  - Routine use of film holders. A patient should only hold a film in position when it is impossible to position the film any other way.

X-rays—practical tips and helpful hints

Practical tips

- When an exposure is made the raised dot on the packet should face the direction of the X-rays. When the processed film is viewed from the side with the raised dot, the patient's right is shown on the left of the film.
- In order of radio-opacity: air, soft tissues, cartilage, immature bone, tooth-coloured fillings, mature bone, dentine and cementum, enamel, metallic restorations.
- View films in subdued lighting against an illuminated background.
- For soft-tissue views (e.g. after trauma) a very short exposure (often below the lowest setting on the X-ray set) is required. A slower occlusal film may be more practical.
- The incisive foramen will have a parallax shift in relation to an incisor apex.
- Routine use of a lead apron is no longer considered necessary (📖 p. 17).
- Dental radiographs are not contraindicated during pregnancy (📖 p. 17).

Processing

Manual Do this either in a darkroom or a daylight processing tank. It is important to always keep the developer and fixer baths in the same order.

Automatic There are several dental types available which can process IO and some EO films. It is faster as the first wash is eliminated and rollers squeeze off the solutions.

Method

Manual regimen:
- Remove packaging and put film carefully in holder.
- Place in developer. Length of time varies according to the manufacturer and the temperature, but is usually 3–4min.
- Rinse.
- Place in fix for twice as long as it takes for film to clear.
- Wash. The recommended time is 10min.

If a film is urgently required the films can be viewed 'wet' after 2–4min in the fixer, but they should be returned for complete fixing.

NB Avoid contamination of the developer with fix and change the chemicals at least once a fortnight.

Self-developing film So called because the developer and fix are contained within a sachet, which also contains the film. Following exposure, tabs are pulled which release first developer and then fixer onto the film. The film is then removed and rinsed. Although this method obviates the need for processing equipment, the results are inferior so do not use it routinely.

Digital detectors allow an image to be viewed and stored on a computer system. Processing time is ↓ and the image can be manipulated to diagnostic yield. Exposure settings should be ↓ to the minimum compatible with the diagnostic quality required of the image.

Film faults

Film dark	• Fogged film: out-of-date or poorly stored film. • Overexposure. • Overdevelopment. • Temperature too high.
Film pale	• Underexposed. • Underdeveloped: impatience, exhausted chemicals. • Temperature too low.
Poor contrast	• Overdevelopment. • Developer contaminated with fix. • Inadequate fixation &/or washing.
Poor definition	• Patient movement.
Blotches	• Dark blotches are due to developer splashes, and white blotches to fixer splashes.

The most common faults are overexposure and underdevelopment. The article by Chadwick discusses the factors affecting b/w, and is recommended.[1]

1 B. L. Chadwick 1998 *BDJ* **184** 80.

Syndromes of the head and neck

Contents

Principal sources and further reading R. J. Gorlin 1990
Syndromes of the Head and Neck, 3 Edn, OUP.

Syndromes of the head and neck

Introduction

The aim of this section is neither to bemuse the reader nor to demonstrate esoteric knowledge, although both may appear to occur. The real importance behind the learning of names associated with conditions which may be of relevance to, or be picked up by, clinical examination of the head and neck, is that, once learned, some difficult diagnostic problems can be quickly solved and appropriate Rx instituted. We have retained eponyms where relevant (although this is not in keeping with current fashion) as they are, we feel, easier to learn and certainly more fun. Examiners have a tendency to remember their favourite eponymous syndrome and it helps to at least agree on the name. We have, however, avoided the use of the possessive when using eponyms because invariably others were involved in describing or elucidating the condition and the syndrome does not belong to the individual(s) associated with it. The following list is in no way comprehensive but takes you through conditions met by the authors either in their clinical practice or in examinations, and which could therefore be considered worth knowing about.

Definitions

Malformation A primary structural defect resulting from a localized error of morphogenesis.

Anomalad A malformation *and* its subsequently derived structural changes.

Syndrome A recognized pattern of malformation, presumed to have the same aetiology but not interpreted as the result of a single localized error in morphogenesis.

Association A recognized pattern of malformation not considered to be a syndrome or an anomalad, *at the present time*.

Syndromes

Albright syndrome (McCune–Albright syndrome) Consists of polyostotic fibrous dysplasia (multiple bones affected), patchy skin pigmentation (referred to as *café-au-lait* spots), and an endocrine abnormality (usually precocious puberty in girls). Facial asymmetry affects up to 25% of cases.

Apert syndrome is a rare developmental deformity consisting of a cranio synostosis (premature fusion of cranial sutures) and syndactyly (fusion of fingers or toes). Severe mid-face retrusion leads to exophthalmos of varying severity. Early surgical intervention may be indicated for raised intracranial pressure or to prevent blindness from subluxation of the globe of the eye.

Beckwith–Wiedemann syndrome consists of exomphalos, macroglossia, gigantism, adrenal and renal anomalies. May have profound hypoglycaemia. Tongue reduction sometimes required.

Behçet syndrome (pronounced behh-chet, after Turkish doctor Hulusi Behçet) is, classically, oral ulceration, genital ulceration, and uveitis. Clinical Δ can be made on finding any two of these. It is, in fact, a multisystem disease of immunological origin, although no hard diagnostic tests are yet available. It tends to affect young adults, especially males and there is an association with HLA-B5. It undergoes spontaneous remission, although a variety of drugs including thalidomide are in use to treat it. See also 📖 p. 404.

Binder syndrome Maxillonasal dysplasia, severe mid-facial retrusion, and absent or hypoplastic frontal sinuses are the main features. There is no associated intellectual defect.

Chediak–Higashi syndrome is a combination of defective neutrophil function, abnormal skin pigmentation, and ↑ susceptibility to infection (leading to severe gingivitis, periodontitis, and aphthae in young children). It is a genetic disease.

Cleidocranial dysostosis (cleidocranial dysplasia) is an autosomal dominant inherited condition consisting of hypoplasia or aplasia of the clavicles, delayed ossification of the cranial fontanelles, and a large, short skull. Associated features are shortness of stature, frontal and parietal bossing, failure to pneumatize the air sinuses, a high arched palate &/or clefting, mid-face hypoplasia, and failure of tooth eruption with multiple supernumerary teeth. Many of the teeth present have inherent abnormalities such as dilaceration of roots or crown gemination. Hypoplasia of 2° cementum may occur. The condition mainly, though NOT exclusively, affects membranous bone.

'Cri du chat' syndrome is a chromosomal abnormality caused by deletion of part of the short arm of chromosome No. 5, resulting in microcephaly, hypertelorism, and a round face with a broad nasal bridge and malformed ears. Associated laryngeal hypoplasia causes a characteristic shrill cry. There is associated severe mental retardation.

Crouzon syndrome is the commonest of the craniosynostoses. It is an autosomal dominant condition consisting of premature fusion of cranial sutures, mid-face hypoplasia, and, due to this, shallow orbits with proptosis of the globe of the eye. Radiographically the appearance of a 'beaten copper skull' is characteristic. The enlarging brain is entrapped by the prematurely fused sutures and ↑ intracranial pressure can lead to cerebral damage and resulting intellectual deficiency. This and the risk of blindness justify early craniofacial surgery to correct the deformity.

Down syndrome (trisomy 21) is the commonest of all malformation syndromes, affecting up to 1:600 births. Risk ↑ with maternal age. Down's children account for ⅓ of severely mentally handicapped children. Facial appearance is characteristic with brachycephaly, mid-face retrusion, small nose with flattened nasal bridge, and upward sloping palpebral fissures (mongoloid slant). There is relative macroglossia and delayed eruption of teeth. Major relevant associations are heart defects, atlanto-axial subluxation, anaemia, and an ↑ risk of leukaemia. Most Down's children and adults are extremely friendly and cooperative.

Eagle syndrome is dysphagia and pain on chewing and turning the head associated with an elongated styloid process.

Ehlers–Danlos syndrome A group of disorders characterized by hyperflexibility of joints, ↑ bleeding and bruising, and hyperextensible skin. There appears to be an underlying molecular abnormality of collagen in this inherited disorder. Bleeding is commoner in type IV, early onset periodontal disease in type VIII. Pulp stones may be seen in all types.

Frey syndrome (Lucie Frey, a Polish physician) is a condition in which gustatory sweating and flushing of skin occur. It follows trauma to skin overlying a salivary gland and is thought to be due to post-traumatic crossover of sympathetic and parasympathetic innervation to the gland and skin, respectively. Its frequency following superficial parotidectomy ranges from 0–100% depending on which surgeon you are talking to, but is almost certainly present in all cases to some degree if looked for carefully enough (use starch–iodine test).

Gardener syndrome This comprises multiple osteomas (particularly of the jaws and facial bones), multiple polyps of the large intestine, epidermoid cysts, and fibromas of the skin. It shows autosomal dominant inheritance. The discovery on clinical or X-ray examination of facial osteomas mandates examination of the lower gastrointestinal tract, as these polyps have a tendency to rapid malignant change. This is a highly 'worthwhile' syndrome.

Goldenhar syndrome is a variant of hemifacial microsomia and consists of microtia (small ears), macrostomia, agenesis of the mandibular ramus and condyle, vertebral abnormalities (e.g. hemivertebrae), and epibulbar dermoids. Also, cardiac, renal, or skeletal abnormalities can occur. Up to 10% of patients may have mental handicap—in other words, 90% **do not**.

Gorlin–Goltz syndrome (multiple basal cell naevi syndrome) 📖 see, p. 512. Consists of multiple BCCs (epitheliomas), multiple jaw cysts (odontogenic keratocysts), vertebral and rib anomalies (usually bifid ribs), and calcification of the falx cerebri. Frontal bossing, mandibular prognathism, hypertelorism, hydrocephalus, eye, and endocrine abnormalities have also been noted.

Graves' disease Autoantibodies to thyroid stimulating hormone cause hyperthyroidism with ophthalmopathy; women 30–50yrs are commonly affected; exophthalmos can be helped by craniofacial approach to orbital decompression.

Heerfordt syndrome (uveoparotid fever) is sarcoidosis with associated lacrimal and salivary (especially parotid) swelling, uveitis, and fever. Sometimes there are associated neuropathies, e.g. facial palsy.

Hemifacial microsomia Prevalence: 1 in 5000 births. Bilateral in 20% of cases. Congenital defect characterized by lack of hard and soft tissue on affected side(s), usually in the region of the ramus and external ear (i.e. first and second branchial arches). Wide spectrum of ear and cranial deformities found.

'Histiocytosis-X' Really three broad groups of diseases with the histological feature of tissue infiltration by tumour-like aggregates of macrophages (histiocytes) and eosinophils.
1) *Solitary eosinophilic granuloma* Mainly affects males <20yrs. Mandible is a common site. Responds to local Rx.
2) *Hand–Schüller–Christian disease* Multifocal eosinophilic granuloma causing skull lesions, exophthalmos, and diabetes insipidus. Affects younger group. May respond to cytotoxic chemotherapy.
3) *Letterer–Siwe disease* Rapidly progressive, disseminated histiocytosis. Associated pancytopenia and multisystem disease; can be fatal.

Horner syndrome Consists of a constricted pupil (miosis), drooping eyelid (ptosis), unilateral loss of sweating (anhydrosis) on the face, and occasionally sunken eye (enophthalmos). It is caused by interruption of sympathetic nerve fibres at the cervical ganglion 2° to, e.g. bronchogenic carcinoma, invading the ganglion or neck trauma. Scores high on the 'worthwhile' rating.

Hurler syndrome is a mucopolysaccharidosis causing growth failure and mental retardation. A large head, frontal bossing, hypertelorism, and coarse features give it its classical appearance. Multiple skeletal abnormalities (dysostosis multiplex), corneal clouding, and serum and urinary acid mucopolysaccharide abnormalities also occur.

Hypohydrotic ectodermal dysplasia hypodontia found in association with lack of hair, sweating, and saddle nose.

Kikuchi syndrome is really Kikuchi disease, histiocytic necrotizing lymphadenitis. Increasing cause of cervical lymphadenopathy. Associations with SLE and haemophagocytic syndrome.

Klippel–Feil anomalad is the association of cervical vertebral fusion, short neck and low-lying posterior hairline. A number of neurological anomalies have been noted, and unilateral renal agenesis is frequent. Cardiac anomalies sometimes occur.

Larsen syndrome is a mainly autosomal dominant condition, with a predilection for females, consisting of cleft palate, flattened facies, multiple congenital dislocations, and deformities of the feet. Sufferers are usually of short stature. Larynx may be affected.

Lesch–Nyhan syndrome is a defect of purine metabolism causing mental retardation, spastic cerebral palsy, choreoathetosis, and aggressive self-mutilating behaviour (particularly involving the lips).

MAGIC syndrome stands for Mouth And Genital ulcers and Interstitial Chondritis and is a variant of the Behçet syndrome group.

Marcus Gunn syndrome aka 'jaw wink syndrome' is unilateral ptosis which opens (not winks) on moving the jaw to the contralateral side. Odd.

Marfan syndrome is an autosomal dominant condition characterized by tall, thin stature and arachnodactyly (long, thin, spider-like hands), dislocation of the lens, dissecting aneurysms of the thoracic aorta, aortic regurgitation, floppy mitral valve, and high arched palate. Joint laxity is also common. This condition is highly prevalent among top-class basketball and volleyball players, for obvious reasons.

Melkerson–Rosenthal syndrome Consists of facial paralysis, facial oedema, and fissured tongue. It is probably a variant of the group of conditions now known as orofacial granulomatosis.

Multiple endocrine neoplasia A group of conditions affecting the endocrine glands. MEN IIb is of particular relevance as it consists of multiple mucosal neuromas which have a characteristic histopathology, pheochromocytoma, medullary thyroid carcinoma, and a thin wasted appearance. Calcitonin levels are elevated if medullary thyroid carcinoma is present. Index of suspicion should be high in tall, thin, wasted-looking children and young adults presenting with lumps in the mouth. Biopsy is mandatory and if histopathology is suggestive the thyroid must be adequately investigated. This is another 'worthwhile' syndrome.

Orofacial–digital syndrome is one of the many CLP syndromes, all of which are associated with hypodontia (laterals especially) and supernumeraries. This one has finger abnormalities as well.

Papillon–Lefevre syndrome is palmoplantar hyperkeratosis and juvenile periodontitis, which affects both 1° and 2° dentition. Normal dental development occurs until the appearance of the hyperkeratosis of the palms and soles, then simultaneously an aggressive gingivitis and periodontitis begin. The mechanism is not well understood.

Patterson–Brown–Kelly syndrome (Plummer–Vinson syndrome) is the occurrence of dysphagia, microcytic hypochromic anaemia, koilonychia (spoon-shaped nails), and angular cheilitis. The dysphagia is due to a post-cricoid web, usually a membrane on the anterior oesophageal wall, which is premalignant. The koilonychia and angular cheilitis are 2° to the anaemia but may be presenting symptoms. The main affected group is middle-aged women, and correction of the anaemia may both relieve symptoms and prevent malignant progression of the web.

Peutz–Jeghers syndrome is an autosomal dominant condition of melanotic pigmentation of skin (especially peri-oral skin) and mucosa, and intestinal polyposis. These polyps, unlike those of the Gardener syndrome, have no particular propensity to malignant change, being hamartomatous, and are found in the small intestine. They may, however, cause intussusception or other forms of gut obstruction. Ovarian tumours are sometimes associated with the condition (10% woman with Peutz–Jeghers).

Progeria is probably a collagen abnormality. It causes dwarfism and premature ageing. Characteristic facial appearance occurs due to a disproportionately small face with mandibular retrognathia and a beak-like nose, creating an unforgettable appearance; death occurs in the mid-teens.

Pycnodysostosis is micrognathia with hypoplasia of the mandibular angle, exopthalmos, dwarfism, short fingers and osteopetrosis. Rarely present for orthognathic/orthodontic treatment. Be aware of the osteopetrosis.

Ramsay Hunt syndrome is a lower motor neurone facial palsy, with vesicles on the same side in the pharynx, external auditory canal, and on the face. It is thought to be due to herpes zoster of the geniculate ganglion.

Reiter syndrome Consists of arthritis, urethritis, and conjunctivitis. There are frequently oral lesions, which resemble benign migratory glossitis in appearance but affect other parts of the mouth. The condition is probably an unwanted effect of an immune response to a low-grade pathogen; however, some still believe it to be a sexually transmitted disease, although there is no hard evidence for this.

Reyes syndrome is not a head and neck syndrome but encephalopathy and fatty degeneration of the liver which can be lethal. Probable association with aspirin and viral illness in children and the reason you don't give aspirin to under 16s.

Robin sequence Named after Pierre Robin (and mistakenly called Pierre Robin syndrome at times). This is micrognathia, cleft palate, and glossoptosis. Huge number of associated anomalies.

Romberg syndrome (hemifacial atrophy) consists of progressive atrophy of the soft tissues of half the face, associated with contralateral Jacksonian epilepsy and trigeminal neuralgia. Rarely, half the body may be affected. It starts in the first decade and lasts ~3yrs before it becomes quiescent.

Sicca syndrome (primary Sjögren syndrome) is xerostomia and kerato conjunctivitis sicca, i.e. dry mouth and dry eyes. There is an ↑ risk of developing parotid lymphoma with this condition. Interestingly, although Sicca syndrome has certain serological abnormalities in common with systemic connective tissue disorders such as rheumatoid arthritis, it does not have any of the symptomatology (unlike Sjögren syndrome).

Sjögren syndrome (secondary Sjögren syndrome) In addition to dry eyes and dry mouth this has both the serology and symptomatology of an autoimmune condition, usually rheumatoid arthritis, but sometimes SLE, systemic sclerosis, or primary biliary cirrhosis. Actual swelling of the salivary glands is relatively uncommon and late-onset swelling of the parotids may herald the presence of a lymphoma.

Stevens–Johnson syndrome A severe version of erythema multiforme, a mucocutaneous condition that is probably autoimmune in nature and precipitated particularly by drugs. Classical signs are the target lesions, concentric red rings which especially affect the hands and feet. Stevens–Johnson syndrome is said to be present when the condition is particularly severe, and is associated with fever and multiple mucosal involvement. Viral infections, e.g. herpes simplex, are the second commonest cause.

Stickler syndrome Perhaps the commonest syndrome associated with cleft palate (20%). Consists of flat mid-face, cleft palate, myopia, retinal detachment, hearing loss (80%), and arthropathy. 30% of Robin sequence patients have Stickler syndrome, therefore examine eyes.

Sturge–Weber anomalad is due to a hamartomatous angioma affecting the upper part of the face, which may extend intracranially. There may be associated convulsions, hemiplegia (on the contralateral side of the body), or intellectual impairment. The risks of surgery are obvious.

Treacher–Collins syndrome (mandibulofacial dysostosis) Basically involves defects in structures derived from the first branchial arch. It is inherited as an autosomal dominant trait with variable expressivity, and consists of downward-sloping (antimongoloid slant) palpebral fissures, hypoplastic malar complexes, mandibular retrognathia with a high gonial angle, deformed pinnas, hypoplastic air sinuses, colobomas in the outer third of the eye, and middle and inner ear hypoplasia (and hence deafness). 30% have cleft palates and 25% have an unusual tongue-like projection of hair pointing towards the cheek. Most have *completely normal intellectual* function, which may be missed because they are deaf and 'funny-looking kids' (how would you like to be called a funny-looking dentist/doctor?). These people may well miss out on fulfilling their potential because of society's (and some professionals') attitude to deformity. This syndrome is a prime indication for corrective craniofacial surgery.

Trotter syndrome is unilateral deafness, pain in the mandibular division of the trigeminal nerve, ipsilateral immobility of the palate, and trismus, due to invasion of the lateral wall of the nasopharynx by malignant tumour. Pterygopalatine fossa syndrome is a similar condition where the first and second divisions of the trigeminal are affected.

Van der Woude syndrome is present in 1–2% of cleft patients, lip pits (which are actually small sinuses to minor salivary glands) associated with cleft lip and/or palate. Autosomal dominant with variable penetrance. Second premolars missing in 10–20%.

von Recklinghausen neurofibromatosis/syndrome Multiple neurofibromas with skin pigmentation, skeletal abnormalities, CNS involvement, and a predisposition to malignancy are the basics of this syndrome. It undergoes autosomal dominant transmission and has a large and varied number of manifestations. Lesions of the face can be particularly disfiguring.

Chapter 19

Useful information and addresses

Contents

Tooth notation

FDI
Permanent teeth

R $\dfrac{18\ \ 17\ \ 16\ \ 15\ \ 14\ \ 13\ \ 12\ \ 11\ \ |\ 21\ \ 22\ \ 23\ \ 24\ \ 25\ \ 26\ \ 27\ \ 28}{48\ \ 47\ \ 46\ \ 45\ \ 44\ \ 43\ \ 42\ \ 41\ \ |\ 31\ \ 32\ \ 33\ \ 34\ \ 35\ \ 36\ \ 37\ \ 38}$ L

Deciduous teeth

R $\dfrac{55\ \ 54\ \ 53\ \ 52\ \ 51\ \ |\ 61\ \ 62\ \ 63\ \ 64\ \ 65}{85\ \ 84\ \ 83\ \ 82\ \ 81\ \ |\ 71\ \ 72\ \ 73\ \ 74\ \ 75}$ L

Zsigmondy–Palmer, Chevron, or Set Square system
Permanent teeth

R $\dfrac{8\ \ 7\ \ 6\ \ 5\ \ 4\ \ 3\ \ 2\ \ 1\ \ |\ 1\ \ 2\ \ 3\ \ 4\ \ 5\ \ 6\ \ 7\ \ 8}{8\ \ 7\ \ 6\ \ 5\ \ 4\ \ 3\ \ 2\ \ 1\ \ |\ 1\ \ 2\ \ 3\ \ 4\ \ 5\ \ 6\ \ 7\ \ 8}$ L

Deciduous teeth

R $\dfrac{e\ \ d\ \ c\ \ b\ \ a\ \ |\ a\ \ b\ \ c\ \ d\ \ e}{e\ \ d\ \ c\ \ b\ \ a\ \ |\ a\ \ b\ \ c\ \ d\ \ e}$ L

Because of the difficulties of putting the grid notation in word processed documents it is common practice to indicate the quadrant by abbreviating the arch and side. Thus the upper right second premolar is UR5 and the lower left second deciduous molar is LLE.

European
Permanent teeth

R $\dfrac{8+\ \ 7+\ \ 6+\ \ 5+\ \ 4+\ \ 3+\ \ 2+\ \ 1+\ \ |\ +1\ \ +2\ \ +3\ \ +4\ \ +5\ \ +6\ \ +7\ \ +8}{8-\ \ 7-\ \ 6-\ \ 5-\ \ 4-\ \ 3-\ \ 2-\ \ 1-\ \ |\ -1\ \ -2\ \ -3\ \ -4\ \ -5\ \ -6\ \ -7\ \ -8}$ L

Deciduous teeth

R $\dfrac{05+\ \ 04+\ \ 03+\ \ 02+\ \ 01+\ \ |\ +01\ \ +02\ \ +03\ \ +04\ \ +05}{05-\ \ 04-\ \ 03-\ \ 02-\ \ 01-\ \ |\ -01\ \ -02\ \ -03\ \ -04\ \ -05}$ L

American
Permanent teeth

R $\dfrac{1\ \ 2\ \ 3\ \ 4\ \ 5\ \ 6\ \ 7\ \ 8\ \ |\ 9\ \ 10\ \ 11\ \ 12\ \ 13\ \ 14\ \ 15\ \ 16}{32\ \ 31\ \ 30\ \ 29\ \ 28\ \ 27\ \ 26\ \ 25\ \ |\ 24\ \ 23\ \ 22\ \ 21\ \ 20\ \ 19\ \ 18\ \ 17}$ L

Deciduous teeth

R $\dfrac{A\ \ B\ \ C\ \ D\ \ E\ \ |\ F\ \ G\ \ H\ \ I\ \ J}{T\ \ S\ \ R\ \ Q\ \ P\ \ |\ O\ \ N\ \ M\ \ L\ \ K}$ L

Some qualifications in medicine and dentistry

BA	Bachelor of Arts
BC/BCh/BS	Bachelor of Surgery
BChD/BDS	Bachelor of Dental Surgery
BM	Bachelor of Medicine
DDPH	Diploma in Dental Public Health
DDR	Diploma in Dental Radiology
DDS/DDSc	Doctor of Dental Surgery/Science
DGDP	Diploma in General Dental Practice
DOrth	Diploma in Orthodontics
DPhil	Doctor of Philosophy
DRD	Diploma in Restorative Dentistry
DSc	Doctor of Science
FDS	Fellowship in Dental Surgery
FFD	Fellow in Faculty of Dental Surgery
FFGDP	Diploma of Fellowship in General Dental Practice
FRCGP	Fellow of Royal College of General Practitioners
FRCP	Fellow of Royal College of Physicians
FRCS	Fellow of Royal College of Surgeons
LDS	Licentiate in Dental Surgery
MBBCh/MBChB	Bachelor of Medicine and Bachelor of Surgery
MCCD	Membership in Clinical Community Dentistry
MCDH	Master of Community Dental Health
MD	Doctor of Medicine
MDS	Master of Dental Surgery
MDentSci/MDSc	Master of Dental Science
MFDS	Member of the Faculty of Dental Surgery
MFGDP	Diploma of Membership of Faculty of General Dental Practitioners (UK)
MGDS	Diploma of Membership in General Dental Surgery
MJDF	Diploma of Membership of the Joint Dental Faculties at the Royal College of Surgeons of England
MOrth	Membership in Orthodontics
MPhil	Master of Philosophy
MRCGP	Member of Royal College of General Practitioners
MRCS	Member of Royal College of Surgeons
MSc	Master of Science
NVQ	National Vocational Qualification
PhD	Doctor of Philosophy

Bur numbering systems

Maximum diameter of bur head	ISO	UK/USA		
		Round	Inverted cone	Flat fissure
0.6	006	$\frac{1}{2}$	$\frac{1}{2}$	
0.8	008	1	1	$\frac{1}{2}$
0.9	009			1
1.0	010	2	2	2
1.2	012	3	3	3
1.4	014	4	4	4
1.6	016	5	5	5
1.8	018	6	6	6
2.1	021	7	7	7
2.3	023	8	8	8
2.5	025	9	9	9
2.7	027	10	10	10
2.9	029	11		11
3.1	031	12		12

File sizes (for endodontic therapy)

Size	Tip diameter	ISO colour
08	0.08	grey
10	0.10	purple
15	0.15	white
20	0.20	yellow
25	0.25	red
30	0.30	blue
35	0.35	green
40	0.40	black
45	0.45	white
50	0.50	yellow
55	0.55	red
60	0.60	blue
70	0.70	green
80	0.80	black
90	0.90	white
100	1.00	yellow
110	1.10	red
120	1.20	blue
130	1.30	green
140	1.40	black

Wire gauges

Size on wire gauge	Diameter	
	Imperial (inches)	Metric (mm)
14	0.080	2.0
19	0.040	1.0
20	0.036	0.9
21	0.032	0.8
22	0.028	0.7
23	0.024	0.6
24	0.022	0.55
25	0.020	0.5
26	0.018	0.45
27	0.0164	0.4
28	0.0148	0.37
29	0.0136	0.35
30	0.0124	0.3

Passing exams

Preparation First, there is unfortunately no substitute for the sheer hard work of revising, and to have a chance of being adequate this should start well before the exam. Beware of those who try to impress by saying they have passed every exam, first time, having only started revising the night before. These people are not super-intelligent (in fact, their behaviour suggests the reverse) they have probably only been lucky ... to date!

Equally well, the human brain is not a computer and revising for hours, day in day out, could result in 'burn-out'. Each person needs to find their own method, but a break of 5–10min every hour and a complete hour off after 3 hours' work, has succeeded for others.

It is important to be sure that you are revising the correct material in sufficient depth. One way of ensuring this is to go over past questions. If some are tackled under exam conditions, this also gives practice in exam technique.

If your nerve is strong enough it is probably wise to stop working 2–3 days before the exams start and have a rest, doing something that you enjoy. Most people baulk at this suggestion, but see the logic as of a marathon runner resting before an important race. Studying the night before is akin to an élite runner going out the night before the Olympic marathon and running 26.2 miles just to make sure he can cover the distance.

Written exams It is important to know beforehand how many questions you have to answer; whether they all have to be tackled or there is a choice. If essay style—work out how long should be spent on each question and, if a choice is permitted, take a few minutes to decide which to answer and in what order. It is better to tackle your best question second, thus allowing the butterflies to settle. Read each question carefully, and periodically stop to check that you are answering the question set, not the one you'd like to answer. A rough plan helps to produce a more logical essay and provides an *aide-mémoire* in case of panic halfway through. Write neatly.

Multiple choice exams are popular with educationalists because they are 'reliable', can be marked by computer and 'number-crunched'. Extended matching questions are a variation on the theme.
- Do the necessary revision; it is impossible to waffle hopefully round the subject in a multiple choice exam.
- Remember that your first instinct is often right so consider carefully before revising your answer to any question.

Objective structured clinical examinations (OSCEs) should be:
Objective—independent and competent examiners should have agreed what skills are being examined, with agreed marking scales.
Structured—have agreed criteria (in advance) for the correct answer for each element of the exam.
Clinical—to test clinical and practical competence, including communication and problem-solving skills.
Examination—this may include evaluation of written responses &/or observation by an examiner.

They usually comprise a series of stations, which test a different skill, often interspersed with rest stations. A set time is allocated to each station. The clinical proficiencies tested may include taking a history from a 'patient' (increasingly actors are used rather than actual patients) and establishing a diagnosis; communication and psychomotor skills. Students may be evaluated by an examiner, who observes and marks their responses and actions at a particular station.

Logbooks are increasingly used to evaluate clinical experience and competencies and often include a reflective learning log.

GOOD LUCK!

Dentistry and the World Wide Web

The Web has permeated all areas of our lives and is a great resource, not only for social networking, but also for finding information and gaining knowledge. Web-based learning is one type of distance education that removes the barriers of time and space—'anytime, anywhere learning'. It is a component of the broader term 'e-learning', defined as: the use of electronic technology and media to deliver, support, and enhance teaching and learning.

In education, the Web is increasingly used both to support lectures (printed course materials) and as a means of delivering online learning programs. These may be interactive, with online activities (such as self-assessments), animations, and simulations, which can be more enjoyable and meaningful to learners. Discussion forums via e-mail, video-conferencing, and live lectures (videostreaming) are all possible through the Web. Another advantage is that Web pages and a virtual learning environment may contain hyperlinks to other parts of the Web, thus enabling access to a vast amount of Web-based information. However, newer technologies are not necessarily better (or worse) for teaching or learning than older technologies, just different. Therefore, it is necessary to pick and choose to find what suits your learning style.

The Web is a fantastic way of finding information quickly and easily. However, the downside is that skill is required to ensure that your search yields a manageable number of relevant sites/pages. Structuring your search using 'rules' that are used by the major search engines will help:

- Search boxes are not case sensitive
- Using **and** will include both words/terms
- Using **or** will include either the word before or the word after
- Placing a **+** sign in front of a word means it must be included
- Placing a **–** sign in front of a word means it will be excluded
- Using quotation marks around a group of words will ensure that phrase is included
- Using a 'wildcard' symbol will include any words with the same stem e.g. dent* will yield dental, dentistry, dentist etc.
- Using **:site** will limit the search to a named domain
- Using **:link** will yield pages that link to the specified web address

The following website is useful as it provides details as to whether a journal is peer-reviewed thus helping the reader to assimilate the value of the results of articles produced by a web-search:
℘ www.ulrichsweb.com/Ulrichsweb/

Glossary

e-conferencing Use of online presentations and discussion forums (in real time or stored as downloadable files on a website) so that participants need not travel.

HTML HyperText Mark-up Language. Is used to write web pages.

Hyperlinks Links in web pages that enable the user to access another web page (either on the same or a different site) with just one mouse click.

Internet service provider (ISP) Links the home user to the Internet. The ISP maintains a network of personal computers that are permanently connected to the Internet.

Intranet A network of computers that share information, usually within an organization. Access normally requires a password and is limited to a defined range of users, e.g. the NHS.

Managed learning environment Provides an integrated function, with administrative tools such as student records, and links with other management information systems.

m-learning Listening to audio-recordings or podcast of a lecture or other learning event(s).

Podcast An audio-recording which can be listened to via a MP3 player or i-pod distributed via a service such as Apple i-tunes. RSS allows users to subscribe to podcasts.

Search engines (such as Lycos, Google) Can be used to find information.

Videostreaming The process by which video images are able to be stored on and downloaded from the Web. This might be done in real time (such as a conference) or the images may be used asynchronously. Also known as webcasting.

Virtual learning environment A set of electronic teaching and learning tools. Principal components can map a curriculum, track student activity, and provide online student support and electronic communication.

Useful websites

The amount of information available on the Web is constantly increasing. Caution is required as there is little guidance out there as to which sites are reputable and reliable—a fact which patients sometimes need to be reminded of. The following sites are, at best, a sampler of interesting sites (we take no responsibility for their content). Please also see the Useful Addresses page. If you have any suggestions for future editions then please let us know.

Acronyms: ℜ www.nottingham.ac.uk/cpcme/edu/Acronym.htm

American Dental Association: ℜ www.ada.org

British Association of Dental Nurses: ℜ www.badn.org.uk

British Association of Dental Therapists: ℜ www.badt.org.uk

British Association of Oral and Maxillofacial Surgeons: ℜ www.baoms.org.uk

British Association for the Study of Community Dentistry:
ℜ www.bascd.org

British Dental Practice Managers Association: ℜ www.bdpma.org.uk

British Endodontic Society: ℜ www.britishendodonticsociety.org.uk

British National Formulary: ℜ www.bnf.org

British Orthodontic Society: ℜ www.bos.org.uk

British Society of Dental Hygiene and Therapy: ℜ www.bsdht.org.uk

British Society for Disability and Oral Health (BSDH): ℜ www.bsdh.org.uk

British Society for Oral Medicine: ℜ www.bsom.org.uk

British Society for Paediatric Dentistry (BSPD): ℜ www.bspd.co.uk

British Society of Periodontology: ℜ www.bsperio.org.uk

British Society of Restorative Dentistry: ℜ www.bsrd.org.uk

Care Quality Commission: ℜ www.cqc.org.uk

Chief Dental Officer: ℜ www.dh.gov.uk/cdo

Chief Medical Officer: ℜ www.dh.gov.uk/cmo

Centre for Evidenced Based Dentistry: ℜ www.cebd.org

Centre for Reviews and Dissemination: ℜ www.york.ac.uk/inst/crd/

Clinical Dental Technicians Association: ℜ www.cdta.org.uk

Clinical evidence: a compendium of research findings on clinical questions:
ℜ www.clinicalevidence.org

Cochrane Collaboration: ℜ www.cochrane.co.uk

Cochrane Oral Health group: ℜ www.ohg.cochrane.org

Committee of Postgraduate Dental Deans and Directors:
ℜ www.copdend.org.uk

Conference of Postgraduate Medical Deans: ℜ www.copmed.org.uk

Confederation of Dental Employers (CODE): ℜ www.codeuk.com

CONSORT (Consolidated Standards of Reporting Trials Statement:
ℜ www.consort-statement.org

Dentanet: ℜ www.dentanet.org.uk

Dental Practice Managers Association: ℜ www.bdpma.org.uk

Dental Technologists Association: ℜ www.dta-uk.org

Equator Network Resource Centre for Research reporting:
ℜ www.equator-network.org

Health Protection Agency: ℜ www.hpa.org.uk

Institute of Healthcare Management: ℜ www.ihm.org.uk

International Organization for Standardization (ISO): ✍ www.iso.org
Kings Fund: ✍ www.kingsfund.org.uk
National Library for Health: ✍ www.library.nhs.uk
National Institute for Clinical Excellence: ✍ www.nice.org.uk
NHS Education for Scotland: ✍ www.nes.scot.nhs.uk
Oral Health Specialist Library: ✍ www.library.nhs.uk/oralhealth
Patient information: ✍ www.informedhealthonline.org
Pubmed: ✍ www.pubmedcentral.nih.gov
Scottish Intercollegiate Guidelines Network (SIGN): ✍ www.sign.ac.uk
Study Skills: ✍ www. asp.wlv.ac.uk/Level3.asp?UserType=6&Level3=542
TRIP database: ✍ www.tripdatabase.com
Voluntary Services Overseas: ✍ www.vso.org.uk

For when it all gets a bit stressful … try the following
✍ www.bbc.co.uk/weather
✍ www.bored.com
✍ www.extremeironing.com
✍ www.lastminute.com
✍ www.locata.co.uk/commons
✍ www.lovelaughs.com
✍ www.multimap.com
✍ www.oofun.com
✍ www.saynoto0870.com
✍ www.tau.ac.il/~melros
✍ www.upmystreet.com

NB All these addresses were correct at the time of going to press.

Useful addresses

Aberdeen University School of Medicine and Dentistry, Polwarth Building, Foresterhill, Aberdeen, AB25 2ZD. Tel: 01224 553015
℘ www.abdn.ac.uk/medicine

Barts and the London Dental School, Queen Mary's School of Medicine and Dentistry, Turner Street, London E1 2AD. Tel: 020 7882 2399. ℘ www.smd.qmul.ac.uk

Birmingham Dental School, St Chad's Queensway, Birmingham B4 6NN. Tel: 0121 236 8611. ℘ www.dentistry.bham.ac.uk/home

Bristol Dental School, Lower Maudlin Street, Bristol BS1 2LY. Tel: 0117 928 9000. ℘ www.dentalschool.bris.ac.uk

British Dental Association, 64 Wimpole Street, London W1M 8AL. Tel: 020 7935 0875. ℘ www.bda-dentistry.org.uk

British Dental Health Foundation, Smile House, 2 East Union Street, Rugby CV22 6AJ. Tel: 0870 770 4000. ℘ www.dentalhealth.org.uk

British Library, 96, Euston Road, London, NW1 2DB. Tel: 0870 444 1500. ℘ www.bl.uk/aboutus/quickinfo/loc

British Medical Association, BMA House, Tavistock Square, London WC1-9JP. Tel: 020 7387 4499. ℘ www.bma.org.uk

Cardiff Dental School, Heath Park, Cardiff CF4 4XY. Tel: 029 2074 2468. ℘ www.cardiff.ac.uk/dentl

Cork Dental School, John Redmond Street, Wilton, Cork, Eire. Tel: 00 353 21 454 5100. ℘ www.ucc.ie/en/dentalschool

Dental Defence Union, 230 Blackfriars Road, London SE1 8PJ. Tel: 020 7202 1500. ℘ www.the-ddu.com/section_Dental_professionals

Dental Practitioners Association, 2nd Floor, 61 Harley Street, London, W1G 8QU. Tel: 0207 636 1072. ℘ www.uk-dentistry.org

Dental Protection, 33 Cavendish Square, London W1G OPS. Tel: 020 7399 1400. ℘ www.dentalprotection.org

Department of Health, Chief Dental Officer, Richmond House, 79 Whitehall, London SW1A 2NL. ℘ www.dh.gov.uk

Dublin Dental School, Dublin University, Trinity College, Dublin 2, Eire. Tel: 00 353 1671 1255. http://web1.dental.tcd.ie/index.php

Dundee Dental School, Park Place, Dundee DD1 4HN. Tel: 01382 660111. ℘ www.dundee.ac.uk/dentalschool

Edinburgh Dental Institute, 4th Floor, Lauriston Building, Lauriston Place, Edinburgh EH3 9HA. Tel: 0131 536 4970. ℘ www.epdi.org.uk/index.asp

Faculty of Dental Surgery, The Royal College of Surgeons of England, 35–43 Lincoln's Inn Fields, London WC1A 3PE. Tel: 020 7869 6810. ℘ www.rcseng.ac.uk/fds

Faculty of General Dental Practitioners (UK), The Royal College of Surgeons of England, 35–43 Lincoln's Inn Fields, London WC2A 3PE. Tel: 020 7312 6671. ℘ www.fgdp.org.uk

FDI World Dental Federation, 13 Chemin du Levant, l'Avant Centre, F-01210 Ferney-Voltaire, France. Tel: +33 4504050507. ℘ www.fdiworldental.org

Fluoridation Society, Ward 4, Booth Hall Children's Hospital, Charleston Road, Manchester M9 7AA. Tel: 0161 918 5223. www.bfsweb.org

General Dental Council, 37 Wimpole Street, London W1M 8DQ. Tel: 020 7887 3800. www.gdc-uk.org

Glasgow Dental School, 378 Sauchiehall Street, Glasgow G2 3JX. Tel: 0141 211 9600. www.gla.ac.uk/schools/dental

Guys, Kings and St. Thomas' Dental Institute, Kings College, London WC2R 2LS. Tel: 020 7836 5454. www.kcl.ac.uk/schools/dentistry

Leeds Dental Institute, Dental and Medical Building, Clarendon Way, Leeds LS2 9LU. Tel: 0113 343 6199. www.leeds.ac.uk/dental

Liverpool Dental School, Pembroke Place, PO Box 147, Liverpool L69 3BX. Tel: 0151 706 5132. www.liv.ac.uk/dental

London School of Hygiene and Tropical Medicine, Keppel Street, London WC1E 7HT. Tel: 020 7636 8636. www.lshtm.ac.uk

Manchester Dental School, University Dental Hospital of Manchester, Cambridge Street, Manchester M15 6FH. Tel: 0161 306 0220. www.dentistry.manchester.ac.uk

Medical and Dental Defence Union of Scotland, 120 Blythswood Street, Glasgow G2 4EA. Tel: 0845 270 2034. www.mddus.com/mddus/CCC_FirstPage.jsp

National Advice Centre for Postgraduate Dental Education, The Royal College of Surgeons of England, 35–43 Lincoln's Inn Fields, London, WC2A 3PE. Tel: 020 7869 6804. www.rcseng.ac.uk/fds/nacpde

National Oral Health Promotion Group, Postern House, Cherry Orchard, Marlborough, Wiltshire, SN8 4AS. Tel: 0672 517632. www.nohpg.org

Newcastle upon Tyne School of Dental Sciences, Framlington Place, Newcastle upon Tyne NE2 4BW. Tel: 0191 222 8347. www.ncl.ac.uk/dental

Peninsula Dental School, The John Bull Building, Tamar Science Park, Research Way, Plymouth, PL6 8BU. Tel: 01752 437444. www.pms.ac.uk/dentistry

Queens University of Belfast, School of Medicine and Dentistry, 73, University Road, Belfast BT7 1nn. Tel: 028 9097 1444. www.qub.ac.uk/schools/SchoolofMedicineandDentistry

Royal College of Physicians and Surgeons of Glasgow, 234–242 St. Vincent Street, Glasgow G2 5RJ. Tel: 0141 221 6072. www.rcpsg.ac.uk

Royal College of Surgeons of Edinburgh, Nicolson Street, Edinburgh EH8 9DW. Tel: 0131 527 1608. www.rcsed.ac.uk

Royal College of Surgeons of England, 35–43 Lincoln's Inn Fields, London WC2A 3PE. Tel: 020 7405 3474. www.rcseng.ac.uk

Royal College of Surgeons of Ireland, 123 St. Stephen's Green, Dublin 2, Eire. Tel: 00 353 1402 2100. www.rcsi.ie

Royal Society of Medicine, 1 Wimpole Street, London W1G 0AE. Tel: 020 7290 2900. www.rsm.ac.uk

Scottish Dental Practice Board, The Scottish Health Service Centre, Crewe Road, Edinburgh, EH4 2LF. Tel: 0131 275 7740. www.shsc.scot.nhs.uk/shsc/default.asp?p=8

Sheffield Dental School, Charles Clifford Dental Hospital, Wellesley Road, Sheffield S10 2SZ. Tel: 0114 271 7801. 🖰 www.shef.ac.uk/dentalschool
UCL Eastman Dental Institute, 256 Gray's Inn Road, London WC1X 8LD. Tel: 020 7915 1000. 🖰 www.eastman.ucl.ac.uk
World Health Organization, Avenue Appia 20, 1211, Geneva 27, Switzerland. Tel: (+41 22) 791 2111. 🖰 www.who.int

All details were correct at the time of going to press.

Index